The Complete
Encyclopedia of
NATURAL
HEALING

REVISED &
UPDATED

The Complete
Encyclopedia of
NATURAL
HEALING

A comprehensive A-Z listing of
common and chronic illnesses and
their proven natural treatments

GARY NULL, Ph.D.

www.BottomLineSecrets.com

The Complete Encyclopedia of Natural Healing,
Revised & Updated
By Gary Null, PhD

Copyright © 1998, 2005, 2006, 2007 by Gary Null

Bottom Line Books® Hardcover Edition
Revised and Updated Edition: October 2005
Published by arrangement with
Kensington Publishing Corp.

Bottom Line Books® is a registered trademark of Boardroom® Inc.
281 Tresser Blvd., Stamford, CT 06901

10 9 8 7 6 5 4 3 2 1

ISBN 0–88723–439–9

This book is intended as a reference volume only, not as a medical manual. The information given here is designed to help you make informed decisions about your health. It is not intended as a substitute for any treatment that may have been prescribed by your doctor. If you suspect that you have a medical problem, seek competent medical help.

Printed in the United States of America

Contents

Preface   ix
Acknowledgments   xii

I. Conditions   1

Aging   3
AIDS   21
Alcoholism   41
Allergies   44
Alzheimer's Disease and Dementia   56
Anemia   64
Arthritis   69
Autism   81
Back and Neck Pain   85
Breast Cancer   96
Breast Implant Reactions   104
Cancer   106
Candidiasis   126
Carpal Tunnel Syndrome   132
Cerebral Palsy   135
Cervical Dysplasia   138
Chronic Fatigue Syndrome   142
Chronic Pain   154
Cold and Canker Sores   167
Colds and Flu   171
Dental Disorders   179
Depression   187
Diabetes   195
Digestive Disorders   202
Dysmenorrhea   215

Ear Infections   221
Eating Disorders (Anorexia Nervosa and Bulimia)   226
Endometriosis   232
Environmental Illness   238
Eye Disorders   244
Fever   251
Fibroids and Uterine Bleeding   254
Foot and Leg Problems   261
Gallstones   273
Headaches   277
Heart Disease   286
Heat Exhaustion and Heatstroke   300
Hemorrhoids   303
Hepatitis   306
Herpes   311
High Cholesterol Level   317
Hypoglycemia   323
Hypothyroidism   328
Infertility   332
Learning Disorders   340
Lupus   351
Lyme Disease   355
Lymphedema   360
Menopause   364
Motion Sickness   372
Multiple Sclerosis   374
Obesity   377
Osteoporosis   386
Parasites   393
Parkinson's Disease   399
Periodontal Disease   404
Phobias   410
Pregnancy-Related Problems   417
Premenstrual Syndrome   427
Prostate Conditions   434
Respiratory Conditions   442
Sickle Cell Anemia   451
Sinusitis   453
Skin Cancer   457
Skin Conditions   461
Stroke   468
Tinnitus   477

TMJ Dysfunction   481
Toxic Shock Syndrome   485
Trauma   488
Urinary Tract Infections   493

II. The Gary Null Protocol and Participant Testimonials   503

The Gary Null Protocol   505
Testimonials   508

III. Treatments and Patient Experiences   573

Acupuncture   575
Alexander Technique   581
Applied Kinesiology   583
Aromatherapy   586
Ayurvedic Medicine   587
Biofeedback   592
Biological Dentistry   594
Chelation Therapy   608
Chiropractic   617
Colon Therapy   628
Enzyme Therapy   636
Herbal Therapy   639
Homeopathy   641
Hypnotherapy   649
Massage Therapy   658
Nutritional Therapy   663
Oxygen Therapies   677
Qi Gong   687
Reconstructive Therapy   693
Reflexology   696
Reiki   698
Rolfing   701
Shiatsu   703
Tai Chi Chuan   705
Vitamin Drips   708

Patients Speak Out on Cancer Therapies that Work   713

Index   741

Preface

Today, more than ever, tens of millions of Americans are seeking alternative opinions on how to treat and prevent disease. What accounts for this major paradigm shift? Orthodox medicine has not lived up to its billing as the be-all and end-all in health maintenance. Sure, traditional medicine does a superb job in certain crisis-oriented spheres (e.g., trauma, strokes, organ transplants and burns). But an objective, detached review of *overall* care paints a different picture. In the management of the chronic conditions that inundate our society (e.g., heart disease, cancer, arthritis, mental illness and diabetes), traditional medicine has fallen short. Orthodox medicine does not preach prevention as fervently as it should. Traditional medicine often uses drastic remedies that result in iatrogenic (induced by the doctor or hospital) illnesses. I have written this book because of this chronic-care situation.

You should consider this book a second opinion—an alternative, if you will—for today's bewildered health care consumer. However, it is not the traditional second opinion—the kind that refers you to beta-blockers or antidepressants, or guides you through the steps of a coronary bypass. Plenty of other sources can provide you with this information.

This work is a revised edition of the original work that was published in 1997. The saying goes that time and tide wait for no one. Well, the same can be said about scientific reports and studies. I have read tens of thousands of such reports and have updated this book with the invaluable information contained therein. I have translated tedious, complicated, double-blind, placebo-controlled experiments into lay language.

This book represents true second opinions. Contrasted with the beliefs of traditional medicine, these second opinions will hit you like breaths of fresh air. The concept presented herein is to look and think outside of the box—the box of traditional medicine—to incorporate nature, and what is natural, into a new healing paradigm.

Keep in mind that I am not your personal health care provider. Thus, I will not advocate anything specifically for your condition. But when you meet with your health care professional to discuss your options, you will be well-armed with true alternatives, not merely regurgitated, recycled traditional treatments. An exhaustive list of choices will literally be at your fingertips.

Finally, I believe it is vital for anyone considering a treatment, whether alternative or mainstream, to hear the words of those who have used and benefited from that particular treatment. Therefore, I have included patients' experiences—in the patients' own words—in this book. These testimonials are from your neighbors, people you may have passed on the street today. They testify to the validity of the Gary Null Protocol, as well as to the alternative treatments presented in this book. These testimonials put human faces on the healing modalities discussed in this book. And, after all, the human aspect of health care is why this field really matters.

The testimonials in this book are from participants in my health support groups. The vast majority of these participants were not treated for a particular condition, but were given an overall overhaul that included distressing, detoxifying, exercise, vitamin drips, chelation therapy and ozone treatment. They were also guided in cleaning up their home and work environments. Over the years, more than 13,000 people, with approximately 100 different conditions, have participated in my health support groups. The protocol, specifically designed to promote the overall healing of the body, has helped each of these conditions. Some of the participants have been in my support groups for 13 years. However, many of the testimonials you will read are from people who were in the program for just three to six months. Yet, these participants saw improvements in disorders such as high blood pressure, high cholesterol levels, chronic fatigue syndrome, AIDS and heart disease.

Mind you, this is not to suggest that traditional medicine does not work or that the Gary Null Protocol should be used as a substitute for orthodox medicine.

It is merely to suggest that by grasping the concepts of proper diet and nutrition that you can become healthier, ward off disease, and enjoy a quality of life that you once thought unattainable. The adage, "You are what you eat," has never been truer. If you eat nutrient-deficient foods, your body and mind will suffer. Conversely, if you furnish your body with foods rich in nutrients (vitamins, minerals, enzymes, water, amino acids, carbohydrates and lipids), your body and mind will benefit. Many people make the tragic mistake of believing that because their bodies are not manifesting outward signs of illness, they are healthy. Nothing could be further from the truth.

Many of us know someone who passed a doctor's physical examination only to drop dead shortly thereafter. Did that person suddenly become sick? No, it's just that the examination did not detect the degree of sickness. No one who is properly examined and given a clean bill of health suddenly drops dead.

In the final analysis, your health is in your hands. To become healthy and to stay healthy, you must become proactive. You choose the doctor you want, as well as the lifestyle you live. You decide whether or not to smoke (knowing that it has been estimated that for each cigarette you smoke, you take a minute off of your life), drink alcohol (which, among other things, kills brain cells) or take drugs. You determine whether to exercise or to become a couch potato. And regardless of which decision you make, you will pay. When I was a child growing up in West Virginia, the adults used to say, "You don't always get what you pay for, but you always pay for what you get." How well that saying applies to your health.

In this book, you will find the most up-to-date information on health and nutrition. By using the information contained here, you are well on your way to optimizing your health.

Gary Null

Acknowledgments

A book of this magnitude could not have been completed without the assistance of some outstanding and gifted researchers and editors. I relied on Doug Henderson, Esq., for his research and editorial skills in arranging the many disparate aspects of this monumental project into a uniform whole. Zoi Florosz worked diligently at providing invaluable research assistance, as did Rani Karnik. Lastly, I want to thank Ann Rickl for her expert suggestions, Sondra Hollander for her work in organizing the testimonials and Ray Wilson for his help.

I.
Conditions

Aging

Himalayan mountain people are famous for their longevity. It is common for the Hunzas to live 120 healthful years due to their intake of mineral-rich water, unpolluted air, and a diet rich in complex carbohydrates, as well as to their active, purposeful way of life. On Pitcairn Island, in the South Pacific, it's not unusual for residents past 70 to labor alongside 20-year-olds. Inhabitants credit their strength and vitality to a natural lifestyle and a menu consisting mostly of grains, fruits, and vegetables. In China, doctors have studied the secrets of rejuvenation for thousands of years, and have long known how to keep sex glands functioning well past the prime of life with herbs, acupuncture, and special exercises called tai chi and qi gong.

Americans have much to learn from these cultures. For the most part, we and the people of other Western nations have become fast-paced and out of step with nature. We manage on devitalized foods, and control failing body systems with multiple medications. In midlife, we stop exercising and lose lean muscle mass. As a result, bone density is lost and metabolism slows down, causing flabbiness and weakness, and setting the stage for osteoporosis. Most seniors are physically feeble, and some are mentally so, due to a lifetime of poor habits.

On the brighter side, scientists are teaching us why we age, and what we can do to slow down, and even reverse, the aging process. Through their efforts, we now know that aging begins at the cellular level with free radical damage, and that antioxidant vitamins, minerals, and enzymes can prevent such destruction. In addition, research confirms the value of natural regenerative remedies esteemed by the ancients and of new "smart drugs" that improve mental acuity.

As this information filters down to the general public, more and more people are attempting to turn back the clock by eating better, supplementing their diets, reducing stress, and increasing their exercise levels. Most importantly, attitudes are changing and people are seeing themselves as youthful at older ages. This is important because "thinking old" creates a physiological response in the body. When we picture ourselves losing strength and vitality with age, that is what occurs. Conversely, when we see time as a friend, we are apt to remain young and vibrant into our 50's, 60's, and beyond. In fact, with today's new knowledge and increasingly positive attitudes, extending our healthful years to equal those of the Hunzas does not seem an impossible goal.

To Fight Aging—Detoxify

The more toxic we are, the faster we age. Cosmetic changes, such as facelifts and hair coloring, may temporarily help us appear younger, but to really regenerate we must detoxify, that is, clean ourselves up from the inside. The youthful appearance that results will be the natural by-product of improved health.

Cleansing practices date back thousands of years. The Essenes, for example, filled gourds with clean river water, and used long reeds to wash "devils" out of their intestines. In the modern, polluted world, internal cleansing is especially important, for no matter how well we take care of ourselves, we still breathe in polluted air, bathe in polluted water, and take in all sorts of chemicals. Once these substances are absorbed, we never fully eliminate them unless we detoxify.

Some methods of detoxification focus on specific systems; others, such as juice fasting and chelation therapy, help the entire body at once.

Juice Fasting

Fasting can be likened to staying home to clean and repair the house. Going on a juice fast allows the digestive system to rest so that it can focus on all the other areas that need healing. At the end of the process, everything works better and the skin takes on a healthy glow.

Fasting seems like an even better idea when you consider that, in the United States, we generally take in from 10 to 20 percent more calories than our bodies need. In fact, most people can benefit from a one- to two-day fast of freshly squeezed juice, protein drinks, pure water and herbal tea. Initially, it would be advisable to get clearance from a physician, one who understands the benefits of fasting. If you are taking medications, you should not stop taking them unless a doctor says it is safe to do so.

Here are a few guidelines: When making your juices, use organic produce whenever possible, as harmful chemicals found in tainted fruits and vegetables become more concentrated after juicing. Obviously, that is counterproductive to your objective to cleanse internally. Drink about eight 10-ounce glasses of juice a day, and you will be treating your whole body to a maximum usable supply of health-giving phytochemicals, antioxidant vitamins and minerals, chlorophyll, and enzymes.

To ensure digestibility, you should understand that the juices of dark green vegetables, such as spinach, arugula, parsley, and watercress, are very concentrated, and should be liberally diluted with more watery juices, such as those of cabbage, celery, or cucumber, or with aloe vera and mineral water. Also, to get the most physical and psychological benefit from juices, drink them slowly, consuming them as you would food as opposed to water. Drinking too fast cheats the mind of taste satisfaction and places unwanted stress on the kidneys and bladder. Finally, remember to come off a fast—especially a longer one—gradually. Eating too much is never a good idea. But it can be especially bad for the system after having not eaten for an extended period of time.

Once these simple rules are learned, the fun of an all-juice diet begins. Alternating between carrot/apple, pineapple/sprouts, and tomato/lemon with a dash of cayenne can keep the taste buds happy all day. Meanwhile, the body is getting vital nutrients to help it function at its best. Here are some beneficial fruits and vegetables from which to choose:

Apple . . . Apple helps to correct skin and liver disorders. It has a laxative effect, and is a valuable aid to digestion and weight loss.

Beet . . . Drink beet juice to nourish the liver, one of the most important organs of the body, as it has hundreds of different functions. If your liver is functioning well, most likely everything else in your body is, too.

Cabbage . . . Cabbage is high in vitamin K, as well as cancer-fighting indoles. It is excellent for alleviating stomach ailments, especially when combined with comfrey.

Carrot . . . Carrot juice is high in the antioxidants, including beta-carotene and vitamins A, C, and E. In addition, it is filled with health-giving minerals and antiaging enzymes. One caveat on carrot juice: Since it is high in natural sugar, this juice should be diluted with water, especially when there is a blood sugar imbalance.

Celery . . . This one is moderately high in sodium, not the bad-for-you salt shaker kind, but the good, natural kind that promotes good cell chemistry.

Melon . . . Melon juices are wonderful kidney cleansers. And did you know that the rind provides a wide range of enzymes, minerals, and chlorophyll? Drink melon juice alone, not in combination with other fruits or vegetables.

Pineapple . . . The juice of this fruit contains bromelain, which has an anti-inflammatory effect. This is especially good for alleviating arthritic symptoms.

Susan Lombardi, founder of the We Care Health Center, in Palm Springs, California, and author of *Ten Easy Steps for Complete Wellness*, recommends a combination of carrot, celery, cabbage, and beet juice, mixed in equal proportions, with a little cayenne for flavor and circulation. This mixture is taken throughout the day while fasting to promote healing in every corner of the body.

Sometimes a person feels temporarily unwell when fasting. This is called a healing crisis, and usually occurs around the third day. This is not necessarily a bad thing, but rather a sign that the body is releasing toxins and probably withdrawing from addictions, if you've been, for example, a habitual consumer of caffeine, sugar, or dairy foods. The best advice is to get plenty of rest and to drink lots of water during this time. After a while, the discomfort will disappear, and the system will be newly recharged. Your health practitioner will give you more guidance on juice fasting.

Chelation Therapy

Chelation therapy has many benefits, all of which add up to a longer, healthier life. While no studies directly relate the treatment to increased life expectancy, several show it to favorably impact the four major causes of death in the United States: cancer, heart disease, cerebrovascular disease, and chronic obstructive lung disease.

During treatment, medical doctors administer a man-made amino acid, called EDTA, via intravenous drip. Once in the bloodstream, EDTA attaches itself to heavy metals, such as lead, cadmium, and mercury, and holds onto these toxic substances until they exit the body through the kidneys. Eliminating these substances prevents premature aging and disease.

In these polluted times, health professionals often recommend chelation therapy for many people over 30. As we get older the toxic metals from the environment, especially lead, accumulate in the skeleton. Even natural calcium can accumulate in the wrong places. Chelation therapy will take calcium out of the heart vessels and place it back into the long bones, thus preventing osteoporosis.

Another benefit of chelation is that it helps the brain work better. As artery blockages are removed, more blood flows to the brain and cognitive abilities improve. And when pathways are kept open, individuals are at lower risk for stroke.

Detoxification for Specific Systems

We have several organs for detoxification—the intestines, kidneys, liver, skin, and lungs. In addition, the lymph glands play a major role. Each area must work optimally to avoid overburdening other systems. The following are some therapies beneficial to these organs:

Intestines . . . The average person carries around several pounds of impacted fecal matter on the intestinal walls, which can create constipation, emotional repression, and an environment conducive to bacteria and disease. To help with this problem, a detoxification drink can be made from ground flaxseeds, psyllium seeds, and bentonite, a liquid clay. This formula is excellent for colon cleansing because the clay absorbs toxins while the seeds expand in water and brush the intestines clean. Certain herbs, such as rhubarb root, buckthorn bark, Ramnus frangula, cascara sagrada, Ramnus purshiana and goldenseal, are powerful laxatives. Furthermore, sanicle roots and leaves help remove poisonous waste matter from the body. Lastly, sumac berry and bark tea is very cleansing to the system.

Another helpful technique is colonic irrigation. This therapy gently but thoroughly washes the intestines by infusing water into the large bowel in small amounts at steady intervals. Water travels the entire length of the colon. In the process, old encrustations of fecal matter are dislodged and swept away. Often this material has been attached to the bowel for many years, and is laden with millions of bacteria. Unless eliminated, this sets up the perfect environment for disease.

Colonic irrigation restores the colon to its natural shape and function so that food is better absorbed and eliminated, skin improves, and irritability, fatigue, and constipation disappear. A healthy colon means a healthy body.

Kidneys . . . The herbs dandelion leaf, echinacea, and corn silk are beneficial to the kidneys. Short fasts, during which apple juice is mixed with small amounts of parsley, also improve kidney health. The uva ursi leaf is a great remedy in cases of kidney infection.

Liver . . . Milk thistle protects liver function and helps this organ expel toxins. That, in turn, promotes health and youthfulness. The herbs licorice, pau d'arco, Tabebuia heptaphylla, stilingia root, prickly ash, St. John's wort (wort means "plant"), wood betony, chickweed, fennel and sassafras leaf and root protect the liver by drawing toxins from the blood, thus helping to avoid blood toxicity.

Lungs . . . With each exhalation, waste products are removed from the system. And one of the best ways to improve lung capacity is through regular aerobic exercise. Of course, exercise has other age-defying benefits; it facilitates lung functioning. Exercise enables us to detoxify, as we sweat, through the outlet of our skin. It allows more blood to flow to tissues throughout the body, which keep cells from dying prematurely. By oxygenating brain cells, exercise prevents or minimizes senility. It also improves metabolism, so that the body can easily maintain a normal weight. Finally, weight-bearing exercises, such as walking, jogging, and weight-lifting, enhance bone density, which helps prevent osteoporosis.

Skin . . . Not only does our skin provide a protective covering, it also expels many toxins daily. But to do this job properly, the pores must not be clogged. One technique for ensuring this is skin brushing. Using a natural bristle brush or loofah, rub the skin all over in a circular motion, to get rid of dead skin that clogs up the pores. Always brush toward the heart, and never brush thin facial skin.

Taking a sauna is a good follow-up to dry skin brushing because sweat expels toxins through the now open pores. Beginners should keep the temperature at around 185 degrees Fahrenheit and start out slowly. There are different types of saunas, and the directions for each type should be followed.

Lymphatic System . . . The job of the lymphatic system is to move disease-causing wastes out of the body. Cleansing herbs, such as burdock root, red clover, echinacea, dandelion, yellow dock, and garlic, can speed up a sluggish lymphatic system. Lymphatic massage and skin brushing also help.

Rebuilding

As we regain health through detoxification, the body becomes more responsive to therapies that rebuild the system, such as a healthy diet and vitamin/mineral supplements. Below are general recommendations for life-extending foods and nutrients. For more precise guidance, a holistic practitioner can make recommendations based on individual test results.

Tests are important because we do not age uniformly; rather, individual organs diminish in energy at different rates. One thing that Western medicine excels at is laboratory analysis, and a full spectrum of tests can determine which systems are out of balance, and thus causing premature aging. Tests can indicate, for instance, whether the adrenal glands are producing enough anti-aging hormones, whether vitamins and minerals are being properly digested, and whether toxic metals are polluting the system. Findings may reveal that one person is anemic due to an iron deficiency, for example, while another is low in folic acid. Results help holistic health practitioners address the unique needs of their patients.

Once you begin a health regimen, subsequent testing shows how well recommendations are taking effect, and adjustments are made accordingly. Some nutrients can be dispensed with once the body starts producing more of its own, while others are needed on a continual basis. Thyroid supplements, for instance, are often needed by patients with low body temperatures until the system catches on, a few weeks later, and starts converting the hormone to a usable form on its own. Some nutrients, like vitamin C, leave the body rapidly and need to be taken several times each day.

Subjective measures of improvement must also be taken into account. This is done through observation of symptoms and appearance. If symptoms diminish and appearance improves over time, it is an indication that therapies are working. And as the body rejuvenates, a person will notice additional improvements, such as increased endurance, enhanced memory, and better body tone.

The Antiaging Diet

The foods we eat should keep us balanced—not too acid or alkaline. One way to keep our systems stable is to place a pH strip in a urine sample each morning. The ideal result should read in the range of 6.8. Deviations from that number mean that the foods eaten the day before were too acidic (downward deviations from 6.8) or too alkaline (upward). Acidic foods are especially harmful as they contribute to numerous diseases. Cutting down on these foods, and eating lots of fruits and vegetables instead, will support the body.

Complex Carbohydrates . . . An antiaging diet is high in complex carbohydrates, such as grains, legumes, fruits, vegetables, nuts, and seeds. Many are eaten raw or close to their natural state, and none are unnecessarily processed or overcooked. Frying is minimized, although stir-frying is acceptable. Very little, if any, animal proteins are eaten, and fats are used sparingly. Only about 10 to 15 percent of calories should come from fat.

Complex carbohydrates help us in several ways. First, they are high in fiber, and can therefore prevent common afflictions associated with aging, such as constipation, hemorrhoids, intestinal diseases, ulcers, high blood pressure and colorectal cancer. They are also rich in phytochemicals, antioxidant substances found in plants that help us prevent everything from cancer, arthritis and heart disease, to wrinkles and age spots.

By eating diets centered on complex carbohydrates, we not only feel healthier, we look better. Most people tend to gain weight as they age because their metabolism slows down. Complex carbohydrates counter this problem because they are digested quickly. Thirty minutes after a meal of rice and vegetables, the body starts to burn up food at maximum speed, a process that continues for 2½ to 3 hours. Of course, this works best when foods are eaten without creamy or greasy sauces. But this does not mean that meals must be bland. Many cookbooks show how wholesome food can be healthfully spiced and dressed.

How can foods minimize wrinkling? Beta-carotene, from carrots and other yellow/orange vegetables, enters the cell's outer membrane, and provides some protection against sun damage. This nutrient's cousin, lycopene, is twice as powerful.

Lycopene gives the watermelon, tomato and pink grapefruit their red colors. It is a powerful antioxidant that enters the membrane of skin cells and provides protection against ultraviolet damage. Recent studies tout it as the new heart attack preventer. Lycopene reduces human DNA damage that can cause cancer.

Polyphenol, a type of phytonutrient, can be obtained from plums as well as any deep-colored berries, such as blueberries, bilberries, grapes and black currants. Color can be used as a guide: the stronger, more vibrant the color, the more nutritional value the fruit or vegetable has. Polyphenol also has a great neuroprotective effect. It reduces neuropathology and enhances neurogenesis and production of new nerve cells. Polyphenol also has an anti-infammatory property, and it is a powerful iron chelator. Iron plays a key role in the development of Alzheimer's and Parkinson's diseases.

Green Foods . . . Greens are rich in chlorophyll, the ultimate blood purifier. Chlorophyll is known to cure various infections in the respiratory tract and can lessen the effects of various pollutants, such as second-hand smoke, diesel fuel, and coal dust. In addition, it can turn an acidic pH more alkaline. Then, food is better absorbed and antioxidants are able to effectively do their job of strengthening the immune system. This, in turn, is a key aspect of slowing the aging process.

Excellent sources of chlorophyll are barley grass and wheatgrass. These are high in superoxide dismutase (SOD), an antioxidant enzyme that scavenges free radicals from the body. Additionally, they're far richer in vitamins, minerals, amino acids, and trace elements than are most other vegetables.

Sea Vegetables and Algae . . . They may not be household words, but you should know that the sea vegetables dulce, kelp, and nori are exceptionally high in minerals, particularly calcium, iodine, potassium, and magnesium, and in trace elements as well. Kelp can rebalance thyroid metabolism, resulting in successful weight management and the reversal of many conditions that are caused by a thyroid imbalance, including stomach and respiratory disorders.

Spirulina and chlorella are single-celled, waterborne algae that are rich in chlorophyll, vitamins, minerals, and amino acids. These foods help protect cells and boost energy levels. By building and strengthening at the cellular level, they protect against the effects of aging.

Garlic and Onions . . . These two are health superstars because they contain sulfur compounds that have an antiaging and anticancer effect.

Water and Juice . . . Pure water is an essential part of a good diet, but most people don't get enough. This is important because suboptimal water intake can dehydrate the brain, causing symptoms of senility in the elderly. Eight 8-ounce glasses daily is a minimum requirement. In addition, fresh, enzyme-rich juices should be a regular part of the diet.

Natural Hormone Rebalancing

How Does the Hormonal System Work? The human body manufactures hormones—such as adrenaline, DHEA, human growth hormone and dozens of others—which are chemical messengers that help regulate the body's functions. Most hormones are produced by glands. However, some are made by organs such as the heart, the stomach and the small intestines. Some hormones seem to be responsible for controlling levels of other hormones. For instance, many hormones released by the pituitary gland signal other glands, such as the thyroid or adrenals, to release other hormones.

Just as your eyes work together, many hormones work in pairs to create balance according to the principle of opposing forces, with one hormone opposing the action of the other. For example, the pancreas produces the insulin-glucagon pair—a pair in which insulin reduces blood sugar. Through the functions of the pancreas, first adding a little of one hormone then a bit of the other, the sugar concentration in the blood is kept nearly constant. It is evident that such a system must be precise in order to maintain a healthy balance. A breakdown in such a sensitive system—one that depends on one reaction triggering a second reaction that in turn triggers a third and so forth—could result in shifts that could be catastrophic to the body.

Why the Hormonal System Breaks Down. The hormonal system may become imbalanced because of toxins from the environment (lead, mercury, cadmium, the amalgam fillings in your teeth, fluoride or chlorine in your water, bacteria, viruses, or even electromagnetic stressors). Hormonal dysregulation may arise, though subtle, and with no apparent symptoms. However, if your metabolism changes, you may see a corresponding decline in your energy level, a risk factor for many serious diseases.

Metabolic rate changes could trigger a dangerous cycle. As the body stores more fat, you may feel more fatigued, which may cause you to lose some of your enthusiasm for everyday activities. Consequently, you may begin to skip regular exercise.

But since exercise combats depression, lack of exercise may cause you to become even more depressed. And because depression may cause hormonal imbalances, as well as the release of stress hormones, effects can spiral.

After a number of years, the body adapts to a reduction in the central hormones and/or an imbalance in the manner in which they are used. An indication of a possible hormonal imbalance is the inability to lose weight no matter what you do—though you must keep in mind that after the age of 40, your metabolism naturally slows down. High protein diets, vitamin supplementation, counting calories, or skipping meals will not correct an underlying hormonal imbalance.

To determine whether you have a hormonal imbalance, you must have a careful examination by a trained professional. If the examination determines that you have a hormone problem, you must undergo a comprehensive detoxification program, followed by a hormonal rebalancing program. When this program is concluded, you may be able to lose weight without dieting, and you may be able to regain energy.

Though not everyone suffers from a hormone imbalance, it is wise to eliminate the possibility of having this condition before beginning a rejuvenation program. In reality, hormone problems are more prevalent than one may think. It is smart to see an endocrinologist who can perform a simple hormone test to determine whether you are producing adequate levels of melatonin, estrogen, thyroxin and other critical hormones. If your tests come back normal, then your problem is not related to hormones. If the tests indicate an imbalance, then the treatment you receive may stabilize your weight and improve your overall health.

Let's look at the most important hormones, and at how you could maximize their effects in improving your health.

HGH (Human Growth Hormone) Replacement . . . The levels of HGH start to decline after age 40. Some people may benefit from the replacement of this very important hormone, but the physician should decide that.

DHEA (Dehydroepiandrosterone) Replacement . . . Called the master hormone, this natural hormone enhances brain functioning and promotes well-being, and could be very important in terms of lengthening the lifespan. It is typical that by the age of 70, DHEA hormone levels are 80 to 90 percent lower than they were earlier in life. The highest levels of DHEA in the blood occur at around age 25 and progressively decrease thereafter. Naturally, there is great interest in restoring DHEA to youthful levels. Oral administration of 50 mg of DHEA daily provides the same benefits as traditional hormone replacement and triggers the release of growth hormone releasing hormone (GHRH), which stimulates the release of growth hormone.

DHEA counteracts cortisol, a hormone released by stress. It protects the brain against aging. Higher DHEA levels help to release acetylcholine, a neurotransmitter that transmits nerve impulses between brain cells. DHEA strengthens the hippocampus by enhancing its activity. This is essential in preventing or improving Alzheimer's disease. It helps to overcome depression, while promoting a stronger immune system. A properly formulated topical preparation of DHEA restores and maintains the proper collagen level of the skin.

Before seeking DHEA replacement therapy, men should check their PSA (prostate specific antigen) level and have a digital rectal exam. Men with prostate cancer or benign prostate hypertrophy should avoid DHEA because it could easily be converted into testosterone and estrogen. Note: Tests of PSA and DHEA serum levels should be conducted every 6 to 12 months.

Women need to check their estogen and testosterone levels periodically in order to determine the dosage of DHEA. Women who have a history of estrogen-dependent cancer should consult their physicians before beginning the DHEA replacement process.

DHEA can promote free radicals in liver cells. When taking oral supplements of DHEA, it is important to take antioxidants to avoid liver damage. It is also suggested that a person take 1000 mg of N-acetyl-cysteine (NAC) and 210 mg of gamma tocopherol daily. It is suggested that men take saw palmetto extract (160 mg twice a day), pygeum extract (50 mg twice a day), nettle extract (120 mg twice a day), and boron (3-10 mg daily). Women should supplement with melatonin (300 mcg-3 mg nightly) and vitamin D3 (1000-1400 IU daily).

Testosterone Rebalancing in Men . . . Low production of free testosterone is not the most important issue aging men have to confront. The pressing problem, in most instances, is the excessive conversion of testosterone into estrogen. Estrogen triggers the production of sex hormone binding globulin (SHBG), which binds active free testosterone into an inactive "bound testosterone." When the testosterone receptors are unable to pick up the bound testosterone, it is useless to the system. Low testosterone elevates the level of the dangerous hormone cortisol, causing immune dysfunction, brain cell injury, and arterial wall damage.

The following are natural approaches that rebalance testosterone in men:

Chrysin is a bioflavonoid that is extracted from various plants. The suggested daily dose is 1000 mg, combined with 10 mg of piperine (a component of black pepper). Originally used by bodybuilders, chrysin is a natural aromatase-inhibitor that increases free testosterone, thereby decreasing excess estrogen. It has a terrific libido-enhancing effect and has antianxiety properties as well.

Nettle (constituents of highly concentrated extracts from nettle root) binds to SHBG in place of testosterone. It thereby decreases the chances of producing bound testosterone.

Muira puama is an herbal extract that increases free testosterone and suppresses excess estrogen. It enhances the libido and boosts energy.

Losing weight is highly recommended.

Natural Hormone Replacement in Women . . . Menopause is not just an estrogen deficiency. Balancing estrogen, testosterone, DHEA, and progesterone is essential. When a deficiency arises, it needs to be corrected. These hormones affect the entire system and are linked to fatigue, brain electrical activity and cognitive function, healthy sexual function, vaginal lubrication, proper sleep, mood, skin, hair, muscle tone and a general feeling of well-being.

Eric R. Braverman, MD, director of the Place of Achieving Total Health (PATH), recommends a testing protocol before natural estrogen therapy is used. The protocol consists of a physical examination with standard blood work, attention testing, memory assessment, analysis of hormone and nutrient levels, allergic and toxic metal screening and cancer screening.

As for men, natural approaches are available to help rebalance hormones in women. Natural estrogen is a phytoestrogen formula manufactured by Life Extension™ made up of different ingredients that improve estrogen synthesis: 20 mg of black cohosh mimics the safe estrogen estriol, 12.5 mg of dong quai helps with estrogen balance and 10 mg of vitex extract creates hormonal balance and prevents the accumulation of excess prolactin. The suggested dosage is one capsule two times a day.

Topically applied natural progesterone cream could also be used. Additionally, it is suggested that one use alpha lipoic acid (250 mg twice a day), calcium citrate (1000 mg a day) to help prevent bone loss, CoQ10 (100-300 mg a day) and essential fatty acids.

Antioxidant Supplements

By reducing free radical damage, antioxidants help us stay young, vital, and productive for as long as we live. Some antioxidants are naturally produced by the body, but to promote regeneration, we need to be taking additional ones in supplement form. Here is a list of nutrients we should be taking on a daily basis:

Vitamin A . . . 1000-3000 IU per meal. Blood tests will determine whether or not a person is getting too much vitamin A, which can be toxic.

Beta-Carotene . . . Up to 25,000 IU per meal. Beta-carotene is a nontoxic precursor to vitamin A that helps slow down aging and lessens cancer risk.

Bioflavonoids . . . A minimum of 75 mg three times daily of grape seed extract, one of the most powerful antioxidant substances available.

Vitamin C . . . 3000-5000 mg, in divided doses throughout the day. To fight disease, higher doses are given orally and intravenously. Vitamin C is a powerful immune system strengthener. When C is combined with vitamins A and E, as well as riboflavin and beta-carotene, there is a lowered risk of cataracts and macular degeneration. The combination of vitamins A and C with a commercial UVA sunscreen topically applied works as a photoprotectant against phototoxic damage.

Vitamin E . . . 400-800 IU per day, taken at the largest meal. Vitamin E is best in its natural form (as a mixed tocopherol or d-alpha tocopherol). Avoid synthetic vitamin E (dl-alpha). Benefits include increased mental activity and reduction in symptoms of Alzheimer's disease and macular degeneration.

Selenium . . . 100 mcg per meal. Selenium is needed to produce glutathione peroxidase, an antioxidant enzyme that protects the body from free radical damage. It is also important in preventing cancer and cardiomegaly, an enlargement of the heart that causes premature aging and early death.

Zinc . . . 30-50 mg daily. Zinc feeds over 100 enzyme systems in the brain, as well as various systems throughout the body. It is essential in the formation of stomach acid; without sufficient zinc, malabsorption syndrome occurs. Most older people are zinc-deficient.

NADH . . . A daily dose of 2.5 mg per day. NADH, short for nicotinamide adenine dinucleotide, is a potent antioxidant that is also called coenzyme Q1. Every living cell contains NADH, and in each one it plays a central role in energy production. Aging is associated with a loss of energy due to an increased incidence of cellular degeneration and death. NADH helps cells survive and thrive. It's recommended to counter memory loss, as well as in the treatment of Alzheimer's disease and other dementias, Parkinson's disease, and Huntington's chorea.

Minerals and Enzymes

Nina Anderson, author of *Over Fifty, Looking Thirty,* stresses the importance of minerals and enzymes as two key antiaging factors. Minerals are found in every part of the body. They are in our tissues, blood, and bones. They assist in hormone production, as well as nerve transmission, and they balance our energy. Very little will work properly without them.

Getting the minerals we need keeps the body in balance, which is important because when we are unbalanced from a lack of essential minerals, the body tends to pick up harmful minerals, such as lead, aluminum, and mercury, in an attempt to compensate for the deficiency. Being balanced also lessens the incidence of degenerative diseases associated with aging, such as arthritis and osteoporosis. Arthritis begins when there is a shortage of calcium, magnesium and electrolytes. Osteoporosis happens as a result of the body leaching minerals out of the bones when minerals are lacking in the blood.

Since a full spectrum of nutrients is no longer available from deficient soils, it is important to take mineral supplements. The best minerals to take are crystalloid. These are very fine and so can permeate the cell wall and shore up the inside of the cell, keeping the shape of the cell round by maintaining its osmotic pressure. This protects the cell against free radical damage.

Even more important are enzymes, catalysts that stimulate all cellular processes, essentially making everything happen. Unless enzymes function properly, vitamins and minerals cannot do their job. Before fat-soluble vitamins A, D, E, and K can be broken down, for example, they need the enzyme lipase. Otherwise, they are partially flushed out of the body. Abundant enzymes are found in raw foods, especially juices. But to increase enzyme levels further, they can be taken as supplements. Remember, the crystalloid form is recommended.

Antioxidant enzymes are produced naturally by the body, and include superoxide dismutase (SOD), glutathione, and catalase. To keep enzyme production high, sufficient minerals are needed.

Herbs

Herbs help us resist disease by strengthening the immune system, so that it can ward off invaders of all types. They are an important part of any antiaging protocol, and can be taken as capsules, powders, teas, or tinctures.

Fo-Ti Tieng . . . This is a blend of Chinese herbs that rejuvenates the endocrine system, keeping sex glands in top working condition well into one's years. This formula also revitalizes nerve cells and keeps the blood pure.

Garlic . . . Garlic has multiple benefits and should be used by everyone. It protects the heart and liver and can prevent cancer. It is antiviral, antibacterial, anti-arthritic, and antiparasitic. By keeping the immune system strong, garlic helps the body fight off degenerative forces.

Ginkgo Biloba . . . The gingko leaf comes from the oldest species of tree on the planet. Its unique properties have allowed it to survive the natural hardships of the ages, and some say that these same traits may help people slow down their own aging process. Specifically, ginkgo is known to improve microcirculation, particularly in the brain. It may therefore be an excellent herb for those with Alzheimer's disease. And according to clinical research, subjects with this condition substantially improved their recall ability when the herb was taken three times daily. Gingko will also address other common symptoms of aging related to poor circulation: headaches, vertigo, tinnitus, dizziness, coldness or numbness of the hands and feet, cramping, and reduced ability to walk distances.

Ginseng . . . The Chinese have revered ginseng for centuries, considering it an outstanding rejuvenator, aphrodisiac, and improver of most conditions. Its ability to help a variety of conditions may be due to the fact that ginseng is an adaptogen, meaning that it works with the body to correct imbalances. For instance, if blood pressure is too high, it helps bring it down; if it is too low, it pulls it up.

There are several types of ginseng on the market today, and it is important to note their differences. Korean (red) ginseng is very hot and is said to be best suited for people with cold constitutions. The herb is also said to increase sexual fire, and, for that reason, is not recommended for people under 45. Chinese (white) ginseng is milder, and American ginseng is cool and helpful for hot, or inflammatory, conditions. American ginseng supports digestion, adrenal function, and overall vitality.

Gotu Kola . . . Elephants, animals known for their excellent memory and long life, browse on gotu kola. Similarly, people who ingest gotu kola can expect greater longevity, good memory, and mental alertness.

Sarsaparilla . . . This herb contains phytoestrogens, plant compounds that resemble estrogen and act as precursors in the production of sex hormones by the adrenal glands and the ovaries or testes. These phytoestrogens also function as precursors in the adrenal glands' production of DHEA, one of our anti-aging hormones.

Astragalus . . . This is a total body energizer, like ginseng.

Bee Pollen . . . This comes from bees and has many healing, rejuvenating, antiaging and disease-fighting properties. It is good for fatigue, allergies and many other conditions.

Black Walnut . . . This is a good source of manganese, important for the brain, nerves and cartilage.

Dock . . . This herb contains more vitamin C than oranges and more vitamin A than carrots.

Eyebright . . . This herb is excellent for inflammations. It also has cooling and detoxifying properties, and helps with memory loss.

Ho Shou Wu . . . A powerful rejuvenator, this herb strengthens the liver and the kidneys.

Propolis . . . This is unique as a natural antibiotic.

Reishi Mushroom . . . This is an antibacterial, antiviral fungus that aids the liver and substantially impacts the immune system, assisting it in fighting diseases and allergies.

Yerba mate . . . This stimulates the mind and the nervous system. It also helps with the production of cortisone. It is a good remedy for allergies and hay fever.

Aromatherapy

Properly used, essential oils can help us overcome many physical and psychological conditions associated with aging. Often, they serve as a sensible alternative to medications, because unlike drugs, which distress the system with unwanted side effects, essential oils are natural substances that the body readily accepts. They benefit us on a physical level, and, at the same time, leave us feeling relaxed and uplifted.

Aromatherapist Shirley Price points out that none of us feel old until we fall sick, and that aromatherapy is one way to feel healthier, and, therefore, young again. She reminds us that when using aromatherapy, it is important to use pure oils from aromatic medicine markets whose distillers obtain organic plant materials from natural sources. She also recommends ordering oils by their Latin names, when possible, to make sure you don't purchase products with similar names whose effects are markedly different. Here are some conditions that commonly plague the elderly, and the essential oils that can alleviate them:

Insomnia . . . The essential oil universally used to help induce sleep is lavender (Lavandula officinalis), which can be vaporized, breathed in on a tissue, or added to a carrier lotion and massaged into the shoulders (about 12 drops per 4 fluid ounces). Other sleep-inducing essential oils are bergamot (Citrus begamia), marjoram (Origanum majorana), Roman chamomile (Anthemis nobilis), lemon (Citrus limon), ylang ylang (Cananga odorata), bay (Laurus nobilis) and nutmeg (Myristica fragrans).

Indigestion . . . Digestion difficulties can often be overcome by taking essential oils by mouth, but this should only be done under the supervision of a clinical aromatherapist. An essential oil tea can be made by adding one or two drops of a specified oil into tea along with one tea bag. Caraway (Carum carvi) is an excellent choice, and can be taken together with bitter orange. Also beneficial to digestion is sweet fennel (Foeniculum vulgare dulce), which is powerful and should only be used in combination with other oils, under the guidance of an aromatherapist. Cumin (Cuminum cyminum), dill (Anethum graveolens) and peppermint (Mentha piperita) also are beneficial.

Arthritis . . . Analgesic, anti-inflammatory oils help alleviate muscular pain and arthritis, and include coriander (Coriandrum sativum), juniper (Juniperus communis), rosemary (Rosemarinus officinalis) and niaouli (Melaleuca viridiflora), as well as clove (Syzygium aromaticum), eucalyptus (Eucalyptus globulus), peppermint (Mentha piperita) and hyssop (Hyssopus officinalis).

Memory Loss . . . Rosemary (Rosemarinus officinalis) and peppermint (Mentha piperita) are gentle nervous system stimulants that are known to increase memory recall. Other good oils include frankincense, rose, and clary sage. Best effects are through inhalation, but these oils can also be added to bath water, or massaged into the scalp, hands, or feet.

Stress Reduction

Stress overtaxes the adrenal system, and is a major contributor to premature aging, degenerative disease, and early death. In these hurried times, we need to make a conscious effort to slow down and find satisfaction in life. Many methods help the mind to overcome stress: deep breathing, tai chi, yoga, meditation, qi gong, mantras, self-hypnosis, hypnosis and Bach flower remedies. EFT (Emotional Freedom Technique) is another method for stress release. By touching or tapping the body's numerous meridian points, we stimulate the flow of energy. Biofeedback uses the body's own signals to help combat stress. In addition, massage is an excellent way to relax.

One of these modalities, reiki, is a powerful tool toward this end. The term is Japanese for universal life force, and reiki, a form of therapeutic touch, works by amplifying and channeling this energy. This technique, like acupuncture, is centered on bodily meridians, or energy paths, and proponents extol its ability to release physical and emotional blockages, promote total relaxation, and enhance recovery from stress and injuries.

Art, when used as therapy, helps an individual calm down. By coloring, dancing and writing, one can find the road to self-discovery and personal fulfillment. Art has spiritual power.

What to Avoid

Keeping young and healthy is a balancing act. We must stay away from, or compensate for, the myriad of factors that disturb our equilibrium, such as foods and chemicals that artificially stimulate energy and wear down the body, like coffee, drugs, and cigarettes; alcohol, which accelerates brain cell deterioration; environmental toxins that compromise the immune system; and medicines that cover up symptoms, such as antacids, diuretics, and aspirin. It is equally important to let go of our preconceived notions of aging and, instead, stay active. Finally, we must remember not to let stress get the best of us.

Treatment Summary

Any method that removes the toxins that we accumulate every day will act to retard aging. Some detoxification methods are juice fasting, chelation therapy, colonic irrigation, exercise, skin brushing, saunas, and the use of herbs.

Laboratory tests can let us know which systems need boosting and thus which nutrients will be most helpful.

The antiaging diet is one that keeps our pH balanced. The best foods: fruits, vegetables, grains, legumes, nuts, and seeds.

Antioxidant supplements keep us young by slowing down free radical damage. These include vitamin A, beta-carotene, bioflavonoids, vitamin C, vitamin E, selenium, zinc, and NADH.

Herbs important to an antiaging protocol include fo-ti-tieng, garlic, ginkgo biloba, ginseng, and gotu kola.

Essential oils may alleviate common conditions associated with aging, including insomnia, indigestion, arthritis, and memory loss.

Stress reduction is essential to slowing down the aging process, and preventing degenerative disease.

AIDS (Acquired Immune Deficiency Syndrome)

There is disagreement over what causes AIDS, how to treat it, and whether or not the condition is curable. The accepted viewpoint is that the human immunodeficiency (HIV) virus causes AIDS. While this may be one factor, the belief that HIV alone is responsible for the massive deterioration that characterizes AIDS is a gross oversimplification. After years of research, there is no solid scientific evidence supporting this virus-as-sole-cause theory. Rather, the virus may be a cofactor, with other factors necessary before a person becomes ill.

AIDS is officially defined by the Centers for Disease Control as the presence of HIV with the manifestation of one or more of a list of over two dozen previously known diseases. So, for example, tuberculosis with HIV is AIDS; without it, it is still tuberculosis. Other diseases on the list are Kaposi's sarcoma, progressive multifocal leukoencephalopathy, disseminated cytomegalovirus, pneumonia and candidiasis.

Nagging questions persist about the HIV=AIDS concept. For one, why are some people with AIDS symptoms actually HIV-negative? And if AIDS is spread by bodily fluids why has it not spread to the general population and why has it not reached epidemic proportions? The fact is that most research outside of the HIV=AIDS paradigm suggests that AIDS can occur only after the immune system is worn down. This can be caused by long-term drug use—either intravenous or oral, and either recreational or prescription; by hepatitis; or by malnutrition. Also, excessive sexual activity can weaken the immune system, and sexually transmitted diseases, acquired before the individual was exposed to HIV, may contribute to immune system breakdown as well. Additionally, multiple infections place an increased burden on the immune system. Yeasts, molds, fungi and a variety of viruses can play a part. Unfortunately, the all too common treatment for infections—antibiotics—suppresses the immune system further.

Symptoms

Initial symptoms can include extreme fatigue, night sweats, fever, chills, swollen lymph glands, swollen spleen, loss of appetite, weight loss, severe diarrhea and depression. As AIDS progresses and the immune system weakens, the body becomes receptive to opportunistic infections. A form of pneumonia (pneumocystis carini) and a rare cancer (Kaposi's syndrome) are commonly contracted. Other forms of cancer associated with the condition include non-Hodgkin's lymphoma and Burkitt's syndrome. A swelling of the lining of the spine (meningitis) or the brain (encephalitis) may also occur.

Treatment

Up until recently HIV and AIDS were considered tantamount to a death sentence. The conventional treatment has relied on powerful drugs taken in the hope of slowing the progression of the disease. The trouble is, such drugs add toxins to an already weakened immune system. Researchers now seem hopeful that new drug combinations can keep the disease under control, and this approach does seem to be helping some patients. At this point, though, no one knows the long-term effects of these drugs.

What we do know is that long-term survivors do not rely totally on pharmaceuticals. Many do not take drugs at all. They alter their diets and lifestyles to maximize the health-giving elements in each. Plus, they make positive affirmations about the future.

Under the guidance of a holistically trained physician, AIDS patients should incorporate multiple healing modalities that stimulate the immune system to a healthy state of activity. Different remedies may be needed at different times, and individuals need to be flexible in their approach. The therapies listed here are immune-enhancing, antibacterial, antiviral, antimicrobial and nontoxic or minimally toxic.

Diet

Everyone needs a good diet, but when people have severely weakened immune systems, high-quality nutrition becomes essential. This means eating organic vegetarian (or mostly vegetarian) foods and drinking lots of filtered water.

Complex carbohydrates should be the mainstay of the diet. Unlike simple sugars, these foods are close to their natural form when eaten, and work to strengthen the immune system. There are plenty of whole grains from which to choose, including brown rice, wheat berries, barley, millet, whole oats, amaranth, quinoa and bulgur wheat.

Vegetables are rich in several important antioxidants, including beta-carotene, vitamin C, vitamin E and selenium, which work together as a team to fight free radical damage. Six to eight cups of various types of vegetables should be eaten daily. Good sources of vitamin C and calcium are kale, collards and broccoli. Squash, almonds and carrots are high in beta-carotene, while wheat germ and nuts are good sources of vitamin E. Because these foods are high in fiber, they stimulate the immune-enhancing cells of our intestinal lining, and cleanse the colon of toxins. Fiber helps prevent intestinal infections as well.

Raw foods are good sources of enzymes, but should not be eaten if there is a problem with diarrhea. Be sure to get your produce cleaned off before eating it. A good way to wash foods is with food-grade hydrogen peroxide from the pharmacy.

Easily digestible proteins are something you should look for. Think in terms of vegetable proteins and sprouts. Fermented food products, such as tempeh or miso, are also easy to digest. A cup of miso soup can be eaten daily.

To keep calorie consumption up, eat avocado, nut butters, almonds and sunflower seeds.

Small quantities of fat are important, but these should come from high-quality sources. A tablespoon of unrefined olive oil can be added to salads. Flaxseed oil and fatty fish, like salmon, are also excellent. Remember that oils need refrigeration to prevent rancidity.

Oriental mushrooms, like shiitake and maitake, boost the immune system. Shiitake mushrooms contain lentinan, a substance that stimulates the body's interferon and helps fight viruses. Soups and teas can be made from these mushrooms and taken daily.

Garlic is another valuable food. It contains allicin, a potent antibacterial and antiviral agent. When garlic is cooked, allicin is lost, so try to take this herb raw or in capsules. Garlic also contains protein, vitamins A and C, thiamin, calcium, potassium, copper and selenium. Note that garlic can be juiced along with your other vegetables.

Sea vegetables, which include dulse, kombu, nori and wakame, contain trace minerals that are no longer found in foods grown on land.

An important part of a health-maximizing diet is juicing. Freshly made juice supplies concentrated nutrients and plenty of raw enzymes, which help the body digest foods, making their nutrients available to our cells. Juices also contain an abundance of antioxidants.

A small amount of greens can be juiced together with carrots, beets, garlic or apples. Greens should be rotated; your choices can include cabbage, kale, broccoli, mustard, collard and dandelion greens, Swiss chard, spinach, watercress, parsley and wheatgrass. All of these are high in chlorophyll, which is antibacterial and a good energy provider. People with digestion problems should start off slowly by diluting a glass of juice with a glass of water. Gradually, they can build up to 4 to 6 glasses of juice a day. A holistic health practitioner can provide individualized guidance on juicing and other aspects of diet.

AIDS researcher Mark Konlee offers this juice recipe for building the immune system, flushing the liver and the lymphatic system, getting nutrients and increasing energy: wash a whole undyed lemon, cut it in quarters, blend in a blender. Add one cup of water and one tablespoon of cold-pressed, extra virgin organic olive oil. The drink can be sweetened with a few tablespoons of orange juice. Blend. Strain and drink the juice. Taking this drink once a day, Konlee reports, can raise T-cell counts, decrease viral load and improve lymphatic drainage.

Supplements

AIDS patients need large doses of immune-building nutrients both orally and intravenously. Particularly important are antioxidants, which provide essential protection against free radical damage. Vitamin C, beta-carotene, vitamin E and selenium are four-star nutrients of the antioxidant group that work best as a team to clean up the system and resist infection. The following supplements and herbs combat AIDS and related conditions. They can be taken individually or in combination.

Vitamin C . . . AIDS patients need considerable amounts of vitamin C, both oral and intravenous, to build immunity and protect against secondary infections. Such high dosages make intravenous administration a necessity. In addition, vitamin C should be taken orally; a buffered form of the nutrient protects the stomach. Vitamin C polyascorbate is the most easily assimilated form of vitamin C and is recommended for people suffering from chronic illnesses. For those with Kaposi's lesions, applying a topical paste is quite healing.

Vitamin C stimulates white blood cell activity, causing cells to surround viruses and place them in vacuoles, so that superoxide dismutase and other substances in the body can fill the space, killing the viruses.

Research supports vitamin C's ability to inhibit the replication of HIV and other pathogenic microorganisms commonly found in HIV-positive individuals, including Rous sarcoma virus, Epstein-Barr virus and cytomegalovirus. This is accomplished in several ways: vitamin C decreases viral production, increases the immune system cells (called monocytes) that fight viruses and stimulates interferon, a natural antiviral, antibacterial substance produced by the immune system.

The power of intravenous vitamin C drips is further enhanced by the addition of antibiotic and immune enhancing herbs, such as garlic, chaparral, red clover, pau d'arco, echinacea, goldenseal, lobelia, ginger, astragalus, ganoderma and licorice root.

Acetyl-L-Carnitine . . . A dosage of 6 g per day could enhance lipid metabolism and immune response in AIDS patients. This demonstrates that L-carnitine is capable of lessening the toxic effects of AZT.

In cases of AIDS-related dementia and senility, 1000 mg of acetyl-L-carnitine per day showed significant improvement.

Acidophilus . . . These beneficial bacteria help rebuild the microflora in the intestine that have been weakened or totally wiped out by repeated antibiotic treatments before other harmful bacteria can take over or yeast super-infection can build up. A weakened digestive system and a breakdown in absorption are the symptoms of AIDS. We can see the value of acidophilus for its general immune-boosting effect, as well.

Alpha-Lipoic Acid . . . This is an antioxidant acid that can increase resistance to HIV.

Vitamin B6 . . . This vitamin, recommended in dosages of 100 mg daily, is important for building up red blood cells and activating natural killer cells. Deficiencies in B6 have been related to suppressed natural killer cell activity.

Beta-Carotene/Vitamin A . . . Studies show that the powerful antioxidant beta-carotene increases T-cell numbers, which protect against infections, and boosts the immune system. Beta-carotene is converted by the body into vitamin A, and is safer in large doses than vitamin A.

Vitamin B12 . . . Hematologic and neurological dysfunction in AIDS patients is connected to B12 deficiency. The low functioning of acid, pepsid and gastric juice causes the decrease in the levels of B12. This results in B12 malabsorption. Normalizing the status of the vitamin by supplementation with 250 mcg in HIV-infected patients significantly improved their cognitive function. Studying the relationship between vitamin B12 deficiency and AIDS dementia complex, researchers found that it may be a reversible adverse synergistic interaction.

Bifidus . . . Bifidus is a supplement that contains B. bifidum. It enhances the intestinal microflora, and has immune-mobilizing, antiviral properties. Research has shown that B. bifidum can decrease acute diarrhea. It also counteracts the negative effects of antibiotics on the digestive system.

Boron . . . Boron is a trace mineral found in many fruits and vegetables. When combined with amino acids, it could inhibit HIV protease.

Bromelain . . . In digesting proteins, bromelain, a group of enzymes, plays an important role. In terms of combating AIDS, supplementation of bromelain boosts T-cell proliferation.

Bioflavonoids . . . These enhance the absorption of vitamin C.

Butyric Acid . . . This nutrient aids in cellular repair and is especially good in treating lymphomas and leukemia.

Citrus Seed Extracts . . . Extracts from oranges, grapefruits, lemons and limes are credited with enormous antimicrobial activity. They are broad-spectrum, nontoxic antibiotics, with antifungal, antibacterial and antiviral properties. Citrus seed extracts can fight off a wide variety of infections, including E. coli, intestinal protozoa, fungi and viruses.

In addition, citrus seed extracts can kill over 30 types of yeast, including Candida albicans. At the same time, citrus seed extracts do not interfere with healthful bacteria that are needed to rebalance the system.

A final benefit of these extracts, sold in powder and liquid form, is that a few drops added to water can be used to clean bacteria from fruits and vegetables.

Coenzyme Q10 . . . AIDS and HIV patients have significant deficiencies of CoQ10. Supplementation with CoQ10 produces energy for cellular functions and increases blood levels of IgG and T4/T8 ratios. Future research will most likely show more beneficial properties of this substance that is found in the human body.

Dioxychlor . . . Dioxychlor is an antiviral, antibacterial, antifungal and antiparasitic agent. More research needs to be done, but in the test tube, this substance disarms HIV as well as cytomegalovirus, herpes and other infectious organisms. In fact, any pathogenic virus moving from one point to another comes under attack. Dioxychlor can be administered intravenously, orally or topically as a gel.

DHEA . . . Studies in journals such as *AIDS Treatment News* and *AIDS Res Human Retroviruses* show that DHEA, the hormone produced by the adrenal glands, kills HIV in vitro and lowers viral load. One investigation suggests that there is an inverse association between DHEA levels and increased HIV progression in patients with CD4 counts below 300. Oral supplementation with DHEA, using an average dose of 75 mg, combined with standard antiviral treatment in cases of HIV-infected patients leads to raised levels of CD4 and CD8 counts.

Egg Lipids (AL-721) . . . AL-721, a formula made from two active phospholipids found in egg yolk, is an adjunctive therapy for the containment of HIV and other viruses. The substance was first developed at the Weitzmann Institute of Science in Israel by a team of scientists, led by Meier Shinitsky. They found this formula effective in treating memory loss and impaired immune function, and in easing the withdrawal effects from alcohol and drug addiction.

AL-721 was also found to prevent human T-cells from becoming infected by HIV. It is thought to work by removing cholesterol from the envelope surrounding the virus, in the process rendering it ineffective. Egg lipids have none of the toxicity problems found in drugs such as AZT.

Essential Fatty Acids . . . Essential fatty acids contain GLA, which is converted by the body into prostaglandin-El. This helps stimulate T-lymphocyte function and has a direct inhibitory effect on the replication of the HIV virus.

Glutathione Peroxidase... This protective antioxidant is naturally produced by the body and is deficient in AIDS patients. Intravenous glutathione protects the organs and the blood cells against damage, especially when used in conjunction with selenium, vitamin C and vitamin E. It also helps to protect the body against viral illnesses, including HIV. Taken as a supplement, glutathione can be helpful in preventing the HIV virus from becoming active. Sometimes N-acetyl-cysteine, which is converted by the system into glutathione, is given in its stead.

Intestinal Flora... Lactobacillus acidophilus, lactobacillus bulgaricus and bifidus bacteria are healthful bacteria that many people lose after taking antibiotics. These flora strengthen the body's infection-fighting power by generating more lymphocytes.

Iodine... Iodine is an element that is needed to make thyroid hormones. Iodine preparations show effective countermeasures against varied infective agents, such as herpes, Candida, different fungal infections and intestinal bacterial infections. Yet, no extensive research has been done to connect iodine with combating AIDS. There is a possibility that iodine will be viewed as an adjunctive agent for treating AIDS.

L-Dopa... This drug converts dopamine, a neurotransmitter chemical, in the brain. The supplementation of L-dopa in HIV-infected children alleviated symptoms of nerve dysfunction.

Melatonin... Melatonin is a substance produced by the pineal gland. Since it has demonstrated great ability to restore depressed immune function, melatonin should be studied more closely by AIDS scientists.

NAC... As mentioned earlier, NAC is converted into glutathione. Glutathione has HIV-diminishing capabilities. Increased levels of glutathione may enhance survival rates among AIDS patients. Also, the number of CD4-positive T-cells in HIV-infected patients goes up as a reaction to higher levels of glutathione. The unique quality of NAC that separates it from the other antivirals is that while it depresses HIV, it also strengthens T-cell function and stimulates growth.

Phosphatidylserine... This organic brain compound could be an excellent candidate for further studies because of its positive impact on AIDS.

Selenium... Selenium, an enzyme-activating nonmetallic element in the body, increases intracellular glutathione levels. A study shows that it could significantly elevate the activity of natural killer cells. Another report proves that supplementation of selenium leads to enhanced immune response.

Vitamin D... One significant study shows that supplementation with this nutrient corrected certain immune system cell damage in AIDS patients that was due to the disease.

Vitamin E... This powerful antioxidant is capable of increasing the cells' antiviral properties. By inhibiting undernutrition and other pathological symptoms, vitamin E might retard the progress of AIDS and help the body ward off the immunological damage caused by the disease.

Vitamin K . . . One study shows that vitamin K compounds stopped HIV replication in vitro.

Zinc . . . An important study shows that normalization of a deficiency in zinc levels might trigger CD4 production and improve immune functions. This study indicates that oral supplementation with 200 mg of zinc sulphate stimulated T-cell production in HIV-infected patients who were asymptomatic.

Shark Cartilage . . . According to research, shark cartilage may be useful in the treatment of AIDS, cancer, arthritis and a variety of other degenerative diseases. It may be particularly effective in stopping Kaposi's sarcoma.

The idea behind the use of shark cartilage is that the skeleton of sharks contain a great amount of anti-angiogenesis factor. Angiogenesis refers to the formation of the local capillary network that sustains a tumor. When that production is stopped, there is no network of blood vessels to feed the tumor. The tumor stops growing and spreading. It may even begin to shrink and disappear.

Herbs

Traditional Chinese Medicine (TCM) holds that the terrain is more important than the germ attacking it. A healthy person easily resists foreign invaders, while a weak one is susceptible to almost everything. Based on this philosophy, certain plants have been used for thousands of years as a fundamental part of Chinese medicine to strengthen the immune system. Now, mainstream Western medicine is getting interested in herbs and opening its eyes to what TCM, Native American and other types of herbs can offer.

Up until now, herbal therapy has been based on empirical evidence, but the recent challenge of AIDS and other modern-day diseases has generated scientific interest in the field. Experimenters ask if herbs can help overcome dreaded diseases. If so, how?

Research does scientifically confirm the value of plant medicines, both alone and in conjunction with other therapies. For example, double-blind studies show that AIDS patients who are given Chinese herbs and AZT consistently do better than patients given placebos in place of the botanicals. Other studies report remission from cancer when astragalus is given alone.

Dr. R.S. Chang, Professor of Medical Microbiology and Immunology at the University of California School of Medicine, has listed Chinese herbs according to their specific actions on the immune system. Ethnobiologist Dr. James Duke has done the same, looking at herbs the world over. Some of the herbs that keep coming up again and again on such lists are astragalus, panax ginseng, ganoderma and ligustrum. Herbs that increase the number of T-lymphocytes, according to Chang, are:

Panax ginseng
Ganoderma lucidum
Coriolius versicolor
Lentinus edodes
Phaseolus vulgaris
Atractylodes macrocephala
Coix lachrymajobi
Polygonatum sibiricum
Asparagus cochinchinensis
Ligustrum lucidum
Epimedium grandiflorum

Duke lists as promoting phagocytosis:

Aconitum	Cynanchum	Matricaria
Adina	Datura	Mentha
Alliurn	Dioscorea	Morus
Althaea	Dyera	Myroxylum
Angelica	Echinacea	Oldenlandia
Aralia	Eleuthero	Panax
Aristolochia	Epimedium	Persea
Astragalus	Eucommia	Petiveria
Atractylodes	Eupatorium	Phytolacca
Aucoumea	Forsythia	Pistacia
Boswellia	Garioderma	Platycodon
Byrsonima	Glycine	Polyporus
Canarium	Glycyrrhiza	Psoralea
Cephaelis	Hedyotis	Rehmannia
Chiysanthemum	Houttuynia	Scutellaria
Clastanthus	Indigofera	Stephania
Codonopsis	Lentinus	Styrax
Commiphora	Ligusticum	Tussilago
Coptis	Lonicera	Uncaria
Curculigo	Manilkara	Vinca

Many of the plants that appear to be most useful belong to a category of herbs known as adaptogens. These work through a wide variety of actions to help create homeostasis or biological balance. So, for example, if the blood pressure is too high, adaptogens help the body lower it; if it is too low, the body responds by raising it. Adaptogens help normalize the system regardless of the pathology.

Studies demonstrate that adaptogenic plants are especially good at stimulating the body's own natural immune functions. For example, they have been shown to increase CD4 counts, interferon production, macrophage activity and natural killer cell action. Adaptogens are often combined for a more potent synergistic effect. An example is astragalus and legustrum; the combination is more effective than either plant used alone.

These herbs may be helpful in an AIDS treatment protocol:

Astragalus . . . Astragalus' membranaceous root has been used medicinally in China for centuries, and indeed, modern scientific research shows the herb to possess powerful immune-strengthening properties. Of particular note is its ability to foster normal immune response in cancer and AIDS patients, to correct T-cell deficiency and to promote antiviral action.

Astragalus increases interferon production as well as phagocytosis, allowing the body to consume more pathogenic microorganisms. It also decreases tumor cell growth and lessens the suppression of the immune system caused by drugs, making it a good adjunctive therapy.

When combined with legustrum, astragalus is even more potent, and is especially good at increasing the activity of spleen cells. These two herbs are sold in combination in extract and capsule form. They can also be bought whole in Chinatown, crushed and then simmered in a small amount of water for several hours. The Chinese prepare herbs in this way and consume them daily.

American Creosote Bush . . . This shrub from the Mojave Desert is a very old plant. The first growth goes back 12,000 years. It has strong antimicrobial properties against organisms such as L. monocytogenes, C. perfiringens and S. dysenteriae.

Angelica . . . From ancient times, this plant is famous for its healing power. Research by Inamori reveals that its root has antibacterial properties against certain pathogenic bacteria. These facts suggest that angelica can be helpful in combating AIDS.

Basil . . . Research suggests that this herb can help regulate the immune system. It has long been known as a friend to the immune system.

Bee Propolis . . . This substance is collected by bees from trees and plants. It has powerful antibacterial qualities. It fights Staphylococcus aureus, Trichomonas vaginalis and herpes simplex I.

Bupleurum Falcatum . . . This Chinese herb contains saikosaponins, which triggers the consumption of foreign cells by macrophages in vivo. It defends the liver by increasing protein synthesis.

Burdock . . . Chemical compounds of some varieties of this plant are proven to be antibacterial, antifungal and tumor-protective, and appear to inhibit cancer-causing agents.

Castanospermine . . . There is an indication that castanospermine, a plant alkaloid, blocks the growth of HIV, possibly by altering the enzyme production of the retrovirus.

Chlorella . . . This green algae is known for its immune-stimulating qualities.

Cruciferous Extract . . . Dithiolthione is a compound extracted from cruciferous vegetables such as cabbage, cauliflower and broccoli that seems to protect normal cells in cancer patients and protects the liver. These qualities may be beneficial to AIDS patients.

Compound Q and Bitter Melon . . . Compound Q is the purified extract of Chinese cucumber. Bitter melon is in the same cucumber family. These vegetables have been popular in China, Indonesia and the Philippines for centuries. They have recently proven effective against HIV activity. The proteins in these herbs can selectively kill HIV-infected cells but do not harm non-infected cells. This combination also helps the immune system to recover.

DASM (dehydroandrographolide succinic acid monoester) . . . This compound from the Chinese medicinal herb, Andrographis paniculata, inhibits the HIV virus's replication in vitro.

Eclipta Alba . . . This herb grows in the Southwestern United States, and, according to herbologist Letha Hadady, it has a stimulating effect on the immune system's white cell production without causing inflammation. Eclipta alba is well known in India. A study conducted by T. Chandra revealed that in a liver that had increased in weight due to damage by carbon tetrachloride, levels of enzymes were restored to normal by using this herb.

Feverfew . . . This herb has sedative qualities and works as an antidote for headaches, according to Dr. Mary Gordon. It is proven to be antiviral, and kills candida in vitro.

Ginseng . . . Both Siberian and panax ginseng boost the immune system by increasing the number and activity of natural killer cells. These herbs work to prevent liver toxicity and are anticarcinogenic. Ginseng is best taken as an extract or a tea.

Garlic . . . Garlic has great antiviral qualities; it works as a natural antibiotic. It has been proven effective against opportunistic microbes, such as herpesvirus hominus type I, crytococcal mycobacterial and candida organisms. It has the ability to suppress human cytomegalovirus in vitro. Garlic works as a free radical scavenger, eliminating toxic oxidation products. In a test with AIDS patients, the impact of the supplementation of 5 to 10 mg of aged garlic extract was studied. The results were very promising. In six weeks, the natural killer cell activity in the patients was restored to normal and they experienced a significant improvement in immune function. The AIDS-fighting qualities of garlic should be studied further.

Ginkgo Biloba . . . This powerful herb, recognized for its memory-enhancing qualities, has shown its ability in coping with some infections like P. carini. It has not been studied in connection with AIDS.

Goldenseal . . . This plant has three major components that are especially valuable. Berberine sulfate shows antimicrobial qualities and stimulates the immune system; hydrastine blocks microbes; and canadine destroys human carcinoma cells in vitro. For its antimicrobial, antiprotozoal and antifungal qualities, goldenseal could be a valuable ally in the war against AIDS.

Bitter Melon . . . This vegetable has been popular in China, Indonesia and the Philippines for centuries, and recently has been proven effective against HIV activity in laboratory studies. Some AIDS patients who use the juice report substantial improvement. It reduces night sweats, helps with weight gain and stops viral replication.

Caterpillar Fungus . . . This Chinese tonic has been used by people recovering from illness since ancient times. Its positive effects include strengthening the kidneys, clearing of the lungs and fortification of the bone marrow, an essential part of the immune system. Caterpillar fungus also inhibits bacterial and fungal infections. It is currently being used in combination with other herbs to treat malignant tumors, anemia, asthma and, most recently, AIDS.

Osha Root and Lepotania . . . These plants are native to the American West and an integral part of Native American medicine. Although scientific studies of their beneficial effects on the immune system have yet to be conducted, empirical evidence with viral diseases strongly suggests their use in a protocol for viral diseases.

Other plant remedies that are not characterized as adaptogens should be considered in a treatment protocol for HIV and AIDS. While there is no one magic bullet against the syndrome, combining several of these nonspecific immune enhancers can make a positive difference:

Aloe Vera . . . Even though aloe vera is over 99 percent water, it is a nutritionally dense substance, with over 200 active ingredients. Aloe vera contains 17 amino acids as well as the minerals calcium, copper, iron, phosphorus, potassium and zinc. It supplies live enzymes and essential fatty acids, which are needed for good health. Additionally, it has substances that stimulate phagocytosis, the process by which white blood cells work to destroy invading organisms. Not all brands of aloe vera are qualitatively equal. Heat-processing destroys vital nutrients. For maximum benefit, look for brands that cold-process the whole leaf.

Carnivora (Venus Flytrap) . . . Carnivora has been proven effective against cancer, AIDS and other chronic pathologies. According to studies, unless the immune system has been damaged by radiation and chemotherapy, many cancers will diminish, or go into remission with its use.

Carnivora works by building the immune components of the blood. It increases the numbers of B-cells, T-cells, lymphocytes, granulocytes, monocytes, phagocytes and other solid components of the immune system. Additionally, it excites inactive blood elements to begin functioning again. The immune system can then mobilize against disease-producing pathogens. They begin to attack and devour cancer cells, much like carnivora swallows and digests flies.

American laws prevent carnivora from being shipped to doctors, but the product can be mailed directly to consumers, who can then hand-deliver it to doctors. Severely compromised AIDS patients may need a two- or three-hour infusion five days a week for three to four months. As an individual improves, the treatment can be given intramuscularly three times a week, for about two years. Carnivora can be acquired from the manufacturer, Edgar Fischer, Manager, Carnivora Forschungs-GmBH, Postfach 8, Lobensteiner Strasse 3, D-8646 Nordhalben, Germany.

Echinacea . . . Echinacea stimulates immune cell production and activity as well as levels of interferon and interleuken-2. The herb is usually sold as a tincture, and the best brands produce a strong tingling and numbing sensation on the tongue.

Research shows benefits to be short-term. Echinacea boosts the immune system to high levels of activity. But to do this continuously would be too much for the body. For this reason, it is best to take the extract for up to four days, and then to rest an equal length of time before starting again.

Cat's Claw . . . This rain forest herb is useful in treating numerous conditions and may be especially important for stimulating immune system activity.

Ligustrum Lucidum . . . Known for its immune-system and vitality-boosting qualities, ligustrum lucidum could be an important herb for stimulating the blood in AIDS patients who were treated with AZT or other antivirals. It is used after chemotherapy or radiotherapy to restore white blood cell levels.

Maitake Mushrooms . . . In vitro tests have shown maitake mushroom powder has an anti-HIV effect. In animal studies, scientists found that it activates effector cells that attack foreign cells such as macrophages, natural killer cells and T-cells, and it potentiates the activity of mediators (such as lymphokines and interleukin-1). It is already used for prolonging the lives of cancer patients.

Mistletoe . . . Combined with lactobacillus, mistletoe can double the number of natural killer cells to destroy malignant cells, and the extract from the herb has anti-HIV, immunomodulating and anticancer properties.

Peppermint . . . Peppermint kills herpes simplex virus and other microorganisms, and it has a soothing effect in cases of irritable bowel syndrome.

Reishi Mushrooms . . . This fungus, known in Japan and China, helps to regulate blood sugar, and protects the body from free radicals and radiation.

Rhubarb . . . This Chinese herb shows significant activity against Bacteroides fragilis, a major microorganism in the intestinal flora of humans. Due to its action on spleen cells, rhubarb enhances immune response.

Royal Bee Jelly . . . This bee product contains a full spectrum of vitamins and minerals. Being a natural source of acetylcholine, which is vital to the transmission of the nerve impulses in the brain and the body, royal bee jelly has unique immune-enhancing properties.

Schizandra . . . One of the most important herbs of TCM, schizandra restores balance to the body's systems. Combined with ginseng, it helps to detoxify the liver.

St. John's Wort . . . This is an established anti-HIV herb that has two potent antiviral chemicals: hypericin and pseudohypericin. St. John's wort is capable of blocking and reducing the spread of the HIV virus in vitro and in vivo. Because of its ability to cross the blood-brain barrier, it can enter the brain and attack viruses. The herb is available worldwide. It is relatively inexpensive.

Tannins . . . Some reputable sources state that tannins can inhibit HIV reverse transcriptase and HIV replication in vitro. Several other credible studies back up this statement.

Turmeric . . . The bright yellow spice that colors curry powder has been getting a lot of attention lately due to its ability to stabilize the mast cells that make up the lining of the intestinal tract and serve as the first line of defense for the immune system. These cells are important for blocking out unwanted materials. In an experiment, turmeric was found to inhibit HIV replication.

Violet . . . Violet is one of the eleven Chinese herbs capable of fighting HIV. It actually can break up HIV growth, as it has demonstrated in repeated experiments.

Licorice Root (Glycyrrhizin) . . . Licorice is the most frequently used herb in TCM. It has been universally studied. It has antiviral effects, and it can inhibit virus proliferation. Of all of the natural detoxifying agents known, licorice is the most broad-spectrum. It gets rid of more than 1200 different toxins from the body without harmful side effects.

Phyllanthius (Life Plant) . . . Traditionally used in TCM, phyllanthius is new to this country where it is now being researched for its antiretroviral and anti-HIV activity.

Phytochemicals

Phytochemicals have been associated with the prevention and treatment of at least four of the leading causes of death in the country—cancer, diabetes, cardiovascular disease and hypertension—according to the American Dietetic Association's journal. Found in different fruits and vegetables, they are the force behind the beneficial properties those foods exhibit. Now that we have the technical skills, we can pinpoint and isolate them in order to use them in treating conditions. Here is a list that indicates which phytochemicals seem to be helpful in various health areas impacted by AIDS:

Antidiarrhetic . . . Red mangrove; rowan berry; arbutus; pomegranate; marshmallow; canaigre; babul; gum ghatti; poison hemlock; sunflower; guava; coconut; nance; emblic; fenugreek; winter's bark; smooth sumac; simaruba bark; and chinaberry.

Antifatigue . . . Lettuce; asparagus; endive; black gram; cowpea; lambsquarter; radish; chayote; Chinese cabbage; purslane; oat; garland chrysanthemum; dill; dandelion; pigweed; cucumber; kudzu; spinach; and borage.

Antiglaucomic . . . Camu-camu; pansy; Japanese pagoda tree; pumpkin; acerola; Chinese foxglove; buckwheat; sang-pai-pi; celery; peegee; bitter melon; American elder; pokeweed; parsley; common smartweed; and warburghia.

Anti-HIV . . . Rowan berry; licorice; poison hemlock; sunflower; coconut; fenugreek; winter's bark; rice; white willow; corn; giant reed; black locust; crab's eye; cork oak; evening primrose; oats; hull husk; lantana; red mangrove; coffee; and mango.

Antiviral . . . Khasi pine; lemon; chilgoza pine; celery; red mangrove; camu-camu; rowan berry; arbutus; pomegranate; emblic; canaigre; babul; gum ghatti; poison hemlock; guava; sunflower; chir pine; celery; coconut; nance; fenugreek; winter's bark; grape; Chinese goldthread; generic goldthread; mango; huang-lia; goldenseal; witch hazel; aleppo oak; barberry; huang po; prickly poppy; strawberry; rhubarb; and soybean.

Bactericide . . . Lemon; chir pine; khasi pine; celery; chilgoza pine; grape; red mangrove; mangosteen; camu-camu; copaiba; Hindi chaulmoogra; rowan berry; arbutus; pomegranate; marshmallow; canaigre; and babul.

Candidicide . . . Clove; grape; cowberry; coconut; allspice; garlic; cucumber; bayrum tree; carrot; cherimoya; common thyme; basil; carrot; cantaloupe; pignut hickory; purslane; spinach; and oats.

Fungicide . . . Parsnip; grape; lemon; clove; coconut; potato; cardamom; oats; coffee; rice; common thyme; celery; java-olive; bayrum tree; winter savory; celery; turmeric; and allspice.

Hepatoprotective . . . Cantaloupe; English walnut; red mangrove; avocado; cucumber; safflower; arbutus; Brazil nut; apricot; sunflower; great scarlet poppy; butternut; canaigre; babul; opium poppy; calabash gourd; pomegranate; gum ghatti; guava; and sesame.

Immunostimulant . . . Chicory; gobo; elecampane; dandelion; licorice; coneflower; costus; leopard's bane; crab's eye; coffee; mugwort; Chinese goldthread; generic goldthread; java-olive; huang-lia; goldenseal; beet; malangra; and lambsquarter.

Other Natural Remedies

The following list of disparate remedies represents a wide range of beneficial treatments. Because of their somewhat anomalous nature, it is impossible to list them in any category other than "Other Natural Remedies." Yet, their effectiveness warrants their inclusion in this book.

DNCB (Dinitrochlorobenzene) . . . This substance works similarly to acupuncture by stimulating the blood flow. Applied to the skin with a cotton ball, it penetrates the skin and triggers a strong immune response that results in full-scale immune system rejuvenation. The DNCB antigen boosts CD4 T-helper-cell production; the aroused immune system is capable of eliminating the HIV virus.

Dysidia and Seaweed . . . One of the compounds of dysidia, an ocean sponge, combats the HIV virus. Ocean seaweeds are also potent antiviral agents.

GE-3-S . . . GE-3-S is extracted from lichen umbilicaria esculenta. It shows antiviral and anti-HIV properties in animal studies and in vitro. It exhibits such strength that further research should be demanded.

Glandular Polypeptide Extract . . . A highly purified extract from animal thymus and spleen can boost CD4 production and decrease the CD8 count in HIV-infected individuals. In a test, oral splenic polypeptide was combined with Siberian ginseng, making a PCM-4 formula that resulted in an increase in CD4 counts, weight gain and cessation of diarrhea. This treatment is approved for treating HIV-positive patients in Tanzania and Uganda.

Lignosulfonate (LS) . . . LS is a water-soluble lignin that is extracted from the waste liquor of pulping wood created during the papermaking process. In vitro, LS exhibits unique antiviral activity against HIV by blocking HIV's ability to kill cells (cytopathy) or clump together (syncytia), as well as by stopping the retrovirus from replicating and locking onto healthy cells. Further exploration of these qualities should be investigated.

Pentamidine . . . A rare form of pneumonia called PCP is one of the most opportunistic infections AIDS patients have to face. Inhaled pentamidine can reduce relapse by 50 percent. Even if it returns, the PCP is mild and much less fatal. The injected form of pentamidine tends to go to the liver and other organs, but not to the lungs. This drug is available by prescription only.

Ricin . . . The chemical ricin is derived from castor oil and works as a biological wrecking ball, seeking out virus-infected cells and killing them. Ricin blocks protein-building, so the cells can't even be manufactured.

Rovital-V (R-1103) and Carciviren-V (C-1983) . . . The nontoxic and antiviral R-1103 and C-1983 are the combination of plant extracts. These substances slow down or even inhibit the progression of HIV from stages I, II, III and IV.

Homeopathy

Homeopathy works on emotional, mental and physical levels. Treating the whole person is particularly important in AIDS and other diseases that are deemed incurable by allopathic medicine, as the shock of the diagnosis often triggers an emotional state that worsens the physical state of the patient.

According to a noted classical homeopath, one appropriate remedy should be chosen for each patient on an individualized basis. As symptoms change and lessen with time, so should the remedy. When using homeopathic remedies, the homeopath advises avoiding mints, perfumes and coffee. These medicines should be taken 20 minutes before eating:

Ignatia . . . The person is silent, brooding, with changeable moods. There is a lot of sighing and sobbing and a great despair of being cured.

Gelsemium . . . Symptoms include listlessness and apathy. The person has a dread of being alone and wants to be with people. There is an apathy regarding the illness. Diarrhea accompanies bad news.

Arsenicum Album . . . Use for the fear of dying. The person has a restless mental state, almost to the point of panic. There are periodic fevers.

Thuja . . . This person has a high sex drive and a history of sexually transmitted conditions, such as discharges, gonorrhea, genital warts and herpes. There is rapid exhaustion with emaciation. The individual has fixed ideas. Often there are feelings of weakness and a feeling that one is weaker and sicker than the physical condition would warrant.

Mercurius . . . The person has a history of syphilis. Fevers and night sweats occur without amelioration. Any type of weather aggravates this person, who never feels comfortable. There are also tendencies to have swollen glands, sore throats, sores in the mouth, and thrush. Mentally, the person is paranoid, especially in the advanced stages.

Arsenicum Iodadum . . . Symptoms for which this remedy is prescribed are similar to arsenicum album, except that the person feels warmer and better in the cold. There is also a tendency to get swollen glands and periodic fevers.

Iodadum . . . This remedy is indicated when there is sudden emaciation with swollen glands. Despite loss of weight, there is a great appetite. Restlessness is characteristic here.

Phosphoric Acid . . . The person is extremely exhausted, feeling apathetic and ready to give up the fight. There is a sadness regarding the future, without fear and anxiety about death. Thinking may be scattered as well.

Medorrhinum . . . Acute diseases manifest as discharges, such as bladder infections and prostatitis. There is restlessness; the person does not sleep well at night.

Syphilinum . . . The person has a lot of pain and suffering, with a great fear of not recovering. The person may have tried arsenicum first, and found that it did not really help. An extreme fear of germs is associated with this one.

Pyrogenium . . . This is a remedy for septic fevers. The whole body aches and there is great restlessness from the fever. Pyrogenium is also associated with offensive odors, such as bad breath. There are sores that don't heal, and the person can go into a septic state.

Baptisia . . . Symptoms here are similar to those associated with pyrogenium, but are less severe.

Carsinonima . . . This may help when Kaposi's sarcoma is present.

Ozone Therapy

This is one of the most important therapies for patients with AIDS or HIV. During treatment, small amounts of medical ozone are introduced into the bloodstream to kill harmful microbes. The therapy activates the immune system to increase CD4 (T4) cells, and has been shown to change the HIV status of some patients from positive to negative.

HIV reversal is no small matter. Nathaniel Altman, author of *Oxygen Healing Therapies* (Health Arts Press), explains: "When I was in Cuba, I interviewed one of the chemists doing research on the subject. She said if a person infected with HIV receives ozone before it gets into the lymphatic and bone systems, HIV can be killed and stopped right on the spot."

Ozone therapy can stop intractable diarrhea, prevent the development of new opportunistic infections and improve blood circulation, thus allowing more life-giving oxygen to reach tissues. It is often given in conjunction with vitamin C to enable patients to better tolerate it. When properly administered, there are no adverse side effects.

Various protocols using ozone have been developed for treating AIDS patients. An anonymous doctor (practicing in a state where ozone users are not safe from prosecution) recommends 12 treatments on 12 consecutive days. He cites dramatic improvement in patients. "Virtually all the people I have treated—and I have treated over 170—have improved their condition within days," he reports. This doctor strongly believes that for AIDS, ozone is the most important modality of all because it removes infections.

Aqueous Penicillin Treatment

According to Dr. Michael Culbert, megadoses of aqueous penicillin, as part of a total AIDS treatment program, have had highly positive effects. Culbert, who treats AIDS patients in his Mexican clinic, utilizing an eclectic treatment approach, reports that advanced AIDS patients with cryptococcal meningitis, toxoplasmosis and advanced PCP, respond favorably to a combination of aqueous penicillin, vitamin C and dioxychlor within a matter of days. This implies, Culbert asserts, that AIDS, in part, may actually be stage IV neurosyphilis, which can be managed by an unpatented old drug. Dr. Culbert can be reached at 1-800-227-4458.

Other Approaches

Naltrexone is a prescription drug that can triple killer cell activity. This inexpensive medication has been used for nine years, and no side effects have become evident in that time. Another promising and low-cost treatment, called DNCB, is a topical agent that promotes natural killer cells.

A totally different kind of approach is found in live-cell therapy. This modality has been used for almost half a century in Europe and is just now being investigated in the United States for its remarkable ability to repair cells. The fetal cells of an animal are injected into a patient. The body takes in this embryonic material, and absorbs it through the macrophages. The living material develops receptor sites, which direct the immune system to take this fresh material to any matching tissue, e.g., spleen to spleen, heart to heart and thymus to thymus.

In terminal end-stage AIDS, live-cell therapy may not be indicated because it may enhance cancers and other pathogens in the patient. But for patients in the early stages, with mild symptoms, this therapy may enhance their chances for survival especially when it is accompanied by detoxification.

Hyperthermia, the administration of an artificial "fever" to a patient in order to burn out a virus, could remind someone of a nineteenth-century "heroic cure." However, recent success stories suggest the opposite. In one case, a patient with advanced AIDS—specifically, Kaposi's sarcoma—lost a lot of weight and had terribly low energy. During the procedure, he had blood dialysis. The removed blood was heated up to 116 degrees Fahrenheit and then put back in his body. It caused a 108-degree fever. Due to the treatment, his CD4 count went up, the KS lesions disappeared and he had incredibly high energy for several years. The conclusion is that hyperthermia could be a powerful way to treat AIDS patients in various stages of the disease.

Regular exercise is important for delaying AIDS-related complications, and in strengthening T4-cell production. Tai chi, a sequence of movements practiced for thousands of years in China, brings the energy of the environment into the system through breathing, thereby strengthening the life energy (chi). Yoga and meditation bring the mind into an awareness of inner energy, allowing it to rebalance and heal on a spiritual level. We can see how important it is to transform stress into understanding through empowering conversations with supportive friends or therapists, through participation in group activities and by practicing techniques to channel and focus one's energy. This enables the life force to be freed, strengthened and enhanced.

Acupuncture is another way to strengthen the chi. This traditional Chinese approach enhances the blood flow and the circulation of the energy. It shows positive impact on AIDS-related diseases. Reflexology is a Western alternative therapy based on the fact that certain areas of people's feet are connected to different parts of the body. Through stimulation of these points, pain can be reduced in AIDS patients. Relaxation and better sleep follow.

What to Avoid

Stay away from anything that weakens the immune system, including drugs, stress, excess sexual activity and poor food choices such as white flour, refined salt, margarine and sugar. Studies show that sugar suppresses antibody activity for hours after consumption, which means that eating sugar regularly compromises immune health. In particular, studies show that sugar paralyzes the phagocytic activity of immune cells, so that these cells become unable to surround and destroy viruses and bacteria. Large amounts of sugar are also associated with thrush. Note that sugar is disguised in many foods as sucrose, fructose, maltose, corn syrup and dextrose; all of these forms are detrimental to good health. There should be no caffeine, alcohol or cigarettes used either. If animal proteins are in the diet, they must be used sparingly. They carry residues of antibiotics and steroids, which weaken the immune system.

Dairy products, especially commercial milk, can be irritating and should be avoided by a person with a weakened immune system.

Treatment Summary

It is important to remember that there are long-term AIDS survivors, and that a variety of holistic approaches exist that can be undertaken with the help of a health care professional.

The AIDS patient must be particularly careful about diet, choosing healthful, life-promoting foods with a concentration on complex carbohydrates. Organic, whole foods should be chosen over processed foods. Of special value are fresh juices, sea vegetables, Oriental mushrooms and garlic.

Herbs exist the world over for strengthening the immune system. Of particular note for AIDS are astragalus, especially when combined with legustrum, ginseng and bitter melon. Echinacea, cat's claw and other herbs are also beneficial.

Homeopathic AIDS remedies can be prescribed according to symptoms.

Large doses of intravenous and oral supplements are usually required.

Antioxidant nutrients are particularly important.

Ozone therapy is one of the best modalities for reversing and overcoming AIDS, when used in conjunction with other treatments.

Live cell therapy is an approach involving cell repair that is widely used in Europe and which is now being investigated in the United States.

Other approaches include treatment with dioxychlor, shark cartilage and aqueous penicillin.

Alcoholism

Alcoholism wreaks havoc on mind, body and spirit. The disease is a long degenerative process, wherein a person gradually drinks more and more until he or she is addicted. It can be characterized by mental disturbances, cirrhosis of the liver, gastritis, nerve damage and hallucinations. Stopping cold turkey, without nutritional support, can cause delirium tremens (a sudden, psychotic withdrawal that can result in death).

It is important to understand that alcoholism affects not just the alcoholic himself or herself but that person's family, friends, coworkers and employers. Those touched by alcoholism also include victims of drunk drivers. Ultimately, the country as a whole is affected by this massive problem, considering both the human and economic losses incurred.

One way of looking at the physiological aspects of alcoholism is to see it as a carbohydrate metabolism imbalance. The late complementary physician Dr. Robert Atkins, of New York, explained that people crave alcohol for the sugar. In fact, many people who give up alcohol become sugarholics, or "dry drunks," as they switch from alcohol to sugar. Orthomolecular physician Dr. Abram Hoffer stresses that nutrient deficiencies add to the problem. People do not eat healthfully and are low in essential nutrients, especially minerals, such as chromium, zinc and manganese.

Treatment

Conventional alcoholism treatment programs combine drugs (such as Antabuse) that make people sick when they take a drink with counseling and other social supports. Many individuals have success with Alcoholics Anonymous (AA), especially with the addition of a good diet and supplemental support. The philosophy behind these modalities is that alcoholism is a lifelong disease that can be controlled but never cured.

The Importance of Nutrition

A natural approach to treating alcoholism sees it as a correctable disease; in other words, through physical and emotional rebalancing a person can overcome the condition. Natural practitioners emphasize that good nutrition is key in combating alcoholism; they note that alcohol robs the system of nutrients, which causes free radical damage and degenerative disease. Heavy drinkers accelerate the process, but even moderate drinkers lose valuable vitamins and minerals. Therefore, anyone who drinks, or who is recovering from substance abuse and attempting to rebuild health, can benefit from a full spectrum of supplements. The ones listed here are particularly important:

Vitamin A . . . Take 25,000 IU daily.

Vitamin B Complex . . . B vitamins work together to restore integrity to the brain and nervous system. Certain members of the B family are especially important for alcoholics; these include vitamins B1, B2, B5 and B6. Pantothenic acid (B5) supports the adrenal glands and helps the body regulate its sugar metabolism.

Vitamin E . . . The suggested dosage of 400-600 IU daily prevents death of the brain cells and lowers the chance of vascular injury caused by alcohol.

Essential Fatty Acids . . . Alcoholics tend to be deficient in these energy-providing substances, which can be taken in capsule form. The suggested daily dosage is 1000 mg.

Amino Acids . . . Two in particular, glutamine and L-methionine, are especially valuable for detoxifying the brain. And their effectiveness is boosted when they're combined with vitamins B6 and C. (Note: Glutamic acid should never be substituted for glutamine, as it does not have the same effect.) Additionally, we have to mention N-acetyl-cysteine, an antidote for acetaldehyde, which protects the physiological proteins. The suggested dosage is 500 mg three times a day. It is also good to take 50 mg of glutathione each day and 500 mg of carnitine twice a day.

Trace Minerals . . . Most people are deficient in trace minerals, a problem more prevalent today than it was in the past, because our agricultural soil is often depleted of these essential substances. Getting enough magnesium, 500-1500 mg daily, manganese, 5 mg daily, chromium, 250-500 mcg daily and zinc are especially important for recovery from alcoholism. Chromium has the special quality of reducing blood sugar levels connected to alcohol cravings.

Vitamin C and Quercetin . . . Vitamin C is a strong detoxification agent, and its ability to heal is greatly enhanced by the addition of the bioflavonoid quercetin. The suggested oral dosage is 2000-10,000 mg daily. High doses of intravenous vitamin C and other antioxidants can also protect the liver and improve metabolism.

Kyolic Garlic Formula 105 . . . Garlic contains S-allyl-cysteine, which helps neutralize acetyldehyde.

Selenium . . . The suggested dosage is 100 mcg.

S-Adenosylmethionine (SAMe) . . . The suggested dosage is 400-800 mg twice a day. This effectively protects the liver against damage caused by ethanol. In case of deficiency of SAMe, liver cirrhosis can occur. Trimethylglycine (TMG) has equal liver-protecting properties. The suggested dosage is 500 mg a day.

Folic acid . . . It is helpful to take folic acid at a dosage of 800 mcg daily.

Probiotics . . . These beneficial bacteria help to recolonize the intestinal tract, preventing liver damage such as cirrhosis.

Fructooligosaccharides (FOS) . . . This is a beneficial supplement for people with chronic liver problems because it reduces the formation of toxic liver metabolites.

Lecithin . . . Lecithin improves functioning of the brain and liver, two organs that alcohol users need to repair.

Herbs . . . In addition to nutrient supplements, herbs are valuable to the recovering alcoholic. Milk thistle, in particular, is important because it aids in repairing and rejuvenating the liver. The active ingredient in milk thistle is silymarin, shown in a recent double-blind study to have a liver-protective effect for those with cirrhosis. Valerian root can aid alcoholics in a different way. This is a nerve tonic that helps to heal the emotional stress and pain accompanying alcohol withdrawal. Siberian ginseng should also be remembered when alcoholism is a problem. This herb supports the liver, and has been shown to reduce the occurrence of people falling off the wagon after going through rehabilitation. Dandelion root, at 1-2 g three times a day, is an effective liver detoxifier. Skullcap (Scutellaria lateriflora) is traditionally a good remedy for hysteria, tension and nervous disorders such as anxiety.

Allergies

An allergy is the result of an overaggressive immune response to a substance that is inhaled or ingested, or that comes in contact with the skin. While one person can walk into a dusty room and have no reaction because her immune system cells (e.g., lymphocytes and phagocytes) are able to engulf or otherwise disable the antigens in the dust, another individual has an allergic response upon entering that same room because her immune system is not as efficient.

Allergies are so common that almost everyone has them to one degree or another. When we hear the word allergy, most of us think of classic, or fixed, allergies, such as hay fever or immediate reactions to certain foods. But we are less familiar with cyclic food allergies and chemical sensitivities. Different types of allergies are described below.

Hay Fever

About 37 million people suffer from this seasonal condition. During the spring and late summer, people react to the germination of trees, grass and ragweed, which fill the air with microscopic particles. These substances enter the body and combine with immune cells known as immunoglobulins (specifically the type called IgE). Then they undergo chemical reactions, ending with the release of histamine. This causes an allergic response and a person experiences sneezing, itching and an obstruction of the nose. If hay fever goes untreated, more serious problems, such as asthma, can develop.

Food Allergies

Sometimes a food allergy is obvious because it causes an immediate response after a food is ingested. For example, strawberries are eaten and an individual breaks out in hives. This is a Type 1, or fixed allergic response, because it occurs each time strawberries are eaten. Other food allergies are more difficult to diagnose, as symptoms do not usually appear right after eating the offending substance but rather hours or days later. Also, reactions may change with age, season, stress and a host of other factors. Further, they can move from one organ system to another. Thus, milk may cause an asthmatic response in a young child, and skin disruptions in the same person as an adolescent.

These masked, or cyclic, allergies are responsible for most reactions. In fact, some reports indicate that as many as 90 percent of common complaints heard by general practitioners are related to food allergies, although they are often not understood as such by mainstream doctors. Seemingly unrelated allergy symptoms can include depression, headaches, joint pains, muscle pains and abdominal complaints.

Chemical Sensitivity

Reactions can be brought on by substances in the environment, such as photocopy machines at work, dust and mold in the home and pesticide residues on foods. Today, people are routinely exposed to thousands of such toxins. As a result, immunity may diminish. The immune system reacts to one thing, then two and then more. Eventually, in the most extreme form of environmental illness, a person can become nonfunctional.

Allergy Tests

Type 1 allergies, the classic type, are IgE-mediated. IgE is an antibody or immune cell that binds to an irritant, such as a food or pollen. High 1gb levels, which are detected by blood tests, are confirmation of Type 1 allergies. However, the type of blood test used does not generally identify cyclic food allergies.

Cyclic food allergies can be identified by both objective and subjective methods. Complementary physicians measure IgG food antibody levels or white blood cell reactions to antigens. Skin testing may also be done to check for reactions to foods, chemicals, pollens, dusts, molds and other agents. Underlying problems, such as parasitic infections, candida and the insufficient secretion of digestive enzymes, may be identified and treated as well because improvement in these areas may improve absorption and lessen reactivity to foods. In addition, patients answer questionnaires to help determine the cause and extent of the problem. The reason behind allergy-like symptoms could be infective dental toxicity. Biological dentistry postulates that allergies can be triggered by hidden infections in root canal-treated teeth, cavitation abscess and periodontal disease, or that they can be implant-related.

I realize that to many the term biological dentistry is alien. Therefore, I feel it warrants further discussion. Biological dentistry involves putting substances in patients' mouths that will not cause the immune system to adversely respond. When a dentist places a "silver amalgam" in your mouth, that filling is about 50 percent mercury. Mercury is the most powerful neurotoxin on the planet. Research suggests that there is a 92 percent chance that the patient's immune system will fight against this mercury.

Biological dentists use materials that are assured to be compatible with the body. Furthermore, these dentists remove all of the metal from the patient's mouth. Surprisingly to many, biological dentists believe that root canals can produce toxins that may poison the patient. These dentists believe that root canal is a procedure that forces the body to accept dead tissue. In fact, they say, it is the *only* medical procedure that forces the body to accept dead tissue. The body rebels against this procedure, then produces toxins in response.

Applied kinesiology is another technique sometimes used as an allergy test. This diagnostic procedure has a patient place a food under the tongue while lowering an outstretched arm against the resistance of the doctor. Difficulty lowering the arm indicates that the food is causing weakness.

Allergies produce stimulating effects, followed by degenerative ones. Doctors rate severity on a scale of one to four. The first level of stimulation, in which a person remains relatively symptom-free, is called +1. The person is active, alert and responsive and behaves normally. At the +2 stage, a person becomes hyperactive, irritable, hungry, thirsty, tense, jittery, talkative, argumentative and overly sensitive. With a +3 reaction, an individual becomes hypomanic, toxic, anxious, egocentric, aggressive, loquacious, clumsy and apprehensive. An extreme +4 stimulation causes mania, excitement, agitation and possibly convulsions.

At the degenerative end of the scale, a -1 reaction gives an allergic manifestation that might include a runny nose, hives, gas, diarrhea, frequent urination or various eye and ear symptoms. At the -2 stage, there are systemic allergic reactions such as tiredness, mild depression, swelling, pain and cardiovascular effects. With a -3 reaction there are depression, disturbed mental processes, confusion, moodiness and withdrawal. Finally at the -4 stage, severe depression and possibly paranoia or even suicide, can result.

Self-Diagnosis

There are several ways to check for food allergies on one's own. One is with the Coca test, based on Dr. Coca's observation that a person's pulse rate increases after eating a food to which he or she is allergic. The test consists of taking your pulse before eating and every 30 minutes thereafter for up to two hours. Normally, the average person's pulse is between 70 and 80 beats per minute. After eating a food to which one is allergic, however, the pulse can increase significantly to a count that's 20 or even 40 beats above the normal level.

Another effective diagnostic measure that can be self-administered is the elimination test. Here, suspected allergy-producing foods are eliminated from the diet for four days. Every fifth day one of the foods is added back in to see if an allergic reaction occurs. So, if, for example, wheat is eliminated, on the fifth day a bowl of cracked wheat can be eaten. (Bread should not be used for this purpose because the person might be reacting to the yeast, sugar or additives.)

Recording Symptoms

It is helpful to keep a food diary to isolate those chemicals and foods that make you ill. Ask yourself: "Do I get bloated? Tired? Headaches?" Even if symptoms are not immediate, write them down. If you are allergic to a food, patterns will begin to emerge. A wide array of symptoms can occur depending upon which systems are most affected:

Adrenal System Reactions . . . Low energy or chronic fatigue is a common reaction, with immune dysfunction being at the most severe end of the spectrum. Another possibility is obesity, which can stem from a tendency to overeat in response to low glucose levels. A hypoglycemic person eats to raise the blood sugar and overcome inertia and exercises too little because not enough energy is available.

Central Nervous System Reactions . . . Brain allergies occur when molecules, breathed in or eaten, leave the blood and enter the brain. These foreign substances can interfere with enzymes and lead to any number of reactions—diminished concentration, impaired thinking, spaciness, anxiety, headaches, aggressive or antisocial behavior, depression, rapid mood swings, insomnia, hallucinations or episodic memory loss. Many children experience hyperactivity or fatigue from allergens. Even serious psychotic problems can result; it is estimated that for over 90 percent of schizophrenics, food or chemical intolerances are contributory factors to their conditions. Unfortunately many allergic reactions, and many psychological problems compounded by allergic reactions, are mistaken for purely psychological problems.

Skin Problems . . . Some people experience rashes, or skin redness, discoloration, roughness or inflammation.

Respiratory System Problems . . . There may be wheezing or shortness of breath, asthma or bronchitis.

Cardiovascular Symptoms . . . These include heart pounding, rapid or skipped beats, flushing, pallor, tingling, redness or blueness of the hands and faintness.

Gastrointestinal Symptoms . . . Numerous symptoms include dry mouth, burping, flatulence, bloating, canker sores, stinging tongue, diarrhea, constipation, nausea, abdominal pain, rectal itching and indigestion.

Other Problems . . . Other annoying, uncomfortable symptoms are muscle aches and joint pain, ringing in the ears and frequent urination.

Unless corrected, subclinical signs can turn into disease states. Most people mask their symptoms with medications instead of addressing the cause of the problem. They do not realize that seemingly diverse conditions such as rheumatoid arthritis, osteoarthritis, asthma, migraines, irritable bowel syndrome, adult onset diabetes and skin diseases, can have food and chemical allergies as an underlying cause.

Treatment

Detoxification

Most allergies can be traced to an impaired digestive system, the result of a toxic buildup within the intestines. Embarking on a cleansing program, then, is a first step in overcoming the problem, and can include the following:

Bentonite Clay . . . Bentonite clay has a negative charge and can therefore attract positively charged particles. Toxins are drawn to the clay and drawn out of the body. Bentonite clay is taken as a part of a drink; use one teaspoon in 10 ounces of water.

Hydrotherapy . . . A series of colonics and enemas cleanse and restore colon function. As a result, many allergic symptoms begin to clear up.

Fasting . . . A short watermelon and lemon fast is a great detoxifier, and will help eliminate allergies.

Detoxifying the home, schoolroom and place of employment may be equally important, and you can work toward that end in numerous ways. The first step is to check the quality of indoor air, to find out what pollutants are being breathed in. It is not that expensive to hire professionals who will come in and measure contaminants.

Air can be vastly improved with a filtration system. Actually, units with three to four filtering systems are best. Those that filter down to a level of 3 microns are able to screen out most bacteria, mold, pollens and animal danders. Placing a filter directly in a window and sealing the sides will limit the amount of pollutants coming into a room. (Many people mistakenly place air filters 3 to 4 feet away from a window, which prevents most incoming air from being drawn into the system.) There are also new technologies to purify water and air (such as ozone disinfection). These can be used to sterilize drinking water, saunas, whirlpools, swimming pools and private bathing facilities. EcoPure disinfection is a unique oxidation technique that purifies air using EcoPure, which is a gas form of activated oxygen.

To recycle water and air, we might consider using fine filtration, membranes, drum filters, disk filters and active carbon filtration.

Plants are inexpensive natural air filters that can be extremely helpful. Spider plants will filter out toxins, including formaldehyde, and produce oxygen in return. Other helpful plants are Brazilian palms, wide-leaf wandering Jews and marigolds.

Diet

A change of diet is often key in overcoming allergies. As mentioned earlier, suspect foods should be eliminated and gradually reintroduced to the diet to check for reactions. The most common allergy producers are sugar, wheat, dairy foods, beef, potatoes, shellfish, eggs, tomatoes, coffee, peanuts, soy, corn, yeast and citrus fruit. Any other food that is eaten daily should be suspect as well.

The best menu for preventing allergies is the rotation diet. This involves eating different kinds of foods each day and not repeating an item for four to seven days. Using grains as an example, if rice is eaten on Monday you might use millet on Tuesday, wheat on Wednesday and oats on Thursday with rice eaten again no sooner than Friday. This type of diet keeps the body from overreacting to most foods although some items will still need to be completely excluded. Milk, for example, may cause a reaction each time it is taken. But the majority of people can safely enjoy most foods with a rotation diet. Note that besides minimizing allergic reactions, a rotation diet provides the added benefit of ensuring that you consume a wide variety of nutrients.

Also, keep in mind that certain nutrients help build up immune response. Such nutrients can be obtained, first and foremost, from freshly squeezed juices, sprouts, grains and legumes.

For mild allergies, a few changes in diet alone may be enough, but sometimes a doctor trained to see relationships between individuals and their surroundings, known as an environmental physician, may be needed to help get to the root of the problem.

Neutralization Immunotherapy

Neutralization immunotherapy is a way of provoking the body to produce antibodies against offending substances. Once an environmental physician, using blood and skin tests, discovers which foods, chemicals, pollens, etc., are causing allergies, allergy vaccines are administered. These are different from the classical allergist's treatment in which all patients are given equal amounts of antigens. Here, low doses of specific dilutions are tailor-made for each individual. When injections are given in small amounts, the body reacts by making antibodies against those allergens. Patients are retested until symptoms disappear. This method is highly effective.

Lifestyle Changes

Many of our daily routines involve the use of commercial products with artificial ingredients that can provoke sensitivities. Fortunately many safe and inexpensive alternatives exist, such as the ones listed here:

Soaps without artificial scents and colors can be obtained in local health food stores.

Shaving cream can be made from a natural soap.

Shampoo can be made with castile soap and olive or avocado oil. A tiny amount of sesame oil can be used as a conditioner.

Toothpaste can be inexpensively made with peppermint extract and baking soda.

Deodorant can be replaced with cornstarch.

Talcum powder should not be used as it may contain asbestos fibers. A good replacement for talc is cornstarch.

Moisturizer can be made from sesame oil, as it contains vitamin E.

Facial scrub can be made from vegetable oil and applied with a soft loofah to remove dead epithelial cells.

Grease remover can be made from butter.

Room deodorizers can be made from lemon juice and vinegar, spritzed into the air. Also effective as a deodorizer is baking soda, which can be placed in a room and changed every six weeks. In addition, boiling peppermint oil will act as a deodorizer. An exhaust fan is useful as well.

Pesticides must be avoided and can be replaced naturally indoors and out. In the house, boric acid can be put down in a pencil-thin line—out of the reach of children and pets—at the baseboards and underneath places where there is moisture or paper, to get rid of roaches and ants. To prevent them from returning, simply apply a line of garlic powder, mixed with boric acid and Borax, around the perimeter of the room. In the garden, a product called Safer Insecticidal Soap can be used on fruits and vegetables. This nontoxic product is made from natural fatty acids and will kill most garden pests without harming beneficial bugs.

Cleansers made naturally are as effective as commercial brands and far less toxic. Glass cleaner can be made by adding three tablespoons of vinegar to one quart of water. Baking powder can be used in place of scouring powder as an abrasive cleaner in the bathroom and kitchen. And Borax mixed with water serves as an excellent all-purpose cleaner.

In the laundry, pure washing soda will remove residues of detergent from clothing, and clothes can then be rewashed using a mixture of washing soda and soap. One cup of vinegar added to the final rinse cycle will serve as a fabric softener and leave no smell. In addition, some natural soaps and detergent can be obtained that are less chlorinated and less toxic than most commercial brands. Some good detergents are washing soda, Borax and Bon Ami.

Dry cleaning should be avoided whenever possible. But when clothes must be dry cleaned, they should either be soaked in cold water afterwards to remove some of the chemicals or aired outside in the sun before wearing.

Supplements

Saturating the system with extra nutrients can be most helpful, especially when allergies are in full bloom. Exact requirements should be given by a complementary physician, but these general daily recommendations can serve as a guideline:

Vitamin A . . . A great supporter of the immune system, it reduces the possibility of developing allergies. The suggested dosage is 10,000 IU daily.

Vitamin C . . . Taking 3000 mg of vitamin C in divided doses throughout the day is excellent for reducing histamine levels in the blood. More can be taken when fighting off an allergy. Vitamin C detoxifies and strengthens the immune system, and helps overcome symptoms of withdrawal at the start of an allergen-free diet.

Vitamin C works best in combination with 100 to 200 mg of the bioflavonoid quercetin and 100 to 200 mg of pycnogenol. Quercetin increases the strength of mast cell membranes. Mast cells, part of our connective tissue, contain histamine, which can trigger allergic reactions. By strengthening their membranes with quercetin, one is preventing their bursting and hence preventing the release of histamine. The action of vitamin C and bioflavonoids is further enhanced by the addition of other antioxidant nutrients, such as vitamin E, beta-carotene and selenium.

Vitamin D . . . For well-controlled calcium absorption, this is a great aid. Taking 600 IU per day has good results.

Vitamin E . . . Among its many benefits, vitamin E strengthens the endocrine system, and by so doing, indirectly builds immunity. Vitamin E is especially important for women with allergies who are experiencing hormonal imbalances. A good natural source of E is soybean oil, which supplies the body with an unestrofied d-alpha tocopherol. People who have difficulty absorbing oil-based natural vitamin E can benefit from an easy-to-digest, water-soluble form. Women with allergies and hormonal imbalances generally benefit from 600 IU a day. Men usually need 400 IU per day. Vitamin E works well together with 100 mcg of the trace mineral selenium.

B Complex . . . B vitamins work as a team to enhance immunity. Pantothenic acid (B5), pyridoxine (B6) and B12 are particularly effective in balancing the immune system. Choline, the primary component of lecithin (frequently referred to as B4), helps to provide proper mental functioning, aids brain development and efficiently breaks down fats. Vitamin B5 is especially important because it is a building block of cortisone, one of the basic defense mechanisms of allergic response.

N-acetyl-cysteine (NAC) . . . NAC is a stable form of the amino acid cysteine and an amino acid precursor to glutathione, a critical antioxidant. It can help to clear the respiratory tract of mucus. NAC strengthens the body's defense against cold, flu and allergies.

Coenzyme Q10 . . . Taking 100 mg per day improves cellular oxygenation and strengthens the immune system.

L-Tyrosine . . . This amino acid has an important function in protein synthesis. Thus, 500 mg a day is recommended.

Alpha Lipoic Acid . . . This is a star nutrient in the antioxidant family. By enhancing the antioxidant function of vitamin C, vitamin E and glutathione, alpha lipoic acid helps to neutralize the damaging effects of free radicals on the system. The recommended dosage is 25 mg a day.

Glutamine . . . This amino acid has a great enhancing effect on the immune system.

Glutathione . . . This powerful antioxidant fights free radicals. Glutathione is considered an important element in the body's defense. It helps to increase certain immune responses and detoxifies the liver.

Ginkgo Biloba Extract . . . Taking 60 mg one to three times a day is recommended.

Goldenseal . . . Native Americans have been using this herb for allergy and infection-induced conditions for many years. Being rich in alkaloids makes it antibiotic, anti-infective and stimulating to the immune system.

Grape Seed Extract . . . This is a natural antihistamine. Its flavonoids inhibit allergic reactions that can cause eczema. The suggested dosage is 100 mg one to three times a day.

Licorice Root . . . This has been used by the Chinese for over 5000 years for fevers, inflammation, cold symptoms and skin disorders. Taking 450 mg one to three times daily offers great support for the adrenal system.

MSM (Methylsulfonylmethane)... MSM contains bio-nutritional sulfur, which plays an important role in the body's functions. Taking 1000 mg one to three times daily improves allergies, asthma, headache and skin problems. It also assists in restoring the immune system to normal, and it supports the respiratory system.

Essential Fatty Acids... Essential fatty acids—found in one tablespoon of flaxseed oil or fish oil, or GLA found in 500 mg of borage, black currant seed, or evening primrose oil—play a primary role in restoring immune function.

Bromelain... Derived from pineapple, the enzyme bromelain is a potent anti-inflammatory that also helps to strengthen the immune system. According to Dr. Susan Lark in *The Lark Letter,* "Allergies are an inflammatory reaction triggered by over-acidity. If you can restore your body's alkalinity, the allergic reaction often vanishes." She recommends taking 1000 mg of bromelain with a cup of spring water and baking soda.

Minerals... The mineral zinc may help correct food allergies when the problem stems from undigested food particles that are the result of insufficient production of hydrochloric acid in the stomach. Another helpful mineral is calcium in the form of 400 to 600 mg of calcium citrate or calcium chelate (increased to 1000 mg during allergic response). Taking potassium citrate or chelate is necessary for adrenal gland function. In the case of asthma, to ease spasms in the bronchial tubes, magnesium could help, as it has soothing effects on some uncomfortable symptoms of allergies. Molybdenum, an essential trace mineral, through its participation in the detoxification of sulfites, might help to prevent sulfite-reactive asthma attacks.

Digestive Enzymes... Digestive enzymes help the stomach and pancreas break down large protein molecules so they can be fully digested. This prevents large peptides from entering the bloodstream and setting off allergic responses.

Herbs

Herbs reduce allergy symptoms in a more gentle way than do most medications. The following are some that may prove helpful:

Garlic... Garlic is the number one herb of all time, and it should be a frequent component of everyone's diet. Garlic builds immunity and also serves as a natural antiseptic agent.

Astragalus... Astragalus is one of the best-researched immune system stimulants now available. It works like echinacea, in that both herbs increase the number and activity of immune cells. However, astragalus concentrates on building the immune system, and unlike echinacea, it can be taken on a daily basis.

Echinacea . . . Echinacea boosts immune system activity and promotes fast recovery, especially when taken at the onset of symptoms. The most potent formulas have a peculiar tingling and numbing effect on the tongue. Since the body cannot sustain such high levels of activity without rest, echinacea should be used for short intervals at a time. In Europe, where echinacea is extensively used, people take the herb in a pattern of four days on and four days off.

Ginseng . . . The Chinese say that ginseng builds stamina and endurance by stabilizing the qi (pronounced "chee"), the energy of the body. Another way of explaining ginseng's ability is that it boosts the immune system.

Wild Cherry Bark . . . This helps hay fever and other allergies by healing irritated mucosal surfaces, including the lungs. It's also soothing to the skin.

Mullein Leaf . . . This herb protects the mucous surfaces, including the throat, esophagus, intestines and lungs.

Horehound . . . This affects respiration by dilating muscles.

Yerba Mate . . . Being a nutritious ancient herb, containing several vitamins, yerba mate is able to help the body adjust to its surroundings, thereby supporting the body's own defense mechanism against allergies.

Ashwaganda . . . This Ayurvedic herb, often referred to as Indian ginseng, is one of the best health tonics and restorative agents for fatigue and exhaustion caused by stress. It has an overall rejuvenating effect.

American Angelica . . . This herb is known for its anti-inflammatory, soothing effect on colds, flu, headaches and other allergic symptoms.

Tylophora Asthmatica . . . This herb is used by Ayurvedic practitioners as an antiasthmatic and antiallergic medication. Tylophorine, the major element in tylophora, is able to interfere with the action of mast cells, the key components in the process of inflammation.

Butterbur . . . This herb, also known as butterdock or bog rhubarb, works as a natural antihistamine. It provides great relief to seasonal allergy sufferers.

Red Eyebright . . . Used as an eyewash, this herb eases burning and itching. As a tea, red eyebright helps with excessive mucus and nasal congestion.

Boswellia Serrata . . . This is an Ayurvedic herb from India. For modern herbal preparations, the purified extract of the gummy resin from the boswellia tree trunk is used for asthma.

Schizandra . . . This adaptogenic herb helps to rebalance the body. It also builds strength, reduces fatigue and protects the liver.

Turmeric . . . This herb is known for its anti-inflammatory qualities.

Other good herbs for allergies include stinging nettle and capsicum.

What to Avoid

Allergies are exacerbated by stress; physical and psychological stressors should therefore be eliminated as much as possible. Stimulants in the form of caffeine, cigarettes and recreational drugs are particularly bad. Nor should the same foods be eaten every day. Too much meat, sugar and refined carbohydrates can lead to a state of acidosis. To neutralize an acidic system and stop an allergic response, a person can take baking soda, buffered vitamin C powder or pantothenic acid in a glass of apple or pineapple juice.

Allergenic chemicals placed on the skin in the form of soaps, lotions and shampoos, and those breathed in and found in the water should be minimized and, when possible, eliminated through the use of natural alternatives.

Treatment Summary

Allergy sufferers often need to improve their digestive health. Recommended measures include a cleansing diet with the help of bentonite clay, hydrotherapy and a short watermelon and lemon fast.

People are commonly allergic to one or more of the following: sugar, wheat, dairy beef, potatoes, shellfish, eggs, tomatoes, coffee, peanuts, soy corn and yeast. An environmental physician can check for problem foods, which should be eliminated from the diet or eaten on a rotation basis, once every four to seven days.

With neutralization immunization therapy, injections of small amounts of specific allergens, tailor-made for an individual's needs, help the body develop antibodies.

Instead of using chemically laced personal and home care products, we can lessen our allergic load by making or purchasing natural ones.

Cleansing the air with a filtration system and plants lessens the amount of inhaled contaminants.

Nutrients that give our immune system an extra boost include vitamin C, quercetin, pycnogenol, vitamin E, selenium, B-complex vitamins, zinc, essential fatty acids and gamma linolenic acid.

Herbs that strengthen the immune system include garlic, astragalus, echinacea, ginseng, wild cherry bark and horehound.

Alzheimer's Disease and Dementia

Approximately 2 million Americans are currently afflicted with some form of dementia, Alzheimer's disease being the most widely publicized form, due to its severity. Alzheimer's is a degenerative brain disease that manifests during the later years of life. It affects the hippocampus and cerebral cortex of the brain, where memory, language and cognition are located, and is characterized by neurological damage and deterioration of the neurotransmitters, which are responsible for nerve communication. In addition, circulation in Alzheimer's patients can be impeded by up to 30 percent.

This condition, and other forms of dementia, develops when the neurons located in the front of the brain perish, resulting in diminished quantities of acetylcholine. Acetylcholine is the neurotransmitter responsible for fast reactions and muscular activity, and its absence can induce symptoms commonly associated with Alzheimer's, including difficulty communicating, memory loss, concentration problems and reduced motor skills.

It should be noted that the symptoms of Creutzfeld-Jakob disease, which in cattle is known as mad cow disease, are sometimes mistaken for those of Alzheimer's. Creutzfeld-Jakob disease has a latency period of 30 years, which means that people who have eaten contaminated beef many years in the past may be infected without even knowing it, and may eventually experience symptoms almost identical to those of Alzheimer's. We should note too that a practice that has developed over the past 20 years in the meat industry does not bode well for beef-eaters' future health. Through a process called rendering, cattle parts that are not used by humans are actually being included in cattle feed. In effect, the cattle are forced to practice a type of cannibalism that propagates the spread of the disease.

Causes

One possible cause of Alzheimer's disease is atherosclerosis, a condition in which the diminished flow of blood within the body affects the brain and produces common Alzheimer's symptoms.

Also implicated in the onset of this condition is heavy-metal toxicity. In autopsies performed on victims of Alzheimer's, an accumulation of aluminum and mercury deposits is usually present in the areas of the brain affected by dementia. Unfortunately, toxic accumulations of metals, especially aluminum, have become quite prevalent in modern society, and our bodies can assimilate excessive quantities of aluminum without our knowing it. Also, despite the attempts of water treatment facilities to purify our water supply, the reservoirs from which we draw tap water continue to be besieged by various pollutants, including pesticides, bacteria, viruses and aluminum. Since our bodies are over 70 percent water, this can obviously have health-compromising consequences. In addition to unfiltered tap water, aluminum deposition within the body can originate from aluminum cookware, antacids, deodorants, antidiarrheal preparations, buffered aspirin and food additives.

Vitamin and mineral deficiencies constitute yet another potential cause of Alzheimer's disease, although the conventional medical community does not acknowledge this. But the fact is that the dominance of processed foods in the typical American diet has deprived us of essential nutrients required for proper brain functioning. Processed foods are often stripped of vital nutrients, which are replaced with processed sugars, such as fructose, corn sweetener and corn syrup. Other unhealthy additives include trans-fatty acids, such as partially hydrogenated vegetable oils. The bottom line is that deficiencies of essential nutrients can lead to a wide assortment of health problems and facilitate the eventual onset of Alzheimer's.

Subclinical hypothyroidism is yet another factor that can contribute to the manifestation of symptoms, or compound an existing condition. Most doctors rely on the results of blood tests to diagnose thyroid problems; but sometimes hypothyroidism is not reflected in a blood test, though it still may be present and contributing to a patient's dementia symptoms.

Treatment

Contrary to the beliefs of most mainstream doctors, safe, natural and nontoxic treatments for Alzheimer's disease and other types of dementia exist. Research has demonstrated that these remedies can aid in preventing the onset of Alzheimer's or alleviating symptoms that have developed. In the past, people allowed their loved ones to wither away before their eyes, citing aging as an uncontrollable force. While we cannot stop time, we can take action to prevent the later years of life from being characterized by rapid degeneration.

Nutrition and Supplements

As people age, their bodies become more susceptible to nutritional deficiencies, and a lifetime of deficiencies can encourage the development of degenerative disorders like Alzheimer's. The upside of this picture is that the cumulative effects of poor dietary habits can be avoided by improving dietary intake early in life.

As we've mentioned, the prevalence of processed and tainted foods in our society is a serious health risk factor for all of us. In order to obtain the nutrients our bodies need, we should try to consume an abundance of non-labeled foods. Whole grains and fresh vegetables are especially healthful. And it is advisable to purchase organic foods, which are more likely than others to contain trace minerals that are vital to the brain, such as chromium, magnesium, selenium and zinc.

If the Alzheimer's disease process has begun, there are a variety of nutritional programs that can be initiated to combat it. Since the severity of degeneration differs from one individual to the next, each patient should be evaluated by a qualified professional so that proper treatment can be prescribed. As we age, the body's ability to produce stomach acid within the digestive system diminishes. Deficiencies of vitamins B6 and B12 and iron commonly develop during the later years, eventually causing symptomatic memory problems.

It is important for those with Alzheimer's disease to receive parenteral (i.e., injected or intravenous) supplements of vitamin B complex. Oral supplements are not usually as effective as internal supplements in reversing dementia symptoms because the necessary levels cannot be absorbed into the bloodstream through the intestines. Of course, the dosage and procedure have to be supervised by a qualified medical practitioner.

To increase the effectiveness of vitamin B complex, add 800 mcg of folic acid, which decreases homocysteine levels.

In terms of homocysteine reduction, S-adenosylmethionine (SAMe) is a powerful agent. A dosage of 400-1600 mg is recommended. This natural metabolite of the amino acid methionine is in virtually every cell of the body. Recent studies indicate that Alzheimer's patients have extremely low levels of SAMe in their brains.

Frequently unnoticed by the general public, the nutrient known as DMAE can augment the body's natural production of energy, enhance the sleeping cycle and improve memory. Although this nutrient can be supplemented relatively safely, excessive consumption can result in insomnia, muscle tension and mild headaches. Therefore, be sure to regulate dosages.

Daily consumption of coenzyme Q10, in quantities of 50 mg, can augment the supply of oxygen to the brain. This is useful in cases of Alzheimer's induced by atherosclerosis, where the blood supply to the brain is impeded and consequently the reduced oxygen supply can exacerbate cognitive deterioration.

Lecithin, which contains a substance known as choline, can enhance production of acetylcholine. Since deficiencies of this vital neurotransmitter have been correlated with the onset of Alzheimer's disease, one tablespoon of lecithin should be consumed daily with food. Lecithin also contains inositol, which can help alleviate anxiety by acting as a natural Valium, minus this drug's adverse side effects.

Supplements of vitamin C are also crucial for older adults. One thousand milligrams of C should be taken three times each day during mealtimes (vitamins are most easily assimilated into the system when they are taken with food).

Vitamin E has beneficial antioxidant properties and should be supplemented in quantities of 400 IU per day.

The mineral magnesium can relax the body by dilating the blood vessels and airways. Magnesium can aid in the treatment of circulatory and respiratory disorders, and so it's unfortunate that an overwhelming majority of the population does not receive an adequate amount of it in their diets. For maximum results, magnesium should be supplemented in the chelated form because the amino acid that it is paired with facilitates absorption into the blood. Between 500 to 1000 mg of magnesium should be consumed daily on an empty stomach, with 200 to 300 mg taken in the morning and the remainder taken before retiring for the evening. Since magnesium is a relaxing mineral, it can aid the sleep cycle. One possible side effect of this mineral is loose stool; so, if this occurs, limit your dosage.

Many people who suffer from dementia have deficiencies of selenium and zinc. Supplements of selenium should be consumed in quantities of 200 mcg daily while 40 to 50 mg of the chelated form of zinc, known as zinc picolinate, is recommended as well. One hundred milligrams of potassium should also be taken as a supplement on a daily basis.

Another nutrient that can aid in the battle against Alzheimer's is acetyl carnitine. The suggested dose is 1500 mg, twice a day. This versatile nutrient is able to transport itself through the blood/brain barrier and stimulates and fortifies the brain's nerve cells. Acetyl carnitine directs fatty acids into the cell mitochondria, which are responsible for creating cell energy. Furthermore, it can act as an antioxidant and can supplement the neurotransmitter acetylcholine.

DHEA is a hormone produced by the adrenal glands, but production declines steadily with age. Clinical studies have indicated that the level of DHEA in a 60-year-old is only 10 percent of the amount in the average 20-year-old. DHEA supplementation during the later years can hinder the onset of an assortment of serious disorders, including heart disease, cancer, arthritis and asthma. It can also aid our mental abilities and alleviate stress. DHEA can be obtained in dosages of 5-25 mg. The suggested dose is 15-50 mg for women and 50-75 mg for men.

The total balance of hormones is extremely important in preventing or combating Alzheimer's. Therefore, the estrogen, testosterone and progesterone levels should be closely monitored. When a deficiency of these hormones arises, damage to the brain cells and immune dysfunction may result. The hormones should be naturally replaced. Estrogen could boost acetylcholine, a chemical important for memory, and it seems to reduce the formation of beta amyloid, which forms in plaques in the brains of Alzheimer's victims. Studies show that most men who develop the disease have low levels of free testosterone. In fact, in some cases, the drop in the levels was detected 10 years earlier.

Supplementation of the "mother hormone" pregnenolone may be important in preventing and slowing down memory loss.

To slow senility, glutamine, a stimulator of human growth hormone, and glutathione could play an important role. The suggested dose for glutamine is 3000 mg.

Flaxseed oil can provide the body with ample quantities of the essential fatty acid omega-3, which is transmuted into another fatty acid and ultimately provides nourishment for the cells in the brain. The recommended dosage of flaxseed oil is one tablespoon daily. Remember to keep flaxseed oil refrigerated, and avoid cooking with it because heat can destroy its nutritional value. The essential fatty acid DHA can be obtained from fish oil. Life Extension makes a product called Super GLA/DHA that could provide the ideal balance of essential fatty acids. The suggested dose is 6 capsules a day.

Melatonin, which is manufactured naturally in the pineal gland, may need to be supplemented during the later years of life when natural production diminishes. Taking 3 mg prior to bedtime can help stabilize the sleeping cycle.

The process called glycosylation (the cross-linking of proteins) strongly contributes to Alzheimer's. During this process, sugar aldehydes reacting with the amino acids on the protein molecule create advance glycosylation endproducts (AGE's). Carnosine has the ability to slow the formation of AGE's. It also seems to change the toxicity in the nervous system that is caused by the presence of copper and zinc, which is characteristic of Alzheimer's. A minimum of 1000 mg of carnosine a day should be considered.

N-acetyl-cysteine (NAC) has antioxidant properties that can promote healthy functioning of the brain, while phosphatidylserine enhances the ability of enzymes in the membranes of nerve cells to relay messages in and out of the cells. Supplementation can improve memory and learning capacity in older adults and can ameliorate symptoms of depression. Phosphatidylserine is especially effective when paired with omega-3 fatty acid supplements. There is a product by Life Extension Foundation called Cognitex that is a combination of phosphatidylcholine, phosphatidylserine, vinpocetine and pregnenolone. These potent brain-boosting nutrients provide the much-needed choline. Choline is crucial for the production of the neurotransmitter acetylcholine. It is also vital for building cell membranes of the brain. In addition, vinpocetine can improve blood flow and the utilization of oxygen.

Taurine is an antioxidant that protects the supply of magnesium and calcium within brain cells. It also enhances nerve cell functioning.

Tryptophan fosters comfortable sleep, which, in turn, enhances brain functioning.

Tyrosine and phenylalanine promote the production of dopamine within the brain, a vital compound responsible for regulating the operation of neurotransmitters.

Due to its rich hydrogen content, nicotinamide adenine dinucleotide (also known as NADH or coenzyme 1) is vital in producing energy within the body. Although NADH is a natural biological substance that should be present in all cells, older adults who suffer from Alzheimer's tend to lack up to 50 percent of the necessary amount of this chemical. When the body engages in rigorous activity, muscle and brain cells can contain up to 50 mcg of NADH per gram of tissue. An ample supply of NADH can allow the body to reap the benefits of an additional power source. Fortunately for Alzheimer's patients, risk-free supplements of coenzyme 1 are now available and can produce miraculous results. Studies have demonstrated that the administration of NADH supplements can halt further development of the disease, and can increase energy and improve functioning within 10 to 12 weeks. Unfortunately, the clinical effects of NADH last only a limited amount of time.

New studies have analyzed why we should look at curcumin (curry spice) from a different angle. A newly discovered characteristic of curcumin is its natural nonsteroidal anti-inflammatory properties, which help to reduce the level of damaging free radicals. The recommended dosage is 900 mg twice a day.

Herbal Treatments

Although the U.S. claims to lead the global community in medical technology in some instances, we actually lag behind the times. As we discussed in the preceding section, some of the treatment modalities that have proven effective overseas are not being utilized to their full potential in our own country. A further example involves an herbal extract derived from the ginkgo biloba tree, used extensively throughout Europe for the past 20 years. This herbal remedy has produced remarkable results in the treatment of Alzheimer's and other age-related degenerative diseases and consequently has become the leading prescribed plant medicine in numerous countries. In fact, in France and

Germany, ginkgo biloba currently ranks in the top five medications used overall. That's not the case here, where, unfortunately, the conventional medical community is generally ignorant of the vast assortment of herbs that possess medicinal capabilities. You have to journey to Europe, where herbal remedies have become an integral part of modern conventional medicine, to understand that the U.S. is not necessarily in the vanguard when it comes to knowledge about health.

The ginkgo biloba herb is valuable because it can alleviate several dementia related symptoms. First of all, ginkgo enhances the circulation to the central nervous system, which frequently becomes impeded in older adults. Furthermore, this herbal extract has a tendency to stabilize abnormal nerve communication in the brain. Within the U.S. pharmaceutical industry, a product known as tacrin has enjoyed the status of being the only medication prescribed for the early stages of dementia. Interestingly, European studies comparing the effects of this product and ginkgo biloba have indicated that ginkgo extract is more effective in enhancing circulation and brain functioning. Furthermore, ginkgo has potent antioxidant properties that are vital in protecting the cells of the central nervous system from free radical damage.

Elderly people, who rely upon ginkgo to combat Alzheimer's disease or other forms of dementia, should consume 240 mg daily, divided into two or three doses while people who are just using ginkgo as part of their daily regimen should take only 120 mg.

The herb ginseng—in particular, Korean ginseng—has also demonstrated its capacity to curb the onset of psychological deterioration. In addition to aiding a patient's mental condition, ginseng can enhance adrenal functioning. Considering that many older adults suffer from deteriorated adrenal capacities, ginseng can prove a valuable supplement to the ginkgo biloba extract.

Huperzine A, a compound isolated from a Chinese herb, increases acetylcholine activity in the cortex and hippocampus sections of the brain. This improves memory, as well as cognitive and behavioral functions.

Kut is a Japanese herbal formula, mixed from 13 different herbs, that also seems to elevate choline acetyltransferase levels. In addition, it stimulates nerve growth factor.

Yet another herb that promotes healthy circulation to the brain is butcher's broom. Enhanced memory and clearer focus can be expected when two to four 425 mg capsules are taken daily.

What to Avoid

Unfortunately, most Americans indulge in an abundance of processed foods, foods stripped of vital nutrients. Unhealthy additives replace vitamins and minerals that are crucial in preventing the onset of Alzheimer's disease as well as other forms of dementia. In order to avert nutritional deficiencies and harmful toxins, we need to limit our intake of salt, processed sugars, red meat and trans-fatty acids and seek healthier sources of nourishment; it is also a good idea to completely avoid meats that are the product of animals given rendered feed. In addition, it is important for elderly adults to avoid accumulations of hazardous metallic toxins within the body. So, limiting the use of aluminum-containing cookware, deodorants, antacids and other preparations is prudent. And since our reservoirs often contain dangerous pollutants, charcoal block filters, which can effectively eliminate harmful toxins, should be installed on all sources of tap water used for drinking or cooking purposes.

Treatment Summary

Contrary to popular belief, Alzheimer's disease and other forms of dementia are not part of the normal aging process and can be prevented or ameliorated by eating a nutritious, organic diet throughout one's life; getting a nutritional evaluation to determine problems with assimilation; and taking various supplements and herbs.

The herb ginkgo biloba is noteworthy for its remarkable results in the treatment of Alzheimer's patients. It is used extensively in Europe for this purpose.

Anemia

Anemia is a medical condition characterized by a deficiency in the hemoglobin content of red blood cells. An insufficient amount of hemoglobin diminishes the ability of the blood to carry oxygen to the tissues and to remove carbon dioxide. Anemia is a common affliction in the United States, which may seem surprising in light of the fact that so many foods are fortified with iron.

According to New York physician Dr. Dahlia Abraham, there are actually three major causes of anemia. First, acute or chronic blood loss could be responsible. Chronic blood loss can stem from a variety of conditions, including hemorrhoids, cancer, menstruation and peptic ulcers. Another cause of anemia is excessive red blood cell destruction, that is, the condition that exists when the destruction of old cells exceeds the production of new ones. This condition can occur as a result of defective hemoglobin synthesis or trauma within the arteries. The third major cause of anemia is a deficiency of vital nutrients, either iron, vitamin B12 or folic acid. This type of anemia—and specifically the iron-deficiency type—is the most common.

Getting enough iron is particularly important during the growth spurts of infancy and adolescence, while women may need additional supplements during pregnancy and lactation. Iron deficiency anemia is quite common in children under the age of two, and in teenagers. Children who eat nutritionally poor foods or do not include enough variety in their diets are the most at risk. Often, teenagers develop a habit of subsisting on junk foods, which do not satisfy their developmental needs. Sometimes supplements do not provide an adequate countermeasure because many people have difficulty absorbing iron due to a lack of hydrochloric acid, which allows the stomach to properly assimilate the mineral. Iron deficiency is especially common in elderly people, who do not produce the needed amounts of stomach acid, and in people who suffer from chronic diarrhea.

Vitamin B12 anemia is often accompanied by folic acid anemia. One of the reasons folic acid is important is that it fosters healthy prenatal development: It is vital in the prevention of birth defects, such as those of the neural tube, and is crucial for proper cell production in the growing fetus. Folic acid is easily consumed by heat; hence, diets that consist primarily of cooked foods, with few raw foods included, often result in this type of deficiency. In addition, young children may develop a folic acid deficiency if they are given goat's milk. (Although superior to cow's milk in many ways, goat's milk lacks folic acid.) Teenagers and adults who are vegetarians may also fall victim to this form of anemia if they do not carefully balance their diets. Finally, folic acid anemia can be caused by alcoholism, which completely drains the body of this nutrient; it can also be caused by the consumption of certain prescription drugs, such as oral contraceptives and anticancer drugs.

New York acupuncturist and educator Dr. Pat Gordon offers an Asian perspective on anemia in women. According to this philosophy, a woman's blood rises and falls in a cyclical fashion. Women can become anemic if they ignore the needs of their monthly cycle, especially during menstruation. In today's fast-paced world though, many women claim they simply cannot ignore their numerous commitments and rest while their body recuperates. In addition, Gordon explains, anemia can result from an incorrect approach to pregnancy. After the termination of pregnancy, whether it is a result of a miscarriage, induced abortion, or birth, women should let their bodies rest for at least a full month, regardless of other responsibilities. Plus, after the pregnancy is terminated, conception should be avoided for at least a year because the body needs to build up blood to sustain another pregnancy.

Symptoms associated with anemia include fatigue and weakness, headaches, irritability, dizziness and sometimes, gastrointestinal distress. In teenage girls, amenorrhea or cessation of menstrual bleeding, is occasionally present. Children who are anemic are usually smaller in height and weight than other children. In older children and adults, B12 anemia may result in nerve damage that is characterized by numbness or tingling in the hands or legs, depression or confusion.

Treatment

Diet

Children should be encouraged to eat a wide variety of whole foods especially leafy green vegetables and legumes. At approximately six months of age, parents should begin feeding their infants beets, broccoli, carrots, applesauce, blackberries, blueberries and cherries. (Not all at once! New foods should be introduced to babies one at a time.) These foods are relatively hypoallergenic and rich in phytochemicals and antioxidants.

Iron-rich vegetable juice can be made from a combination of beet juice, parsley, spinach, beet greens and watercress. Green juices should be dispensed in small quantities as a quarter of a cup a day can improve a child's condition in a relatively short period of time. The juice should be diluted 50 percent with water or apple juice and sipped slowly.

A vegetarian diet rich in vitamins includes sprouts, raisins, kale, prunes, parsley, watercress, dandelion greens, beets and blackberries. Seaweeds, such as hijiki, wakame and dulse, are also excellent nutritional sources and can be added to soups and salads. Vegetarian sources of B12 include fermented soy products, such as soy sauce and tempeh, yogurt, cottage cheese and eggs. Some sources of folic acid are legumes, orange juice, oatmeal, spinach, beets, broccoli and Brussels sprouts. Protein should be part of everyone's daily consumption, especially if it is derived from vegetarian sources such as grains, legumes and soy milk. If meat is consumed, it is important that the animals were raised in a healthy manner.

Supplementation

Supplementation to counter anemia makes sense only when it is keyed to the specific form of anemia that a person is suffering from, which is why you should be guided by a competent health professional. Remember that some forms of anemia do not involve iron deficiency. In these cases, iron supplements are not appropriate and can become dangerous if taken in excess.

Iron . . . If a nursing child is iron-deficient, the mother should take a chelated form of the supplement so that her milk becomes enriched with the mineral. Typically, breast-fed babies do not develop an iron deficiency unless the mother suffers from the deficiency. A product known as Floradix, which can be found in most health food stores, offers a valuable source of iron. The liquid form of the product is recommended over the dry form.

Bee Pollen . . . One ounce of bee pollen daily can serve as an additional combatant of iron-deficiency anemia.

Vitamin B12 . . . Vegetarians need to supplement their diet with B12 daily to prevent a deficiency. Although the condition takes three to four years to develop, it can become serious and potentially lead to nerve damage. Supplementing is especially important for pregnant mothers who expect to raise vegetarian children. In case of pernicious anemia, the methylcobalamin form of B12 could work, orally or sublingually, at 2000-4000 mcg daily. Methylcobalamin has another great feature; it protects neurotransmitters and supports cognitive function. If there is no significant improvement, injections of

B12 are recommended for patients with pernicious anemia, the form that's more common in older people and which is caused by a deficiency of intrinsic factor that is needed to properly process the vitamin.

Spirulina . . . One teaspoon of spirulina provides the body with a useful amount of vitamin B12 and chlorophyll.

Folic Acid . . . Since folic acid is a vital nutrient for proper fetal development, pregnant women require 800 mcg of this nutrient daily, regardless of how good their regular diet is. Because it is water-soluble, excess folic acid in the body is simply washed out. Parents feeding their children goat's milk should add about 800 mcg of liquid folic acid to the milk.

DHEA . . . The supplementation of this steroidal hormone could help decrease the levels of pro-inflammatory cytokines, which cause inflammation and damage red blood cell-forming proteins. The suggested daily dosage for women is 15-25 mg; for men, 50 mg.

DHA . . . This essential fatty acid can be obtained from fish oil. DHA, like DHEA, reduces inflammation.

Vitamin K . . . Taking 10 mg daily could protect against pro-inflammatory cytokines.

Additional Supplements . . . Supplements of hydrochloric acid and intrinsic factor are sometimes needed by people who lack these chemicals for the nutrient absorption process. Certain trace minerals have the tendency to support the red blood cells in oxygen transportation. These trace minerals are zinc (30-60 mg daily), selenium (200 mcg daily), and copper (2-3 mg daily).

Melatonin . . . A deficiency of melatonin could indicate anemia. The recommended dose is 3-10 mg at bedtime.

Herbs

Dandelion root, gentian, yellow dock and blackstrap molasses are effective treatments for iron-deficiency anemia. Other useful herbs include alfalfa, parsley, burdock root, comfrey root, ginseng, red raspberry and nettle leaves. Herbs can be taken separately or combined in capsules or tea. In addition, the Chinese herb dong quai contains phytoestrogens that aid women who become anemic as a result of heavy menstruation. The herb contains vitamins A, E and B12, and can be taken during most days of the month, until menstruation starts.

For people having difficulty absorbing B12, a combination of goldenseal, gentian and wormwood powder taken in capsule form will help increase the level of hydrochloric acid, which will aid the stomach in digesting the vitamin. This formula should be taken only temporarily, for a couple of weeks at a time. In the absorption of iron, herbs such as mint and linden flowers can be helpful in tincture, juice or tea form. To treat anemia, the following herbs may also be useful: aloe vera, apple, astragalus, black locust, Chinese angelica, elder, horseradish, horsetail, maidenhair fern, meadowsweet, plantain, thyme, walnut and spirulina.

Homeopathy

Before prescribing a remedy, an experienced homeopath takes into account the individual person. For iron deficiency, ferrum phosphoricum may be recommended. In a case of poor digestion, or cold hands or feet, calcarea phosphorica may help.

External Treatment

Alternating warm and cold water in showers, 30 minutes before, or two hours after, meals and brushing dry skin with a loofah brush can be useful as adjunctive measures in overcoming anemia. In addition, deep breathing exercises assist with the intake of oxygen and the elimination of carbon dioxide.

What to Avoid

Stay away from refined foods, salt and too much meat. Also, caffeine and alcohol are injurious to healthy blood and should be eliminated.

Treatment Summary

Before anemia is treated, its cause should be medically determined. Anemia stemming from nutritional problems can be due to a shortage of iron, vitamin B12 or folic acid. Iron-rich foods include green, leafy vegetables, legumes and vegetable juices. Good sources of B12 (a nutrient especially important for pregnant women) are fermented foods, such as soy products, tempeh and yogurt. Folic acid can be obtained from orange juice, oatmeal, spinach and beets.

Good supplementary sources of iron include a product called Floradix, and bee pollen. Vitamin B12 can be obtained from a B-complex vitamin or from spirulina.

Sea vegetables, green vegetable juice, dandelion root, gentian and yellow dock are herbs useful in countering iron deficiency.

Alternating hot and cold showers, skin brushing and deep breathing exercises are useful supplementary treatments.

Arthritis

Forty million Americans experience the painful, crippling effects of arthritic diseases. Of that number, about 16 million have osteoarthritis and 7 million are afflicted with rheumatoid arthritis. Many others suffer from less common forms of the condition.

Osteoarthritis, the most common form of the disease, is the form that usually plagues older people or develops after either overuse of the joints or an accident. This is an inflammatory condition affecting any of the 68 joints in the body. It occurs as the spongy cushioning at the end of the bones, known as cartilage, breaks down. Cartilage is encapsulated in a structure called the synovium. The synovium's function is to lubricate the area between the bones and to nourish cartilage. As cartilage wears away, it ceases to act as a shock absorber. Bones touch one another, resulting in stiffness, swelling and painful friction.

Rheumatoid arthritis is more of a systemic disease than osteoarthritis. It is also characterized by painful, swollen joints, but differs from osteoarthritis in that the synovial membrane becomes inflamed and extra fluid leaks into the joints. The result is pain and swelling. Sometimes the whole body—not just the joints—is affected; early signs can include fatigue, weakness, mild fever and anemia. Women between 20 and 50 are this condition's prime targets, although 25 percent of those affected are men. At times, onset is sudden and symptoms are severe; on other occasions, no symptoms manifest. At its worst, rheumatoid arthritis can be crippling.

Less common forms of arthritis include **gouty arthritis,** which occurs when excess uric acid crystallizes and settles into the joints and tissues. The condition affects mainly men who experience pain and inflammation in the joints, accompanied by fever and chills. The disease can become crippling, and, if untreated, can lead to joint breakdown. **Psoriatic arthritis** is a form of rheumatoid arthritis that affects the bones, often occurring in the joints of the fingers or toes. **Juvenile rheumatoid arthritis** generally attacks the large joints of children, and may result in bone deformity. Ankylosing spondylitis is an inflammation of the vertebrae that causes back pain and stiffness, especially in young males.

Causes

Allergies

Arthritis is usually an allergic reaction to foods and substances in the environment. Generally, the foods people eat all the time are the ones to which they are allergic. Many people, for example, eat milk, beef, corn or wheat just about every day. And many react to materials breathed in, such as dust, mold or pollen. Since exposure is continual and invisible, and the effects are not always immediate, most people do not make the connection and thus do not know how to eliminate problem-causing substances.

Why do allergies in some people affect the joints while in others they affect the lungs, the stomach or the skin? The reason has to do with genetic predisposition. Different people have different areas of weakness. So when the body becomes weak from an allergy infection, yeast or some other cause, the most vulnerable area is the one that suffers. Sometimes more than one system becomes affected at once. For example, after drinking milk, a person may experience both arthritis and asthma.

Environmental Toxicity

The body can weaken from continual exposures to poisonous substances in the environment, such as pesticides, artificial colorings and preservatives in foods, and chlorine and fluoride in water. These substances enter the bloodstream and cause autotoxemia, which leads to arthritic changes. An invisible enemy is electromagnetic radiation, which can trigger an arthritic reaction.

Chronic Infections

A proliferation of pathogenic bacteria, viruses, yeast or fungi can be a cofactor contributing to arthritis. Fats and carbohydrates ferment and create an environment that invites Candida albicans, unhealthy bacteria and parasite growth. Some of the bacteria produce toxins that attack joints. The result is acute inflammation, or a slow destruction of joint cartilage. Chronic infections are also the result of heavy metal poisoning, from lead, cadmium and the mercury that leaches out of dental amalgams.

Symptoms

Symptoms of osteoarthritis increase as the disease progresses. In the beginning, there are no indications. The first sign to appear is usually joint pain, and it is commonly associated with exercising or the carrying of weighty items. Other signs may include inflexibility when getting out of bed in the morning and when the weather is cold and damp. As the disease advances, swelling and inflammation of the joints may occur. If muscles are underused from a lack of exercise, there may be fatigue, loss of motion and leg cramps.

The signs of rheumatoid arthritis also worsen gradually. At first there are vague feelings of ill health. Later, symptoms specific to the disease appear, such as joint pain, stiffness, swelling and redness. Joints may become warm to the touch, and stiffness may follow periods of inactivity. Weakness and deterioration can eventually spread to the heart and lungs.

Treatment

Conventional Treatments

Orthodox medicine consistently maintains that arthritis is an incurable disease. Therapies for osteoarthritis are therefore geared toward alleviating symptoms only, not to stopping degenerative processes. Treatments can include rest, exercise, heat, surgery (including joint replacement) and rehabilitation. Mostly though, conventional medical practice relies on various drugs.

Arthritis medications are primarily painkillers or anti-inflammatories, which can have serious side effects. Even aspirin, which is routinely given to patients in large doses on a constant basis, can be dangerous, resulting in dizziness, ringing in the ears, intestinal tract bleeding, kidney damage and lowered immunity (aspirin destroys vitamin C).

As aspirin fails to work, nonsteroidal, anti-inflammatory medications, such as Motrin, are generally given in its place. Although less harmful than steroidal drugs containing cortisone, these produce many of the same side effects as aspirin including gastrointestinal bleeding, peptic ulcers, ringing in the ears and dizziness. In addition, there may be nausea, nervousness and vomiting.

When nonsteroidals fail, drugs that contain cortisone, such as Prednisone, are given. These medications are notorious for their severe side effects. They interfere with the immune system directly, leaving a person defenseless against infections and other diseases thereby making healing difficult.

Some rheumatologists give gold injections. At one time, this treatment fell out of favor because it was considered too dangerous. Unfortunately, more and more doctors are using it again. The intent with using gold is to destroy the immune response. Doing so, however, can lead to massive infections.

These treatments totally miss the mark. Not only do they fail to reach the cause of arthritis, but they are also becoming increasingly expensive, invasive and toxic.

Natural Treatments

Natural medicine reports much success in reversing arthritis because it addresses the cause of the problem as opposed to just masking the symptoms. The consumer should be aware that not all claims for natural arthritis treatments are valid, but that a number of them do work, and can be scientifically validated. Some methods that can produce favorable results are described below:

The Anti-arthritis Diet . . . To prevent and combat arthritis, the types of foods that should be eaten most often are complex carbohydrates with lots of fresh fruits and vegetables. There should also be a small amount of high-quality proteins and fats. These foods are especially protective:

> Foods rich in folic acid, such as lentils, split peas, barley alfalfa, soy and oats.
> Garlic and onions; their high sulfur content stops inflammation.
> Deep-sea, cold-water fish such as salmon, trout, tuna, sardines and mackerel. These contain omega fatty acids that lubricate the joints. Olive oil, avocado, nuts and seeds are good for their oils, as well.
> Soy products, such as tofu, tempeh and miso; they are high in the amino acid methionine.
> Foods that break apart and eliminate uric acid, such as dandelion greens, parsley and alfalfa.
> Plenty of pure drinking water, up to a gallon each day.
> Juices from red, yellow and green fruits and vegetables, six to eight times a day. This is the best way to get high amounts of phytochemicals. (Some recommended juices are listed later in this chapter.)

Recommending Diet by Blood Type . . . There is evidence to the effect that a person's blood type determines the type of arthritis expressed and the kind of treatment needed. This observation was first made by a naturopathic doctor, James D'Adamo, over 25 years ago. He noticed that people with type A blood usually developed puffiness, which could be termed rheumatoid arthritis, while those with type O blood were more prone to a granular or gritty type, associated with the more common osteoarthritis.

The first group responded better to a strictly vegetarian diet, while the second group tolerated lean animal proteins but no dairy. People with type B or AB blood benefited from a more individualized approach. Today, Dr.

D'Adamo's son Peter employs this diagnostic and treatment strategy in Greenwich, Connecticut.

Juices . . . Fresh juices can make an important contribution to any anti-arthritis program. Here are some recommendations:

> Pineapple Juice. The stem of the pineapple contains bromelain, which, when juiced, provides the body with important enzymes helpful against arthritis. This juice is better yet when some juiced alfalfa sprouts are added.
>
> Potato Juice. One raw potato can be juiced, diluted with water and taken in the morning.
>
> Combination Vegetable Juice. Aloe vera (from the bottle) can be mixed with organic red cabbage, cucumber, dandelion, celery mint, apple and carrot.
>
> Star Fruit Juice. Juice from this sweet-tasting fruit can be blended with equal parts of pure water. Drinking this three times a day lessens or eliminates inflammatory joint pain.

Green juices are particularly healing, but are too strong to be taken straight. A good proportion is 2/3 green to 1/3 carrot or beet juice. Those just starting on a juice regimen may want to dilute their green juices with filtered water.

> Cabbage Juice. This is one of the best juices for helping arthritic patients. It can be mixed with carrot for flavor and aloe vera for better cleansing effects.
>
> Chlorophyll Combination. Two ounces of liquid chlorophyll can be mixed with diluted apple or carrot juice and taken daily.
>
> Other Good Greens. These juices can be taken in any combination: celery, broccoli, zucchini, cucumber, kale, parsley and spinach. Ginger root, apple or carrot can be added for flavor and extra nutritional benefits.

Herbs . . . Many natural aids can be grown right in your own backyard. Here are some good ones to consider if you're concerned about arthritis:

> Alfalfa. Alfalfa is rich in chlorophyll, making it an excellent blood purifier. By eliminating uric acid, it helps relieve joint pain. If you're taking this in tablet form, about 20 tablets can be taken each day for the first month; then decrease the amount to 6 to 10 per day.
>
> Aloe Vera. By cleansing the intestines, aloe vera rids the body of toxins that can cause arthritis.
>
> Boneset. As its name implies, this herb can relieve aches and pain in the bones.

Boswellia. Many consider this botanical to be the best natural remedy for treating arthritis. In fact, its healing properties are recorded in Ayurvedic medical literature, dating back thousands of years. Boswellia works much like nonsteroidal anti-inflammatory compounds without the side effects. Additionally, it stimulates repair by increasing circulation to the joints.

Burdock Root. This is a blood cleanser that is especially good for helping patients with gout.

Cayenne. This is a popular arthritis remedy used worldwide. It can be taken internally in a capsule, as a tea, or as a tincture. And it can be used externally in liniments. If used as a spice, cayenne should be sprinkled on food after cooking to prevent irritation.

Comfrey. Comfrey promotes healing of the bone's fibrous coverings.

Devil's Claw. One of the best herbs for helping joints. It removes deposits and helps eliminate uric acid from the body.

Ginger. Traditionally used as an Ayurvedic herb, it is capable of relieving pain caused by arthritic joints.

Nettles. Nettle leaves can be crushed and made into a poultice to stop rheumatic pain.

Prickly Ash Bark. Good for rheumatism and arthritis. As a blood purifier, it gets rid of deposits in the joints.

White Willow Bark. Nature's aspirin; it alleviates joint pain.

Yucca. Research suggests that vaccines from yucca may be valuable for alleviating symptoms of rheumatoid arthritis.

Supplements

We have been told that nutrients do not make a difference in treating arthritis. In actuality, a large body of scientific literature demonstrates that they do. The fact is that arthritis patients can benefit from a full range of nutrients with an emphasis on the ones listed below:

Antioxidant Vitamins . . . Vitamins A, C and E counter inflammation and stop free radical damage to joints. Among its many benefits, vitamin C is an essential nutrient for joint and cartilage repair, especially when taken in combination with glucosamine. Bowel tolerance doses can be taken daily, or in divided amounts throughout the day. (Total daily dose may range from 2000-20,000 mg.) Generally, 400 IU of vitamin E and 50,000 IU of vitamin A or beta-carotene each day help to reduce arthritic pain. In cases of advanced arthritis, patients benefit from intravenous megadoses of these nutrients.

Niacinamide . . . This form of B3 helps both osteoarthritis and rheumatoid arthritis. For the best results, 150-250 mg should be taken before a meal, three or four times daily. Effects are not immediate, but result in a gradual reduction of symptoms and improved range of motion over time. Niacinamide is not to be confused with niacin, which is used for lowering cholesterol.

Pantothenic Acid (Vitamin B5) . . . This one is especially helpful for people with gout.

Other B Vitamins of Note . . . Include a B-complex supplement with approximately 150 mg of vitamin B6, 50 mg of B2 and 15-50 mg of B1.

Chondroitin Sulfate . . . Chondroitin sulfate is a molecular cement that holds together cartilage, allowing collagen proteins to form actual tissue. It both prevents damage from arthritis and stimulates repair.

Cod Liver Oil . . . In generations past, this was a well-known remedy for arthritis. Although its popularity has declined, the remedy still works.

Gamma Linoleic Acid (GLA) . . . GLA is rich in prostaglandins that turn off pain and stop inflammation. It is contained in evening primrose, borage and black currant oils. All forms are equally beneficial, but some are less expensive than others. Six capsules of evening primrose oil, or one capsule of borage oil, provide the needed 240 mg of GLA.

Glucosamine . . . This is one of the most important nutrients for repairing joint cartilage and tissue damage. It is sold as glucosamine sulfate and glucosamine hydrochloride, and both work equally well. Since glucosamine is a substance that each cell in the body naturally manufactures on its own, it is perfectly safe to use. Studies suggest 1500-2000 mg should be taken each day, divided into two or three doses.

Grape Seed Extract . . . Grape seed extract is rich in the antioxidant pycnogenol. It is known to strengthen collagen and support capillaries and veins.

Omega-3 Fatty Acids . . . These are anti-inflammatory, making them especially useful in the treatment of rheumatoid arthritis. Salmon oil is one good source. A vegetarian source is flaxseed oil, which is also rich in important omega-6 and omega-9 fatty acids, making it complete in polyunsaturated acids. Three capsules each day are generally recommended. If omega-3 fatty acids are taken as an oil, a tablespoon can be added to salads, but should not be cooked.

Minerals . . . Adequate supply and absorption of calcium, phosphorus and magnesium are essential for the formation of healthy bones, while zinc and selenium are important for the immune system. Also, new findings suggest that three to six milligrams of boron may actually reverse symptoms of osteoarthritis. Other needed nutrients are potassium, copper and manganese. It's important to note, that since the typical American diet does not contain adequate minerals, taking it can eventually result in damage to the joints. A whole-foods diet, on the other hand, that is rich in raw fruits, vegetables, fresh juices, nuts, seeds and grains, in combination with a multivitamin/mineral supplement, can make a positive difference.

Superoxide Dismutase (SOD) . . . SOD should be taken on an empty stomach, with water, about a half hour before meals. This enhances energy and reduces pain and inflammation. SOD's benefits are enhanced by the addition of vitamin E.

SAMe (S-Adenosylmethionine) . . . This is an activated form of methionine that seems to restore T-cell activity in the synovial fluid by reversing glutathione depletion. SAMe also inhibits damage of the cartilage, and even stimulates cartilage growth. Doses range between 400-1200 mg daily.

MSM (Methylsulfonylmethane) . . . After water and sodium, MSM, a natural sulfur, is one of the most significant components in the body. Taking 2000-3000 mg a day could reduce inflammation and muscle spasms, enhance blood flow and help the immune system to normalize itself.

DHEA . . . Recent studies have reported that DHEA (and other adrenal hormones) is significant in treating rheumatoid arthritis. Reports indicate that adrenal hypofunction may be a precursor to rheumatoid arthritis. This is more so in women than men. This is noteworthy because the vast majority of those suffering from rheumatoid arthritis are women. Therefore, replacing DHEA in women suffering from this condition is crucial.

Vitamin K . . . 10 mg daily could add to the protection against inflammation in the body.

Nexrutine . . . This natural anti-inflammatory plant extract helps to relieve aching in stiff and sore joints.

Copper . . . Studies show that in terms of anti-inflammatory capabilities, copper surpassed aspirin. It should be taken in small amounts. *Caution*: Too much copper produces adverse effects.

Curcumin . . . Extracted from a plant similar to ginger, curcumin is successful in blocking autoimmune activation and decreasing tissue distraction. A small amount of piperine enhances the bioavailability of curcumin.

Inflacin . . . There has been much research focusing on getting at the heart of the causes of arthritis and other inflammatory disorders. These studies not only seek to attack inflammation from within, but also desire to fight it from without. The latter approach has resulted in the discovery (by scientists at BioZone Laboratories, Inc.) of a new group of compounds called Inflacin. When Inflacin was topically applied to patients, it relieved the pain normally associated with arthritis.

Allergy Testing for Problem Foods

Since allergic responses to foods are a major cause of arthritis, skin and blood allergy tests, administered by a complementary physician, can be of value in that they reveal problem foods and chemicals. The foods to which people are highly sensitive must be completely eliminated, at least for a while. Later, some of these foods can be returned to the diet. Foods that cause less of a reaction can be eaten infrequently on a rotation diet, in which the same food is not eaten more than once every four to seven days. So, for example, if wheat is eaten on Monday, it is not eaten again until Friday, at the earliest.

Sometimes, people are allergic to every food they eat. In these instances they are given low-dose allergy vaccines. Unlike typical allergy shots, where patients are uniformly given similar doses of a substance, these vaccines are prepared for the individual's unique requirements. Small doses of antigens are given to stimulate enzyme systems. Enzymes are particularly important as they help break down circulating immune complexes that lead to disease. With insufficient enzymes, these circulating immune complexes build up, enter the synovial membrane of a joint, and establish themselves there. The result is swelling, pain and arthritis. When enzymes are active, food is metabolized and the body does not react to it as if it is a foreign substance. Then there is no inflammation and no disease.

Detoxification

Cleansing the body and the external environment are necessary to overcome arthritis. These are some methods to consider:

Chelation Therapy . . . Chelation, a treatment that gets rid of toxic heavy metals and plaque, is an adjunctive therapy that, by improving overall circulatory functioning, and lessening free radical damage, can lessen arthritic symptoms. This therapy is particularly good for alleviating the crippling effects of rheumatoid arthritis. Scientists hypothesize that the chelation drug EDTA has similar chemical properties to penicillamine, a drug rheumatologists use to treat the disease.

Colon Therapy . . . Many arthritic patients have constipation from an accumulation of toxins in the body. As a result, they have inflammation and suffer autotoxic reactions, in which the body reacts to the poisons. This can exacerbate any disease, including arthritis.

Colonic irrigation opens the digestive tract and thoroughly removes accumulated wastes, getting rid of harmful bacteria. A series of treatments leaves a person feeling lighter, cleaner and more alive. When colon therapy is combined with an improved diet and supplementation, proper balance is restored. As a result, mobility increases and arthritis may even disappear.

Balanced Hormonal Treatment

This treatment was developed by Dr. Robert Liefman, a Canadian physician, who devoted his entire life to understanding the cause of arthritis, and who helped more than 30,000 individuals in his lifetime. After treatment, many were able to lead normal, pain-free lives.

Dr. Liefman and his associates began their research in the 1940s, when cortisone was being hailed as a miracle cure. It soon became apparent that the hormone produces dangerous side effects when used alone, but that it is less harmful when used concurrently with estrogens, and, better still, when testosterone is added. Dr. Liefman developed formulas consisting of various amounts of these three basic ingredients.

According to the proponents of this therapy, it is anti-inflammatory and healing, with minimal side effects, because the substances are in balance with each other. Effectiveness is further enhanced because it is adjusted to the individual needs of each patient, and is used in conjunction with a healthy diet and an exercise program.

Chiropractic

Chiropractic care is a gentle, safe and noninvasive way to offer patients relief from osteoarthritis. During treatment, spinal adjustments are given to release nerve pressure. This allows nerve energy to flow properly. Circulation increases to the joints, enabling them to function better and to heal.

People not helped by this method are those in the advanced stages of the disease, where joints are fused together, causing nerve passageways to be blocked.

Chiropractic treatments increase range of motion, alleviate pain and lengthen the spine, allowing the person to stand straighter and appear taller. Also, by encouraging proper posture, chiropractic treatments minimize pressure on the joints.

Homeopathy

Homeopathic remedies for arthritis, like those for other ailments, are keyed to very specific conditions.

Rhus Toxicodendron . . . Used for pain that worsens at night and in the morning, upon awakening. Pain is worse in cold, damp weather and before a storm. The person feels better with heat and motion.

Rhododendron . . . For joint pains that feel worse in the morning, before a storm or weather change and in heavy winds. Symptoms are alleviated with heat and motion.

Calcarea Carbonica . . . For pain that is worse in cold, damp weather, when there is exertion and motion and when the limb is hanging downward.

Aconitum Napellus . . . For pain and inflammation, especially when the skin is hot and dry.

Reconstructive Therapy

To stimulate the healing of ligaments, tendons and cartilage, reconstructive therapy is sometimes used. Treatment involves low doses of nutritional substances that are injected into the ligaments. The substances vary according to the area being treated, but may include vitamin C, glutathione, shark cartilage and glucosamine sulfate. As a result, ligaments become stronger, enabling them to support the vertebrae and joints with greater ease.

By correcting the root of the problem, symptoms naturally fade. Reconstructive therapy strengthens the structural foundation of the body and pain dramatically disappears.

IntraArticular Growth Hormone (IAGH)

Orthopedic surgeon Dr. Allen Dunn has developed a new method to deal with joints that threaten to deteriorate completely. In order to stimulate the growth of the cartilage, human growth hormone is injected directly into the affected joint spaces, which increases the production of collagen. The Intra-Articular Growth Hormone procedure has proven effective on hips, knees, ankles, shoulders and elbows.

Neuromuscular Therapy

Neuromuscular therapy uses touch to balance the muscular and nervous systems. The therapist improves skeletal alignment, thereby allowing energy to run freely throughout the joints. This is important because when energy is locked in place, blood and other fluids become stuck and pain occurs. Arthritis can be a response to such stressors, according to neuromuscular therapist Sara Vogeler, who explains that postural distortion can cause pressure on the bones, which, in turn, can create stress and compression, causing the formation of bony spurs. A bony spur can aggravate surrounding soft tissue, and cause pain to travel to other parts of the body. Neuromuscular therapy helps to diminish pain by improving postural alignment and teaching correct ways of moving.

Exercise

An exercise routine is important for restoring mobility function and muscle mass. However, people should not push themselves beyond their limits. Pain is a warning signal to slow down, and people should wait until they are comfortable enough to engage in activities.

Walking is excellent for the total body and a good way for the novice to begin. It can improve circulation in the hands, knees, shoulders and fingers, areas frequently affected by arthritis. Another type of exercise that benefits people of every age is yoga. Slow stretches lubricate joints and increase flexibility, while special breathing techniques expel toxins in the joints and muscles.

Other Therapies to Consider

A comprehensive program incorporates several modalities for complete healing. In addition to the approaches mentioned above, those suffering from arthritis might consider acupressure, acupuncture, aromatherapy, Ayurvedic medicine, Bach flower remedies, biological dentistry hydrotherapy, light therapy, massage, meditation, oxygen therapy, ozone therapy, physical therapy, qi gong, tai chi and vitamin drips. Combining a number of treatments is the best way to meet the unique needs of each patient.

What to Avoid

As mentioned previously, most any food, especially those eaten on an everyday basis, can cause an allergic response that produces arthritis. But certain foods and chemicals are common triggers. Highly acidic foods have been associated with the exacerbation of arthritis symptoms. Saturated fats found in meat, dairy and fried foods, as well as alcohol and aspirin, produce prostaglandin-E2, which suppresses the immune system, causing inflammation and pain. Pork is one of the worst offenders, whether it is in the form of ham, bacon or any food cooked in lard (a hidden ingredient in some restaurant foods).

A small percentage of people with arthritis need to avoid the nightshade family of vegetables: tomatoes, potatoes, eggplant and bell peppers. You can tell if these foods affect you by staying away from them for 30 days and then eating all of them in one day. If you do not feel any worse after challenging yourself in this way, then you need not worry. If pain in the joints worsens, stay away from these foods.

Other substances to avoid include coffee and tobacco (both members of the nightshade family), caffeinated tea, sugar, and salt, as well as artificial colors, food additives, and preservatives. Carbonated drinks are high in phosphates, which change the mineral balance in the body. Margarine is unhealthful because of the partially hydrogenated trans-fatty acids, which our bodies cannot digest. Overcooked and processed foods rob the body of essential nutrients and can pave the way for arthritis. Anti-inflammatory medications may appear helpful initially but in the long term, they are destructive.

Another thing to avoid, for those with arthritis, is the prolonged immobility of a lengthy car or plane ride. To prevent the increased knee, ankle, or foot pain that can result from such a ride, travelers should try to exercise periodically during the trip, if this is at all possible.

See also: Allergies, Acupuncture, Chiropractic, Oxygen Therapies, Reconstructive Therapy, Vitamin Drips.

Autism

During the first month of life, newborns do not know that a world beyond themselves exists. As children grow, so do their interactions with the world. But in some instances, a child's ability to interact with the environment and people stays limited. This severe behavioral problem is known as autism.

Autistic children are extremely withdrawn and tend to live in their own fantasy worlds. They are often unable to express themselves verbally, and do not make eye contact. According to studies performed by the Autism Research Institute in San Diego, autistic children tend to have weak immune systems, which causes decreased resistance to infections, particularly upper respiratory and ear infections, as well as autoimmune problems.

Causes

Studies indicate that autism may be the result of adverse reactions to childhood vaccinations. Dr. Alan Cohen, an environmental physician from Connecticut, notes that high levels of autism and attention deficit disorder (ADD) did not occur until the mandatory use of childhood vaccinations, and suggests that there may be a connection between certain vaccines and the onset of these conditions. A recent FDA statement concludes that children are exposed to unsafe levels of mercury through vaccines containing Thimerosal, which has been linked to autism. Thimerosal in vaccine form is 50 times more toxic than plain mercury. Since infants are unable to excrete mercury, it accumulates in the brain cells, nerves, gut and liver, causing symptoms of poisoning. Lipoic acid appears to draw mercury back into the bloodstream in order for it to be chelated from the blood.

Antibiotic overuse can lead to an inability to properly digest nutrients, known as malabsorption syndrome. What happens is that antibiotics destroy healthy bacteria in the gut, with a concomitant proliferation of yeast.

Many autistic children suffer from food allergies. Certain foods produce inflammatory compounds that travel to the brain and cause brain allergies, which are manifested as psychological disorders. Food allergies are actually easily tested for and treated; sadly, though, this is an area often neglected by mainstream medicine.

Autism can be related to biochemical abnormalities. Autistic children may be low in sulfur amino acids, which are needed by the liver for detoxification. When these amino acids are absent, the liver is unable to effectively purge harmful molecules taken in from the air, food and water. As a result, poisonous substances reenter the bloodstream and circulate to the brain, where they can then cause behavioral, focusing and memory problems.

Children with autism also tend to suffer from heavy metal toxicity. Hair analysis and other tests that detect this problem often show that autistic children have excessive amounts of antimony, aluminum, arsenic, lead and cadmium. This may be related to the disordered sulfur chemistry just mentioned, which prevents heavy metals from being excreted from the body. Supplying sulfur amino acids can sometimes eliminate this problem.

Autistic individuals also tend to have vitamin and mineral deficiencies, particularly shortages of zinc, selenium, vitamin B6 and magnesium. Fortunately, it is easy to test for these problems and to correct them.

Sometimes autism is the result of subclinical hypothyroidism, a problem not detected by blood tests, but by temperature. If low body temperature is accompanied by cold hands and feet, dry skin, memory and concentration problems, subclinical hypothyroidism may be at the root of the problem.

Treatment

Orthodox medicine approaches autism from a psychiatric perspective, and treats patients accordingly, with behavioral modification programs and medications. Although autism does manifest as a psychological disorder, the brain is a physical entity, whose functioning can be significantly improved through nutritional therapies. Environmental physicians, doctors who study the relationship between patients and their environment, see positive changes when nutritional protocols are followed. While exact recommendations should be made by a medical professional, and based on sound tests, some general guidelines can be offered.

Nutrition

Autistic children should be eating a variety of fresh foods that are free of additives and preservatives. A diet of organic food assures that what is eaten is pesticide-free. This is important for anyone, but especially for these children who have difficulty eliminating toxins.

In addition, autistic children are often low in vitamin B6 and magnesium, two nutrients that, when taken as supplements, can produce vast improvements. Several studies show that between 30 to 40 percent of autistic children respond to B6 replacement.

The herb ginkgo biloba is good for anyone who needs to enhance brain functioning because it strengthens circulation to the brain. Ginkgo effects are further amplified by the addition of coenzyme Q10, an enzyme that gets more oxygen to all parts of the body, particularly the brain. Dimethylglycine, an over-the-counter, vitamin-like compound that is taken sublingually, has a similar effect. Bee pollen can be wonderful for improving focus, if the child is not allergic to bee stings. It is especially high in B vitamins, which are essential for good mental health. Vitamin E with selenium aids circulation, as do choline and inositol. Moreover, vitamin C, an effective free radical scavenger, builds the immune system and improves circulation. Research suggests that the amino acid L-glutamine is helpful for anyone with mental and emotional problems. Autistic children can benefit from papaya and pineapple enzymes to a degree, when there are digestive problems related to a difficulty in breaking down protein. Autism caused by subclinical hypothyroidism can be corrected with a natural thyroid medicine, available by prescription, called Armour Thyroid. Garlic, citrus seed extract and caprylic acid can help keep down the growth of yeast. For the latter problem, antifungal medications, such as Nystatin or Diflucan, can also be beneficial.

Most autistic children can benefit from a multivitamin and from essential fatty acids, found in flaxseed oil, fish oil, primrose oil, sesame seed oil, almond oil and walnut oil. It is important to remember that children need smaller doses of nutrients than do adults. Exact amounts depend on the age and size of the child, and supplement intake should be prescribed and monitored by a health practitioner, but we can offer general ranges for daily doses:

Vitamin B6 . . . The recommended dosage is 50-200 mg, although some physicians prescribe more.

Magnesium . . . The recommended dosage is 200-300 mg.

Zinc Picolinate . . . The recommended dosage is 20-40 mg.

Selenium . . . The recommended dosage is 100-200 mcg.

Calcium . . . The recommended dosage is 200-500 mg.

Vitamin E . . . The recommended dosage is 200-800 IU.

Taurine . . . A dosage of 500 mg of this amino acid could provide enough sulfur, which is typically low in autistic children.

Glutamine . . . It is a precursor to the antioxidant glutathione. A dosage of 500 mg a day is recommended.

Glutathione . . . It could be supplemented orally. It provides help in replenishing the gastrointestinal tract.

Carnosine . . . The suggested dose is 400 mg twice a day. It enhances neurological function.

Melatonin . . . To help with sleep 0.3-5.0 mg could be used nightly. Although it is safe, it is still a hormone, so it should not be overused. Additionally, melatonin protects against mercury.

DMSA . . . This heavy metal chelator could help to expel mercury from the system.

In order to maintain a normal pH level, lemon water may be used. When there is an elevated pH level, cranberry juice and/or nonbuffered vitamin C can be added.

What to Avoid

Pollutants, and food additives and preservatives should be avoided as much as possible. Foods containing yeast and mold should also be avoided in the diet of the autistic child because yeast overgrowth in the intestinal tract can lead to worsening of the condition. Autistic children must also stay away from any foods that provoke brain allergies. Often there is a sensitivity to gluten, found in grains, and to casein, the main protein component of milk and milk products. Other common foods that produce allergies include corn, soy products, eggs, tomatoes, beef and peanuts. The specific foods responsible for causing reactions can be detected through food allergy tests.

Treatment Summary

Eating organically grown fresh foods is especially important for the autistic child, so that chemicals added to foods will not set off unwanted brain reactions.

Nutrients that can improve brain function include vitamin B6, magnesium, the herb ginkgo biloba, coenzyme Q10, dimethylglycine, bee pollen, and the amino acid L-glutamine.

See also: Allergies.

Back and Neck Pain

Our prehistoric ancestors' switch from quadrupedism to an upright, two-legged posture was a great achievement. Unfortunately, this advance had a price attached: It heralded the beginning of human back and neck pain. Studies have shown that even ancient civilations, such as the Egyptians, were plagued by these pains; in fact, they devised forms of spinal manipulative therapy using their hands and other parts of the body as levers. Today, approximately 80 percent of all people will experience back pain at some point during their lives. While neck pain is not quite as common as back pain, the two together are responsible for millions of lost work hours and billions of dollars of lost earnings, not to mention untold human unhappiness.

Back ailments are especially problematic in the industrialized nations of the world, where people have lost touch with natural ways of working and using their bodies and are thus more prone to overexertion and injury. Backaches become a recurring affliction in over a million people in the U.S. who have been disabled by back pain. One study revealed that, yearly, there are approximately 19 million patients who visit doctors with this complaint.

Who is the typical back pain patient? Most people with back discomfort are age 30 or older. And people who are overweight, especially in the abdominal region, are more likely than their slimmer counterparts to be afflicted with lower back pain because of the greater amount of pressure and strain being placed upon this region. If there is a variance in the length of a person's legs, with one leg being ½ or ¾ of an inch shorter than the other, there is often an imbalance, or mechanical dysfunction, in the person's gait and distribution of weight, which can lead to back pain. Other causes of back pain can be spinal curvature, as well as poor muscle tone in the lower back and abdominal regions. Finally, a major characteristic associated with the onset of back pain is the presence of unusually high stress, which can be caused by anxiety, tension, fatigue, or depression.

The workplace is often not a back-friendly place. Over half of back-related injuries are caused by the lifting of equipment or products on the job.

Vibration of factory equipment tends to traumatize the spinal cord, while driving can severely aggravate lower back pain. Industrial workers who engage in prolonged bending, twisting, heavy manual labor, and repetitive processes are prime candidates for backaches. For both blue-collar and white-collar employees, the maintenance of continuously static postures at the workplace is yet another cause of back pain. And for both, stress related to dissatisfaction with working conditions can contribute to the physical pain.

Back injuries can have lasting financial and psychological effects on workers, in that employees who miss work for prolonged periods as a result of backaches often do not have a job to return to. Furthermore, studies have shown that, of disabled workers who are out more than three months, those with back problem suffer more from emotional distress than do those forced to stay out as a result of injury to the extremities. Some employers, who stand to lose millions of dollars in disability payments and lost hours, have instituted "back schools" at the workplace to teach their employees how to properly bend, lift, and stand.

Symptoms

Back and neck pain can vary widely in severity, ranging from mild sensation to excruciating suffering that warrants immediate medical attention. Usually, the appearance of certain symptoms requires medical attention. A burning or tingling sensation, or numbness in the arms, back, or legs accompanying back pain warrants a visit to a medical practitioner. Also, increasing severity of pain in the back or neck, or a lack of improvement in your condition despite the application of self-help remedies, is an indication that professional advice should be sought. The concomitant appearance of a fever, with or without a headache, is yet another indicator, as is complete immobilization.

The Importance of Seeking Treatment

When the proper therapy or combination of therapies is used, back pain patients can usually experience significant improvement in their physical condition. As there are an infinite number of possible ways to injure your back, so there is not one single treatment approach that can be applied to everyone. However, generally a patient's lifestyle needs to be looked into when he or she is being treated for back pain, because this often reveals why the problem has arisen in the first place.

Many times people, especially men, ignore back problems until they are in severe pain, and only then seek medical attention. This is not the model to follow. If the patient deals with the problem at its onset, extraordinary pain will probably never develop. And while studies have been conducted indicating that people with backaches are capable of recovering on their own after several months, these reports neglect the fact that people who recover are likely to experience recurrences of greater severity at a later time. In addition, people who initially recover as a result of exercise and then discontinue their exercise programs can also experience severe recurrences. It is important to note too that a lack of symptoms does not necessarily signify that the underlying condition no longer poses a threat. In short, evidence indicates that people who follow medical advice recover more quickly and suffer from fewer recurrences.

Professional Assistance

There are numerous people one can consult when suffering from back pain, but only some are capable of offering suitable treatment. Most individuals who seek professional help initiate their treatment with a medical doctor, such as an orthopedic surgeon, but eventually turn to non-medical practitioners after experiencing unsatisfactory results. This is usually due to the medical establishment's failure to acknowledge exercise as an alternative treatment, or stress as a possible cause of the pain.

Orthopedic doctors, who specialize in injuries related to the muscles, joints, bones, tendons, and ligaments, are often inexperienced with conservative methods of treatment and are sometimes too willing to engage in unnecessary surgery. The problem is that surgery has limited long-range benefits and is completely unnecessary for many lower back pain sufferers. When confronted with pain caused by a factor that does not show up on an X ray, an orthopedist will generally refer the patient to another professional. If you are going to an orthopedic specialist for advice on back pain, it is recommended that you see one who does not reflexively advocate surgery or prolonged reliance on prescription drugs.

Internists and general practitioners are generally more versatile than orthopedists in their approach to helping patients cope with back pain. They're more apt to delve into their patients' lifestyles and exercise habits, and more willing to initiate a wide variety of treatments that do not involve dependence on prescriptions. Internists often have a close relationship with their patients and are truly interested in helping them solve their problems. Also, an internist or general practitioner may be more open than an orthopedist to making a referral to an alternative practitioner, such as an acupuncturist.

Neurosurgeons rely on surgery and drug prescriptions to alleviate back pain, but the surgical alternative should be resorted to only when all others have failed. If a neurosurgeon suggests an operation as a back pain cure, it is a good idea to get several other opinions, both from other neurosurgeons and from doctors in other fields. When making a decision on surgery versus alternative methods of coping with the pain, one must factor in the risks of the surgery and the difficulty of rehabilitation. **Neurologists** should also be approached with caution because of their reliance on prescription drugs, such as antidepressants, which can have adverse side effects.

Physiatrists, who specialize in rehabilitative medicine, are dedicated to helping their patients discover the cause of their pain. They generally investigate all aspects of their patients' lives until they find the source of pain, are quite responsive to the needs of their patients, and do not rely heavily on drugs. What they do is develop special treatment programs for their patients, which may involve a variety of techniques such as hydrotherapy, ice, exercise, heat, and even manipulation. Unfortunately, there are fewer than 2000 physiatrists in the entire United States.

Acupuncturists can be quite helpful in alleviating back pain, and they provide virtually risk-free care. Because acupuncture is not a part of orthodox Western medicine, many Americans are reluctant to try it, but those who have are often impressed with the results.

Rheumatologists' specialty is treating pain that is a result of arthritis. Back pain with a gynecological basis can sometimes be treated by an **obstetrician** or **gynecologist,** but their expertise in regard to general pain is also quite limited. **Sports medicine specialists** have achieved some short-term success with athletes suffering from chronic pain, but generally, they are not recommended for long-term relief.

Chiropractors have enjoyed widespread success in treating back pain and, consequently, have become the primary source for nonmedicinal care in this area. Chiropractors treat approximately 60 million patients annually. Their therapy consists mainly of a variety of manipulative reflex techniques, from low-force and low-velocity manipulation to powerful and deep manipulation, depending on the needs of the individual. Evidence has indicated that gentle manipulation of the spine contributes to the release of endorphins, which are opiates produced by the body that help it cope with pain, including spinal pain caused by disk disease. Also, chiropractors often use nutrition as part of their treatment, because patients' eating habits can be directly connected to their strength and ability to recover. Clinical evidence reveals that patients who are malnourished will not effectively respond to manipulation.

Chiropractors can be expected to study the lifestyles of their patients, as this often reveals the cause of pain. They usually design exercise programs for their patients, which is crucial for maintaining relief over the long term. On the other hand, they generally regard drug therapy as useless in the treatment of lower back pain, feeling that it can even be dangerous.

Physical therapists are helpful in treating an assortment of back problems, but they can only treat after they receive consent from a licensed medical doctor. In addition to exercise and education, their healing arsenal includes electrical muscle stimulation, ultrasound, and transcutaneous electrical nerve stimulation (TENS). Physical therapists are qualified in aiding patients who suffer from weak or tight muscles and can correctly evaluate posture and sleeping position. Sometimes, they offer at-home service for patients who are in serious pain.

A non-medical method of coping with back pain is participation in yoga, exercises that use the strengthening and stretching of muscles, ligaments, and tendons crucial to long-term rehabilitation. Despite yoga's helpfulness in alleviating back pain, inexperienced participants should be warned that engaging in yoga while experiencing pain could complicate back problems further. People interested in yoga should find a qualified instructor; the personal touch here is much superior to an instructional video.

Although **massage therapists** trained in Swedish massage may offer immediate relief and pleasure, they usually are not trained to offer self-care advice, and do not provide the long-term rehabilitation program that is essential. **Shiatsu,** a 20th-century Japanese massage technique that is like acupuncture without the needles, can be used in the treatment of minimal lower back pain, but is too complex to try on your own. Relatively controversial is the technique called **Rolfing,** which involves using fingertips, knuckles, and elbows to deeply probe the muscles in order to relieve them from tightness, adhesions, and malfunctions. The **Alexander technique,** which was devised by 19th-century actor Frederick Mathias Alexander, is based on the philosophy that back pain is a result of misusing the body. This abuse may be caused by physical elements, such as standing or moving incorrectly or by emotional factors such as stress. The Alexander technique can be a useful treatment for maintaining rehabilitation, but initial treatment by another trained professional is suggested.

TENS

Transcutaneous electrical nerve stimulation, or TENS, is a short-term pain relief procedure based on the fact that the nerve impulses going up the spinal chord have a hierarchy. The theory is that with a small pulsating current of electricity, these nerve impulses can be confused for a while, thus providing temporary relief.

O'Connor Technique

This technique addresses back and neck pain caused by a physically displaced intervertebral disk of the spine. The sequence involves simple, specific and sequential postural movements of the body.

Magnets

Using magnets is a most effective form of noninvasive pain management. The magnetic field enhances blood flow and circulation, thus accelerating healing and helping the body to flush out the unwanted, toxic waste materials.

Herbs and Essential Oils

Essential oils can help relieve pain and stress. The combination of 3 drops of the following essential oils for every 6 ml of massage base oil or moisturizing lotion may do the trick: camellia, lavender, juniper, peppermint and water inhaled from a diffuser. Menthol and peppermint oil massaged into the muscles is helpful as well.

Herbal packs made of St. John's wort oil, lavender oil, castor oil and horsetail oil have a great soothing effect on tense muscles. Hot baths with 5 drops each of arnica, comfrey and thyme essential oils help stimulate blood flow.

Different forms of the following essential oils (in capsules, powders, teas, glycerine extracts or tinctures) can be used three to six times a day to relieve aches: black haw, jamaica dogwood (both are great relaxants), petasites, valerian, wild yam and lobelia (all are good for muscle spasm). Turmeric, white willow bark, devil's claw and leopard's bane are anti-inflammatories.

Chinese Herbal Combinations

To lubricate joints and to relieve discomfort, a combination of 31 Chinese herbs could be the answer. The formula is called chien pu hu chien wan. D hou ji sheng wan, a different formula, consists of eucommia and codonoposis, and slows down age-related joint and muscle pain. Other formulas, such as guan jie yan wan, te xiao yao tong ling (blend of eucommia and morinda), xiao hou lou dan (blend of aconite and arisaema), yao tong pian, and aka anti-lumbago (mixture of angelica and eucommia), provide fast-acting relief.

Bach Flower Remedies

In cases of sudden, agonizing pain caused by a slipped disk, Bach Flower remedies—such as Rescue Remedy, which includes cherry plum, clematis, star of Bethlehem and rock rose—are recommended.

Homeopathy

Several homeopathic remedies could produce positive results. For stiffness, rhus toxicodendron is suggested. For cramping, colocynthis may be the remedy. In case of burning pain, lycopodium is useful. For sciatica that is accompanied by numbness, gnaphalium can bring relief.

Self-Help

When suffering from back pain, you should use ice during the initial 24 to 48 hours, applying it, wrapped in a towel if this is most comfortable, for 20-minute periods. Heat should not be used during this initial period because it will increase the inflammation, but it can be used after the first 48 hours of pain. Sometimes you can vary your treatment with four minutes of a hot compress followed by one minute of cold.

After your back has recovered, do not immediately resume exercise. Many times people engage in full range of motion (ROM) exercises immediately and continue to do so even after feeling recurrences of pain. If you feel pain while performing ROM exercises, this signifies that you are not ready to do these exercises and should regress to an easier form that does not cause pain.

Nevertheless, do remember that regular exercise should serve as the basis for a proper self-help regimen. If you exercise consistently your body will be able to recover more quickly from an injury and there will be less chance of a recurrence. After receiving care—and your initial exercise go-ahead—from a health care professional, it is important to maintain your rehabilitation by adhering to an exercise program that suits your needs. Exercise that creates bodily aggravation should be immediately discontinued, and warm-up and cool-down exercises should be integral parts of your routine. Strenuous exercise immediately after you awaken is not recommended because your body lacks nutritional sustenance and your muscles are not prepared for any type of vigorous action at that particular time. Your routine should consist of a careful balance of light exercise, such as biking or swimming, and more difficult exercises. If you are lifting any type of heavy weight, forward bending—a common irritant of back problems—should be avoided.

Before commencing your regular exercise, it is imperative to stretch smoothly and gently avoiding jerky motions. Muscles need to be warmed up before they engage in rigorous activity and a proper warm-up routine will enable the muscles to effectively respond to the body's increasing demands. Some people need more time to warm up than others, but in general, each stretching exercise should last at least 15 to 20 seconds.

When stretching the muscles, ligaments, and tendons, concentrate on the movements your body is making and be alert to any subtle twinges of pain. Be aware too that when stretching tight muscles, you shouldn't overexert your body by stretching past the point of joint resistance, as this will only cause discomfort later. Stretching can be quite therapeutic, but only if you are aware of the signals your body is giving you. Feelings of pain, fatigue, or stiffness should provide an instant cue to stop what you are doing. Some popular stretches include trunk rotations, extension lifts, cat stretches, elbow props, pelvic swings, hip rolls, knee-to-chest rocking exercises, back leg swings, and hand and knee exercises.

Stretching properly can provide a multitude of advantages for the body First of all, it can improve the body's full range of motion because the muscles loosen up and become increasingly more mobile. As you become proficient in stretching, the amount of pain associated with the body's movement will decrease as a result of increased circulation throughout the muscles. The muscles will begin to pump additional blood, causing improvements in your pulse rate, blood pres sure, and overall strength. Stretching also contributes to the detoxification of the body because it increases venous drainage.

Once you've stretched, beneficial exercises include brisk walking while swinging the arms and breathing deeply, swimming and bicycling. All of these exercises help to improve circulation, which is important for the healing process. Since a strong abdominal region is vital to increasing back strength, pushups and knee pushups, which strengthen both the upper body muscles and abdomen, are also advantageous. People with a history of back ailments should start out doing three to five repetitions of each exercise and work their way up to doing ten. But if pain is experienced during the performance of an exercise, the exercise should be discontinued immediately. Remember not to strain your body and do not hesitate to seek professional advice if pain persists.

According to chiropractor Dr. Allen Pressman, athletic activities can be divided into three categories as a guide for back and neck patients. The first group, low-risk activities, includes water aerobics, ballroom dancing, cycling, horseback riding, ice skating, basketball, the martial arts, skiing (without the falling aspect), soccer, swimming, and yoga. Medium-risk activities are badminton, baseball, jogging, sailing, squash, racquetball, tennis, volleyball, and wrestling. Some medium-risk activities, notes Pressman, should be considered high-risk for people with especially injury-prone backs or necks. The high-risk category includes such activities as aerobics, ballet, football, gymnastics, rowing, track and field, diving, weight training, and surfing. People with back or neck problems should avoid activities in this final group or they should be performed under close supervision. Aerobics and jazzercise are quite popular, and they can be a lot of fun, but they often involve bending, twisting, and jerky motions, which can aggravate an injured back. So if you want to move on to these advanced forms of exercise, be sure to build up your fitness level at an easier low-impact level.

A final caveat concerning your exercise regimen: Rest, as well as movement, is an integral part. In order to fully reap the benefits of stretching and exercise, the body requires rest and relaxation after its workout to allow time for the muscles to repair themselves and grow.

To Prevent Reinjury

To prevent reinjury to your back, there are several guidelines people who partake in athletic activities should obey. First, don't overtrain. This can cause the body to behave as if it were in a constant state of stress. Eventually this stress will become too difficult for the body to handle, and an injury will result. The definition of overtraining varies from individual to individual, with people in better shape able to sustain more vigorous activity. People who have had a history of back problems should beware of participating in contact sports, as this type of activity is notorious for provoking reinjury. And remember to avoid fatigue, which will hamper your ability to correctly perform your stretches and exercise.

Eating a healthy diet is an important factor in avoiding reinjury; it also enables the body to heal quickly from back or neck pain. A nutritious diet with the correct amount of calories will prevent infection and the loss of muscle, and note that people who become involved in difficult training routines sometimes need to increase their caloric intake by up to 200 percent. A proper diet consists of at least 50 to 60 percent complex carbohydrates, such as fruits and vegetables, potatoes, pasta and rice, and requires few or no simple carbohydrates, such as sugar. Those who suffer from injuries will need to increase the percentage of protein in their diet to approximately 18 to 20 percent.

Be aware of your nutrient status. Deficiencies of iron, zinc and antioxidants should be avoided because an insufficient intake of these nutrients can impair the body's ability to heal, cause a breakdown of connective tissue and prolong the inflammation period. It's a good idea to take 25,000 IU of vitamin A and 30 mg of zinc per day to aid in tissue repair. In general, 50 mg of B-complex vitamins daily is recommended, and a minimum of 1000 to 2000 mg of vitamin C can be especially helpful for healing back injuries. When taking vitamin C, remember to apportion your intake so that you are not taking more than 1000 mg (1 g) at a time. Calcium and magnesium in a 1:1 ratio, and 10-50 mg of manganese per day are additional nutrients that can aid the healing process. Taking 400 IU of vitamin E daily and 250-500 mg of bromelain three times a day, combined with turmeric, helps the body to recover faster.

Reinjury frequently occurs as a result of a person's inability to correctly perform a particular exercise or stretch. Many people like to watch television while exercising, which causes them to be distracted and prevents them from concentrating on the body's movement. During the healing process it is imperative to be wary of exercises that have caused or might aggravate an injury. Allow ample time for the body to readjust to your exercise regimen. It is also important to wear the proper attire while training. Sneakers that do not fit right do more than hurt the feet; they can cause a multitude of injuries to different parts of the body especially the joints. Clothing that is too tight will prevent proper movement, in addition to not allowing sweat to evaporate.

What to Avoid

Preventing a back or neck injury from occurring in the first place is preferable to having to deal with one once it happens. First, be aware of proper lifting technique. Although the act of lifting may seem quite simple, if improperly done it can cause an astounding number of injuries. The correct method involves bending the knees and using the quadriceps and hamstring muscles in your legs to support the weight of the object. Thus, the lower back is spared strain.

Second, to minimize the chance of neck and back problems, see if you can reduce the amount of prolonged stress in your life. If reducing your stress level is out of the question, try to find outlets to cope with the stress, so it will not have physically adverse effects. Also, correct posture is vital to averting back and neck pain, so try to refrain from slouching and slumping. People who suspect that they have a posture problem should have their posture evaluated by a trained professional, such as a chiropractor. And since a significant portion of back injuries are caused by foot or ankle problems, people involved in athletic activities such as running or walking should wear footwear that provides adequate support. Also, women should be wary of continual use of high heels.

When working out at the gym or at home, be sure that your clothes are loose-fitting. When walking with a briefcase or gym bag, do not overload it, and shift the bag from one side of the body to the other periodically to avoid a weight imbalance. An overweight body places a tremendous amount of strain on the lower back region, causing eventual pain and suffering, so keeping trim is a good back-preserving strategy.

If you're sitting or driving for long periods, support your back with a rolled-up towel or other supportive material. In addition, avoid sitting in uncomfortable chairs or chairs that are too soft, and make sure that your wallet is not causing an imbalance in your posture. It is important to shift your weight frequently because continuously sitting on the same place can lead to injury. Finally, avoid crossing your legs for extended periods; instead, maintain a straight posture with your feet flat on the ground. People who have had back problems in the past should try not to sit for more than a half hour without getting up to stretch.

When you are about to stand up from a seated position you can follow a simple procedure that will prevent you from irritating your bad back. First, push yourself gently to the edge of your seat, with one foot placed carefully in front of the other. Remember to use the quadriceps and hamstrings in your legs to lift yourself, refrain from leaning forward, and keep a vertical center of gravity when rising.

Driving can easily aggravate an injured back, so when you are experiencing back pain you should try to stay away from your automobile. If you do have to drive, bring your seat as close to the steering wheel as possible, allowing the knees to rise above the hips. After 30 minutes of diving you should pull over to the side of the road and allow your body some time to stretch. At break time, passengers suffering from back pain should lie down on the backseat, bend their knees, and try to relax their bodies.

When purchasing a mattress, back pain sufferers should stay away from extra firm ones as well as from overly soft mattresses and waterbeds. A medium-firm mattress is your best bet. In the morning, you should move your body to one side of the bed, shift onto your side, pull your knees upward, drop your feet carefully to the ground, sit up slowly and finally stand up using the proper technique previously described. Be sure to avoid bending at the waist when rising as this can be detrimental to an injured back.

Treatment Summary

People who follow medical advice recover more quickly from back pain and have fewer recurrences.

Surgery should be used only after other methods of dealing with back pain have failed.

In addition to mainstream medical practitioners, acupuncturists and chiropractors can offer significant help to those suffering from back and neck pain.

The Alexander technique may be useful in maintaining rehabilitation after an injury.

First aid measures taken immediately after an injury can prevent inflammation and reduce pain.

To prevent reinjury, athletes need to remember to rest, not to overtrain, and to perform stretches correctly.

Eating a nutritious diet speeds up the healing process.

Breast Cancer

While in 1950 only one in 20 women suffered from breast cancer, today this figure has risen to one in eight. Although the medical establishment has recommended early diagnosis via periodic breast examinations and mammograms, less stress has been placed on possible causes of the disease and preventive measures. Yet, it's these last areas of understanding that hold the most promise.

Causes

A family history of breast cancer does put one at higher risk for the disease. But there's so very much more that comes into play. Medical evidence indicates that prolonged exposure to the female sex hormone estrogen as a result of either an early onset of menstruation or a late menopause increases the chance for acquisition of breast cancer. In addition, women who have not had children or have not breast-fed are at higher risk of developing breast cancer, suggesting that the female sex hormone progesterone can serve as a preventive agent. Estrogen and progesterone are usually equally balanced, but when the amount of estrogen increases or the amount of progesterone decreases, an imbalance, known as estrogen dominance, is created. Increased levels of estrogen are associated with a high alcohol intake, being overweight, and consuming a lot of fatty foods. Also, people who eat large quantities of meat are more susceptible to breast cancer due to the estrogen-stimulating hormones that are frequently used to improve the texture of meat products.

A diet that is high in fat has other adverse effects upon the body. One is that when a person consumes a large amount of fatty food the membranes of body cells can become damaged by the fat. After this occurs, the cell can either die and eventually be replaced by another cell, or it can attempt to repair the damage that has been done. During the latter process it is possible for the damaged cell to transform itself into a cancer cell while attempting to fix itself.

The liver, which is responsible for the elimination of estrogen and other hazardous materials, is often overwhelmed by the abundance of toxic substances that find their way into the human body each day. Problems with the breakdown of estrogen by the liver can also be compounded by the presence of excessive amounts of sugar or alcohol.

The presence of foreign chemicals in the body known as xenoestrogens can be troublesome. While forms of xenoestrogen that are derived from plant foods can have positive effects on the body, forms that originate from synthetic materials such as fuel, pesticides, or plastics have proved to be carcinogenic.

Another possible cause of breast cancer is a dysfunction in the lymphatic system, which is responsible for the drainage of toxic substances from the tissues. The lymphatic system is essential to the body's immune system and aids in the removal of the xenoestrogens that can accumulate in the fatty tissue of the breast. The flow of lymphatic fluid, which carries the body's toxins and waste products away from the cells, is not analogous to that of blood, as it can be interrupted by muscle contraction and external force. It is important to note that an excessively constrictive bra can be a cause of lymphatic blockage, and that eventually the accumulation of harmful materials within the breast can lead to cancer. Studies have indicated that wearing a bra for more than 12 hours a day is correlated with an increased incidence of breast cancer; therefore, it is advisable to limit the wearing of a bra as much as possible and to beware of bras that may constrict the flow of waste products from the breast.

The absorption of excessive amounts of radiation, such as medical X-rays, can be a causal factor in breast cancer. Years ago doctors were ignorant of the dangers of radiation because the manifestation of harmful side effects can take decades. Consequently the amount of "rads" a patient received was not a cause for concern, and many treatment procedures, such as fluoroscopic examinations, exposed patients to excessive radiation numerous times a year. Excessive exposure to harmful rays can lead to chromosomal damage, and eventually, to various forms of cancer. Dr. John Gofman of the University of California at Berkeley who investigated the correlation between X-rays and breast cancer, has asserted that up to 90 percent of all cases of breast cancer can be attributed to overexposure to X-rays. It is true that during the past few decades radiological facilities have been forced to lower their dosages dramatically but there is still substantial room for improvement. Dr. Gofman feels that pressure should be applied to the medical community to further reduce dosages. And he recommends that people alert themselves to the potential dangers of medical X-rays and insist that when they receive an X-ray a low dosage be administered.

Studies have demonstrated that excessive absorption of electromagnetic radiation, which can be emitted from common household objects like televisions, digital clocks and microwave ovens, contributes to the development of breast cancer in men and women by preventing the production of melatonin in the pineal gland during the sleeping cycle. Numerous tests have been conducted in this field, including one that revealed a cancer rate directly proportional to the use of electric blankets.

Other factors that are contributory to breast cancer are use of alcohol and tobacco products. Nicotine is the second largest cause of breast cancer (after elevated estrogen levels due to dietary and environmental factors). And the consumption of only two to three alcoholic beverages a week increases breast cancer risk significantly.

Symptoms

Early symptoms of breast cancer are thickening of the breast, a lump, and dimpling of the skin. The person may experience pain, ulcers, nipple discharge and swollen lymph glands under the arm at a later time.

After the manifestation of any of these symptoms, you should immediately seek professional assistance. When a diagnosis of breast cancer is confirmed, there are several facts that one should be aware of. First, the survival rate is dependent on whether or not the cancer has spread to the regional lymph nodes, on the size of the cancerous region within the breast, on how fast-growing the tumor is and finally on whether or not the cancer has spread to other parts of the body. During the initial, very localized, stage of breast cancer known as stage zero, the five-year survival rate is approximately 90 percent. If the cancer has spread to the lymph nodes above the collarbone or to other vital organs (stage four), the five-year survival rate is only 10 percent. This is why early diagnosis is stressed.

Treatments

The mainstream medical establishment often prescribes mastectomy radiation and chemotherapy to treat breast cancer, an approach that has been described as a slash-and-burn strategy. This approach may be in for a reappraisal with the recent insight by the medical world that breast cancer is actually three different diseases, with indistinct boundaries, rather than one. In other words, only some breast cancers fit the image of a disease that is fast-growing and fast-spreading. Two other categories of this condition exist, the slowest-growing of which may never spread or be life-threatening at all. With this realization comes the idea that giving everyone with breast cancer chemotherapy may be unnecessary. Considering the harmful effects of chemotherapy, the belated nature of this realization is disturbing, to say the least.

Diet and Supplements

One of the most important steps to take in preventing breast cancer is to avoid a diet that is high in animal fat while at the same time increasing consumption of fruits, vegetables, beans and whole grains. The abundance of fiber in vegetarian diets helps the colon dispose of unnecessary estrogen, while the low fiber and high iron content of beef and processed foods can damage cells and encourage the spread of cancer. In addition, some foods, such as lima beans, soy beans, and other soy products, seem to have medicinal capabilities because of the presence of isoflavones and phytoestrogens, or plant estrogens. These substances actually curb the activity of the excess estrogen in the body tissues. Phytoestrogens can also be found in other vegetables and in fruits, along with useful amounts of nonsoluble fiber, beta-carotene and selenium. Flaxseeds and certain types of fish, including salmon, tuna, sardines, mackerel and herring, contain omega-3 fatty acids, which have an anticancer effect. Life Extension provides the formula Mega EPA (with DHA), which provides 3200 mg of EPA and 2400 mg of DHA. It should be taken orally.

The consumption of broccoli, cauliflower, Brussels sprouts and other cruciferous vegetables is also recommended to combat cancer. A phytochemical isolated from these cruciferous vegetables called indole-3-carbinol (I3C) helps turn the "strong" estrogen, estradiol (which could trigger cancer cell formation), into the "weak" estrogen, estriol. It also elevates the levels of 2-hydroxyestrone (2-OHE), another metabolite of estrogen, and inhibits the formation of 16-a-hydroxyestrone (16-OHE), which could be dangerous because it sends growth signals to breast cancer cells. I3C is also capable of blocking the development of cancer cells and stimulates them to kill themselves, a process called apoptosis. I3C is also a free radical inhibitor, which works especially well with radicals that are responsible for the oxidation of fat. The suggested dose is 200 mg twice a day for women under 120 lbs, 200 mg three times a day for women weighing 120-180 lbs and 400 mg twice a day for women over 180 lbs. It is not recommended for pregnant women because estrogen is essential in the growth of the fetus.

Curcumin, the extract from the spice turmeric, may be a powerful agent in fighting cancer. It confuses the growth signals in cancer cells and inhibits the development of new blood vessels into the tumor (antiangiogenesis). Supplementation of four 900-mg capsules three times a day (for a total of 10.8 g) is suggested. Caution should be exercised in cases of chemotherapy.

Another great antiangiogenesis agent is green tea. Its effects come from epigallocatechin gallate, which enables green tea to block vascular endothelial growth factor (VEGF is crucial in new tumor blood vessel growth). Green tea is established as a preventer of cancer, and new research finds it a potent agent for treating cancer. Oral supplementation of five 350-mg capsules is suggested three times a day. This enables one to get the needed amount of 5.25 g, which is difficult to obtain in liquid form. Caffeine enhances the anticancer effect of tea polyphenols.

A compound of beef and milk, conjugated linoleic acid is essential for the transport of dietary fat into cells. It is believed to have protective properties against metastasis. The suggested dose is 3000-4000 mg daily, combined with 300 mg of guarana. Further, the daily addition of acidophilus and approximately an ounce of wheat fiber to the diet can further enhance the colon's ability to eliminate estrogen. An adequate amount of wheat fiber can be obtained by taking 2 tablespoons of raw wheat bran per day. Finally evidence has shown that reishi, shiitake and maitake mushrooms can serve as formidable opponents of cancer cells.

Supplements of vitamin D can protect the body from breast cancer, especially if one is deficient in phosphorus; however, do not exceed 800 IU per day without medical supervision. Medical evidence has indicated that the prevention of breast cancer may also be related to consuming the proper ratio of calcium to phosphorus. The optimal ratio is 1.5:1, but most people have a greater phosphorus intake because of the presence of meat in their diets. Although meat products contain calcium, the phosphorus content can push the calcium out of the tissues and into the bloodstream, where it eventually lodges in the walls of the arteries and in the joints. Damage to breast tissue can be avoided with the proper intake of antioxidants. Many doctors are currently recommending the following nutrients to prevent breast cancer: between 10,000 and 50,000 IU of beta-carotene, with monthly blood testing to avoid toxicity; 100 mg of coenzyme Q10 three times a day; 2000 mg of coenzyme A, which is a crucial catalyst to utilize CoQ10, twice a day; NADH and other energy-producing metabolic enzymes; the mineral germanium; DMG (dimethylglycine); two capsules of garlic three times a day; 400 IU of vitamin E daily; 10 mg of vitamin K daily; and up to 10,000 mg of vitamin C, taken in divided doses throughout the day.

Other doctors stress that the body requires the proper amounts of calcium, magnesium, selenium, chromium, alpha linoleic acid and molybdenum, all of which can be supplemented when a deficiency exists. The naturally occurring selenium (Se-methylselenocysteine) has an enhancing effect on cancer cell destruction (apoptosis) and inhibits cell proliferation. The recommended dose is 200-400 mcg a day.

Borage, evening primrose and black currant seed oils contain a cancer-fighting agent known as gamma linoleic acid. Gamma E tocopherol/tocotrienol, from Life Extension, is a great antioxidant that protects against free radical damage. A dosage of 200 mg of palm-oil tocotrienol may lower tumor formation. For bone support, 6 mg of silicon daily is recommended. For the protein SOD to function correctly and prevent oxidative cell damage, it is essential to avoid deficiencies of zinc, copper and manganese. A nutritionally oriented physician can help you decide which nutrients are most important for you.

Herbs

Numerous herbs are protective against breast cancer. The Venus flytrap has become quite popular in Europe. On this side of the Atlantic, the Native American herbal formula called Essiac is used to prevent cancer and treat cancer that is already present. Cat's claw, an herb used by Peruvian Indians, is another known cancer combatant. Xiao Yao Wan, a Chinese combination of digestive herbs that people take to improve circulation, build blood and treat fibroids, is often used to combat breast cancer as well. Astragalus can aid in preventing and treating breast cancer by enhancing the immune system, and is especially useful for people undergoing chemotherapy who need to regain strength. One teaspoon of the herb should be added to purified water and consumed once or twice daily. Other herbal solutions for avoiding breast cancer use echinacea, pau d'arco, sassafras, red clover and burdock, which improve the immune system and purify the blood. Studies have also shown that extracts of mistletoe can be of use for immunity enhancement.

Detoxification

Activities that detoxify the body can further reduce the chance of acquiring breast cancer. For instance, aerobic exercise assists in lymphatic drainage and induces sweating, which is a natural way for the body to eliminate waste products. And exercise has in fact been shown by studies to be correlated with a lowered breast cancer risk. The removal of hazardous waste products by the lymphatic system can be aided by manual lymphatic drainage, which involves a light massage that stimulates the lymph nodes and enables them to properly dispose of waste. As mentioned earlier, the blockage of the lymph fluid in the breast, which can occur after the performance of a mastectomy, allows potentially dangerous substances to collect in the breast, eventually leading to cancer.

Psychoneuroimmunology

A new branch of science, known as psychoneuroimmunology, studies the integration of thoughts, emotions and physical reactions at the cellular level. When a person feels depressed for extended periods of time, this state of mind can have an adverse effect on the body's ability to fight off disease and to heal itself. On the other hand, positive emotions can aid in maintaining or regaining physical health.

According to Dr. Carl Simonton, director of the Simonton Cancer Center in California, women who are diagnosed with breast cancer should work to overcome the stereotypes associated with cancer. Women in this position are often under the impression that their cancer can easily overwhelm and destroy their health, and that their bodies will be severely victimized by harsh treatments. If a person has this defeatist attitude, then her body will read these signals and act accordingly. It is important for patients to evaluate their thoughts about the disease, the treatment and their chances of recovery, and to remain confident.

One way to improve one's psychological and physical health, and to lessen one's chance of breast cancer, is through meditation. Studies report this fact, and give the explanation that women who meditate have more melatonin in their blood than women who do not. This is the case because the pineal gland, which secretes melatonin, is sensitive to psychological processes, and in turn, is important because melatonin is known to inhibit estrogen, and breast cancer is associated with higher levels of estrogen in the body.

What to Avoid

There are a multitude of precautions we can take to prevent breast cancer. First of all, it is utterly foolish to abuse tobacco and alcohol products, as medical evidence has linked these directly to various forms of cancer, including breast cancer. Furthermore, we know that estrogen is a risk factor, so fatty food, which increase levels of this hormone, are to be avoided. Also, consider that an excessively fatty diet can induce free radical production, resulting in the damage of healthy cells and their eventual conversion to cancerous cells. Be especially careful to curtail processed meat products, margarine and other saturated fats. Beware, too, of excessive intake of hot, spicy foods, oily foods, foods high in sugar and stimulants such as coffee, tea and recreational narcotics. Another precaution we can take is to avoid unnecessary exposure to X-rays and other forms of radiation. And remember to try to limit your use of bras to less than 12 hours per day and do not purchase a constrictive bra that may impede lymphatic drainage. Finally, be aware of the quality of the water that you consume, as many urban and suburban water supplies require filtration of fluoride and chlorine.

Treatment Summary

There is a proven correlation between high-fat diets and breast cancer. Conversely, populations that eat more fruit, vegetables and legumes, with an emphasis on soy products, have lower incidences of the disease. Extra protection from breast cancer can be obtained with vitamin C, vitamin D, a proper ratio of calcium to phosphorus (higher in the former) and antioxidant nutrients.

Herbs provide extra protection from breast cancer; especially noteworthy are the Venus flytrap, the herbal formula Essiac, cat's claw, astragalus and pau d'arco.

Aerobic exercise and manual lymphatic drainage rid the body of stored-up wastes that can otherwise lead to cancer.

The new field of psychoneuroimmunotherapy stresses positive emotions and meditation as health and healing promoters.

Breast Implant Reactions

Are breast implants safe? The answer is that anything placed within the body has a good chance of poisoning it. Silicone is not compatible with human body tissue, and will cause everything from mild irritation, fatigue and depression to severe pain. Such silicone reactions show up as abnormal immunological responses on blood tests. In time, breasts that were once soft and supple turn into hard lumps, and well-shaped ones become grotesquely deformed. Even so-called safe saline implants are contained within a silicone sack. Pieces of silicone mix with tissue, even when the capsule remains intact.

Women usually shun the idea of implant removal, fearing that their breasts will look worse than before. Their surgeons tell them that their breasts are too stretched out for corrective surgery. Indeed, it is true that up until recently, most operations resulted in gross breast deformity.

Treatment

Obviously prevention—not having implants put in in the first place—is the best course to take. But in a society that judges women by their appearance, actresses, models and even average young women often feel pressured into getting implants, especially when they are not warned of the potential dangers.

Breast Conservation Surgery

Fortunately, there is a new procedure for removing breast implants without ruining a woman's appearance. Dr. Vicki Hufnagel has pioneered a surgical technique using an argon beam to remove implants without having the breasts cave in. The beam sprays heat to the area and is able to shrink tissue without burning the body. The technique also restores the healthy growth of breast tissue. Hufnagel reports great success and spends much of her time educating doctors on this method.

If you have implants, it is best to have them removed. Use a doctor with a high success rate; speak with that doctor's former patients. And whether or not you decide to have the implants removed, it is important to report any problems from breast implants to the Food and Drug Administration. This will help other women in the future.

Treatment Summary

With everything we know today about the dangers associated with breast implants, the best course of action is to avoid getting them. A new surgical technique uses an argon beam to remove breast implants without causing a deformity.

Cancer

Cancer refers to a group of diseases in which cells deviate from the usual controls that regulate cellular growth and reproduction. They begin to multiply more rapidly than is normal, invading and destroying other body cells. Cancerous cells can spread, or metastasize, from their primary site to other parts of the body through the bloodstream and lymphatic system.

The most common form of cancer is the carcinoma. This is a tumor that originates in the skin, in the epithelial tissue that lines the body, or in glandular tissue, such as the breast or prostate gland. Another type of cancer is the sarcoma, affecting connective and supportive tissue, such as bone, muscle, cartilage and fat. Melanomas are a type of skin cancer; lymphomas affect the lymphatic system; and leukemias are cancers of the blood-forming organs.

Causes

Cancer is largely attributable to the cumulative impact of toxins on our systems. External factors, such as polluted air, water and food, play a major role, as do microscopic pathogens in our internal environment, such as parasites, fungi, bacteria, viruses and toxic chemicals, including heavy metals. Genetic tendencies and immunological weakness come into play, and psychological factors are also believed to affect the incidence and course of cancer.

Lifestyle Factors

Over half of all cancers have been linked to lifestyle factors, with some estimates as high as 70 percent. Prime among these factors is the altered state of our nutrition. More than 60 percent of all women cancers and 40 percent of men's have been attributed to nutritional losses incurred as a result of modern farming and food industry practices.

Before the 1940s, most food was organically grown. Then, the widespread introduction of pesticides, fertilizers, antibiotics and mono-crop farming changed the face of agriculture forever, and with it, the health of consumers. These changes were coupled with the increased promotion of processed foods designed for long shelf life and addictive tastes, but filled with empty calories. Today, chemically grown and denatured foods and drugs are the norm. These include such poisons as processed meats, caffeinated tea and coffee, soft drinks, liquor, tobacco, meat, white sugar, white flour and margarine.

Modern diets create a state of chronic toxicity and slow down the organs of elimination: the bowels, kidneys, liver, lungs and skin. Poisons eventually accumulate around the weakest organs and set the stage for the development of cancer. Three ways an inadequate diet harms the system are through nutrient depletion, free radical damage and a shift in pH levels.

Nutrient depletion may be the result of gross deficiency of certain nutrients over long periods of time. An analogy can be drawn between the body nutrient supply and a reservoir of water. Ideally a reservoir should be full and able to trickle over slightly. When levels are lower, people can still fish and boat quite comfortably. But at a certain point, the water is too low for these activities. The same is true in terms of a person's nutrient reservoir. It can be significantly reduced without producing any symptoms, but once it reaches a certain level of depletion, the disease process begins.

The average American diet lacks sufficient nutrients to keep the reservoir full. A healthful diet is high in potassium and low in sodium, for example, but processed foods reverse this ratio. People need only between 600 and 700 mg. of sodium a day, but one fast-food meal supplies them with over 5000. Also missing from the average diet are enough essential fatty acids, such as omega-3 and gamma linoleic acid (GLA), found in deep-sea fish and unsaturated oils such as flaxseed oil. Instead, people get an excess of arachidonic acid from too many animal proteins. This combination of factors sets the stage for the development of cancer.

Modern farming practices may make agribusiness more efficient, but they have depleted essential trace elements from our soils. A lack of selenium, zinc, chromium and magnesium in foods grown today has been implicated in increased incidences of cancer. Without these protective nutrients, free radical damage goes unchecked in our systems, and abnormal cell reproduction can lead to cancer.

Genetic Predisposition

Heredity plays a role, albeit a limited one, in determining who gets cancer. Researchers have shown that some people are more prone to the disease than others because their cancer-causing genes, known as oncogenes, are more readily triggered.

It should be stressed that while a genetic tendency predisposes a person to a condition, it does not mean that the condition will necessarily be manifested. Educating oneself about factors that increase the likelihood of cancer can lead to lifestyle decisions that decrease the chance of cancer's appearance. While rules of good health are universally applicable, a person genetically predisposed to cancer would be especially wise to abstain from smoking, to eat a whole-foods diet supplemented with anticancer nutrients and to learn to deal with anger constructively.

The Psychological Connection

Experts in the study of mind/body connections, a field known as psychoneuroimmunology, find that depression, hopelessness, a perceived lack of closeness to parents and an inability to cope with life are associated with increased cancer risk. Some researchers even talk about a type C personality. They describe this cancer-prone type as someone who feels that he or she is living the life that others have dictated for him or her, rather than the life he or she would like to be living. Emotions are suppressed and anger is held inside. Of course this is a generalization, and should not be used as a fatalistic explanation of cancer, or as a way of blaming the victim.

Symptoms

The American Cancer Society states that people who treat the disease early have a better chance of survival. Their list of seven early warning signs in adults includes a change in bowel or bladder habits, unusual bleeding or discharge, a thickening or lump in the breast or elsewhere, an obvious change in a wart or mole, a nagging cough or hoarseness, a sore throat that does not heal and indigestion or difficulty swallowing. For children, indications are marked change in bowel or bladder habits, nausea and vomiting for no apparent reason, bloody discharge and failure to stop bleeding, swelling, lumps, or masses anywhere in the body, unexplained stumbling, a generally rundown condition and pains or persistent crying for no apparent reason.

Treatment

The Conventional Approach: Chemotherapy

A patient is diagnosed with cancer, and told that chemotherapy is his or her only hope of survival. Frightened and confused, the individual places full confidence in the doctor's expertise, and undergoes a costly therapy that can produce side effects worse than the cancer itself. The hope is that the ends will justify the means as the tumor shrinks and disappears, never to return. What the patient does not realize is that, in most instances, his/her assumptions are not based on sound studies supporting chemotherapy's effectiveness.

Historically chemotherapy has helped patients overcome a small number of cancers only. It has prolonged the life of children and young adults with rare cancers, such as childhood leukemia and later-stage Hodgkin's disease. Some effectiveness has also been seen in certain common cancers, such as ovarian cancer in women and testicular cancer in men, as well as Duke's C, a form of colon cancer that has spread to regional muscles and lymph nodes. In small-cell lung cancer, life can be extended from several weeks to several months. But outside of these instances, there is no proof that chemotherapy increases life expectancy.

Chemotherapy's use far exceeds its proven effectiveness. The number of cancer patients cured by chemotherapy is in the range of 2 to 5 percent, but about 50 percent receive this treatment. The logical question to ask would be, if chemotherapy has such a low rate of success, why is it used so often? Dr. Ralph Moss, author of *Questioning Chemotherapy*, explains that most people confuse decreased tumor size with disappearance of disease. The association appears logical, but no proof exists to support the connection.

Interestingly, alternative therapies are criticized for not demonstrating patient success according to scientific standards. But why are conventional therapies exempt from the same rigorous expectations of alternative treatments? The answer appears to be economics. While the cost of natural protocols is usually nominal, chemotherapy treatments can run into the six figures. Bone marrow transplants, for example, which combine high doses of chemotherapy and radiation, cost an average of $150,000. While the patient may not benefit from chemotherapy the drug company investor surely does. From a business point of view, chemotherapy is a profitable commodity and so the more people who use it the better.

Alternative Approaches to Prevention and Treatment

For well over 50 years, billions of dollars have been poured into cancer research. Commensurate results haven't been forthcoming, though. Today one in three people get the disease, and in the near future, it is predicted that two out of five individuals will be affected.

Reversing the trend will require taking an entirely new approach to research and treatment. Instead of continuing to view cancer as a single disease in need of a single cure, cancer must be addressed as a complex phenomenon, since multiple factors are involved. As oncologist Dr. Michael Williams, chief medical officer of the Cancer Treatment Centers of America, explains, the reductionist, scientific model of testing A versus B will not get to the root of the problem. Rather, attention needs to be focused on environmental, nutritional and body/mind considerations.

Diet

Eating an organic, whole-foods diet and drinking plenty of pure water ensures us valuable nutrients and keeps the bloodstream pure so that cancer is unlikely to develop. If cancer is already there, these foods give the body the best support for overcoming the condition and preventing recurrence. The following foods are particularly important for their cancer-fighting properties:

Alkaline Foods . . . Eating alkaline foods balances the pH of the blood, which, in turn, inhibits the proliferation of cancer cells. Alkaline foods keep the blood pH in its ideal range of between 7.2 and 7.4, which is important for the prevention and treatment of cancer.

Ideally, the diet should consist of 80 percent alkaline-forming foods, such as those available from many raw fruits and vegetables, as well as nuts, seeds, grains and legumes. Among recommended alkaline-forming fruits are berries, apples, apricots, avocados, bananas, currants, dates, figs, grapefruit, grapes, kiwis, lemons, limes, mangoes, melons, nectarines, olives, oranges, papayas, peaches, pears, persimmons, pineapple, quince, raisins, raspberries, strawberries, tangerines and watermelon. Lemons—contrary to what you might think—and melons are the most alkaline-forming foods. A good idea is to eat some melon first thing in the morning, and then to wait 20 to 30 minutes before eating other foods.

Among the recommended vegetables are artichokes, asparagus, sprouts, beets, broccoli, Brussels sprouts, cabbage, carrots, cauliflower, celery, collards, corn, cucumbers, eggplant, endive, ginger, horseradish, kale, kelp, seaweeds, mustard greens, okra, onions, parsley, bell peppers, potatoes, pumpkin, radishes, spinach, squash, tomatoes, watercress and yams.

In addition, there are a variety of whole grains, seeds and nuts from which to choose. Alkaline-forming beans include green beans, lima beans, peas, soybean products and string beans. Grains such as rice, quinoa, amaranth, barley and oats are good. The most alkaline-producing nuts and seeds are almonds, chestnuts, coconuts and pignolias. Seeds, such as alfalfa, chia, radish and sesame, are excellent, especially sprouted.

Cruciferous Vegetables . . . Vegetables in the cruciferous family—kale, mustard greens, collards, broccoli, cabbage, cauliflower and Brussels sprouts— contain compounds called indoles that act as detoxifying agents. Indoles are believed to remove cancer-causing substances from the body.

Fiber . . . This isn't a food itself, but it's an important component of grains, fruits and vegetables; it's actually the structural support of these plants, and we need it for its ability to facilitate the transit of foods through our system. Unfortunately fiber is often lost when food is processed. The typical American diet includes about five grams of fiber each day, which is not nearly enough for cancer prevention. Studies show that 30 g a day significantly reduces the risk of colorectal cancer. Good sources of fiber are fruits, vegetables and whole grains; initially increasing the fiber in your diet may create gas and abdominal discomfort, but this problem usually clears up.

Olive Oil . . . Olive oil is composed of monounsaturated fatty acids, which studies show have a protective effect against breast cancer, especially in post-menopausal women. Olive oil should be used in moderation and eaten raw for maximum benefit. One tablespoon of extra virgin, cold-pressed olive oil can be added to salads.

Flaxseed Oil . . . One to two tablespoons of flaxseed oil daily may be protective against cancer.

Primrose, Borage and Black Currant Oils . . . These provide gamma linolenic acid, an omega-6 fatty acid important as a cancer preventive.

Green Foods . . . Wheatgrass, barley grass, alfalfa, blue-green algae, chlorella and spirulina are rich in blood-purifying chlorophyll and important nutrients for detoxifying the system and rejuvenating the organs. Chlorophyll has strong antimutation factors.

Soybean Products . . . Soybeans, soy milk, tofu, miso and tempeh contain phytoestrogens that help prevent many forms of cancer. Indeed, Japanese women, who eat soy on a daily basis, have the lowest incidence of breast cancer in the world. Because soy products are high in protein, they make excellent replacements for meat.

Juices . . . Freshly squeezed juices provide valuable enzymes and antioxidant nutrients that are easily digestible. One of the most potent juices for liver detoxification is blueberry juice, while cabbage juice may help to prevent stomach and colorectal cancer. Carrot juice is valuable for its high beta-carotene and vitamin A content, but should be watered down as it is also high in sugar, and can adversely affect blood sugar. Adding a teaspoon of vitamin C to juices makes them into a real preventive tonic.

Green Tea . . . The Chinese, who have low incidences of cancer, routinely drink this beverage instead of coffee. Green tea counters the effects of radiation, keeps the pH of the blood balanced and is high in antioxidants. The substances called polyphenolic catechins found in green tea are actually stronger than vitamin E in fighting free radicals.

Mushrooms . . . Several mushrooms have extraordinary healing properties. The maitake mushroom kills cancer cells by enhancing the activity of T-helper cells. Scientific studies report this food's effectiveness in controlling cancers of the breast, lung and prostate, and in minimizing the side effects of chemotherapy. Shiitake and reishi mushrooms, also called ganoderma mushrooms, exhibit anticancer properties as well, and are used by Asians to enhance longevity. Animal research done in Japan showed a highly significant rate of tumor elimination in animals fed extracts of maitake, shiitake and reishi mushrooms.

Enoki mushrooms are the long, thin mushrooms grown in an area of Japan known to have the lowest incidence of cancer in the country.

MGN-3 . . . MGN-3 is a polysaccharide composed of the hemicellulose-B extract of rice bran modified by enzymes from shiitake mushrooms. It has a unique ability to sustain immune alertness for a long time without becoming less responsive. Outside of natural killer cells, it activates T-cells and B-cells. When MGN-3 is combined with interleukin-2 (IL-2), IL-2 can continue to be given at the desired small dosage, otherwise it has hazardous side effects.

Macrobiotic Foods . . . Proponents of macrobiotic eating claim that cancer patients following this approach lead longer and better-quality lives. In several instances, patients deemed incurable have reported full recoveries. Success may be due to high levels of antioxidant nutrients and low amounts of fat. In fact, the total percentage of calories from fat in macrobiotic diets is approximately 10-12 percent, a 30 percent drop from the average American diet. Best results with the macrobiotic diet are seen with endocrine-related cancers, such as cancer of the breast, prostate, pancreas, uterus and ovaries. This is because, with these cancers, too many fat cells produce or synthesize estrogen and androgen hormones that contribute to the disease; reducing the amount of dietary fat lessens hormone production.

Seaweed . . . Chinese medicine recognizes the value of seaweed for treating cancers as it softens hardened tumors.

Antioxidant Supplements

The value of antioxidants, particularly beta-carotene; vitamins A, C and E; flavonoids; selenium; glutathione; superoxide dismutase; coenzyme Q10; and grape seeds cannot be overestimated in disease fighting and prevention. Antioxidants attack free radicals before they do irrevocable damage. Many clinical studies confirm their protective effects, while other research shows that antioxidants increase a patient's tolerance of chemotherapy and radiation.

Vitamin C . . . Vitamin C is the prime nutrient when it comes to overall support of the immune system. When fighting cancer, large quantities are required both orally and intravenously. Orally, bowel-tolerance levels are recommended: that is, one should take an amount that almost causes diarrhea. (Most people can tolerate up to 12 g daily of vitamin C, dividing this dose throughout the day.) But for best results, intravenous vitamin C drips are needed, as well. Research indicates that this method supplies the greatest healing effects because more of the vitamin can be easily tolerated. Patients are often given between 50 and 100 g of intravenous vitamin C, which is an excellent jump-start to any health protocol. This treatment relieves pain and nausea, often making painkilling drugs unnecessary. High doses of intravenous vitamins C and A are associated with long-term survival of a variety of cancers, even after they have metastasized.

Alpha-Lipoic Acid . . . This is a powerful antioxidant that scavenges the hydroxyl radical as well as other free radicals. It boosts glutathione, which combats the damaging cytokines and regenerates vitamins C and E and coenzyme Q10. The recommended dose is 250-500 mg a day. One can maximally take 500 mg three times a day.

Essential Fatty Acids (EFAs) . . . Omega-3 and omega-6 fatty acids block important causes of cancer. Omega-3-rich fish oil can suppress a cascade of dangerous cytokines, as well as the stress-induced pro-inflammatory cytokines IL-6 and IL-10. In addition, it reduces the risk of colon cancer. The suggested doses of the fatty acids are 1000 mg of perilla oil, which provides 550-620 mg of linoleic acid; 1000 mg of flaxseed oil, which is rich in omega-3-fatty acid, seven times a day; and 4 capsules of the formula MegaEPA (available from Life Extension), which contains 2800 mg of EPA/DHA. Cancer patients can take up to 8 to 12 capsules per day combined with 4 Mega GLA softgels.

Vitamin A . . . Vitamin A reduces infections and tumors, and is especially noteworthy for its ability to clear the lungs of smoke and other pollutants. Emulsified vitamin A comes from fish oil and is easy to digest. Vitamin A also comes from nonanimal sources, such as lemongrass, wheatgrass and carrots. Since vitamin A is fat-soluble and not excreted by the body, excessive intake can be dangerous. But huge quantities of vitamin A (about 100,000 IU taken daily for three years) are needed for this to happen. Four thousand to 7000 IU of vitamin A, from supplemental and food sources, are recommended daily—less if beta-carotene is taken.

Beta-Carotene . . . The liver converts beta-carotene to vitamin A as needed, making it a safe source of the vitamin, especially for women of childbearing years, as no fetal problems are associated with it. (Note: People with liver problems may be unable to convert beta-carotene into vitamin A.) In addition, beta-carotene itself stimulates T-helper cells, which prevent the development of cancer, and studies have, in fact, shown that the substance protects against lung and colon cancer. Fifty thousand international units taken daily may prevent cancer in cigarette smokers. For general purposes, 20,000 to 30,000 IU of beta-carotene is extremely helpful.

Carotenoids . . . With oncology, mixed carotenoids are important as free-radical scavengers. For instance, lycopene is associated with low risk of breast, prostate, digestive tract and colon cancers. There is an inverse relationship between beta-carotene and thyroid carcinoma. Beta-carotene also acted as a radio-protective agent in children exposed to radiation by the Chernobyl nuclear accident. Lutein offers protection against breast cancer in premenopausal women. Suggested doses are 9-20 mg of sulforaphane, 10-30 mg of lycopene and 15-40 mg of lutein, along with a mixed carotenoid blend containing alpha- and beta-carotene.

Flavonoids . . . Bright colors in fresh fruits and vegetables are usually indicative of flavonoids, phytochemicals (or plant chemicals) that are efficient free radical scavengers. Citrin, hesperidin, quercetin and rutin are names of some of these disease-fighting substances

Vitamin E . . . Much like vitamin C, vitamin E prevents cancer by preventing free radical damage, and activating immune system cells against tumors and infections. In clinical studies, 400 to 1200 IU daily have been shown to help patients with breast or cervical cancer. Vitamin E works especially well when taken in conjunction with 200 mcg of selenium.

Selenium . . . This trace element, which is involved in DNA metabolism and the health of all cell membranes, has antioxidant properties, promotes apoptosis, acts as an immunological response modifier and plays a part in cancer prevention and treatment. Supplementation of selenium can improve the quality of life during aggressive cancer therapies. The suggested dose is 200 mcg a day; the optimal dose could range from 200-400 mcg daily.

Silibinin . . . The major active constituent of milk thistle is a long-recognized antioxidant that has recently discovered anticarcinogenic qualities. Milk thistle is an adaptogenic herb. It produces repair where it's needed or shuts down cell production in tumor cells. Silibinin encourages differentiation in malignant cells, blocks the activity of COX-2 and, by cutting off the vascular network of the tumor, inhibits the growth of drug-resistant breast and ovarian cancer lines. For cancer patients, six capsules of Silibinin Plus (1950 mg a day) is the suggested dose. For protection, one to two capsules (325-650 mg daily) could be helpful.

Glutathione Peroxidase . . . Glutathione is found in every cell of our bodies, where it plays a major role in defending our systems. Studies show that low levels of glutathione increase the risk for cancer, AIDS and chronic fatigue syndrome. To stimulate glutathione production, L-glutathione and N-acetyl-cysteine (NAC, a precursor of glutathione) should be taken.

Superoxide Dismutase and Catalase . . . Much like glutathione, these antioxidants are frontline defenses against free radical damage, and are especially protective of the heart, brain, lungs, kidney and liver.

Coenzyme Q1O . . . Coenzyme Q10 works in conjunction with other enzymes in the body to optimize energy. Specifically, Q10 improves oxygen utilization, acts as a stimulus to the immune system and serves as an antioxidant.

According to studies, its concurrent use with the chemotherapeutic agent Adriamycin prevents the latter from harming the heart.

Grape Seed Extract . . . Grape seeds contain pycnogenol, a powerful disease fighting antioxidant. Pycnogenol, among its various age-retardant capabilities, slows cell mutation.

Dimethyl Sulfoxide (DMSO) . . . By suppressing TNF-alpha and NF-kB, DMSO blocks the production of damaging cytokines. The combination of shark cartilage, vitamin C and DMSO was reported to heal basal cell carcinoma.

Glutamine . . . Studies suggest that glutamine may decrease tumor progression. It also may stabilize weight loss by allowing better nutrient absorption. The recommended dose is 2 or more grams daily.

Insitol hexaphosphate (IP-6) . . . The combination of one of the B vitamins and phytic acid does not kill cancer cells, but it has cancer-fighting abilities that come from its skill at enhancing the body's defense mechanism. IP-6 is a sugar, like glucose, except it has six phosphates attached to its molecules. It activates natural killer cell production, and increases the effectiveness of the tumor suppressor gene p53. It encourages cancer cells to either normalize or kill themselves. The suggested dose is 1-3 g. In general, larger doses can be taken in powder form (one scoop twice a day is equal to 16 capsules, or 6.4 g).

Additional Supplements

DHEA . . . Although DHEA is naturally produced, we tend to produce less of this important hormone as we age. This decrease is connected to a number of degenerative conditions, including cancer. Taking DHEA has been shown to reverse many illnesses.

Melatonin . . . The pineal gland, located in the brain, produces this hormone, which is not only vital in regulating sleep cycles, as most of us have heard by now, but is immune-enhancing as well. As with DHEA, levels of melatonin decrease as we age, so supplementation can be helpful. Melatonin increases the activity of our T-helper cells, and aids our natural killer cells in getting rid of tumors. Supplements seem to extend the life, and the quality of life, of patients with inoperable brain tumors and metastatic gastric, colon and breast cancer, as well as advanced endocrine tumors.

Enzymes . . . Enzymes, which are catalysts for all life processes, are found in abundant supply in raw fruits and vegetables. Studies show that enzymes modulate inflammation, and that they may have a direct effect on controlling soft tissue cancers. Types of enzymes needed by cancer patients include trypsin, tyrotrypsin, pancreatin, bromelain (from pineapple), papain (from papaya), amylase and lipase. The bioflavonoid rutin may be of additional benefit when combined with these enzymes.

Conjugated Linoleic Acid (CLA)... This trace fatty acid is extracted primarily from dairy products. It enhances apoptosis (cancer cell destruction) and blocks the growth and metastatic spread of tumors. It suppresses arachidonic acid, which triggers inflammation. In combination with beta-carotene, CLA increases lymphocyte production and cytotoxicity. A relatively small dose (3-4 g) may prevent breast cancer. For cancer patients, a dose of 1000 mg of CLA six times a day is recommended.

Lactoferrin... Lactoferrin is a milk protein that displays antibiotic, anti-inflammatory and immune-modulating properties by acting against the bacterium Helicobacter pylori, which induces gastritis, ulcer and cancer. Lactoferrin inhibits the development of blood vessels to feed the tumor. It also binds iron and scavenges free radicals in fluids and inflamed areas. Lactoferrin is found in the milk of cows, humans, sheep and goats. It can be orally supplemented at a dosage of 300-900 mg a day.

Folic Acid... This vitamin is especially helpful for patients with a history of breast cancer, cervical dysplasia and smoking. For smokers, it cuts down on the adverse effects of nicotine on the lungs.

Modified Citrus Pectin (MCP)... This complex polysaccharide, obtained from the peel and pulp of citrus fruits, is able to bind tightly with galectins, thereby inhibiting tumor cells from clumping together. Due to these characteristics, MCP-3 can decrease metastasis. The typical adult dose of this soluble fiber is 6-30 g. No pattern of adverse reaction has been recorded.

N-Acetyl-Cysteine... N-acetyl-cysteine, or NAC, reduces free radical damage in the body and helps metabolize carcinogens. This immunity-enhancer also helps prevent bladder hemorrhage from cancer drugs.

Shark Cartilage... When tumors begin to form, they establish their own blood vessels. Shark cartilage contains anti-angiogenesis factor, a protein that inhibits the growth of these new blood vessels. As a result, small masses never enlarge and the immune system has an easier time destroying them.

Shark Liver Oil... Shark liver oil contains alkyl glycerols, substances that have antitumor effects. Studies show that when alkyl glycerols are given to women with uterine cancer prior to radium and X-ray therapy, the damage from these treatments is reduced.

Resveratrol... This compound is one of the phytoalexins that are produced in plants during times of environmental stress, such as insect, animal or pathogenic attack. Mulberries and the skins of red grapes are particularly rich in resveratrol. It is a very powerful antioxidant that provides greater protection against DNA damage than vitamins C or E, or beta-carotene.

Resveratrol also inhibits COX-2, due to its anti-inflammatory effect. It also blocks the formation of cancer. The cellular development called differentiation is the process in which abnormal cells become more normal when cancerous cells start to destruct; resveratrol has the ability to promote such destruction. By inhibiting angiogenesis, resveratrol reduces tumor volume, weight and metastasis. The suggested dose is 7-50 mg a day.

Bindweed . . . A common garden weed, it is 100 times more effective than shark cartilage at inhibiting angiogenesis.

Zinc . . . Zinc provides the body with a wide range of immune system functions. It supports the T and B cells in fighting infection and producing antibodies, and works to promote healing and reduce infection.

Chromium . . . This mineral acts like a hormone in the body in that it helps to regulate our blood sugar levels. When blood sugar is normalized, immune function, and hence, cancer resistance, is improved. This is why chromium supplements may be helpful in the prevention and treatment of cancer.

Genistein . . . Along with daidsein, genistein is a phytoestrogen from legumes that has antioxidant, anti-"bad"-estrogen and antitumor properties. The suggested dose for cancer patients is five 700-mg capsules four times a day of a soy extract that provides a minimum of 40 percent isoflavones. For prevention, 135 mg of 40 percent soy isoflavone extract once a day may be helpful.

Arginine . . . Positive studies show that L-arginine enhanced natural killer cell activity and lymphokine cytotoxicity in breast cancer. It also increased the levels of the white blood cells. At the same time, there are controversial views about nitric oxide, a molecule synthesized by arginine.

Herbs

Herbs can help the immune system in three ways. They can stimulate immune defense reactions, suppress immune overreaction and stimulate specific functions for short periods of time. The following herbs have multiple benefits, and are particularly noteworthy for their anticancer properties:

Aloe Vera . . . Aloe vera is antiseptic, antimicrobial and anti-inflammatory. It supplies the system with amino acids and minerals, such as calcium, copper, iron, phosphorus, potassium and zinc. Aloe vera contains live enzymes, including amylase, lactic dehydrogenase and lipase, as well as the essential fatty acids needed for optimum health. Its role in treating tumors, research shows, is due to its ability to stimulate phagocytic activity.

Astragalus . . . Although new to the West, astragalus is a time-honored Chinese remedy. In fact, Traditional Chinese Medicine medical literature from 4000 years ago says astragalus has the ability to strengthen resistance to disease. Modern scientific research confirms these claims, demonstrating that cells damaged by cancer and radiation are stimulated to full function with the introduction of this herb. Astragalus is considered a life energy or qi (pronounced "chee") tonic that strengthens vitality, and increases white blood cell and phagocytic activity. It is safe to take on a daily basis, making it an ideal preventive tonic.

Ginkgo Biloba . . . This antioxidant herb, long used by the Chinese, works to counter a substance in the body called platelet activation factor, or PAF, which may act to encourage tumor growth. By interfering with PAF, ginkgo may fight cancer.

Echinacea . . . When taken for short periods, echinacea revs up the immune system, stimulating the production and mobilization of white blood cells. It also stimulates cells in the lymphatic system, as well as important immune compounds, including interferon and tumor necrosis factor.

Garlic . . . There are numerous advantages to taking garlic, including anticancer benefits. Garlic makes cancer more recognizable to the immune system and interferes with the beginnings of tumor development. In addition, it stimulates immunity against formed tumor cells. The National Cancer Institute recognizes a connection between garlic, onions and related plants and a lower incidence of stomach cancer.

Ginger . . . Ginger will alleviate nausea associated with chemotherapy. It can be taken as a tea, or a small (½- to 1-inch) cube can be added to 10 ounces of juice.

Turmeric . . . Part of the ginger family and an ingredient in curry powder, turmeric—or its main active component, curcumiri—is a powerful antioxidant that seems to work against skin cancer. Curcumin inhibits COX-2 directly. It has also anti-inflammatory effects, and it is known that chronic inflammation is a cause of colon cancer. Curcumin also inhibits, and even reverses, oxidative damage, and it protects the DNA. To increase bioavailability, a small amount of piperine should be added. The normal dose is 900 mg daily, but cancer patients can take as much as four 900-mg capsules three times a day for a 6-to-12-month period. *Caution:* This should not be used in large quantities.

Ginseng . . . Studies associate the use of ginseng with lower incidences of all forms of cancer. It contains ingredients called saponins that encourage macrophage and natural killer cell activity.

Theanine . . . This is a component of green tea that is structurally similar to glutathione, and its presence confuses cancer cells. Glutathione acts by blocking the ability of cancer cells to neutralize cancer-killing agents, resulting in the death of the tumor cell. Theanine enhances the antitumor effect of Adriamycin (doxorubicin); the combination produced a 60-percent tumor reduction in animal studies. The suggested dose is 500-1000 mg theanine daily, taken with doxorubicin.

Lentinan . . . This extract of the shiitake mushroom acts as an immune modulator and can help reduce the side effects of chemotherapy. Peer-reviewed journals report that lentinan also helps colorectal, stomach and breast cancers.

Red Clover . . . Red clover checks free radical damage and protects DNA, which, in turn, helps to prevent mutations.

Essiac . . . Taken in tea form, Essiac is an herbal formula that has been used for years to fight cancer. Among its immune-enhancing ingredients are burdock, Indian rhubarb, sheep sorrel and slippery elm.

Hoxsey Herbs . . . Lymphoma and skin cancer have responded well to treatment with this herbal formula, which contains red clover, buckthorn bark, stillingia root, barberry bark, chaparral, licorice root, cascara amarga and prickly ash bark, along with potassium iodide.

Berberine-containing herbs . . . These herbs include goldenseal, barberry, goldthread and oregon grape. Berberine inhibits an enzyme prominently involved in the cancer process. It is a potent antitumor agent due to its apoptosis-enhancing effect. It is effective against bladder, colon, skin and brain cancer, and leukemia. The suggested dose of goldenseal is 250 mg three times a day.

Feverfew . . . This is an anti-inflammatory herb that inhibits the production of several potentially damaging cytokines. The suggested dose is 1 to 2 capsules a day that contain 600 mcg parthenolide.

Other anticancer herbs to consider include African cayenne, bilberry, bloodroot, comfrey, dandelion root, goldenseal, pau d'arco and suma. Goldenseal should be taken for short periods of time, and not taken during pregnancy.

Ozone

Not to be confused with atmospheric ozone, medical ozone is pure and concentrated, and has unique healing properties. Unfortunately medical use of this nontoxic molecule is legal in only a few of our states, although Europeans and Cubans have been benefiting from ozone treatments for years.

Ozone is used both prophylactically and as a treatment for a wide variety of diseases, including cancer. An antineoplastic substance (one that inhibits the growth of tumors), ozone stimulates the production of white blood cells and increases production of alpha interferon, interleuken-2 and tumor necrosis factor. It has also been found to enhance the action of various antitumor drugs.

According to the naturopathic physician Dr. Stanley Beyerle, prostate cancer patients often respond quite well to ozone treatment if the cancer is left encapsulated (that is, not biopsied). Other types of cancer that Beyerle has seen major improvements with, using ozone, are tonsillar, throat, ovarian, colon and breast cancer.

One mode of delivery of medical ozone is autohemotherapy in which a portion of the patient's blood is mixed, outside the body with a dose of ozone/oxygen, and then reintroduced into the circulation. Other methods used are rectal insufflation and drinking ozonated water.

Other Treatments

Individualized Vaccines ... When some of a patient's own cancer cells are combined in a laboratory with some of his or her white blood cells, it's now possible—experimentally and in certain cases—to create a personalized vaccine that works to stimulate the patient's immune system to destroy the cancer. Dramatic results have been seen in Europe with this new approach. The extent of its applicability still has to be determined.

Coley's Toxins ... This is another, older, vaccine approach to cancer. Dr. William Coley who practiced in the early part of this century found that certain inactivated bacteria could be given to patients to energize their immune systems against cancer. It was as if, by first fighting against the weaker opponent, the bacteria, the body built up its defenses and became more able to fight the cancer. Research has shown this treatment to be of significant value, although a perceived drawback is the fever that develops shortly after the vaccine is given. This, explains proponents of Coley's treatment, is actually a sign that the vaccine is working, and should not be suppressed.

714X ... Nitrogen-rich camphor and organic salts are used to make this substance, which is given to render the immune system more efficient in its battle against cancer cells. Results of 714X treatment, which usually consists of a series of injections into the lymph nodes of the groin, include tumor shrinkage, weight gain, a lessening of pain and extended survival time. People receiving this treatment are cautioned not to take vitamins E or B12 at the same time as 714X treatment, because they may counter its effects.

Interferon ... This natural protein, or lymphokine, is produced by our bodies in response to foreign substances.

Pancreatic Enzymes ... These are a type of proteolytic, or protein-degrading enzymes that are useful in digesting the protein coating of cancer cells. This is important because it's a necessary step before the cancer cells are destroyed by the body's immune cells. What's more, pancreatic enzymes can stimulate anti-cancer factors in the blood, i.e., natural killer cells, T-cells and tumor necrosis factor.

Hydrazine Sulfate ... This experimental treatment shows promise as it helps cancer patients regain lost weight. It seems to improve appetite and feelings of well-being, and may help to shrink tumors.

Thymus extract ... The thymus is responsible for a number of immune system functions, including the important production of T lymphocytes, which are a kind of white blood cell that is in charge of "cell-mediated immunity." This simply refers to the immune mechanisms not controlled by antibodies. Cell-mediated immunity is vital in warding off infection by specific bacteria, yeast (including *Candida albicans*), fungi, parasites and viruses (including herpes simplex, Epstein-Barr and the viruses that cause hepatitis). Furthermore, cell-mediated immunity is essential for strengthening the system so that it can fight against the development of cancer.

Ukrain . . . The plant celandine is combined with thiophosphoric acid to create ukrain, a substance used by so-called terminal cancer patients to block tumor growth and rev up their immune systems.

Indosin . . . Indosin, a nonsteroidal medication, acts to slow the growth of tumors.

Carnivora . . . A treatment for skin cancer, carnivora is a mixture of the juice of the Venus flytrap, alcohol and purified water. This preparation, applied topically, stimulates T-helper cells.

Iscador . . . This is a mistletoe derivative given by injection. Presently, it's not approved for sale in this country but it has been shown effective in the treatment of breast, cervical, bladder, bronchial, ovarian and skin cancers.

Vitamin K . . . A vitamin K analog, compound 5 (CPD 5), has shown great promise in treating primary liver cancer, which is resistant to chemotherapy. In vitro, it was also effective in combating melanoma and breast cancer. CPD 5 kills cancer cells by producing a fatal, excess amount of phosphate. The new vitamin K is not in clinical testing at this time. For updates, clients and physicians can call 800-237-4PCI or 412-624-1115. The suggested dose of vitamin K is 10 mg daily.

Larch Arabinogalactan . . . This is a substance derived from the Western larch tree. It's used in the form of a powder called Larix, or Ara-6, which stimulates immune cell activity and raises patients' energy levels.

Antineoplastin Therapy

A procedure developed by Dr. Burzynski uses antineoplastons, small peptine and amino acid derivatives fed to the body intravenously. His theory is that cancer occurs when the genes responsible for cell growth, including oncogenesor and tumor-suppressor genes, become dysfunctional. Antineoplastons help restore cellular control by reducing rampant cell division and enhancing the tumor-suppressor genes. This protocol is particularly successful in cases of non-Hodgkin's lymphoma, as well as in two brain cancers, glioblastoma multiforme and astrocytoma, all of which are very difficult to control by conventional therapy.

Radiofrequency Ablation (RFA)

According to researchers, this is a treatment that might replace surgery and radiation therapy. It uses high-frequency electric current to internally heat tumors. It is non-invasive, low risk and a relatively cheap protocol that has a high success rate in cases of bone, liver, kidney, prostate, breast and brain cancers. Doctors, using MRI, access the tumor through a needle puncture, then apply enough heat, generated through a titanium electrode, to kill the tumor cells. For information, contact the M. D. Anderson Cancer Center in Houston, Texas at 713-792-2121, or the University Hospitals of Cleveland in Ohio at 216-844-1000.

Psychological Factors

It's been theorized, as mentioned earlier, that people who tend to suppress anger are more prone to cancer than are others. While learning how to release emotions in a constructive way is important for everyone, those concerned with or confronted by cancer may want to pay particular attention to this issue. Part of what's involved here is addressing one's own personal needs, as opposed to living according to other people's expectations.

Also, for those being treated for cancer, creative imagery used in conjunction with standard counseling can be an important adjunct to physical treatments. Dr. Carl Simonton, medical director of the Simonton Cancer Center in California, and coauthor of *Getting Well Again* and *The Healing Journey*, has written extensively on this. Focusing on what is right with an individual and helping the person get in touch with goals, aspirations, creativity and purpose, provides a sense of connection and a will to live that enhances inherent healing mechanisms.

What to Avoid

Meat

Meat should be avoided, and this is especially true of meat from animals raised on factory farms, because these animals are given high levels of hormones. Estrogenic compounds are routinely injected into commercially raised animals to fatten them up. Once eaten, these hormones are stored in gonadal tissue, whether it be ovarian, testicular, or prostatic, where they overstimulate the body's own hormones, and lead to cancer. If you must eat meat, small quantities of meat from animals raised naturally is a safer alternative. Also, removing the fat from meat gets rid of some estrogen.

Dairy Products

Dairy products contain large amounts of estrogen. One reason Japanese women do not get breast cancer as frequently as American women do may be that milk is not a staple in the Japanese diet. Dairy products also contain the chlorine-based pollutant dioxin. A recent Environmental Protection Agency report on dioxin concludes that common levels of exposure may threaten human health by causing cancer, as well as fetal, immune-related and reproductive problems. Adverse reactions can occur at very low concentrations, and minute quantities found in food are implicated. Anywhere from 4 to 12 percent of a person's lifetime accumulation of dioxin could come from breastfeeding during the first year of life. The largest sources of human exposure are generally milk, animal fat, fish and eggs. Over the past few years, the banning of PCPs and 245T herbicide and other highly toxic compounds has resulted in a lowering of dioxin in the environment and in people's bodies.

Antibiotics

Antibiotics are not just overprescribed for us; they are routinely injected into livestock and thus become part of the food we eat. These drugs adversely affect the immune system by diminishing white blood cells needed to fight disease.

Pesticides

In the 1960s, science writer Rachel Carson alerted the world to the life-destroying properties of pesticides in her highly acclaimed book *Silent Spring*. Sadly, the world has not heeded her warning and is paying dearly for it. Recent studies associate indoor and outdoor pesticide use with sharp increases in childhood cancer, particularly soft tissue carcinoma, a cancer originating in bone and connective tissue. Common pesticide ingredients, such as chlordane, heptachlor, Diazinon and chlorpyrifos are also associated with lymphomas, brain tumors and non-Hodgkin's lymphoma.

Tobacco

Everyone knows that smoking is a prime cause of the most prevalent form of cancer, lung cancer. And more people are becoming alerted to the dangers of secondhand smoke. Studies now confirm that 17 percent of lung cancers occur in people exposed to secondhand smoke between the ages of three and fifty, but who have never smoked themselves. Cervical cancer is also associated with the inhalation of secondhand smoke. Chewing tobacco is not a good alternative to smoking; it can lead to mouth cancer.

Alcohol

While two to three alcoholic beverages weekly is considered moderate drinking in some circles, this amount has been associated with a fourfold increase in breast cancer. (One drink is considered 12 ounces of beer, four ounces of wine, or 1½ ounces of hard liquor.)

Radiation

X-rays should be taken only when absolutely necessary, as even low levels are implicated in cancer. In addition, radiation from overexposure to sunlight can cause skin cancer. A hole in the ozone is believed responsible for the increasing incidence of melanoma, and thus sunscreens, sunglasses and hats are wise precautions.

Electromagnetic Radiation (EMR)

According to studies, people living close to high-tension wires are more apt to develop leukemia and breast cancer than the general population. Low-level emissions of electromagnetic radiation from these wires over long periods of time are responsible. Electrical workers have an especially high incidence of leukemia.

In the home, EMR comes from various appliances, such as microwave ovens, electric blankets and digital clocks. It is therefore important to unplug these items before going to sleep if they face the bed, even when they are behind a wall.

Promiscuity

Women who engage in sexual intercourse before age sixteen, especially with uncircumcised partners, have higher than usual rates of cervical cancer. Penile cancer is the equivalent condition in promiscuous, uncircumcised men.

Hormone Replacement Therapy

This popular prescription is offered to postmenopausal women by medical professionals who commend it as a way of reducing osteoporosis and cardiovascular disease. What they fail to emphasize is the relationship between hormone replacement therapy and an increased risk of cancers of the breast and uterus.

Oral Contraceptives

Birth control pills deplete anticancer vitamins and minerals, and are associated with an increased incidence of breast cancer. If oral contraceptives are used, additional supplements are needed to make up for the losses.

Denatured Foods

Sugar, salt, processed foods, cured or smoked foods, fatty foods, hydrogenated oils, food additives, pickled foods, foods cured in salt and caffeine should be avoided. A high-protein diet, and foods high in cholesterol, are also linked to cancer.

Treatment Summary

Cancer is a complex phenomenon, necessitating attention to environment, nutrition, and body/mind considerations, rather than a search for a single cure.

A diet containing vegetarian, organic whole foods and lots of pure water provides valuable nutrients and keeps the bloodstream pure, both important factors in the prevention and treatment of cancer.

The anticancer diet contains alkaline foods, cruciferous vegetables, fiber, flaxseed oil, olive oil, green foods, green tea, fresh juices, seaweed and soybean products.

Antioxidant supplements prevent cells from becoming cancerous and can increase a patient's tolerance for chemotherapy and radiation; vitamins C and A are especially important as they are associated with long-term survival of cancer patients.

While many herbs stimulate appropriate immune response against cancer, astragalus is particularly powerful for that purpose and can be safely taken on a daily basis.

Ozone therapy inhibits the growth of tumors, stimulates the production of white blood cells and increases the production of natural cancer-fighting agents.

Creative imagery, in addition to standard counseling, can be an important adjunct to physical treatment.

See also: Breast Cancer, Cervical Dysplasia, Prostate Conditions, Skin Cancer, Treatments and Patient Experiences.

Candidiasis

Candidiasis is a disorder caused by an overgrowth of the yeast Candida albicans within the body. Given that yeast resides in the skin, mouth, genital tract and gastrointestinal tract, it can affect almost every organ. It is important to note that a certain level of candida yeast is a useful, natural part of the human system, helping to balance normal body function. However, when there is an abnormal increase in the amount of yeast, it can secrete a large volume of toxins into the body that may weaken the immune system.

Once this happens, a self-perpetuating cycle can develop. The longer the yeast is in the system, the weaker the immune system becomes. The weaker the immune system, the higher the tolerance it has to the yeast itself. This allows the yeast colonies to continue to propagate, releasing more toxins and further impairing the immune system. The result, as described by Dr. Marjorie Siebert of New York, is a variety of conditions at different levels of severity and discomfort, experienced by over 60 million Americans each year. Candidiasis occurs in both males and females, although it is more prevalent among females.

Causes

Oral antibiotics are a common cause of increased yeast production. While fighting harmful bacteria, they also kill off much of the normal bacteria in the system as well. Dr. Siebert submits that since yeast has a different biochemical structure than bacteria, it is not affected by the antibiotics. Therefore, when these medicines destroy bacteria, the yeast is left with more room to spread and food upon which to grow. This is a significant point because as the candida yeast may manifest itself in various conditions, antibiotics are often used for symptomatic relief of those conditions. The antibiotics then allow the candida to reproduce elsewhere, causing recurring infections and other maladies.

There are certain physical conditions that make it easier for candida to spread. Pregnancy and menopause create an environment in which estrogen levels vary greatly from the norm, and this may cause a higher rate of infection. And, in general, women are more susceptible at the end of each month's menstrual flow. Diabetes can also lead to increased risk for candidiasis. Other factors that weaken the immune system and create the perfect environment for candida overgrowth are stress, and a diet containing large amounts of sweets and processed foods. Oral contraceptives can further promote yeast growth.

Symptoms

Since candida can cause multiple systemic illnesses, a whole gamut of symptoms, ranging from the general to those affecting specific areas, are possible. These include low energy and fatigue, irritability, anxiety, fear, depression, "brain fog," memory loss, headaches, lightheadedness, muscle and joint pain (arthritis), sensitivity to chemicals, poor circulation, resulting in consistently cold hands and feet, urinary tract infections, rectal itching, white coating on the tongue or esophagus (thrush), heart palpitations and irregular pulse.

Symptoms that show up in the digestive tract include gas, bloating, periodic constipation and diarrhea, indigestion and intestinal cramps.

In the respiratory tract, problems caused by candida range from chronic postnasal drip and coughs to sore throats, colds and asthma.

The skin can be affected too, with eczema, itching, rashes, acne and fungal infections.

A variety of gynecological symptoms are possible with candida, the most common one being a vaginal yeast infection characterized by itching, redness, irritation and a cheesy white discharge.

Treatment

Rectifying immediate and local symptoms is relatively easy. There are many nonprescription corrective measures that can be used, including natural remedies. However, treating local infections does not address the root of the problem, and the overall condition really should be treated so that yeast-related maladies don't continue to occur.

Currently there is no test that can precisely determine whether a person has a yeast-related illness or not. However, some tests are considered helpful indicators. A stool study will show whether a person has an abnormally high amount of yeast, since the intestines are a petri dish for yeast growth. Along these lines, the Heidelberg test for gastrointestinal secretions is very effective. A skin test may also suggest a yeast-related allergy. When dealing with vaginal infections, an analysis of the discharge may help to ascertain the presence of a yeast infection.

However, since these tests are not completely accurate and will zero in only on a local infection, natural, nondrug remedies that are mild to the system can be tested to see if they alleviate a variety of symptoms.

Diet

A person's approach to food is important, for it can either inhibit or accelerate yeast-related problems. In using the diet to cope with candida overgrowth, a restricted diet should be followed for several weeks. Actually, this diet can be followed for an indefinite period of time. Foods can eventually be added back, but they should be added in a gradual, one-at-a-time manner. Doing so will enable you to determine a specific food's effect. If symptoms recur after a particular food is reintroduced, that food should be avoided. To test for food allergies, the ELISA-ACT test may be used as well.

The main thing to remember when following an anti-candida diet is to exclude sugar. The concept is to guard against the continued growth of yeast and to strengthen the immune system. Since sugar is a main food source for yeast and does not benefit the immune system, it has to be eliminated. However, don't just eliminate granulated sugar. Also be wary of honey, corn and maple syrup, fruit, maltose, artificial sweeteners, fructose, cornstarch, sodas and lactose (a milk sugar found in dairy products).

A second rule of thumb: Follow a yeast-free diet in order to avoid additional yeast-induced problems. You should eliminate fermented and yeast- and mold-containing products such as breads (muffins, cake, cookies and other refined carbohydrates); fruits (fruit juice and dried fruits); cheese; vinegar; pickled and smoked foods; alcohol; mushrooms; tomato sauce (unless fresh tomatoes are used); nuts; and any foods with monosodium glutamate (MSG) and hydrolyzed vegetable protein.

You should eat natural, healthy foods, including whole grains (brown rice, millet, amaranth, quinoa and barley); fresh vegetables; tofu; miso; plain yogurt; lean meats; fresh fish; and eggs from free-range hens. Organic extra virgin olive oil may also be effective in treating yeast problems.

Supplements

In addition to diet, natural supplements are effective in combating yeast-induced illnesses.

Special flora can be taken in order to build up the body's beneficial bacteria, which then decrease the yeast. These probiotics are lactobacillus acidophilus (in powder form or as part of sugar-free yogurt, it fights candida in the upper intestinal tract—150 ml of yogurt each day assists in recolonizing the friendly bacteria in the rectum or the vagina) and lactobacillus bifidum (restores the healthy bacteria in the lower intestines).

Antifungal, anti-yeast agents can be used to remove excess yeast from the body. Among these are citrus seed extract, Kyolic garlic, caprylic acid, berberine and biotin. Many people have found that combining odorless garlic concentrate, caprylic acid, biotin, acidophilus and fiber controls the growth of candida in the intestines.

Prescription remedies such as Nystatin may also be helpful.

The homeopathic candida extract, when injected directly into the body, thereby introducing yeast into the system, can help reverse damage to the immune system caused by yeast infection.

In cases of vaginal yeast infection, garlic suppositories have proven effective.

To improve overall health, multivitamin and mineral supplementation is highly recommended. This will increase immune function and deter continued yeast-related infections. The following specific supplements may also be tested to see if they are effective:

Essential Fatty Acids . . . The recommended dosage is 3000 mg of evening primrose, borage, or black currant seed oil daily, in three even doses, or one tablespoon of organic flaxseed oil. (Flaxseed oil should never be cooked and should be kept rcfrigerated.)

Vitamin C . . . The recommended dosage is 3000-15,000 mg daily, in three even portions, to fight infections. The intravenous administration of 50 g vitamin C one to three times a week could speed up recovery.

B Complex . . . Used to alleviate stress, the recommended dosage is 50-100 mg with each meal.

Chlorophyll . . . This can help by cleaning the intestines. Six 8-ounce glasses of vegetable juice are recommended.

Lactoferrin . . . A dosage of 300-600 mg daily of this subfraction of whey protein combats yeasts and certain intestinal parasites, such as C. albicans.

Herbs

Herbs can also be instrumental in inhibiting yeast, particularly in the digestive system. There are several that may prove helpful:

Garlic . . . One of thc star herbal performers, garlic is exceptional for warding off infections. It can be ingested raw, lightly cooked, or in capsule form.

Black Walnut Tincture . . . This can be added to water; the recommended dosage is 30 drops three times daily.

Shark Liver Oil . . . Five capsules of shark liver oil with 200 mg of alkyl glycerol help the body fight candidiasis by promoting healthy blood cell production. Shark liver oil is not recommended for people with too many blood platelets (thrombocytosis).

Oregon Grape and German Chamomille . . . These herbs, when made into teas, are beneficial to the immune system. Aloe vera, rosemary, ginger, alfalfa, red clover, goldenseal, barberry and fennel produce similar effects.

Goldenseal (Hydrastis Canadensis) . . . Outside of the tea form, it could be taken as an oral supplement. A dosage of 4 three times a day provides help against yeast overgrowth.

Digestive Harmony . . . This is an Oriental bitter-herb combination that works as an anti-yeast agent systemically.

Herbastatin . . . This gets rid of yeast caused by mucus.

Yudaiwan . . . A Chinese treatment, yudaiwan helps to eliminate cheesy vaginal discharges.

Ku Shen . . . This Oriental herb is used in a wash to cleanse the vagina.

Oregano oil . . . Taking one capsule on an empty stomach three times a day has antifungal effects.

Homeopathy

While homeopathic formulas are chosen according to the symptoms that manifest, they do more than just suppress particular symptoms; they arouse the body's own healing capacity. These particular formulas may activate recovery responses in individuals with candida:

Pulsatilla may be indicated where there is a thick, creamy yellow or green vaginal discharge. The woman feels weepy and craves sympathy.

Silica should be used when the vulva or vagina itch and are sensitive to touch, with a thin or curdly discharge.

Kreosotum is for severe symptoms. There are heavy discharges, profuse burning, a foul odor, violent itching, and a burning and swelling of the labia. Discharges may be yellow and watery.

Hepera sulph is used for symptoms that resemble those associated with silica, but they are more chronic. There is an itching of the vagina, especially after intercourse, and an odor similar to that of old cheese. Both hepera sulph and silica can be used to treat sores or cysts, especially Bartholin cysts.

Colon Therapy

According to colon therapist Tova Finman-Nahman of New York, colon therapy will help to produce clean internal surroundings and calm an irritated colon. Furthermore, in combination with colonics, psyllium can be taken orally. This moisturizes impacted stool in the colon, which further aids cleansing. Finman-Nahman suggests that a person may take as many colonics in a series as necessary in order to get candida under control.

Tea Tree Oil

Tea tree oil, an antifungal, anti-yeast and antiviral agent, can be used to treat vaginal yeast infections. One tablespoon of the oil mixed with a pint of water and used as a douche will help to abolish yeast infections. This can be followed with the insertion of acidophilus tablets or capsules into the vagina to reestablish appropriate vaginal bacteria.

As a topical treatment, tea tree oil can be used successfully against dermatological candida.

Everyday Habits

Incorporating good habits into one's daily routine is an important way of guarding against yeast infections. Overall, stress needs to be minimized, since it can lead to impairment of the immune system. Other particular lifestyle strategies that work specifically to decrease the incidence of vaginal yeast infections, are as follows: Allow air to circulate in the genital area by wearing cotton crotch underwear and avoiding pantyhose and tight clothing; keep anal bacteria from entering the vagina by wiping from front to back; and avoid "feminine hygiene" sprays and powders which can cause irritation. Also, you should understand that douching is not necessary, as a healthy vagina is naturally clean.

Treatment Summary

Diet either inhibits or accelerates yeast-related problems. Three dietary anti-yeast strategies are: excluding sugar, eliminating fermented or yeast- and mold-containing products and eating only natural, health-giving foods.

Supplements can either specifically target yeast-induced illnesses or help sustain balanced overall nutrition. The following are recommended: appropriate flora, antifungal and anti-yeast agents, multivitamin/mineral supplements and chlorophyll.

Herbs that aid in expelling yeast from the system include garlic, black walnut tincture, aloe vera, rosemary ginger, alfalfa, red clover, goldenseal, barberry fennel, the formula Digestive Harmony, Herbastatin, Yudaiwan and Ku shen.

Homeopathic remedies that may activate a healing response in individuals with candidiasis include pulsatilla, silica, kreosotum and hepera sulph. Also, homeopathic candida extract is sometimes used.

Colon therapy can aid in getting candida under control.

Tea tree oil can be used to eliminate vaginal yeast infections. Also effective are garlic suppositories.

Habits to develop to guard against yeast infections are: minimize stress, wear clothes that allow air to circulate in the genital area, employ good bathroom hygiene and avoid products that produce irritation.

Carpal Tunnel Syndrome

Repetitive trauma disorders, of which carpal tunnel syndrome is one, constitute the most frequent type of work-related illness in the U.S. today. Carpal tunnel syndrome (CTS) stems from pressure to the middle nerve in the channel in the wrist that houses nerves and tendons. It can occur after many years of work involving repetitive use of the hands, as on a computer keyboard, or it can occur more suddenly, after a blow or swelling. CTS can also be brought on by rheumatoid arthritis, and sometimes the fluid retention of pregnancy is a contributory factor.

The syndrome is characterized by pain in the wrist and hand, especially when the thumb is bent toward the palm. Sensations include a burning, tingling, or aching that may spread to the forearm and shoulder. Pain may be persistent or intermittent, and is frequently experienced at night. When the condition is severe, the muscles of the hand stop functioning, and may waste away.

Treatment

Orthodox medical treatment for CTS includes wrist splints and surgery. But there are other approaches that can be tried. One is pressure point therapy, a self-administered treatment that has the advantages of being safe and easy to learn. Surprisingly, most of the pressure points for treating carpal tunnel syndrome are not in the hand or wrist itself, but by the elbow.

Try this: Place the index finger two inches below the crease of the elbow. Press this spot for 10 to 15 seconds. If carpal tunnel syndrome is present, this spot will feel quite tender at first, but relaxed at the end of the treatment.

In mild or moderate cases, transcutaneous electrical nerve stimulation (TENS) could be a solution. During the procedure, an acupuncturist points a red-beam laser light pen to the acupuncture points of the forearm and the shoulder area of the patient. That might reduce inflammation and provoke healing of the painful area.

Reconstructive therapy is another approach that syndrome patients have had success with. Performed by osteopathic physicians, who specialize in musculoskeletal disorders, this therapy involves injection of saline solution into muscle/ligament groups to stimulate the formation of new blood vessels. With new blood vessel formation in the ligaments, a variety of nutrients, vitamins and growth factors that enhance tissue repair and growth can be delivered.

Studies indicate that the swelling of the synovium, the connective-tissue membrane necessary for the movement of the wrist, is associated with a vitamin-B6 deficiency. B6 acts as a diuretic, helping the body to get rid of unnecessary fluid. Supplementation of 50-200 mg of vitamin B6 could ease symptoms with the support of other nutrients, such as one capsule of gamma E tocopherol (a fat-soluble form of vitamin E) that helps expel peroxynitrate, a toxic chemical inflammation product. Other antioxidants, such as 2000 mg of vitamin C and 10,000-25,000 IU of vitamin A can balance out the free-radical damage. Taking 400 IU of vitamin D and 200 mcg of selenium can enhance the healing effect.

Essential fatty acids are also important in lowering the possibility of blood clot forming, which encourages swelling of tissues. Docosahexaenoic (DHA), gamma linoleic acid (GLA), alpha linoleic acid, (ALA) and the omega-3 fatty acid EPA are powerful anti-inflammatories and should be part of the diet of CTS patients. Curcumin from turmeric reduces inflammation, as do boswella and ginger. The following protein-digesting enzymes have the same effect: protease, bromelain, trypsin, lipase, pancreatin and papain. These enzymes could be supplemented from two Super Digestive Enzymes capsules before each meal and ⅛-¼ tsp of bromelain or papain powder before eating. Taking 500 mg of elemental magnesium is important for arterial health. Phosphatidylserine (PS) enhances neurotransmitter function; the suggested dose is 100 mg daily. To decrease pain, try 1500-3000 mg of D and L-phenylaline, an endorphin-level booster that could be helpful.

Another way to increase endorphin and serotonin levels in order to achieve better pain tolerance is to use cranial electrical stimulation (CES). One CES device is Liss Body Stimulator, a Walkman-size machine designed for home use that also helps to electroporate the anti-inflammatory nutrients to the swollen area.

Prevention

The best way to combat carpal tunnel syndrome and other repetitive strain injuries is not to get them in the first place. Susan Fulton is a New York City journalist who sustained computer-related injuries and went on to develop prevention training. She delineates four physical factors in the workplace that can contribute to the development of CTS: repetitive activity, awkward positions, static posture and excessive force. Her recommendations include taking breaks from repetitive work and varying your tasks. For instance, phone calls can be an opportunity to move away from the computer. Or try computer "take-a-break" software programs.

Rearrange your work area and furniture with an eye to minimizing sharp angles in your joints that will pinch and irritate internal tissue. Ask yourself these questions about your desk posture: Are my hands angled up from my wrists when I type? If so, try raising yourself or lowering the key surface. Am I bunching my shoulders down because the table's too low? Make appropriate adjustments. Am I pinching the phone handset between ear and shoulder? Use a headset. Am I pushing my head forward to see the monitor? Move it closer and lower it. Am I reaching for a phone that's too far away, stressing my shoulder? Move the phone closer.

A good idea to keep in mind during the workday is to stretch and move around as much as possible. Fulton notes that sitting in one position actually takes work in that your muscles have to hold you in place. They get tight and less supple in the process.

Using less force in your work is a concept that might not come to mind if you're an office worker. But try holding the pencil less tightly. At the computer, don't squeeze the mouse and pound the keys.

Treatment Summary

Pressure point therapy that can be self-administered, can alleviate carpal tunnel symptoms.

Reconstructive therapy, administered by osteopathic physicians, stimulates new blood vessel growth, so that healing nutrients can reach the area.

Prevention of repetitive strain injuries starts with understanding the ergonomic risk factors: repetitive activity, awkward positions, static posture and excessive force.

To protect yourself from CTS and related problems, rearrange your workspace, vary tasks and take breaks, stretch and move when possible and monitor your work habits for excess muscle tension.

Cerebral Palsy

Cerebral palsy is a broad term used to describe brain-related motor problems. Injury to the cerebrum, occurring at birth or soon afterwards, results in a muscle/nerve dysfunction that is manifested as a lifelong paralysis of one or more parts of the body.

Causes

Usually cerebral palsy is associated with a lack of oxygen during birth, a premature birth, or low birth weight. Low birth weight is related to premature delivery; for this reason, mothers who experience early contractions may be placed on medications to prolong their pregnancy. In recent years, it has been shown that low birth weight may be related to the expectant mother smoking or taking drugs. There is an especially high risk of cerebral palsy in babies of drug-addicted mothers.

Symptoms

Symptoms range in severity, from a mild paralysis of the extremities on one side of the body to an extreme loss of muscle control, speech and vision. Hearing disorders and mental retardation can occur as well. Signs of abnormal breathing, sucking and swallowing may be noticeable at birth or soon afterwards, although they are sometimes overlooked for several months. Later, the child's gross and fine motor development will be spastic and slow to develop. Delayed walking and acquisition of bowel and bladder habits may be present, as well as overly strong reflexes, slurred speech and slow movements of the face.

Treatment

Successful treatment depends on when the diagnosis is made and on the severity of the disorder. The earlier the problem is identified and treated, the greater the effect of the treatment. Orthodox treatment programs may consist of exercise, braces, corrective surgery and drugs that relax muscles and prevent seizures. As a result of therapy, many patients lead independent lives; those severely affected often improve to the point of being able to learn activities of daily living.

One of the most promising directions of treatment is stem cell research. Stem cell research has targeted three different ways to repair the injured brain: replace the damaged or dead cells, or correct the injured axons (brain cell processes), both to enhance the transmission of the nerve cell impulses; or instruct the brain to develop new pathways, to take over the function of the injured cells. All three use embryonic, or stem, cells injected either to the vascular system or directly to the brain. Stem cells are capable of multiplying and differentiating in the brain; the question is how much they can integrate and improve function. Animal studies and clinical experiments show temporary success, and although stem cell research is still in progress, it is suggested that in the near future brain injury will be repaired or the brain restructured, and patients with cerebral palsy could recover from damages.

The administration of a combination of amino acids is a procedure developed by Alexander Khokhlov, a Russian professor. It has a stimulating effect on nerve cell function, resulting in improved motor function.

Another way to repair brain damage is to give oxygen to patients under elevated atmospheric pressure in a hyperbaric oxygen chamber. The treatment, called hyperbaric oxygen treatment, makes oxygen available to help rebuild capillaries and stop plasma leakage and swelling, so that the normal blood flow is restored and cell electrical activity works well again.

To improve oxygen-carrying capacity, stimulate assimilation of nutrients and speed up waste removal, magnetic molecular energizing (MME) treatment is a great choice. It offers a new model of healing. The magnet delivers 3000-5000 gauss pulses (it is best to sleep overnight under the magnet), and it shows improvement after around 200 hours of treatment. It enhances the effects of stem cell therapy.

Pulsed electromagnetic therapy uses intermittent bursts of safe magnetic waves to stimulate the development of nerve cells.

To release muscle contraction and trigger muscle growth, threshold electrical stimulation uses stimulation by electrodes applied to the skin of the atrophied muscle.

To relax contracted muscles, good therapies include a deep tissue massage called Rolfing, foot massage and reflexology. Acupuncture is therapeutic for cerebral palsy patients, restoring the flow of the energy, called the qi. Stimulation of the paralyzed body parts sends stimulating signals back to the damaged areas in the brain.

To improve flexibility and ease of movement the Alexander technique is an effective method that enables patients to relearn patterns they naturally followed as children, but have since lost. By reacquiring their old patterns, the patients become more in line with their center of gravity. Yoga stretches and helps to realign the spine. Therapeutic horseback riding improves balance and coordination. Combination therapies deal with different aspects of the disease. Recreational therapy uses deep breathing, concentration, sports, dramatics, arts and crafts and games to reduce stress, connect physical activities to spirituality and play out a wide range of emotions. Conductive education helps children with cerebral palsy to become more independent by teaching them how to conduct basic activities, such as eating and dressing; develop skills in basic and fine manipulation, such as grasping and releasing; and keep a relaxed position for a longer period of time. Dolphin-assisted therapy involves doing motivational recreational activities with dolphins, and constrained-induced movement therapy retrains the injured brain in cases of partial paralysis to use the affected limb by using the unaffected limb. Biofeedback helps reprogramming by allowing the person to visually see the signal of the movement produced in the brain. Brain gym involves exercises that set up new connections between the mind and the body.

The so-called Ilizarov technique works on lengthening the limbs and reprogramming hip movements using two rings that encircle the arm and leg, and that have wires attaching them together.

The device called the Spider, uses a unique suspension system of elastic cords, enabling the patient to do voluntary controlled movements with greater precision.

Selective dorsal rhizotomy is a procedure that cuts some of the sensory nerve fibers connecting the muscles and the spinal cord to create more balanced activity of the nerve cells in the spinal cord and thus reduce spasticity.

In addition to conventional treatment, herbs can help the patient with cerebral palsy. Many herbal teas nourish the muscles and nerves with valuable minerals and enzymes. When highly diluted, they are gentle enough for infants and children. Some herbs act as antioxidants; they help fight the free radicals that are prevalent in this condition. These herbs include rosemary, ginkgo biloba and ginger. In addition to being an antioxidant, ginger improves circulation to the extremities. Other herbs to consider are yellow duck, watercress and milk thistle. It is important to work with a knowledgeable health practitioner, especially when treating children.

What to Avoid

Expectant mothers should stay away from drugs and cigarettes. They should also be careful to avoid exposure to pesticides, as the chemicals breathed in enter the placenta, where they can harm the muscles and nerves of the developing fetus.

Cervical Dysplasia

Cervical dysplasia is an abnormal growth of cervical tissue. It is caused by the sexually transmitted human papilloma virus (HPV), the same virus responsible for cervicitis, genital warts and cervical cancer. These conditions are detected with a Pap smear.

The conventional medical approach typically does nothing for mild dysplasia and genital warts. The attitude is usually one of "Let's see if the body takes care of itself." In the later stages, the preferred conventional treatment uses an electrical wire to cut out abnormal tissue. In advanced disease states, a hysterectomy may be the only way to save a woman's life.

But much can be done to avoid cervical problems. Prevention is always the best policy and it is particularly so with this condition. Women should understand that cervical dysplasia, genital warts and cervical cancer are sexually transmitted diseases that can be eliminated with safe sex, and improved by healthy lifestyle. Also, if you take birth control pills, it is advisable to take folic acid and vitamin C. Be sure to have a yearly Pap smear to detect the condition early. Statistics show that the longer a woman waits between Pap smears, the higher her chances of getting cervical dysplasia and cervical cancer.

Diagnosis

Before treatment, it is essential to get fully diagnosed to determine the stage of the illness. If a woman has an abnormal Pap smear, her partner needs to be examined by a urologist for warty tissue. Otherwise, they will be passing the virus back and forth and reinfecting each other. Diagnosis by a licensed, well-trained, alternative practitioner will determine if a woman is a candidate for natural treatments only or whether she needs to integrate these approaches with conventional methods.

Naturopathic Treatments

Women with cervical dysplasia often have excellent results using naturo-pathic approaches. Dr. Tori Hudson of Portland, Oregon, notes, "In the re-sults of a research study that I conducted at the College of Naturopathic Medicine, we had 43 cases of all degrees of cervical dysplasia. Through my treatment protocol, 38 of the 43 reverted to normal, three partially improved, and two had no change, meaning they didn't get better and they didn't get worse." Dr. Hudson's protocol consists of three types of treatment: systemic, local and constitutional. An overview of her therapy is outlined below:

Systematic Treatment

Beta-Carotene . . . It is the precursor of Vitamin A. The recommended dosage is 25,000 IU daily.

Vitamin C . . . Low levels of vitamin C are linked with cervical dysplasia. A dosage of 2000-6000 mg daily could prevent or reverse the disease.

Vitamin A . . . The recommended daily dosage is 5000-25,000 IU daily.

Vitamin B6 and Vitamin E . . . Oral contraceptives deplete vitamin B6 and vitamin E. Therefore, the recommended dosage for women taking contracep-tives is 50-250 mg of vitamin B6 daily and 400-800 IU of vitamin E daily. These vitamins should be taken at different times because B6 neutralizes the effect of vitamin E in certain situations.

Indole-3-Carbinol (I3C) . . . This anticancer agent found in cruciferous vege-tables can prevent or inhibit the development of cancer in the cervix. The rec-ommended dosage is 200 mg two to three times a day.

Folic Acid . . . A daily dosage of 800-2000 mcg can help to keep or restore the health of the cervical tissue when taken along with 10-30 mg of lycopene. Alpha-carotene could also be added.

Selenium . . . Taking 200-400 mcg of selenium can be part of cancer pre-vention.

Zinc . . . Taking 15-50 mg of zinc a day enhances immune functions.

One scoop of whey protein also has immune-boosting effects. It helps to build lean body mass by increasing the body's production of muscle protein. In addition, it appears to inhibit the proliferation of cancer cells and provide protection against free radical damage while enhancing the immune system.

Local Treatment

Vitamin A Suppositories . . . Treatment with topical vitamin A in the form of retinoids has been examined and determined to have positive results for both cervical dysplasia and cervical cancers (Graham et al. 1986; Weiner et al.

1986; Meyskens et al. 1994; Ruidi et al. 1997). A number of the studies were performed using topical vitamin A treatment via vaginal suppository inserts. In these studies the vitamin A was applied directly to the cervical tissue with a cervical cap and sponge (Graham et al. 1986; Weiner et al. 1986; Meyskens et al. 1994) or a vaginal suppository (Ruidi et al. 1997). It was concluded that when using a cervical cap and sponge the successful and complete response rate was about 50 percent in subjects who had mild to moderate forms of cervical dysplasia.

Herbal Suppositories . . . Naturopathic doctors have been using a varied approach to treating cervical dysplasia and getting impressive results. One such treatment involves the application of specific herbs, enzymes and herbal suppositories for six weeks. Specific nutrients that have demonstrated their ability to assist the cervical cells in returning to their normal structure are recommended.

Constitutional Treatment

Dietary Changes . . . Many nutritional factors are linked to the development of the disease. While many nutrients by themselves may be crucial in warding off cervical dysplasia (for example, beta-carotene and vitamin A, folic acid vitamin B6 and vitamin C), one must understand that 67 percent of those with the disease have nutritional deficiencies.

Use of Condoms . . . Condoms should be used during sexual intercourse to avoid unprotected contact with a partner who has genital warts.

Avoidance of Smoking . . . Women should avoid smoking, which is the most important co-factor in developing cervical dysplasia.

A diet that optimizes immunity is low in fat and high in whole grains, vegetables and fruits. Immune-system inhibitors such as coffee, sugar, alcohol and fat are omitted.

At the end of three months of treatment, it is very important to follow up with a health practitioner, and to obtain another Pap smear. Sometimes a biopsy is also needed.

Cervical dysplasia means that abnormal cell growth on the cervix exists. It is generally a precancerous condition.

Women who have low vitamin C levels are seven times more likely to develop cervical cancer than women with adequate levels of vitamin C.

What to Avoid

Cervical dysplasia increases with sexual activity at an early age; women who have intercourse at a young age are more vulnerable because of the nature of the cervical cells at that time. Smoking is another factor in acquiring cervical dysplasia. If you smoke and are exposed to the virus, you are more likely to develop dysplasia and cervical cancer. Nicotine actually lodges in the tissue of the cervix. Then, when exposed to the virus, the DNA can become abnormal. Smoking may also cause genital warts to be cancerous.

Treatment Summary

Preventive measures include safe sex, regular Pap smears and a healthy life style, with no smoking. Also, if you take oral contraceptives, you should take folic acid and vitamin C.

A multifaceted naturopathic approach will often reverse cervical dysplasia.

Chronic Fatigue Syndrome

Everyone experiences fatigue time to time, but when exhaustion perseveres for extended periods, it's called chronic fatigue syndrome (CFS). During recent years chronic fatigue has become an increasingly prevalent condition, although conservative elements of the medical establishment continue to question its legitimacy as a distinct syndrome. In fact, federal health agencies, which are appropriated large sums of money to study and treat emerging infectious diseases, have virtually ignored this burgeoning problem.

The condition first became prevalent during the 1980s, when clusters of CFS cases were reported in various parts of the country. In 1988, the Centers for Disease Control finally acknowledged the existence of the condition, designating the term "chronic fatigue syndrome" to describe a constant state of exhaustion. Since then, conservative estimates have put the number of Americans affected at 2 million. A study performed at Harvard University concluded that 3 out of every 1000 people in the U.S. suffer from the syndrome.

Although it is not a fatal disease, chronic fatigue syndrome can be devastating to those who live with it. Most CFS sufferers are young, previously, seemingly, healthy individuals. (While chronic fatigue affects a broad spectrum of people without regard to age, national origin and sex, recent studies have indicated that a significant percentage of sufferers are in their midthirties, while the ratio of women to men who are affected is approximately two to one.) Since symptoms of the syndrome tend to be more felt than visible, CFS can be quite frustrating for people experiencing it, who have to convince family members, friends, employers and doctors that the problem truly exists.

The U.S. is not alone in facing this health problem, as nations throughout the world have reported increased incidence of the condition during the past few years. In Japan, the condition is labeled low natural killer syndrome, or LNKS, while in Great Britain chronic fatigue has been dubbed myalgic encephalomyelitis. Chronic fatigue has become common in several other countries, including Canada, Australia and Holland, where a variety of support groups have been established to help people cope with the condition.

Causes

Research has correlated the onset of chronic fatigue to a breakdown in the immune system that permits viral or bacterial infections—such as Epstein-Barr, herpes, cytomegalovirus, mycoplasma, or candida—to become stronger in the body. When immune system function falters, the body is left susceptible to previously present but previously non-threatening organisms, and to overgrowth of friendly organisms. Chronic muscle dysfunction can be involved; fibromyalgia, which sometimes accompanies chronic fatigue syndrome, is a painful musculoskeletal disease characterized by the thickening and tightening of muscle fibers.

In the majority of cases, chronic fatigue isn't something that hits a person out of the blue, but is, rather, the result of years of bodily assault in the form of poor health habits. During those years the person probably suffered from general fatigue a good deal of the time, but he or she may have considered that normal, as many high-powered, ever-on-the-go Americans do. Years of chronic stress, with its concomitant adrenal overload, often precede the onset of CFS. A person may go along for decades never really relaxing, gulping down coffee and sugary snacks, smoking cigarettes, eating fatty and processed foods, taking excessive antibiotics and indulging in other unhealthy habits, without thinking that he or she is paying much of a price beyond a low energy level. Weakened immunity may not show up at this point. But then a major stress introduced into the person's life can tip the balance in favor of previously dormant viruses within the body. The result—chronic fatigue, which may seem like it struck from out of nowhere but was actually the result of a way of life. This is not to blame the victim, but to say that there are often complex underlying cofactors, besides microorganisms, involved in this condition.

An occupational group that has a high level of chronic fatigue syndrome is flight attendants. People with this job constantly have their systems assaulted. Their workplace is one of contained and contaminated air, pressure changes, atmospheric radiation and high stress, not to mention less than ideal food. It's no wonder that flight attendants tend to age prematurely and to experience CFS more than the general population does.

Some scientists have attributed the onset of chronic fatigue to the administration of vaccinations. Several members of the scientific community have reinforced this argument against vaccinations by establishing a correlation between Gulf War syndrome, which is predominantly characterized by chronic fatigue, and the vaccination program carried out by the military during the Persian Gulf War. Although the federal government denies this, doctors have implicated the administration of multiple inoculations as a partial cause of Gulf War syndrome, asserting that it was responsible for immune system debilitation in numerous servicemen and women. Also, chemical and biological warfare agents—some newly engineered—that our Gulf War troops came in contact with, as well as highly toxic pollutants, such as those from burning oil wells, made our Gulf service people prime candidates for CFS.

General Fatigue

When a person initially experiences fatigue it is important to identify the cause, as most cases of exhaustion are brought on by factors other than viral infections. Viral-induced fatigue is usually accompanied by an assortment of other typical viral symptoms, while with general fatigue these additional symptoms are absent. General fatigue is frequently prompted by exposure to excessive stress, or by sleeping disorders. Insomnia, often worsened by stress, can have a serious effect on the body that is deprived of proper rest time and will inevitably experience fatigue. Sleep disorders can be quite frustrating and debilitating for their victims. Therefore, it is important to control them before they take their toll on the body.

General fatigue is often caused by poor dietary habits, which can include a lack of calories. And although most Americans tend to consume a more than adequate supply of calories, often these calories lack nutritional value. Studies have revealed that people who have an excessive intake of sugar and other simple carbohydrates, eating, for instance, a lot of pastries and white bread, will usually experience some degree of fatigue. A typical pattern is fatigue that hits in the mid-to-late morning, after a short-lived caffeine-and-donut-induced energy surge has dropped away, then again right after a heavier than necessary lunch and then again in the late afternoon or early evening. A poor diet often prompts the onset of hypoglycemia, a condition characterized by a disturbance of blood sugar patterns and insulin production. And hypoglycemia frequently induces fatigue subsequent to mealtime, when the oversecretion of insulin adversely affects the central nervous system.

Another common cause of fatigue is hypothyroidism, or low thyroid function. Hypothyroidism, which can also cause constipation, weight gain, dry skin and menstrual irregularities, can cause fatigue even when it's of marginal severity. Unfortunately, doctors often fail to diagnose it and consequently mistakenly attribute the patient's fatigue to other factors, such as depression or poor dietary habits.

A significant cause of general fatigue is caffeine withdrawal. Since millions of Americans have caffeine addictions, caffeine-related fatigue is a common problem. When a person accustomed to large quantities of caffeine suddenly limits his or her intake, the result will be fatigue, probably accompanied by a headache. Eliminating dependence upon coffee and other caffeinated products is crucial to maintaining health and avoiding debilitating bouts with fatigue.

Symptoms of Chronic Fatigue Syndrome

Ordinary fatigue comes and goes, and people can function with it. But the predominant symptom of chronic fatigue syndrome is an overwhelming, unrelenting exhaustion. The severity of chronic fatigue is unrivaled by the usual amount of exhaustion that a person has after hard work or athletic competition. Victims of chronic fatigue frequently experience difficulty when trying to get up from a prone position. Sometimes they have no desire to rise, and they remain in bed for a prolonged period. Unfortunately, chronic fatigue tends to plague its victims for years. It can completely alter an active person's daily routine. Sometimes, the onset of CFS occurs suddenly; in other cases, it sneaks up gradually.

In addition to a debilitating fatigue, an abundance of secondary symptoms are associated with CFS. The early stages of the syndrome are frequently characterized by acute flu-like symptoms. Depression, irritability, headaches, low-grade fever, sharp muscle pain and weakness can develop later into fibromyalgia, swollen glands, sore throat and diarrhea. In addition, chronic fatigue is often accompanied by cognitive impairment, consisting of memory loss, confusion and difficulty concentrating. Sometimes the patient will be unable to recall the simplest details of everyday life, such as his or her name or why he/she went into another room.

Another common attribute of CFS patients is an inability to cope with emotional and physical stress. Sleep disturbances are also quite prevalent among chronic fatigue patients; many people feel as if their energy level is not being replenished overnight. Often, the person will be unable to fall asleep, while at other times he or she will be frequently interrupted by nightmares. Additional symptoms commonly associated with CFS are numbness or tingling sensations, moodiness, ringing in the ears, rashes, impotence, susceptibility to candida and viral infections such as herpes.

Treatment

Prior to initiating a holistic treatment regimen, it is important for a doctor to examine the chronic fatigue sufferer in order to assess the severity of the situation and to determine possible causes. Often patients will undergo a variety of tests designed to ascertain the presence of any food allergies that may have fostered the debilitation, or the existence of a thyroid, pituitary or adrenal dysfunction.

Diet

People suffering from chronic fatigue, and from less severe fatigue as well, should incorporate an abundance of complex carbohydrates into their diets.

These are used slowly by the digestive system, and consequently provide a good, steady source of energy for the body to use. Whole grains, as well as vegetables, nuts and seeds, are good sources of complex carbohydrates.

In addition, juices, especially juices containing dark vegetables, such as collards and dandelion, are essential for the chronic fatigue victim because they provide an ample supply of immune system–boosting enzymes. These green, chlorophyll-rich juices should be taken liberally, six 10-ounce glasses per day are not too much. Aloe vera can be a valuable component of these juices, as well as celery, cucumber and lemon. Purification and stimulation of the spleen and lymphatic system can be enhanced by consuming fresh dandelions, sprouts, asparagus, mustard greens, radishes and cruciferous vegetables—such as broccoli and cauliflower. Sea vegetables—including kombu, wakame, hijiki, arame and dulse—are beneficial for the maintenance of bone marrow and the thymus gland.

People with CFS should incorporate high-quality protein derived from vegetarian sources into their diets. Some good examples of vegetarian sources of protein include tofu, tempeh, fortified soy milk and legumes. Since fish contain a rich supply of omega-3 fatty acids, small quantities of fresh fish may also be advantageous, but be sure that the fish that you consume are obtained from an unpolluted source and are not submerged into chlorine during preparation. If you eat animal protein, consumption of this type of food should not exceed eight ounces daily. Also, keep in mind that since many animals raised in factory farm conditions are exposed to harmful hormones and pesticides, organic supplies of animal protein are recommended.

There is an immune-enhancing soup created by the Chinese that can help weakened individuals regain energy. The recipe consists of a mixture of a whole astragalus root with onions, garlic, ginger and either organic poultry, fish, tofu or tempeh. Brown rice and fresh green vegetables can also be added. After the soup reaches the boiling point, it should be allowed to simmer. Finally, miso is added to further boost nutrition and enhance flavor.

Drinking a sufficient amount of purified water can help proper maintenance of the immune system along. During the colder months, unsweetened herbal tea, such as echinacea tea, can provide additional benefit. Since cold liquids tend to shock CFS patients, warm ones are preferable.

It is important for people with hypoglycemic-induced fatigue to alter their diets, incorporating high-fiber, protein-containing complex carbohydrates, such as oatmeal, into their meals, and consuming nutritious snacks during the mid-morning and afternoon. Complex carbohydrates and high-protein (from fish and vegetable sources) diets can also be useful in combating fatigue resulting from caffeine withdrawal.

Supplements

A variety of nutritional supplements can help the immune system function properly. Since many CFS victims suffer from deficiencies of magnesium, chromium, zinc and other nutrients, a multivitamin and multimineral supplement can help restore the immune system.

People with chronic fatigue syndrome should try to consume 5000-20,000 mg of vitamin C daily. Vitamin C is crucial for the immune system and the thymus gland to work properly. Because vitamin C is emitted from the body during excretion (it's water soluble), taking vitamin C over the course of the day is wise. Higher dosages of vitamin C can be administered through intravenous drips under the supervision of a physician. Intravenous supplements are quite successful in treating chronic fatigue syndrome. Often 150,000-200,000 mg of vitamin C is dispensed intravenously, while the patient continues to consume quantities of oral supplements, up to bowel tolerance. (Under medical supervision, these high IV dosages of therapeutic vitamin C are gradually built up to, and then stepped down from, over the course of many weeks.)

Vitamin E is another powerful antioxidant and should be supplemented in amounts of 400-800 IU per day from mixed gamma or a mixture of tocopherol with 150 mg of tocotrienol. In addition, 100 mg of vitamin-B complex should be consumed daily. Vitamin B3 (use the non-flush kind), also known as niacinamide, is useful in correcting blood sugar abnormalities, while B6 tends to protect the thymus gland from free-radical damage.

Zinc picolinate can significantly supplement the body's supply of zinc when consumed in amounts of 35-50 mg daily. The picolinate element of the supplement aids in transporting it into the cell. However, do not take excessive quantities of zinc. Amounts above 50 mg have been found to adversely affect the immune system.

Chromium supplements, in either the GTF form or the chromium picolinate form, enable the body's supply of insulin to carry blood sugar into the cells.

Magnesium is also crucial to the production of energy. Unfortunately, many adults overlook it. Magnesium can be found in 300 different enzyme systems, and it aids in the synthesis of ATP, an all-important compound manufactured at the cellular level. It activates B vitamins and relaxes muscles. Often, women who supplement with calcium to fight osteoporosis neglect to consume equal quantities of magnesium. Consequently, they are victimized by fatigue.

Unfortunately, the presence of a magnesium deficiency is difficult to determine, as the standard blood tests fail to take into account actual mineral levels within the cells. To supplement 500 mg of magnesium would be beneficial.

Supplementation of antioxidants, such as glutathione (250-500 mg), N-acetylcysteine (600-1200 mg), or alpha-lipoic acid (500-750 mg), should be considered in combating free-radical damage. Glutathione levels are boosted by taking SAMe; the recommended dose is 200-1600 mg. Whey protein can raise glutathione levels as well, and is also known as an immunity enhancer. For those who have a nutritional deficiency, two scoops are suggested.

NADH, commonly known as coenzyme 1, is a relatively new therapy that has demonstrated an ability to alleviate chronic fatigue without harmful side effects. Coenzyme 1 is a natural substance that can be found in every cell within the human body; it is essential in the production of bodily energy. The amino acid tyrosine also enhances the production of energy by aiding in the functioning of brain hormones and neurotransmitters. A dosage of 1500 mg of tyrosine can improve cognitive functions. It is not recommended, though, for those suffering from melanoma or schizophrenia.

Coenzyme Q10, which works within mitochondria (our cells' powerhouses), acts as an energy stimulant and potent antioxidant. It can be effectively supplemented in quantities of 75-300 mg per day, while a minimum of 1 gram of the amino acid glutamine can increase energy. In addition, 2000 mg of acetyl-L-carnitine works as an energy booster.

Essential fatty acids are helpful when CFS is virus-induced. Many people have found that supplementing with a combination of borage oil and fish oil extract helps when this condition exists.

In cases where chronic fatigue syndrome depletes adrenal functions, DHEA (the hormone produced by the adrenal glands and the precursor of estrogen and testosterone) can be helpful. Women can take 15-50 mg; men's doses typically range from 25-50 mg. Careful monitoring is suggested.

A folic acid deficiency is connected with chronic fatigue syndrome; supplementation of 800 mcg daily is suggested. Note: One must take vitamin B12 with folic acid in order to prevent excessive intake of folic acid from masking a B12 deficiency.

Herbal Remedies

Although there are a variety of herbal remedies that can be useful in combating fatigue, consumption of herbs should be supervised by a qualified professional who has the knowledge to determine which herbs are best for your unique needs. Some medicinal herbs are not ideal for general use because they can cause adverse side effects if used improperly. Others are safer to use on a daily basis. Adaptogenic herbs, which are mild tonics, fall into the second category, and can be useful in alleviating fatigue because they enable the body to naturally create more energy. Examples of popular adaptogenic herbs are astragalus, panax ginseng, Siberian ginseng, lonicera and glycyrrhiza (also known as licorice root).

The herb astragalus has been thoroughly researched and is available from an abundance of sources. Studies show that astragalus enhances immune function and treats a wide variety of illnesses, from the common cold to cancer. Instead of directly attacking infectious organisms, astragalus aids the body by strengthening the immune system. The herb can be taken daily, and is especially effective when paired with the Chinese herb legustrum.

Tulip poplar bark, which Western cultures have borrowed from traditional Native American medicine, is yet another energy stimulant.

Originally used by the Chinese, Siberian ginseng and panax ginseng effectively stabilize the energy levels within the body by boosting vitality during the day and encouraging relaxation during the night. Furthermore, ginseng strengthens the immune system by increasing the quantity and the performance of disease-fighting cells. The recommended dosage of Siberian ginseng is 200-300 mg per day, while the suggested dosage of panax is slightly less. Ginseng can be consumed either as a tea or as an extract.

The herb echinacea can increase the number of immune cells and promote increased cell functioning when taken three to four days out of the week. Echinacea is widely available in tincture form and as a tea, or it may be supplemented at 500 mg twice a day. High-quality sources of the herb display a tendency to produce a tingling sensation and a numbing effect on the tongue.

Fresh oats are a nervous system rejuvenator, and are used to counter chronic fatigue syndrome. In addition, fresh oats can quell recreational drug, cigarette and coffee withdrawal symptoms. *Remember:* Fresh oats should not be confused with rolled or quick oats, as they possess their own distinct qualities and benefits.

Tea brewed from mate (Ilex paraguayensis) may combat mental and physical fatigue, and may be taken as coffee substitute. The suggested dosage is 1 gram per cup, up to 4 grams daily. It is also available in tablet (one per day), tincture (5 drops) or globules (10 globules three times a day).

Garlic is yet another immunosupportive substance that can be used to combat the body's susceptibility to infectious organisms. It aids the immune system by promoting activity of the body's natural killer cells, which eliminate infectious viruses and tumor cells. When garlic is taken in tablet form, two capsules should be consumed with every meal.

Popularized by the Chinese and Japanese, ganoderma—also known as the reishi mushroom—is a general energy stimulant that also possesses cancer-fighting abilities. It is particularly effective when used along with astragalus and legustrum. Licorice root aids in arousing adrenal energy and has powerful antiviral qualities. It is useful in cleansing the blood and the liver. Supplementation of 250 mg three times a day is recommended. Cayenne pepper is useful in eliminating mucus and purifying the blood.

A fungus commonly used by Asians, poria cocos, purifies the blood and increases stamina. Also, usnea and lomacium have antiviral characteristics, and have also demonstrated an ability to quell chronic fatigue.

Finally, stinging nettle and common burdock root have proven useful in fortifying the immune system.

Homeopathic Remedies

In addition to medicinal herbs, a wide range of homeopathic remedies are available to help alleviate chronic fatigue. Some of these are listed below, along with the types of symptoms—and types of patients—they are considered effective for.

Anacardium is prescribed by homeopathic practitioners for chronic fatigue with brain fog, forgetfulness and fixed ideas.

Arsenicum album is a remedy for exhaustion accompanied by anxiety. The person may fear death and disease and feel despair over lack of recovery. There may be burning symptoms in the stomach as well as hay fever, and thin, watery excretions. Other symptoms include weight loss, shortness of breath with exertion and dry rough, scaly skin. The patient has great thirst and tends to crave ice-cold water.

Baryta carbonica is prescribed for people with a slow mental grasp. There is a lot of confusion and difficulty learning, and there may be chronically enlarged tonsils. These people tend to get colds easily.

Gelsenium is for extreme tiredness and muscular soreness, even with very little exertion. The patient wants to remain in bed all the time. Eyelids droop heavily and blurred or double vision is common. A band-like headache may occur and there is fever without thirst.

Kali phosphoricum is considered useful for anxiety, fear and brain fog—when the person can't recall names or words and has other problems with memory.

Lycopodium is for brain fog, weak memory confused thoughts, dyslexia, an inability to find the right words and indecisiveness. There are also abdominal symptoms, noisy flatulence (especially after eating), bloating, excessive hunger and desire for sweets.

Munaticum acid is a homeopathic remedy designed specifically to extinguish fatigue with physical origins. Usually, the physical fatigue victim is emotionally and mentally healthy but the body is simply unable to function properly and constant bed rest is necessitated. If the patient does not receive immediate attention the fatigue can extend to the person's mental capabilities. This particular homeopathic remedy is used to combat fatigue that commonly accompanies chronic diarrhea, gastrointestinal disorders, such as chronic colitis or liver dysfunction and the HIV virus.

Nux vomica helps with impaired liver function, especially when liver damage is due to toxins, such as drugs, chemicals, meats and fats. It is also for the patient with irritable bowel syndrome and constipation alternating with diarrhea.

Phosphoric acid is quite helpful in alleviating fatigue induced by extraordinary emotional events, such as a difficult divorce, a bad relationship, or an accident. In these cases the patient typically becomes withdrawn from others, stays in bed for long periods, refuses to eat, avoids talking and, in general, seems to be frozen at all times. In addition, this remedy is prescribed to alleviate fatigue brought on by too much sexual activity, as well as fatigue associated with cancer, drug abuse, or mononucleosis.

Ticitum acid is commonly used by homeopaths to treat fatigue induced by mental exhaustion, a state that has become prevalent in many professionals due to overwork. Indications of mental fatigue include an inability to perform even the most simple functions, general confusion and difficulty with the elements of everyday life.

Exercise

Although it doesn't come naturally, chronic fatigue patients should push themselves to exercise, as incorporating a regular aerobic exercise program can produce remarkable results in terms of boosting the body's energy level. A sustained, repetitive, total body activity aids functioning of the adrenal glands and helps release stress. Ideally, an exercise routine should be performed for 20 to 30 minutes, five days a week, although a patient with severe fatigue will obviously have to build up to this level. Actually, the diminished strength of a chronic fatigue patient can be dramatically enhanced by participating in relatively gentle exercises. For instance, walking in a swimming pool and gradually building up to a power-walking level of exertion, is quite beneficial.

Outdoor exercises are especially advantageous, as they allow the patient to assimilate fresh air into the system. Walking on cold winter days can be quite invigorating, but remember to bundle up! Tai chi, qi gong and yoga are also recommended for chronic fatigue patients because of their salutary effects on the endocrine and immune systems.

Relaxation

Studies have shown that a significant percentage of chronic fatigue patients have encountered an inordinate amount of stress in their lives. Prolonged exposure to intense stress can debilitate the immune system, and indeed contribute to the onset of CFS. That's why people suffering from chronic fatigue may benefit from engaging in meditation as a way of calming the mind and eliminating stress. Twenty minutes, twice a day is the meditation schedule often recommended. Engaging in breathing exercises and being generally cognizant of breathing patterns during everyday activities can also be beneficial in eliminating anxiety. Other relaxation techniques that may be helpful are creative dance and yoga. Focusing on the positive aspects of life and nurturing an optimistic outlook will reduce the effects of stress upon the body and aid the individual in coping with and improving his or her condition.

Detoxification

Victims of chronic fatigue syndrome have usually accumulated poisonous waste products within their bodies; hence, it is important to regularly detoxify the system for one to two months. The detoxification protocol can include colonics, which should be performed once a month for three months; and enemas, performed once a week. Furthermore, wheatgrass and other green juices can cleanse the blood, while bitters can aid in eliminating bodily impurities and stimulating liver and kidney function. The detoxification process should also incorporate lymphatic stimulation, which can be achieved with acupuncture or massage.

Pressure Point Therapy

Pressure point therapy is another approach that has proven helpful in treating some CFS patients. Pressure points for increasing energy are situated primarily in the chest region. The first point can be located by placing the hand on the notch above the chest in the throat region. Do not press here, but instead slide your fingers approximately two inches below the notch. Once you have reached this lower point, press for 10 to 15 seconds.

Another pressure point is located one inch directly below the first. While these points may appear tender at first, applying firm pressure can alleviate sensitivity and tension. This particular method of pressure point therapy is also quite useful in quelling fatigue induced by jet lag.

What to Avoid

Chronic and general fatigue can be compounded by a variety of factors, and most important among these are poor dietary habits. Foods that should be avoided include coffee and other caffeinated products, dairy products, meat and refined foods. In addition, stress can contribute to the onset of fatigue, so stress reduction is recommended. Also, since vaccinations have been implicated as a potential causal factor in CFS, it is advisable to seek out information on alternatives to vaccines and to weigh the risks and benefits before getting them.

Treatment Summary

Prior to following a holistic treatment regimen, the chronic fatigue sufferer should be tested by a doctor for specific causes of the condition, such as food allergies, hypothyroidism, or adrenal dysfunction.

The diet should contain complex carbohydrates, as these foods provide energy slowly and steadily; enzymes from raw juices stimulate the immune system to health; protein from vegetarian sources and unpolluted fish is advantageous.

Herbs stimulate the immune system and enhance energy.

A multiple-vitamin/mineral supplement should be included, as many chronic fatigue sufferers have nutritional deficiencies.

Vitamin C is needed throughout the day, and is particularly beneficial when taken intravenously under a physician's supervision.

A wide range of homeopathic remedies can help counter chronic fatigue.

Regular exercise will augment the body's natural energy supply.

Relaxation techniques can reduce stress levels, thereby benefiting the immune system.

Detoxification is essential for the elimination of poisonous waste products that slow down body systems, contributing to chronic fatigue. For example, one of the most common findings in persons with CFS is gastrointestinal overgrowth of Candida albicans.

Stimulation of pressure points is a technique for releasing energy, as it is important in helping to relieve tension that frequently contributes to CFS.

Chronic Pain

Constant or long-term pain is a widespread problem. If we listen to the mass media, the painkillers manufactured by large pharmaceutical companies are the way we should seek relief. But there are alternatives to these products, and the Americans who suffer from chronic pain would do well to stop obeying the commands of their television sets. Although running to the medicine chest and swallowing a few over-the-counter or prescription pills may provide immediate comfort by eliminating the perception of pain by the brain, the underlying causes are not addressed, and overall health has not been improved in any way. By contrast, a wide variety of natural treatment modalities exist that can aid the body in coping with chronic pain at a more fundamental level.

Causes

Pain is a signal that something is wrong with the body. It may be triggered by a myriad of factors, ranging from diseases, such as rheumatoid arthritis and cancer, to injuries from exercise or accidents, to food allergies, which can, for example, provoke migraines. While the causes of pain are many, the mechanisms used by the body to produce pain are similar. When the body experiences pain, a nerve impulse travels from the injured site up through the spinal cord, and to the brain. At this point the brain reacts by registering the pain in our consciousness.

When the body experiences pain, inflammation usually results. Inflammation is characterized by swelling, redness, heat and pain, and if left untreated, partial or complete loss of function of the affected area. During inflammation, protease, an enzyme that aids in the assimilation of protein, is liberated in the injured region, initiating a chain reaction that compounds the problem. Small particles of protein, known as bradykinins, are also released and interact with the nerve receptors, resulting in the perception of pain. In addition, the bradykinins summon the immune cells to the region and widen the blood vessels.

Treatment

Nutrition

One of the most effective methods of combating chronic pain is saturation. This can be effectively achieved by consuming eight six- to eight-ounce glasses of water per day. For the elderly this is especially important, as recent medical research reveals that dehydration can play a major role in the onset of chronic pain due to the spinal disks drying out. Note that when the body feels sensations of thirst, partial dehydration has already occurred. Therefore, we should try to quench the body need for liquid prior to actually feeling it.

In addition to water, organic fruits and vegetables, and certain juices create an acid/base balance within the body that is important for diminishing pain. Excess acidity encourages the stimulation of peripheral nerves and increases our perception of pain. By alkalinizing the body this type of stimulation can be prevented. Furthermore, juices derived from plant sources provide abundant sources of phytochemicals and antioxidant vitamins, minerals and enzymes.

The acidity of the body can have a profound effect upon health. According to the late Dr. Emanuel Revici, a renowned health educator and researcher who dedicated a great portion of his life to devising treatments for pain, pain sensations can be substantially alleviated by altering our dietary habits. In his research, Dr. Revici succeeded in eliminating severe pancreatic cancer pain by raising the pH level in his patients. While an excess of acidic foods can contribute to the accumulation of hazardous waste products within the system, recent studies of the average American diet have revealed that 80 percent of our dietary intake is acidic, while only 20 percent is alkaline. In a healthy diet these figures should be reversed. Some good examples of alkaline foods are soybeans, potatoes, melons and lemons—these foods aid the body in eliminating harmful accumulations. It is important to note that beneficial forms of acid do exist and can be derived from coconuts, Brazil nuts, filberts, macadamias, pecans and walnuts. And although a variety of beans—black beans, adzuki beans, chickpeas, kidney beans, lentils, mung beans, navy beans, red beans, white beans and pintos—register on the acidic (low) side of the pH scale, they too can be considered healthy acids. The same principle applies to oats, rice and whole wheat. Negative acids generally register extremely low on the pH scale, meaning that they are highly acidic. Red meat falls into this category. If the bulk of your dietary intake lies on the acidic side of the pH scale, you should neutralize your body by concentrating on more alkaline foods.

Supplements

Our body can block the sensation of pain with endorphins, which are natural proteins manufactured by the pituitary gland in the brain. Endorphins are an effective alternative to typical conventional treatments and, fortunately their production within the brain, can be facilitated with a nutritional approach.

DL-Phenylalanine (DLPA) . . . The substance DLPA can be part of this approach. This essential fatty acid is crucial in preventing the breakdown of endorphins by enzymes in the brain. These enzymes are secreted by the brain to prevent the body from becoming addicted to its own endorphins. By slowing down this process, the body will experience reduced amounts of pain. Studies indicate that four grams of DLPA administered a half hour before a tooth extraction can reduce pain by up to 50 percent. DLPA has also been shown to be quite effective in alleviating chronic lower back pain. It is important to remember that this product will not completely eliminate all pain; however, it can increase the pain threshold significantly in most individuals and can serve as a safe, natural alternative to conventional painkillers. The generally recommended dosage is 500 mg, three or four times per day, to substantially reduce the perception of pain.

B Vitamins . . . Clinical evidence indicates that injections of B vitamins, especially B1 (thiamin) and B12, can ameliorate severe pain induced by headaches, arthritis and dental surgery. Deficiencies of vitamin B12, which are often responsible for the onset of neuropathies, can be eliminated with intramuscular injections. Patients can receive injections of one milligram in their doctors' offices, and symptoms of neuropathy will disappear within several days. Many times blood tests do not provide adequate evidence that a B12 deficiency exists, and consequently the patient is told that intramuscular injections are not needed. However, it is important to realize that there is not a direct correlation between the amount of B12 in the blood and that within the nerve cells. An injection of B12 is completely safe and can produce dramatic results.

Vitamin C . . . Vitamin C will alleviate the problem of sensitive gums, and recent clinical evidence reveals that most patients with this problem benefit from taking vitamin C supplements to bowel tolerance, the point just before experiencing diarrhea. These patients receive help even after they have exhausted all other alternatives, including painkillers, nonsteroidals and even cortisone. While some people can only tolerate 10 g per day others are able to absorb 50 g of vitamin C. On average, the tolerable oral dosage is 20 g. Much higher doses can be taken intravenously and can provide substantial pain relief.

Protease . . . As mentioned earlier, proteolytic enzymes cause inflammation after injury and, thus, pain. By halting the production of protease, the effects of inflammation can be reduced. But since the healing process and inflammation are linked, it's not advisable to eliminate inflammation altogether. Doing so may inhibit the body's ability to heal itself. Basically the objective of protease supplements is to obtain a limited amount of inflammation that will not hinder the healing process.

In the past, studies have correlated the injection of protease with allergic reactions, but oral supplements are now recommended. They have the ability to promote healing and expedite the inflammation period. The enzymes are eventually assimilated into the bloodstream, where they are transported to injured areas and aid the body's natural protease. Protease supplements have established their effectiveness in ameliorating sports-related injuries, bruises, episiotomies, tooth extractions, sunburn and sciatica in a large number of clinical studies. Supplements of protease can accelerate the healing process and diminish the severity of pain by up to 50 percent. If you normally take a week to recuperate from an injury your recovery time can be reduced to three days.

Unlike typical painkillers, such as aspirin, proteolytic enzymes do not completely block out all pain. This is actually a positive effect because the inflammation that manages to develop stimulates the body's natural healing agents. Although a large body of medical research has substantiated the role of protease in the healing process, the public is still by and large unaware of its potential benefits. The reason is that nonsteroidal anti-inflammatory medications, such as ibuprofen, appeared on the marketplace at the same time that protease supplements were first being accepted. Unfortunately the painkillers assumed a dominant role in the medical market because, although they did not aid the body in naturally healing its wounds, products like ibuprofen could provide total relief, while protease supplements could only ensure partial pain alleviation.

People interested in natural protease supplements should follow several basic guidelines. First, protease should be consumed on an empty stomach, in order to prevent digestion by our other natural enzymes. In addition, it is advisable to take supplements three to four times daily. They should be consumed before meals and before retiring for the night. Furthermore, it is important to purchase a product with high potency. Sometimes this is difficult because the information on package labels can be extremely vague. Also, the potency of protease can deteriorate with time, rendering year-old packages completely useless.

Protease supplements can be obtained from most health food stores in a variety of products. One example is bromelain, which is derived from pineapples, while another common source is papain, which originates from papayas. Animal sources of protease are found in trypsinlchymotrypsin. Since the potency of protease supplements is characterized by inconsistency, you should select a product with the highest possible protease content. If this particular product is ineffective, try another package or a completely different product.

Methylsulfonylmetane (MSM) . . . The organic form of sulfur can help repair damaged and worn cartilage, offering pain relief to arthritis patients. It can also reduce muscle soreness and cramps. In addition, glucosamine enhances the effectiveness of MSM.

Glucosamine sulfate . . . This amino acid triggers the production of new tissue in joints, ligaments and cartilage—especially when used with chondroitin, a larger molecule found in cartilage. It is important to remember that glucosamine is a *sugar* that can raise blood sugar levels in diabetics.

Calcium . . . Calcium is used primarily to prevent and reduce arthritic pain, but works effectively with pain from premenstrual syndrome.

Magnesium . . . It has long been used to treat migraine headaches because of its muscle-relaxing qualities.

Essential Fatty Acids . . . To achieve pain-free health, the supplementation of essential fatty acids—such as gamma-linolenic (GLA) and alpha-linolenic (ALA)—could be important. They could reduce the severity and duration of migraine attacks.

Herbal Remedies

The following are some of the many herbs that can be used to treat pain from common sources. Remember, though, that before initiating herbal therapy it is a good idea to seek professional supervision. A trained herbalist can provide the necessary expertise and assistance.

For Menstrual Pain . . . The most common treatment for menstrual cramps is dong quai, although a mixture of other remedies can also be used. Herbalist Christopher Trahan recommends a tincture of equal quantities of angelica sinensis, viburnum opulus and the Chinese herb corydalis for treating severe cramps. The muscle relaxant American wild yam, also known as dioscorea, is incorporated into the tincture, along with a small amount of black haw, also known as viburnum. Additional herbs that can be included in an anticramps mixture are Chinese cinnamon, wild ginger and cassia. If taken as a tincture, the herbs listed above are taken in a dosage of 15-30 drops every half hour during acute pain. These herbs can also be brewed as a tea. Another Chinese herb, shao fu zhu yu wan, offers pain relief by invigorating the blood and thereby warming the uterus. Ge xia zhu yu wan has similar qualities.

For Premenstrual Syndrome . . . Premenstrual problems can be treated by dong quai, as well as by the American herb dandelion root. The latter is especially versatile. The Chinese herbs bupleurum, cypems and melia are said to enhance the energy flow and to be particularly good for alleviating pain in the breast region. Salvia, which is the Chinese version of sage, is said to enhance qi, or life energy, and can be used to treat the heart and chest area.

For Headaches . . . The American herbs valerian and skullcap are commonly used to treat painful headaches. The two herbs can be quite effective when taken together. A tincture of the two, consisting of 15 to 30 drops, or several capsules of each herb, can be taken. Be aware, however, that although valerian can be useful in reducing pain, nervous conditions and insomnia, this herb can have adverse side effects, such as overheating and heart palpitations. Scullcap by contrast, is a relatively safe herb and can successfully eliminate head pain. It can be used by people who suffer from Parkinson's disease, twitching and tremors.

The herb feverfew is used to effectively combat the onset of migraine headaches by altering blood vessel functioning and cellular magnesium transfer. (Headaches induced by stressful situations or muscle tension cannot be treated with this particular herb, only true migraines.) Wild ginger can be used to alleviate head pain, while the versatile dong quai soothes muscle tissue. After a workout, dong quai can be taken along with either ginger or mint. Only small amounts of ginger should be taken at a time, though, and one should be especially careful on hot days, because ginger has a warming effect. Mint, on the other hand, is cooling.

The Chinese herbs tian ma gou teng yin and tian ma mi huan su have positive impact on migraine headaches by lowering the blood pressure and relaxing muscle spasms.

White willow bark can be useful in alleviating headache pain. Aspirin, a product that most of us are familiar with, is actually a derivative of an ingredient in white willow bark, salicylic acid. Natural sources of this compound, though, are safer than the synthetic versions prevalent in most stores because their potency is lower. Several grams of white willow bark are required to obtain an aspirin-like effect.

For Stomach Pain . . . Mint is used for stomach pain and is often paired with either slippery elm or licorice root. Also, the Chinese herb corydalis can be applied to a wide variety of pains, including uterine and stomach pain. For stomach pain, as for other types of pain, a health care professional should be consulted.

For Urinary Tract Infections . . . Pain from urinary tract infections is typically treated with herbs that contain the alkaloid berberine. Sometimes goldenseal is appropriate, but Oregon grape root is used more often due to its potent concentration. Another herb commonly used is barberry bark. The Chinese herb coptis, which resembles goldenseal, is extraordinarily potent and can be used as an antibiotic or antiseptic. Since coptis is so powerful, the soothing effects of marshmallow are frequently employed after its consumption.

For Arthritic Pain . . . Chinese herbal medicine offers a great deal of pain relievers for swollen and painful joints, stiffness and inflammation. These pain relievers include du huo ji sheng, kang gu zheng sheng, tian qi du zhong, china tung shueh, guan jie yan wan, fang ji huang qi wan, tian ma wan and san bi tang wan. A licensed practitioner should decide which one is the most effective in each individual case.

For General Pain . . . Kava kava, which can be found on Fiji and several other South Pacific islands, is especially effective in combating chronic pain because of its ability to bind to nerve receptor sites and numb the brain's perception of pain. The effects of kava kava mimic those of drugs, without the addictive element. This relatively safe herb can also promote relaxation and reduce anxiety.

Additional herbs that can aid the treatment of chronic pain include wood betony and rosemary. Wood betony, which has been used for centuries by folk healers, can also serve as a sedative and carminative, and is a useful remedy for diarrhea, and severe cases of gout. Rosemary, which many know as a culinary herb, has strong analgesic qualities and is particularly beneficial when used as a massage oil for muscle aches or headaches. Rosemary oil is commonly paired with a diffusing agent, usually either almond or olive oil.

The herb blue vervain contains anti-inflammatory and analgesic properties, and finally, curcumin, which is a bright yellow compound derived from turmeric and curry, is another nutritional substance that can be used to treat pain. Like the drug indomethacin, curcumin reduces the inflammation of arthritis and other conditions. But curcumin does not induce adverse side effects, such as the burning of stomach lining holes. The recommended dosage of curcumin is 1200 mg daily.

The Chinese herbs qi ye lian, jin gu shang wan, dang gui si ni wan, juan bi tang wan, hou lou xiao ling wan, sao yao cao wan and shen tong zhu yu wan successfully alleviate pain by promoting circulation and increasing blood flow.

To lessen pain after stroke or paralysis, or to ease numbness, xiao huo luo dan may be a good choice. Pain that accompanies traumatic injuries, fractures, broken bones and strains can be eliminated by jin gu shang wan, and arnica has a similar effect due to its anti-inflammatory qualities. Tian qi wan can stop bleeding and ease pain in minor injuries; ginkgo biloba seems to reduce leg pain. Ching wan hung is commonly used for pain caused by burns, and cong rong bu shen wan is a traditionally used solution for lumbago-related pain. Cayenne, which contains capsaicin, helps to block pain signals by stimulating endorphin release. The anti-inflammatory chamomile can relax the lining of the digestive tract.

Exercise

People who are experiencing extremely severe pain are obviously not candidates for a regular exercise program. In many instances, however, moderate exercise can be quite beneficial in the pain treatment process. When a person engages in exercise, endorphins—which act as natural opiates—are released by the body. This is one reason athletes are often able to continue partaking in athletic events after they are injured. In these situations, sensations of pain are not experienced during participation due to the constant release of endorphins. It is only after the event is finished that the pain is felt.

In addition to the release of endorphins, moderate exercise promotes the release of natural cortisone. Also, since pain and discomfort are frequently accompanied by excessive anxiety the stress-relieving aspect of exercise can be quite beneficial. Furthermore, exercise can normalize sleep patterns and enhance self-confidence, both of which can be useful in treating pain. Moderate exercise includes activities like brisk walking, biking and swimming. The idea is to choose something pleasurable that one can look forward to doing, and stick with.

There are a variety of stretches and exercises that can aid in the healing process and alleviate a number of painful disorders:

For Sciatica . . . People suffering from acute sciatic pain, which is characterized by numbness or tingling in the thigh, buttocks, calf, toe, or groin, should lie on their back and carefully pull their knee toward their chest. This activity can alleviate symptoms of sciatic pain by opening the lower lumbar disks. In addition, treatment for sciatic pain can be performed by lying on one's side and assuming the fetal position.

For Neck Pain . . . Habitual poor posture while sitting at a desk or computer, and sleeping on one's stomach, commonly result in neck tension and eventual pain. A stretch that can be performed to alleviate these problems involves gentle rotation of the head and holding it in place in each direction.

Remember that a sedentary lifestyle can result in the onset of chronic neck, back and leg pain. It is important to take a short break every hour to stretch the muscles and reduce susceptibility to chronic pain.

For Arthritis . . . Studies have indicated that arthritis, which can involve the increasing proximity of spinal-column bones and eventual pinching of the nerves, can be effectively combated with regular stretching, exercise and chiropractic adjustments. Swimming for 30 to 40 minutes, three or four times a week, can be particularly advantageous. The buoyancy of the water prevents injury to arthritic joints.

For Leg Pain . . . Chronic pain in the legs can be treated by placing the injured leg on a chair and bending forward from the waist. This exercise will enable the patient to stretch out the muscles of the legs. While performing this exercise, one should remember to stretch using the waist and avoid using the lower back. Next, the patient should attempt to bend over while in a seated position. These stretches are especially useful for people who are constantly seated at a computer or desk.

Chiropractic Care

Studies have demonstrated that chiropractic care is a most effective means of treating chronic pain, especially when it involves the lower back region and arthritis. Chiropractors are able to alleviate pain by eliminating subluxations, or pinched nerves. They work through manipulation of the spinal column, eschewing drugs and surgery. Some are involved with nutrition.

Home Remedies

Severe headaches and neck tension can be combated by placing a few tennis balls in a sock and positioning the "package" at the base of the neck. After one remains in this position for approximately 20 minutes, the neck muscles tend to relax, thus eliminating the neck pain and any accompanying headaches. Often, headaches that occur during neck pain are caused by compression in the cervical spine that is alleviated with the technique.

For muscle spasms, ice can be applied to the affected area for 10 to 15 minutes, and then removed for an hour. This procedure should be repeated several times. Ice works for muscle spasms because it limits the signals being sent to the brain, hence, decreasing pain awareness.

Psychological Health

People who experience chronic pain are often plagued by bouts of depression. This can be extremely detrimental to the recovery process because negative emotions can actually expedite the onset of adverse symptoms. Then, pain and depression can become a vicious cycle. The other side of the coin is that people can improve their psychological outlook and, consequently, aid the healing process by engaging in relaxation and meditation, or by increasing the flow of endorphins through exercise. Depression can also be lifted through nutritional protocols. Doctors who tailor such programs to a patient's specific needs are known as orthomolecular physicians. By avoiding depression, when possible, and having a positive outlook, we can contribute to the treatment of chronic pain by allowing the brain to secrete chemicals that actually aid the healing process.

Acupuncture

The Chinese concept of qi (pronounced "chee") pertains to the flow of energy within our bodies that is responsible for life. In general, qi can be described as the sum of all physiological processes, metabolism and consciousness. According to Chinese beliefs, clinical disorders can be explained by a deficiency of qi, while pain is commonly a product of blocked qi. Thus, chronic pain often necessitates eliminating blockage and strengthening the qi, which can be achieved with acupuncture. The therapy involves placing extremely thin needles into the skin along a series of lines, called meridians. These facilitate ionic transfer and encourage the generation of cellular energy.

Acupuncture is used in a wide variety of situations. It can serve as an analgesic, a sedative and a muscle relaxant. It can improve immune functioning, increase circulation and strengthen the lymphatic system. In addition, acupuncture can promote production of dopamine within the brain, improve our psychological state and aid motor recovery after an injury.

Frequently muscle strains and sprains can lead to the onset of chronic pain. Even if the injury occurred several years back, the body can enter a vicious cycle of pain. The muscle tone in the injured region can become imbalanced and muscle spasms can manifest. Acupuncture can aid the body in defeating chronic symptoms by acting as an anti-inflammatory agent.

Finally acupuncture can be used to treat joint injuries that elude the tools of modern science, including orthopedic examinations and MRIs. Numerous cases have been documented in which acupuncture has remedied an "untraceable" condition.

Following the traditions of Chinese medicine, a qualified acupuncturist does not merely block pain, but instead, treats the overall structure of the body. The Chinese believe that a single symptom cannot develop by itself; it must be accompanied by a wider variety of problems, and hence the entire system needs to be treated. Furthermore, when treating a patient, the person's entire medical history is taken into consideration by the acupuncturist. Although it is difficult for most medical professionals and patients in the West to accept, the concept of balancing the qi within the body can produce dramatic results in the treatment of chronic pain.

Biofeedback

Biofeedback uses scientific instruments to help patients determine for themselves when their body is stressed and when it is relaxed. Biofeedback instruments register an aspect of physiology such as muscle tension, fingertip temperature, or brain waves. When the body experiences anger or fear, for example, our extremities drop in temperature. Irregular breathing often results from stress.

The idea behind biofeedback is that people can learn to relax by altering their body processes. Breathing patterns can be analyzed and then altered, to create a calmer state. Muscle tension can be lessened, reducing pain. The highly advanced equipment that is employed can measure even the most subtle body changes.

A wide variety of pain-oriented problems can be effectively treated with biofeedback, including neck and shoulder pain, muscle strains and extremity pain. In addition, biofeedback can be used to remedy chronic tension headaches. For patients seeking treatment for headaches, the initial visit to a biofeedback specialist will consist of a stress analysis test to determine stress tolerance. Also, the specialist may request a detailed medical history, in order to ascertain the presence of any conditions that may exacerbate the headache. After the preliminary information is obtained, the biofeedback equipment is attached to the patient. There are several devices that can aid in evaluating a headache patient, including instruments that measure muscle tension and nervous perspiration. The patient sits in front of the output monitors, and watches as the instruments read electrical signals from the skin surface. Then the specialist instructs the patient to close his or her eyes. After observing the patient's ability to relax, the specialist tries to recreate a stressful event that occurred in the past. The biofeedback instruments measure any variations in perspiration, muscle tension and breathing patterns. Learning to change these is the next step.

Numerous biofeedback sessions are required to measure a patient's progress. A key element to biofeedback therapy involves a patient's personal commitment to practicing relaxation techniques at home.

Magnetic Healing

It is not a generally recognized therapy, but proponents of magnetic healing are convinced of this modality's efficacy, and explain that magnets are helpful in overcoming pain because they repolarize the cells of the body. This allows more nutrition and oxygen into the cells, and greater amounts of toxins out.

When pain is systemic, magnetic bed pads are used, with the idea of bathing the whole body overnight in a beneficial magnetic field. This is to oxygenate all the cells. In addition, a 2- x 4-inch, or 4- x 6-inch magnet, placed above the headboard, is used to bathe the pineal gland, which is a small but powerful gland in the center of the head. Among other things, the pineal gland is responsible for melatonin production, which helps us get restorative sleep.

Magnets can also be placed on the site of the pain. During the day magnets can be wrapped over an affected area. Another method sometimes advocated is to use 2- x 5-inch bar magnets or neodymium round magnets. These are very powerful magnets, and it is recommended that they be worn for short periods of time, approximately 30 minutes a day.

Some words of caution: Do not sleep on a magnetic bed pad for more than eight to 10 hours a night. Also, those practiced in this area explain that the body should touch the north, or negative side, of the magnet, as this produces healing effects. The southern pole, or positive side, is said to have the opposite effect, exacerbating pain and disease.

Therapeutic Touch

Therapeutic touch is a method of healing that involves the conscious transfer of energy from the hands of the healer to the body of the client. The technique is an ancient one; in fact, it is documented in cave drawings. In the 1970s, therapeutic touch was reintroduced by Dr. Dolores Krieger, a professor of nursing at New York University.

This modality can help a variety of conditions, particularly those involving pain and anxiety. This approach can help alleviate chronic pain because it relaxes the person, and helps the movement of energy.

During a session, the practitioner centers his or her body, mind and emotions. Then the hands are placed two to four inches from the body of the client, and the entire body is scanned for energy imbalances. Basic cues are tingling, pressure, static, heat and cold. Treatment is carried out administering the law of opposites. In other words, if heat is picked up, the practitioner might balance that energy by sending cool energy and visualizing the color blue. Conversely if cold energy is picked up, the practitioner might send a warm energy to that part of the body and visualize the color yellow. Other techniques, practitioners explain, involve pulling out static and congested energy from the body and "aura brushing," which cleanses the aura and places negative energy that is pulled off into the ground. The therapeutic touch practitioner uses calm, rhythmic movements from head to toe, with the aim of clearing all imbalances.

Massage and Aromatherapy

Massage is a potent technique in treating pain. In cases of muscle tension and stiffness, muscles are deprived of oxygen. Massage improves blood circulation, bringing in the needed oxygen and nutrients, and resulting in a decrease of pain. Massage may also interfere with pain-signal pathways, inhibiting pain signals from reaching the brain by sending different impulses toward the nerves. The process is called the gate theory control. The use of essential oils distilled from plants and flowers to lessen pain goes back to ancient times. These can be applied directly, can be added to baths, or can be used as room fragrances. They can also occasionally be used as internal medication.

What to Avoid

As discussed earlier, the pH level of the body can be directly correlated with general health. Studies have shown that people with an exceedingly acidic diet are more likely to suffer from pain. When searching for a protein source it is important to avoid heavy proteins, such as red meat, because they are extremely acidic. Additional acid-forming foods include gelatin, vinegar, mayonnaise, mustard, table salt, soy sauce and ketchup. Sugar, alcohol, coffee, carbonated sodas and even black tea are acidic, and consequently should not be consumed in excess. Although moderate consumption of some acidic foods is acceptable, the typical American diet significantly surpasses the moderate threshold.

People also need to beware of invisible, but detrimental, electromagnetic fields that come at us from constant exposure to computers, digital clocks, microwave ovens and electric power lines. These aberrant fields can throw our systems out of balance.

Treatment Summary

Saturating the body with water may prevent pain caused by the drying out of spinal disks. An alkaline diet of mostly fruits, vegetables and fresh juices prevents the stimulation of peripheral nerves that causes pain sensations.

Endorphins, proteins naturally produced by the body, help us feel good and are enhanced by certain nutrients, particularly DLPA.

The B vitamins have an analgesic effect, and vitamin C alleviates gum sensitivity.

Taking protease orally will speed up recovery from injuries and diminish the severity of pain.

Numerous herbs have pain-relieving properties specific to different conditions. Examples are dong quai for menstrual cramps, feverfew for migraines and white willow bark for regular headaches.

A moderate exercise program will produce endorphins to help alleviate pain.

The practice of chiropractic care can correct problems that are at the root of chronic pain, especially when they relate to the spine and nerves.

Working to overcome the depression that often accompanies chronic pain may speed up the healing process.

Acupuncture, a time-honored Chinese system of healing, alleviates pain by releasing blockages to energy flows throughout the body.

In biofeedback, scientific instruments are used to teach people how to relax, and thus minimize their sensations of pain.

An increasing number of individuals are discovering that magnets can be effective against pain by correcting polarity imbalances at the cellular level.

Therapeutic touch, which involves the transfer of energy from practitioner to patient, can relieve pain and anxiety.

Cold and Canker Sores

Cold sores, also known as fever blisters, are caused by the herpes simplex virus (HSV1). The virus lodges in the nervous system, and occasionally manifests in short-lived, but painful, fluid-filled blisters on the skin and mucous membranes, particularly around the mouth and nose. It is important to know that the lesions of the herpes outbreak are highly contagious; therefore, good hygiene is crucial in avoiding herpetic whitlow, infection of the fingers, or ocular herpes (the eye infection that can become severe or even lead to blindness). In some people, primary herpetic gingivostomatitis could develop when the patient's mouth and throat are covered with painful ulcers.

Canker sores are similar, though they are not contagious. They can be brought on by the herpes virus, as well as by allergies, anemia, or poor intestinal flora. Some women experience canker sores with hormonal changes.

Cold and canker sores reflect a weakened immune system. When exhaustion or stress set in, the virus expresses itself. This is one more reason why it is important to keep the immune system functioning optimally at all times.

Treatment

While there is no cure for the herpes virus, it can be kept under control. Ice is an external treatment that can relieve swelling and pain during an outbreak. In addition, a lot can be done internally, with supplements and herbs. The most effective treatment for herpes remains fortifying the immune system, which is the key to preventing and controlling the infection.

Supplements

Beneficial bacteria, such as those found in yogurt, lactobacillus and acidophilus, promote the digestive processes necessary for the maintenance of a healthy immune system. Zinc gluconate, vitamin C, bee propolis and beta-carotene provide further immune support. Between 4000-10,000 mg of vitamin C will treat an inflammation of the nerve endings, and works especially well with the bioflavonoid quercetin. The amino acid L-lysine can effectively quell an outbreak. At least 500 mg are needed two to four times a day (some sources suggest 1000 mg three times per day). Including brewer's yeast in the diet may be beneficial. B vitamins counteract biochemical stress and therefore are good as preventive medicine. One good source of B vitamins is bee pollen, unless there is an allergy to bee stings. Other good sources are green algae and the bioflavonoid pycnogenol. Taking 60 mg of pycnogenol daily also has the side benefit of keeping the skin healthy and young. Vitamin A is healing to the skin as well, and preventive against infections. Another important nutrient is coenzyme Q10, which provides oxygen to the tissues, helping them to heal. DMSO (dymethyl sulfoxide) topically applied twice a day penetrates to the center of the herpes infection and stops the growth of the virus. *Note:* Cold sores may indicate a calcium deficiency.

Herbs

There is an abundance of herbs that support the immune system before or during an outbreak. Echinacea, goldenseal and chaparral are especially effective at stopping symptoms from worsening when they first begin to manifest. Cayenne has lots of immune-enhancing vitamin C, and relieves pain and itching when taken internally or applied externally in a cream. Another effective topical application is tea tree oil, which has natural antiseptic qualities. It can also reduce the severity of and shorten the outbreak.

Cornstarch paste is another option. Topically applying camphor—or the extract of the mint family herb Melissa officinalis (melissa cream)—with a cotton ball may reduce the symptoms. Clinical research confirms that aloe vera is as effective as orthodox medicine in combating herpes in tissue cultures, with no side effects. Red clover blossoms and burdock root cleanse the blood and are good to take as a tea. The tea is made from sage and, when combined with one teaspoon of powdered ginger, may clear up the sores. Garlic is gentle to the system and can be taken daily as a preventive or during an attack. Chewing on licorice root may also be beneficial.

Health food stores sell many of these herbs in salves, which quickly soothe skin inflammations. Some combinations to look for contain goldenseal, comfrey, bee propolis, aloe vera and vitamin E.

Elagen is a formula that contains the active ingredient of an Asian plant related to ginseng, called eleutherococcus senticosus, which can support the immune system. The extract from lomatium traditionally used by Native Americans is antiviral and a potent infection fighter. The combination of the tinctures of echinacea, calendula, oats, burdock and lomatium (half a teaspoon taken four or five times daily) enhances the immune system and helps expel toxins. It is aniviral and antibacterial. Rubbing an ice cube on the sore could ease the pain. It may also prevent the virus from moving from the nerve to the skin. Sucking on zinc lozenges and using a mouthwash with sage and chamomile may help ease the symptoms of canker sores.

Homeopathy

Homeopathy offers a couple of choices to lessen the symptoms of a herpes outbreak. Natrum muriaticum (Nat mur) is suggested during the early stages of herpes. Before the fluid-containing sores appear, the mouth and the lips are dry and chapped. Nat mur is recommended in cases where the patient is emotionally upset.

For the burning and itching phase of herpes, when vesicles have appeared, rhus toxicodendron (poison ivy) is recommended. It also can help with the crusting of the tissue, the other characteristic of the outbreak. Sepia (cuttlefish ink) offers relief when eruptions occur around the lips, at the corners of the mouth or on the nose. It can also provide relief for the patient who is exhausted and depressed.

People who have a thick, brown crust with reddish borders, which may bleed, could use dulcamara (bittersweet). These people might find that the symptoms appear parallel to weather changes—from warm to cold and damp— or are due to hormonal changes.

Herpes vesicles can become infected. To avert the need for antibiotics, take hepar sulphuris (calcium sulphide), which may control the infection.

What to Avoid

Cold and canker sores usually surface when stress appears. While this cannot always be avoided, it is important to note what situations create stress and to address those issues. Stress can also be minimized through relaxation techniques, such as meditation and biofeedback. Foods that stress the system should be avoided in general and especially during an outbreak. Sugar and caffeine should not be used. Also, acidic foods such as meat, tomatoes and oranges can be problematic. Chocolate, peanuts and other nuts, grains, peas, seeds, oatmeal and whole-wheat products contain the amino acid arginine, which can trigger a herpes outbreak. Canker sores may be decreased by avoiding the use of toothpaste with SLS (sodium laurylsulfate).

Treatment Summary

External application of ice is helpful. Various nutrients and plant remedies will boost the immune system to aid healing, relieve inflammation and pain and even prevent cold and canker sores from appearing in the first place.

See also: Herpes.

Colds and Flu

People sometimes confuse colds and the flu. The latter is characterized by a swift, severe onset, prostration, high temperature, chills, extreme fatigue, sore throat and a severe, hacking cough. A cold, on the other hand, has a slow onset and is not always accompanied by high fever. Symptoms tend to be localized in the upper respiratory tract, and include hoarseness, stuffiness, watery eyes, runny nose, sneezing, listlessness, mild fatigue, chest discomfort and generally a sore or burning throat.

Treatment

Diet

People who get lots of colds during the winter should cut down on acidic foods, and eat more fruits and vegetables. These foods are high in antioxidants, which give the body the tools it needs to fight off colds on its own.

Once you have a cold, it is a good idea to cut down on or get rid of the gluten in your diet, as well as dairy foods, meat, sugar and refined carbohydrates, and to focus, instead, on plant foods high in antioxidants, phytochemicals and chlorophyll. Juices are particularly recommended; if at all possible, these should be freshly made from organic vegetables and fruits.

Herbs

Astragalus . . . The Chinese have been using astragalus for thousands of years for immune-system strengthening. Studies have proven that this herb can reduce the frequency and duration of colds and the flu by boosting the immune system rather than by killing viruses directly. Astragalus can be taken as an extract, or the root can be added to soups.

Echinacea . . . Taking echinacea at the first sign of a cold or flu often results in the disappearance of all symptoms the very next morning. This extract of the purple coneflower was well appreciated by Native Americans and was used by early American doctors before the widespread use of drugs.

Now echinacea is enjoying a well-deserved renaissance, and is once again America's top herb. The reason is simple: It works. This is how: Echinacea revs up the immune system at the cellular level. First, it stimulates the bone marrow to increase phagocyte production. Then, it facilitates the release of these phagocytes into the bloodstream and lymphatic system. Once there, these fighter cells seek out and destroy cold- and flu-causing microorganisms with a greater than normal intensity.

Since heightened immunity can last for only a short period, echinacea should be used for no longer than four days. If the need for it continues, the immune system should rest for another four days before the herb is employed once again.

Goldenseal . . . Goldenseal has powerful antiseptic qualities, enabling it to destroy a number of microorganisms, including parasites, bacteria and viruses. It has a soothing effect on mucous linings, and is therefore an excellent remedy for sore throats.

Formulas that combine goldenseal with echinacea are especially good for treating colds in progress, as well as influenza that affect the respiratory area. Like echinacea, goldenseal should be taken for short stretches of time only.

Ginger . . . Ginger is an excellent bronchial decongestant. As an expectorant, it helps clear out mucus from the bronchi due to chest colds. And unlike the foregoing herbs, ginger can be taken every day. It can be grated and taken as a tea, used in powder form, or taken in liquid extract form. One squirt of ginger extract into the mouth will clear the bronchi in a few minutes' time. This is also an excellent stomach remedy that counteracts nausea and alleviates the symptoms of stomach flu.

Green Tea . . . Green tea has great cleansing properties and should be taken throughout the day for influenza.

Slippery Elm . . . To soothe a scratchy, tired, or sore throat, or help stop a dry cough, slippery elm can be taken as a lozenge, tea, or tincture. To make the tea, pour a pint of boiled water over one ounce of powdered bark, stir, and simmer for 15 minutes.

Combination Remedy for Colds and Sore Throats . . . One teaspoon of bee propolis in a homeopathic solution is combined with extracts of red clover and licorice root. Ten drops of colloidal silver are added. Gargling with this formula and then swallowing it, every four hours, can help knock out local bacterial and viral infections in the throat and trachea.

Other Cold-Fighting Herbs . . . These herbs, taken as teas, tinctures, or capsules, also help prevent or stop colds: elderflower, elecampagne, eyebright, sage, peppermint, wood betony, angelica, yarrow, gentian, hyssop, masterwort, sarsaparilla, saw palmetto berries, horehound, usnea and lomacium.

Cold- and Flu-Fighting Nutrients

When cold season comes, it's important to keep the following nutrients in mind:

Vitamin C . . . If you find yourself craving grapefruits and oranges when you're sick, think of this as the body's call for extra vitamin C. Among its many functions, this nutrient strengthens the immune system, accelerating its ability to combat harmful substances. Bowel tolerance doses can be taken orally (this is the amount taken just before getting diarrhea), and more can be taken without this effect when administered intravenously.

Bioflavonoids . . . These water-soluble substances enhance vitamin C's protection of cells against viral and bacterial invasion. That's why bioflavonoids and vitamin C are always found together in nature. Excellent food sources of bioflavonoids include grapes, rose hips, prunes, oranges, lemon juice, cherries, black currants, plums, parsley, cabbage, apricots, peppers, papaya, cantaloupe, tomatoes, broccoli and blackberries, as well as the inside white parts of grapefruits.

Gamma-Linoleic Acid (GLA) . . . The GLA found in evening primrose oil, black currant seed oil and borage oil helps relieve fever and muscle soreness associated with the flu. It has an anti-inflammatory effect and reduces sensitivity to pain.

DHEA . . . The adrenal hormone offers immune-enhancing qualities and helps fight viruses. Supplementation of 20 mg twice a day may prove beneficial.

Zinc Gluconate . . . Two zinc gluconate lozenges (24 mg of elemental zinc per lozenge) dissolved in the mouth every few hours can help inactivate cold viruses, reducing the duration of cold symptoms.

N-acetyl-cysteine (NAC) . . . This amino acid can help expel mucus and is capable of fighting viruses directly. A dosage of 600-1200 mg of NAC can help reduce cold symptoms.

Alpha-Lipoic Acid . . . The "universal" antioxidant boosts glutathione levels. When plagued by the flu, two 250-mg capsules twice a day may support the immune system by fighting free radicals and reducing inflammation.

Shark Liver Oil . . . By boosting the production of virus-fighting cytokines, alkylglycerols make shark liver oil a potent antibacterial, antiviral, antifungal and antiparasitic force. For prevention, try supplementing with one or two capsules.

Curcumin . . . Extracted from the spice turmeric, curcumin is a powerful antioxidant that also has unique antiviral effects. The suggested dose is four 900-mg capsules with bioperin.

Melatonin . . . Apart from providing good sleep and killing free radicals, melatonin has antiviral properties. This is because of its ability to trigger T-helper-cell production. T helper cells are necessary for recognizing cancer cells, viruses, bacteria and fungi that have entered the body. Supplementation of melatonin for people with the flu is 3-20 mg before bedtime; for general maintenance, 300 mcg-6 mg is suggested.

Medicinal Mushrooms . . . Mushrooms—such as maitake, shiitake and reishi—are powerful immune boosters due to their beta-glucan content. They can combat viruses from the common cold to HIV and cancer.

Digestive Enzymes . . . Wobenzyme and Vitalzym are digestive enzyme combinations. Taken without food, they show anti-inflammatory effects, which may reduce the symptoms of a cold. Three capsules taken three times a day between meals may be effective.

Whey protein . . . By stimulating glutathione production, 2 tbsp of whey protein two times a day may support the immune system.

Garlic . . . Garlic is traditionally valued for its antiviral, antifungal and antibacterial properties. By stimulating natural killer cell production, it helps the immune system overcome conditions such as the flu.

Beta-carotene . . . Taking 200 mg of beta-carotene may help support the immune system.

Zinc . . . A dosage of 25 mg of zinc can be taken when flu symptoms appear.

Sauna

Researchers found that the only way to kill colds and flu viruses is to heat them up to 7,000 degrees Fahrenheit. An experimental treatment called microwave sauna destroyed the viruses 100 percent of the time. The only problem is that the human body cannot take heat over 100 degrees Fahrenheit. It is certain that using the sauna and steam room is a good way to avoid getting the flu. The reason is the air inhaled in the sauna is hotter than 80 degrees, and that temperature is already too hot for cold and flu viruses to survive. Even the use of a facial sauna (inhaling the steam of boiled water and vinegar vapor) can help. Also, the body heats up and sweats during aerobic exercise, resulting in greater resistance to viral diseases.

Rest

When a cold or the flu has gotten you down, lie down, if at all possible. Don't try to keep up with a strenuous workout routine. Take the day off from work or school if you can, get under the covers with a good book and a supply of fresh juice nearby, and give yourself a physical and mental stress break. You'll be giving your immune system its best fighting chance.

Homeopathy

In deciding which remedy to use, the homeopathic physician analyzes several factors, including the speed of onset of symptoms, sensation, how the patient looks and his or her mental state.

For the early stages of a cold:

Aconite or Aconitum Napellus . . . This is for the first stages of a cold or flu that appears suddenly. It is worse in dry heat and cold wind and often appears when the weather first turns chilly and people turn on the heat, causing the air to get very dry. The coldness outside combined with the dryness inside causes the sudden onset of a cold and fever. This remedy is often prescribed for robust people, as well as those who eat meat. Three 30c pellets, under the tongue, are often all that is needed to get a cold or the flu to disappear just as quickly as it materialized.

Belladonna . . . This remedy is for serious symptoms of colds, the flu, infections and sore throats that suddenly appear. If it does not take effect within a few hours, professional help should be sought.

Ferrum Phosphoricum . . . This formula is prescribed for people with weak immune systems who tend to drag, but whose actual cold and flu symptoms never fully manifest. Symptoms are vague, but uncomfortable. There might be a slight earache, a clear, runny nose, a mild sore throat, or a low-grade fever. The person tends to be anemic. Three pellets are placed under the tongue every few hours when discomfort first appears.

For colds in mid-stage:

Allium Cepa . . . People are given allium cepa when their eyes are watery and clear but their nose is red and irritated. Other symptoms include violent multiple sneezes and burning nasal discharge. A person feels worse in a warm room, and better in the fresh air. A good way to remember allium cepa is to think of the red onion from which it is derived. Onions make the eyes tear and this remedy is for watery eyes.

Euphrasia . . . Symptoms are similar to indications for allium cepa. There is a lot of sneezing. Eyes and nose have watery discharge, but here, eyes are red and swollen, not clear.

Natrum Muriaticum . . . The person has a thick, clear, fluid discharge that resembles raw egg whites. Lips are dry and cracked, with cold sores on the inside or outside of the mouth. Often the person catches a cold after suffering grief.

For advanced colds:

Arsenicum Album . . . This is for a cold or flu in its late stages with symptoms that include burning eyes and sinuses; irritation in the nose, causing sneezing; extreme chill; restlessness; weakness; fever; and exhaustion. If a cough develops, it can sink into the chest and develop into bronchitis. The person feels worse at night and better in fresh air.

Mercurius Vivus . . . Here the cold is already advanced and the immune system is weakened. There is a sore throat that feels worse with swallowing, as well as sneezing, nasal discharge, foul-smelling breath, bad cough, profuse saliva and night sweats.

Hepar Sulph . . . This mineral remedy helps deep colds and the flu when these turn into infections and sinusitis. The person may have tried antibiotic treatments, which did not help. The person is very chilly, and there is often mucus in the lungs with a thick, yellow discharge. The emotional portrait is of a person who is extremely irritable and explosive, even toward people who try to help him or her. This is because the nervous system has become affected by the infection.

For the flu:

Eupatorium Perfoliatuin . . . This remedy is made from the herb boneset, and as its name implies, it is for a flu with achiness in the limbs, muscles and bones, especially the long bones of the legs. The person has recurring fever with chills, preceded by thirst.

Nux Vomica . . . This one is important for the stomach flu. The picture here is of someone who is very chilly but who feels better in the open air. The person is worse after eating and has a dry tickling feeling in the nose and throat. Emotionally, there is extreme irritability. But the main feeling here is: If I could throw up or have a bowel movement, I would feel better. This remedy often helps the person to let go and feel much better.

Gelsemium . . . This remedy is often indicated for acute flu. A key symptom for this remedy is fever with absence of thirst.

For coughs:

Antimonium Tartaricum . . . This is important for people who have very loose, rattling sounds in their chest during or after a cold. The cough is moist and the person coughs to expel mucus but finds that it remains. This remedy helps the type of cough that elderly people get in winter, the type that lasts all season. As with the other remedies, if this one does not help, it is advisable to consult with a health professional.

Dulcamara . . . Dulcamara is needed for coughs that get worse when weather begins to turn cold and damp. It is also for coughs that come on after the feet get wet. A typical time to take dulcamara is in the autumn.

Rhumex Crispus . . . This is for a dry hacking cough that remains after a cold, particularly when the person keeps losing his or her voice. Typically it is worse in the evening and upon arising in the morning. It also worsens when the weather changes from cold to warm or vice versa.

Ignatia . . . The cold and cough for which ignatia is prescribed follow an emotional upset. The cough is tickling and irritating, and the person can cough until exhaustion.

For blocked sinuses:

Kali Bichromicum . . . This remedy is for people who exhibit thick green or yellow mucus. There is pain at the root of the nose, in between the eyes. There can also be pain in small spots in the face, which feel better when pressed.

Pulsatilla . . . Here the mucus can be blown out easily. These people usually feel better in fresh air with movement. The cold is worse in the evening or at night.

Aromatherapy

Inhaling the volatile oils of eucalyptus and thyme can relieve lung congestion in that the oils act as expectorants, helping us to cough up mucus and pollution. Other helpful oils include garlic, lemon, pine, rosemary lavender, peppermint and hyssop. Aromatherapist Valerie Cooksley author of *Aromatherapy: A Lifetime Guide to Healing with Essential Oils,* describes how to do this, through steam inhalation: Add the oil to a ceramic or glass bowl of water that is hot, but not boiling. Then close your eyes, and hold your head about eight inches from the bowl with a tent made from a towel over your head. Inhale slowly and deeply for five to 10 minutes. The process can be repeated two or three times a day, when needed.

Aromatic baths with essential oils can be helpful, too. Lavender, geranium and hyssop are recommended for this purpose. Be sure to use a carrier, such as Epsom salt, sea salt, honey, or cream. Otherwise, the oils will just float to the top.

As a preventive measure, mists of essential oils can be sprayed into our living quarters to kill harmful bacteria in the air. Oils with antiseptic qualities include lemon, orange, bergamot, citronella, eucalyptus, juniper, lemongrass, peppermint, pine, rosemary, sandalwood and tea tree oil.

Treatment Summary

Alkaline fruits and vegetables are rich in nutrients that help the body fight off colds and the flu.

Herbs have immune-enhancing properties, especially when taken at the first sign of a cold or flu.

Vitamin C, bioflavonoids and GLA strengthen the immune system, thus helping us counteract colds and the flu.

Getting enough rest is an important strategy in fighting off these illnesses.

Homeopathic remedies for alleviating colds and flu are given according to symptoms and stage of illness.

Applying pressure to points on the feet can speed up recovery.

Inhaling essential oils can help clear up congestion, and when sprayed into the air, mists of these oils have a germ-deactivating effect.

See also: Fever.

Dental Disorders

Going to the dentist is often considered an unpleasant experience. Most people associate the dentist's office with pain, jarring sounds and medical devices that contribute to patient anxiety just by virtue of their appearance. Of course, much of this apprehension is due to the many common dental problems a person will probably experience at some point in life, such as cavities, root canal problems and gum disease.

What many people do not know is that these conditions, which are commonly viewed simply as uncomfortable, anxiety-producing annoyances, can actually lead to a variety of infections in the body. The potentially harmful consequences are little known because conventional dentistry treats the mouth as if it were separate from the rest of the body. The assumption is that once the problem is corrected there is no further cause for concern. Biological or holistic dentistry on the other hand, supports the view that infections of the teeth, gums and other areas in the mouth can spread bacteria, viruses and other toxins. This can depress the immune system, which, in turn, can lead to disease.

Teeth contain tubules, and these can harbor billions of germs. These microorganisms can then spread to infect the lymph, blood and nerve networks to activate severe illnesses anywhere in the body including the heart, kidneys, joints, endocrine system, nervous system and brain. Biological dentists therefore devote part of their attention to eliminating toxic dental materials, ensuring that infections do not emerge or remain in areas where they often go unnoticed, and minimizing other stresses to the immune system. Of course, they also deal with common dental ailments.

Common Problems

Cavities

Most people experience tooth decay that begins as small holes in the teeth. When a cavity occurs, it is important to get it filled, as decay progresses and

179

can get larger, leading to more severe loss of tooth structure. However, the substances used as fillings for cavities can be harmful. The most common type of filling, which has been used for over 150 years, is the silver amalgam filling. What many people do not know is that it contains a large percentage of mercury which is a material known to be more toxic than lead. It is believed that vapors from the mercury in fillings are released at low levels and can enter the body through inhalation. The material can also be ingested, as tiny portions of the metal may dislodge.

Periodontal Disease

The first stage of periodontal, or gum, disease is gingivitis, which is an inflammation of the gum tissue due to bacterial infection. If left unattended for a long time, gingivitis can evolve into a more serious form of periodontal disease called periodontitis. In this condition, the bone underneath the gum begins to dissolve. Not only can this cause pain and eventual tooth loss, it has the capability of spreading bacterial infection to the rest of the body.

Cavitations

These are chronic infections within the jawbone. This condition is generally a result of diseased tissue or infected bone that is left after teeth have been removed. Circulation is then impeded and proper healing cannot take place. This situation can be corrected by cleaning the lesion.

Bruxism

This is the condition popularly known as grinding the teeth. It is not uncommon and it occurs most often at night. The reason this condition is a cause for concern is that when people grind their teeth, it places abnormal pressure on the teeth and on surrounding areas. This can create an environment that leads to more serious dental problems, such as toothaches, periodontal disease and infections.

Causes

Poor diet and lack of proper nutrients constitute a major reason for tooth decay infection and bruxism. All the refined foods in today's American diet, particularly sugar, fuel bacteria, and our resistance to the bacteria is at the same time lowered by the sugar, so they are able to grow and spread. Hidden food allergies, which increase chances of infection, can also be a problem.

Stress is another cause of dental disorders. It affects our bodies in a few ways. It can overactivate the adrenal glands, which allows for too much calcium in the bloodstream. That calcium is taken from bones, causing them to be weakened and damaged. Stress can also negatively impact the immune system, lowering resistance to overall infection and disease.

There are also lifestyle considerations, oral habits and environmental factors that will contribute to an increased amount of bacteria in the mouth. These include smoking, chewing tobacco, heavy metal contamination, swallowing incorrectly, biting lips or nails, breathing through the mouth, thumb sucking, chewing gum, poorly fitting bridges, crowns (caps) and chemicals such as pesticides and drugs. The teeth may also be filled with toxic metals and other dental materials, which are poisonous. Other factors in dental health include the resistance level of the individual (if it's low, infection can take hold more easily) and skeletal deformities, either congenital or due to trauma, which can necessitate dental work. In addition, electrogalvinism, electrical currents created by dissimilar metals in dental fillings and on different teeth, can create health problems.

Symptoms

When dental problems extend their effects to other parts of the body, they do so by contributing to such conditions as high blood pressure, chronic fatigue, heart problems, epilepsy, multiple sclerosis, brain tumors, arthritis, some forms of cancer (e.g., osteosarcoma and thyroid cancer), vision impairment and pain in the face, head, or joints.

The major signs of advanced cavities are pain and extreme sensitivity to heat and cold, since the nerve is more exposed. When fillings are too old, material will get worn and change shape. Teeth can break, causing fillings to fall out. Then food can wedge in the hole causing constant irritation.

Bacterial infection in the gums is characterized by bleeding, puffy gums, gum erosion at the base of the tooth and bad breath. When gum infection advances to a more serious stage, it can be marked by bone loss in addition to gum loss, toothache, loose teeth and nerve sensitivity.

Cavitations may cause no symptoms or, at the other extreme, severe discomfort. This can manifest as chronic facial pain, persistent pain in the eyes and distress in other areas of the body.

Treatment

The Conventional Approach

Drilling . . . This is usually an accepted part of several procedures used to correct a wide variety of dental problems. While drilling is helpful in removing decay, patients should be aware that it could also cause a variety of difficulties. For instance, if a drill is used improperly or at too high a speed, it can cause trauma to the tooth, resulting in inflammation and infection. As in all areas of health care, it is important to choose your dentist carefully, seeking someone recommended by satisfied patients.

Root Canal Therapy . . . This is a procedure performed to salvage a badly damaged tooth where the nerve is affected. In the root canal process, the dentist will remove the contents from the pulp chamber (nerve and other debris), and then seal the root canal space. One problem with root canal therapy is that thousands of tubules can harbor bacteria. Doing the root canal does not remove bacteria from these tubules. Further, since antibacterial drugs cannot eliminate the bacteria from the tubules in the root of the tooth, these bacteria can eventually discharge toxins into the bloodstream.

Fluoridation . . . Fluoride has generally been considered beneficial for preventing tooth decay. It is contained in toothpastes and in some communities' tap water. The problem is, though, that fluoride is actually a toxic chemical. Studies have shown that areas using fluoridated drinking water have a higher percentage of hip fracture and cancer cases among their populations than do neighborhoods with non-fluoridated water.

Prevention

We've all heard it, but it bears repeating: The best treatment for dental problems is prevention. And this starts with a good dietary foundation. To maintain a healthy mouth, make sure your meals are centered on whole fresh foods and include a high-protein breakfast. Products rich in calcium, such as milk, cheese, yogurt and green, leafy vegetables, will help to produce strong teeth. Raw fruits and vegetables are particularly important because of their ability to enhance enzyme functioning.

Supplements and Herbs . . . Vitamins E, A and D are beneficial to healthy teeth and gums, and vitamin C (500 mg four times daily) is important for gum health and will help fight plaque. In order to properly fortify the bone, which is the foundation of the teeth, the following are suggested: silica and zinc, to ensure adequate bone formation; manganese, to maintain the ligaments that surround the teeth; and magnesium and calcium, which are crucial to ensuring the strength of the bones. Potassium, selenium, phosphorus and iron are nutrients that also support the system. Essential fatty acids, including EPA and DHA, are also beneficial because they facilitate the transport of calcium and magnesium through the cell membrane. Other recommended supplements include bioflavonoids and coenzyme Q10 (100 mg per day), which aid in cellular respiration; garlic and chlorella, which neutralize and eliminate some of the contaminating heavy metals and strengthen the immune system; and GLA, which enhances prostaglandin production and possesses anti-inflammatory cytokines.

Taking a vitamin B complex daily, L-glutathione two times per day and grapefruit seed extract three times a day helps combat gum disease. Folic acid could be supplemented (800 mcg a day) or used in a solution as a mouth rinse to fight infections and combat periodontal disease. Also good are herbal preparations, mouth rinse and toothpaste containing the following herbs: bloodroot, which prevents bacteria from sticking to newly formed plaque; the anti-inflammatory calendula, for swollen gums; and goldenseal, which contains berberine, myrrh and tea tree oil, and that has antibiotic qualities. In addition, sage oil, chamomile and caraway oil can be used. The supplementation of an herbal formula containing rose hips, bilberry and sea buckthorn supports the immune system and assists in fighting infections due to its antioxidant properties. A combination of herbal and vegetable oils—such as rosehip seed oil, borage oil, black currant seed oil, grape seed oil, evening primrose oil, wheat germ oil, natural vitamin E oil, plantain oil extract, carrot seed oil, essential oil of lemon, laurel, caraway and fennel—might stop gum bleeding and promote restorative functions.

Proper Dental Hygiene . . . Tooth brushing should be made a part of any daily routine. And one should not forget to include the tongue in the brushing routine. The tongue houses germs that can cause dental problems, and rinses are not generally effective against these bacteria. It is recommended that a person brush gently with baking soda as it is a germ-fighter. A paste consisting of 3 parts pharmaceutical-grade baking soda, 1 part BioSalt, and 1 part ionic/colloidal silver, can be applied where the gum meets the tooth (sulcus). Use a vibrating motion of the toothbrush. This combination can neutralize the acid environment in the sulcus and can keep harmful bacteria away; the bacteria don't like oxygen or silver water.

One of the most effective toothpaste combinations consists of calcium carbonate baking soda, silica, myrrh extract, peppermint oil, anise oil, menthol crystals, eucalyptus oil, clove oil, echinacea, organic tea tree oil, aloe vera gel, calendula, bloodroot, bee propolis and grapefuit seed extract. A mouthwash containing 1½-percent food-grade hydrogen peroxide, clove oil, menthol, spring water, cchinacea, goldenseal, aloe, grapefruit seed extract, cherry essence, tea tree oil, vitamin C, essential oil of spearmint, olive leaf and xylitol has extremely powerful natural antiseptic qualities and inhibits bacteria build up, thus eliminating bad breath.

Brushing the teeth with an electric toothbrush could be twice as effective in removing plaque. Just remember, don't brush too long or too hard. The ideal approach to using an electric toothbrush is a light touch for two minutes. Additionally, flossing and cleaning with a hydromagnetic oral irrigator should be done on a regular basis, since these techniques can get to the plaque between teeth, where brushing can't. Massaging the gums using a stimulator with a rubber tip can help with circulation in the gum tissue. One should also remember that regular professional cleanings in a dental office are imperative, since they can better remove the hardened material around the teeth. The dentist can also check to see if there are any emerging problems in order to prevent their worsening.

Biological Dentistry

If a problem already exists, there are many treatments that can be considered. In the case of cavities, both conventional and holistic dentists, biological dentists will agree that fillings need to be placed. However, given the potentially harmful effects of the silver amalgam filling, it is important to discuss the other options available with the dentist. Biological dentistry will ensure that the patient receives the type of filling that is best suited to his or her needs. The dentist will test the patient for biocompatibility of the materials that are to be used. Often, people have several types of metals in their mouth, from fillings, crowns and other dental work. Dissimilar metals in the mouth can block energy and incite illnesses in the body. Therefore, ensuring that the metals in the mouth are compatible is an important practice that most conventional dentists do not perform.

With regard to infection and inflammation, conventional dentistry will tend to focus on cleaning and removing the bacteria and their source. The affected tooth may be removed so that infection doesn't persist and negatively impact the immune system. While these surgical treatments are often necessary, the holistic dentist also stresses consideration of natural solutions, either in addition to or instead of conventional treatments. The relation of the mouth to the rest of the body is a main tenet of biological dentistry.

Homeopathic Dental Remedies

Aconite . . . A dosage of 30-200c can be given to a person for an abrupt rush of intense pain (commonly due to cold air). Aconite can also be used for panic, fright and general restlessness.

Apis Mellifica . . . This remedy helps decrease inflammation after injection, and is usually given in 30c potency three times a day.

Arnica . . . This can be used after trauma in general, particularly where there is bleeding. Specifically, it is a good remedy for drilling. The recommended potency for arnica is 30c.

Arsenica Album . . . This is used in doses of 6-30c for delicate, bleeding gums or a toothache that is alleviated by warm water.

Belladonna . . . This is prescribed for early dental abscess characterized by redness and irritation in dosages of 30-200c. It is also beneficial for the pain associated with bruxism.

Calendula . . . This topical solution can be used as a general disinfectant to heal injuries and reduce pain. (However, to guard against closing the wound before the infection has had time to drain, it should not be applied where an infection exits on broken skin.) It can also be used as a mouthwash.

Coffea Cruda . . . This has a tranquilizing effect and is often used for a toothache that gets worse with heat but is relieved by cold water or ice. It can be given in doses of 30-200c.

Ferrum Phosphoricum . . . Given in doses of 12-30c, this medicine is used for throbbing pain or gums that bleed after brushing.

Hepar Sulphuris . . . Cases of ulcerated infection benefit from this remedy.

Hypericum . . . This is another good remedy for trauma, particularly for easing sharp pain associated with tender gum tissue. Not only does hypericum decrease pain and swelling, it fosters the regeneration of disjoined nerves. It is given at a 30c potency.

Mercurius Solubilis . . . This is used for festering gum tissue, indicated by a coated tongue and bad taste in the mouth.

Staphysagria . . . This is good after surgery or incision wounds.

Silica . . . This is used to drain out an acute abscess.

Other Approaches

Also, an herbal preparation that works to minimize inflammation is a paste consisting of a bit of myrrh and peppermint oil combined with goldenseal root powder. Place directly on the infected area.

Acupuncture can be used in dental treatment; research shows that this ancient technique is effective in relieving pain after dental surgery.

What to Avoid

It's most important that sugar and sugary foods be eliminated from the diet (particularly soft drinks which can remove calcium from the teeth). The consumption of processed foods should be restricted, and it is also important to refrain from alcohol, caffeine and diuretics.

Treatment Summary

To prevent dental problems, eat a good diet consisting of whole, fresh foods and products rich in calcium. Consider taking a variety of vitamin and mineral supplements and using the herbal extract aloe vera as a mouthwash. Practice proper dental hygiene, including brushing with baking soda and hydrogen peroxide, flossing and getting regular cleanings by the dentist.

Biological dentistry warns about the use of silver amalgam fillings and supports checking the biocompatibility of metals in the mouth in order to determine the right filling substance for a particular person. For infection and inflammation, conventional dentistry normally chooses to remove the bacteria and possibly remove the tooth.

A paste of myrrh, peppermint oil and goldenseal root can be placed directly on an infected area to minimize inflammation.

Acupuncture is effective in relieving pain after dental surgery.

Homeopathic remedies can be used in dental treatment.

See also: Periodontal Disease.

Depression

There is virtually no person who is immune to depression. Becoming depressed is a normal response to certain situations that arise as part of our daily lives. However, when low or blue feelings hinder our normal functioning in society for an extended amount of time, they can be classified as a clinical depression requiring some type of treatment.

The incidence of depression has risen dramatically over the past several years; the condition affects over 30 million Americans. Its impact can range from mild—suggesting that the affected individual has the ability to defeat the illness through a variety of self-care techniques—to severe, a state that requires attention from a trained medical professional.

Depression can actually be classified as one of the three types. Reactive depression is a consequence of a painful or anxiety-producing incident, such as the death of a loved one, the loss of a job, or an illness, or family or relationship crisis. This is the most common type of depressive disorder, one that can affect anyone at any time of his or her life. A person suffering from a reactive depression generally displays a loss of interest in those things that used to provide pleasure, but is usually still able to function at a basic level.

A physically based depression originates from an imbalance of chemicals in the brain. This type of depression tends to affect people after midlife, although this is by no means always the case. There may be a genetic predisposition to this type of illness. It is characterized by a severe loss of interest or pleasure in almost everything, and the condition has the capacity to negatively impact normal everyday functioning in a significant way.

The last major type of depression, also physically based, is manic depression. This is manifested as severe mood swings. A person with manic depression will fluctuate between periods of extreme energy and vivacity and those of complete hopelessness.

Regardless of how the disease originates, the way it manifests itself, or the degree of severity, depression should generally be considered both a mind and a body disorder. Both realms should certainly be addressed when planning treatment.

Causes

When depression is externally caused, any type of extremely distressing situation may trigger it. Simply being exposed to depressed people can even be an influence, since children learn by imitation. While these are normal reactions, the condition can perpetuate itself when it affects the internal workings of the body, preventing the person from overcoming his or her pain. When it persists, the condition becomes clinical depression.

There are a number of nutritional factors that can affect a person's mood, contributing to depression. Vitamin deficiencies can play a part. The B vitamins are clearly related to the healthy maintenance of the brain. The level of folic acid, in particular, bears an inverse correlation to the severity of depression: the lower the level of folic acid in the blood, the higher the degree of depression. The mineral magnesium is also a substance found to be deficient in depressed people. Large amounts of fluoride, on the other hand, may lead to the onset of depression. These types of nutritional factors should not be surprising, even in the case of reactive depression. Once depressed, the person might lose interest in exercising and eating healthfully—or eating at all. Furthermore, the person may be under a great deal of stress, which not only perpetuates poor eating habits but also causes the more rapid loss of important nutrients.

Chemical imbalances in the brain can also be either the cause or effect of depression. Dopamine is the chemical that produces anxiety stress, nervousness and aggression. When the level of dopamine is elevated, a person may develop feelings of insecurity, paranoia and fear. Serotonin is another important chemical in the brain that can affect a person's mental well-being. Individuals with low serotonin levels are usually controlled personalities who display mood swings and some sort of compulsion, such as alcoholism, overeating, or being a workaholic, perfectionist, or procrastinator. A serotonin imbalance can produce not only depression but also internal anger.

Depression can also be linked to other physical factors, such as hypothyroidism and food or environmental allergies.

Symptoms

Depression is manifested both physically and emotionally. The classic physical signs of depression are headaches, fatigue, digestive problems, hyperactivity, sleeping disorders (these can be difficulty in falling or staying asleep or the need for an inordinate amount of sleep), loss of concentration and distorted eating patterns—either the urge to consistently overeat or loss of appetite. A significant change in weight is often evident. The emotional side of depression can include excessive crying, pessimism, a sense of worthlessness, guilt, or self-pity, loss of self-esteem, loss of enjoyment from normally pleasurable activities, decrease in sex drive and suicidal tendencies. It is important to note that anyone who talks of suicide should be taken seriously and professional help should be provided.

While many of the physical and emotional symptoms of depression are things that can be a normal part of everyday life, when several of these symptoms are experienced for any prolonged length of time (a few weeks or more), they may be an indication of depression, and, again, professional help should be sought.

Treatment

The conventional medical approach to depression is either drug therapy, psychotherapy, or a combination of the two. Drug therapy—antidepressants such as Prozac—can help people feel better, but there are negative side effects to these drugs, and we do not know the ramifications of long-term use. And while psychotherapy is a good outlet for depressive emotions, and may help some patients, it is also important to treat the body as well as the mind.

Natural approaches that treat both the mind and body gently are another avenue to try. Powerful, long-term results have been shown with these. Further, it's always a good idea not just to treat symptoms, but rather to focus on overcoming fundamental causes of a condition and to shore up long-term physical and mental health. Most importantly, a depressed person should speak with his or her doctor, as every individual's situation and needs are unique.

Exercise

Activity is not only an important factor in preventing depression; it can help people overcome it. Exercise can increase a person's energy level with lasting effect. As a result, the individual is left with a feeling of revitalization and accomplishment. The biggest problem in introducing any type of exercise regimen into a depressed person's routine is overcoming the difficulty of getting started. When one is depressed, it is very hard to begin any type of activity; the tendency is rather to withdraw. One suggestion, then, in getting started in an exercise routine is to begin with simple movements. First, just getting out of bed and going for a walk can start to afford the person a sense of well-being. Mild stretching exercises and active hobbies are also a way to introduce exercise into a person's life. As the activity begins to positively affect the mind and body it can then be increased to a level and type appropriate for that individual.

Diet

Getting the proper amounts of amino acids in the system is very important. Therefore, the type of foods one should concentrate on are fresh raw vegetables and a balance of protein foods. Complex carbohydrates are particularly important for the individual who has a low serotonin level. A problem in getting the depressed person to eat healthfully is to overcome the feeling of not wanting to be bothered thinking about diet or not having the energy to prepare a nutritious meal. One suggestion is to make easy meals in quantity once a week. A large amount of salad, for instance, can be stored in the refrigerator. This will help an individual to eat wholesome food for several days without too much fuss.

Supplements

Nutritional status plays a key role in how we feel emotionally, and there are many recommended supplements one can take to optimize that. It is essential to get all the B-complex vitamins, since they work together to balance proper brain functioning. In addition, take 400 mcg of folic acid, another B vitamin, individually, in cases of deficiency, which could lead to elevated homocysteine levels. The essential fatty acids, such as omega-6 and omega-3, as well as magnesium and niacin, are of particular importance. Note, though, that niacin dosages and the length of time it should be taken will need to be carefully monitored, as this nutrient can impact liver functioning. Vitamin C is important as an immune-enhancing antioxidant. It is also significant in the production of serotonin, as well as to SAMe (S-adenosylmethinine), a natural substance in the body. Low SAMe levels in the brain are associated with depression.

SAMe is present in every cell and is a precursor for glutathione, coenzyme A, cysteine, taurine and other essential compounds. Supplementation of SAMe can have a fast-acting antidepressant effect. The suggested dosage ranges from 400-1600 mg. It is recommended that one raise the dose gradually.

To combat depression, 5-hydroxytryptophan, a needed component in serotonin production, may be helpful. It is more popular in Europe, where it's prescribed along with carbidopa, a decarboxylase inhibitor, which prevents 5-HTP from converting into serotonin before it reaches the brain. Serotonin conversion in the blood can lead to excess serotonin levels, which are dangerous in cases of coronary artery disease (when the brain would not be adequately supplied with proper levels of serotonin).

In cases of low DHEA hormone levels, natural rebalancing could improve depression. DHEA, the precursor for estrogen and testosterone, can enhance mood and help menopausal women have a better sense of well-being. The suggested dose is 15-75 mg a day. Supplementation should be decided and monitored by a health practitioner.

The critical sex hormone progesterone tends to decline after age 25. Deficiency can cause premenstrual discomfort, night sweats, hot flashes, anxiety and depression. Natural progesterone cream applied to the skin, to the soft tissue areas—such as the chest, breast, inner thighs and underarms—has the advantage of bypassing the liver and going directly to specific places on the body.

Low levels of the hormone pregnenolone, produced by the adrenal glands, are also associated with depression. The dose of 50-200 mg could improve one's ability to handle stress. Due to hormonal changes, free testosterone levels might also drop, which would cause a person to have a passive attitude, general tiredness and other unwanted symptoms of depression. Lots of problems can be solved with the natural replacement of testosterone. In some people, 1000 mg of the amino acid acetyl-L-carnitine twice a day alleviated depression. In other cases, 5-10 mg of NADH (nicotinamideadenine dinucleotide) had a similar effect. Evidence suggests that supplementing with the precursors of neurotransmitters has therapeutic effects in treating depression. Tyrosine and phenylalanine (amino acids that are precursors to dopamine and norepinephrine) should be taken.

DMAE (dimethylaminoethanol) is a nutrient found in sardines. It is a powerful brain stimulant that increases acetylcholine, which is also a neurotransmitter involved in regulating mood and energy levels. The suggested dosage ranges from 300-900 mg. Choline is also involved in the production of acetylcholine, which is important in memory and learning. A dosage of 2000 mg could be supplemented in divided doses, or it could be obtained from food, such as brewer's yeast and soybeans. The potassium in bananas and peas—and 1000 mg twice a day of inositol, a relative of the vitamin B family—can also alleviate depression. Vitamin D at a dosage of 400 IU a day can improve the all-too-familiar winter blues.

Social and Lifestyle Factors

Trying to persuade a despondent person out of his mood may be futile. However, distracting the depressed mind has proven beneficial. Interaction with other people is extremely important for a depressed person because it can get his or her mind off negative thoughts. In particular, doing things for other people, such as volunteer work, is a great way to get a depressed person out of his own dark thoughts and into something that will feel rewarding.

Herbs

There are herbal extracts that have properties similar to those of the conventional antidepressant drugs, but that are gentler and without the drugs' side effects. Prime among these is St. John's wort, which is very popular in Europe. Clinical double-blind, placebo-controlled studies exist to support the efficacy of St. John's wort. Ginkgo biloba helps with the circulation of the brain and protects nerve cells; hence, it is promising in depression treatment. Ginger, due to its adaptogenic qualities, helps with rebalancing the system. Also consider valerian, skullcap, hops, kava kava root, passionflower, Chinese schizandra berry, wild oats and calamus root.

Light Therapy

According to Dr. Michael Norden, author of *Beyond Prozac,* light therapy has shown positive results in overcoming mild depression associated with the winter season (called seasonal affective disorder, or SAD). The body chemistry of many individuals is thrown off by the decrease in the amount of daylight during this time. But treatments have been designed that utilize bright light to overcome this kind of depression. One of the newest treatments is called dawn simulation. A special lighting system in the bedroom is manipulated to mimic the sunrise. This technique has been proven to increase energy and help overcome difficulty in getting out of bed during this time of year.

Homeopathic Remedies

The following are the most common homeopathic treatments for acute, more temporary cases of depression. In cases of chronic depression, homeopathic remedies, while still beneficial, will need to be utilized in conjunction with other therapies. Always work with a qualified health care professional.

Aurum Metallicum . . . This remedy is prescribed by homeopaths to alleviate feelings of worthlessness, low self-esteem and despair. It can help provide hope for a person with reactive depression, and is said to be particularly beneficial to those generally hardworking individuals who have had life-altering events that they feel suggest failure on their part. This type of person is usually idealistic and goal-oriented.

Ignatia . . . In instances of depression caused by an event that produces profound sadness or grief, such as the loss of a loved one, and in which those feelings of deep sorrow are obvious, ignatia is prescribed.

Natrum Muriaticum . . . This treatment, like ignatia, is also used when depression is caused by an event that generates profound bereavement and distress. However, the difference is that this one is used for those individuals who cannot show their feelings. This is for people who appear strong and controlled and suffer in silence.

Sepia . . . This remedy is used mainly for women going through menopause. While depression associated with menopause often appears and disappears at random, or for no apparent reason, the depression the woman feels is quite real and intense. She may feel disconnected from everything that once gave her pleasure, including family and friends. This type of depression can be characterized by irritability and indifference to others.

Pulsatilla . . . This is generally used for people who show signs of manic depression.

Other Options

Depressed people are typically withdrawn and physically inactive. Exercise boosts circulation and promotes a sense of well-being, leaving the person feeling more energetic and ambitious. Relaxation techniques, such as yoga and meditation, help a person better cope with stress. Aromatherapy, with its knowledge accumulated over thousands of years, can rebalance people. Suggested essential oils are lavender, basil, jasmine, rose, bergamot, sandalwood, neroli (oil of the orange blossom), ylang-ylang, marjoram, clary sage and chamomile. These can be used in baths or inhaled. Applying essential oils directly to the skin is not recommended; they should be mixed with carrier oils.

Art forms—such as music, dramatic arts and visual art—give individuals a chance to voice the suppressed feelings, fear, anxiety and uncertainty that may be the underlying reason for their depression.

Realizing that our environment tremendously affects us, we can see the value of feng shui, an ancient Chinese way of rearranging surrounding objects. In feng shui, every little detail matters: colors, shapes and materials all have a certain energy that can bring our mood up or down. Feng shui restores the flow of the life energy, the qi. Clutter in the workplace or home usually results in confusion, unclear thinking and frustration, and is clearly depressing. For instance, the fiery colors of red, pink and purple suggest dynamic attitude; green soothes the soul. We can say that our environment is a reflection and extension of our emotional, spiritual and intellectual state—that it mirrors our focus and tells a lot about our relationships. Adjusting these factors can have a miraculous effect in fighting and overcoming depression.

What to Avoid

Our diet not only plays an important role in good health, it can also negatively impact emotions and result in depression. The following foods should be avoided to prevent a nutritional or chemical imbalance that could cause or contribute to depression: fast foods, simple carbohydrates (this is particularly important for people with low blood sugar), alcohol, artificial sweeteners, white flour products and caffeine.

Treatment Summary

Psychotherapy may be helpful, but it should be used in conjunction with other approaches in order to address both the mind and the body.

Traditional drug therapy while common, can produce negative side effects and tends to treat symptoms rather than causes of depression, something that is important for the long term.

Exercise can increase a person's energy level and produce feelings of revitalization and accomplishment. A person who is having difficulty getting started can begin with simple movements. Once the effect of the activity is felt, it can be increased to a level and type appropriate for that individual.

A diet centered on raw, fresh vegetables and fruits, and a balance of proteins is recommended to ensure that the proper amounts of amino acids necessary for proper brain functioning are being ingested. Complex, rather than simple, carbohydrates (like sugar), should be the focus.

B-complex vitamins, niacin and magnesium are important in preventing and overcoming depression.

Interaction with others may help to overcome depression. Volunteer work, in particular, can help distract the person, as well as get him or her into something rewarding.

Some herbs have effects similar to those of antidepressant drugs, without drug side effects. St. John's wort is widely used in Europe for this purpose, and double-blind studies have supported this herb's antidepressant effect. People have also had success with valerian, skullcap, hops, passionflower, Chinese schizandra berry wild oats and calamus root.

Light therapy can aid in the mild depression associated with the winter season.

The homeopathic remedies aurum metallicum, ignatia, natrum muriaticum, sepia and pulsatilla are used for cases of acute temporary depression.

Diabetes

Diabetes mellitus affects 14 million Americans and claims over a quarter of a million lives each year. The problem has grown increasingly worse, with a threefold increase in the past three years. The escalation in diabetes corresponds to a rise in heart disease, and both conditions have been associated with a greater concentration of refined carbohydrates in Western diets.

Diabetes is traditionally viewed as a failure of the pancreas to release enough insulin for sugar metabolism (insulin is the hormone needed to move sugar out of the blood and into tissues). Newer thinking in the field sees an insulin deficiency as but one of three possible causes, the other two being insulin resistance and insulin insensitivity.

Juvenile diabetes, also known as type I, is generally characterized by a true insulin deficiency. This most serious form of the disease is believed to affect children and teenagers after their pancreas has been damaged from viral infections or extreme toxicity. It may also be genetically acquired. Juvenile diabetics must receive insulin regularly and generally for life.

In most adult-onset, or type II, diabetes, the body produces sufficient insulin, but the cells do not respond to it. Normally, insulin enters the cells at points known as receptor sites. When receptor sites become clogged up by fat and cholesterol they become insensitive to insulin, and insulin cannot enter cells. Glucose remains in the blood, creating a condition of hyperglycemia or high blood sugar. This excess sugar is diagnosed as diabetes. In this scenario, there is a need to increase insulin sensitivity; taking more insulin will not accomplish this.

Insulin resistance is a closely related concept in which there is also sufficient insulin. Here, allergic responses to specific foods keep insulin from doing its job by disturbing carbohydrate metabolism. The foods creating the problem vary from person to person. Wheat may create high blood sugar in one individual, while corn may adversely affect someone else. Allergy-provoking foods can be determined on an individual basis with food allergy tests.

Adult-onset diabetes is much more common than the juvenile type. It tends to be an acquired disease, precipitated by overweight, poor diet and lack of exercise. It may also be caused by frequently eaten foods in the diet that result in insulin resistance. Most of these cases can be controlled by addressing biochemical and nutritional needs.

The beginning stages of type II diabetes are often asymptomatic, although the prediabetic state can be accompanied by obesity, especially around the waistline. Classic diabetes symptoms are more often experienced by type I sufferers and include frequent urination, especially at night, great thirst and hunger, fatigue, weight loss, irritability and restlessness. As diabetes progresses, the eyes, kidneys, nervous system and skin become affected, and infections and hardening of the arteries can develop. In type I diabetes, a coma can result from the lack of insulin.

Treatment

Conventional Medical Approaches

After its discovery in the 1920s, insulin was deemed a miracle cure. Indeed, it has prevented suffering and saved countless lives. Before that, diabetics were given a bleak prognosis and suffered terribly from disease complications such as blindness, gout and gangrene. Insulin has extended the lifespan of childhood diabetics from months to decades. Today, many diabetic children live normal, productive lives.

The problem with insulin is that it is prescribed universally, not just to those with true insulin deficiencies. Giving this hormone to a person with already sufficient levels does nothing to correct the underlying problem. Furthermore, its use can be counterproductive. This is because insulin stimulates the development of antagonists in the body that counteract its blood-sugar-lowering effects. When a diabetic receives too much insulin, and his or her blood sugar falls too low, the body immediately responds with an output of growth hormones and epinephrine. These hormones keep blood sugar levels elevated. The result of overly aggressive insulin therapy then, is a rebound effect.

Constant fluctuations in blood sugar can lead to a wide range of disorders. Another problem with diabetes is that it may contribute to inner arterial wall damage and lead to cardiovascular problems. In fact, the incidence of heart attacks and strokes is five to eight times greater among diabetics than in the general population. Seventy-five percent of all diabetic mortality is due to heart disease brought on by hardening of the major arteries.

Other complications from diabetes are the result of damage to microvascular vessels, particularly those leading to the eyes, kidneys and peripheral nerves.

As these arteries become thick and brittle, it is more difficult for blood to pass through them, and they become less functional. In the eyes, sudden surges of blood sugar put extra stress on the retinal blood vessels. The repeated stresses that diabetics often experience cause these vessels to hemorrhage and break down. After several hemorrhages, blindness is a likely outcome. Following glaucoma this is the second most common cause of blindness in older people. In the kidneys, similar events can cause renal insufficiency, so that nitrogen wastes can no longer be eliminated from the body efficiently. Interference with blood circulation in both large and small vessels is responsible for the high incidence of neuritis and gangrene, which begins with peripheral sensations of tingling and ends with loss of feeling. A frequent outcome of this problem is amputation.

Insulin is not the only diabetic treatment of choice in orthodox medicine; there is also a group of oral medications that stimulate insulin secretion. Some of these drugs increase the sensitivity of receptor sites so that there are more locations for glucose to enter the cell.

In spite of their seeming benefits, oral agents, with names such as Orinase, Diabinase and Tolinase, are a cause for concern because of their potential for adverse side effects. Most worrisome is an increased susceptibility to heart attacks. Diabetes, itself, makes a person more prone to heart disease, and diabetic drugs add to the likelihood of this event.

Orthodox medicine also pays some attention to dietary modification, but again it may be missing the mark. In addition, allergic responses to foods are not taken into account.

Unlike simple sugars, complex carbohydrates may be beneficial to diabetics. Although both are broken down into glucose, the latter do not go directly into the bloodstream. Complex carbohydrates go through a long digestive process, and release sugar into the blood gradually. Rather than contribute to high blood sugar levels, complex carbohydrates stabilize blood sugar levels and improve health.

Diabetics are advised to eat high-protein diets, which can cause several additional problems, especially when protein is derived from animal sources. Foods rich in animal proteins tend to be high in fat, making the person more prone to cardiovascular disease. Receptor sites become clogged from fat and cholesterol, leading to greater insulin resistance. The inevitable rise in blood sugar results in the prescription of more medicine. Too much protein is also related to kidney damage. Since protein cannot be stored by the body, it needs to be immediately processed. A high-protein diet stresses nephron cells, causing diabetics to suffer from kidney deterioration. Many patients must receive dialysis or a kidney transplant as a result.

Natural Approaches

Diabetes is often reversible with the aid of a healthy lifestyle, diet, supplements and exercise. When making these types of changes, it is important not to immediately stop taking any medication. Instead, a complementary physician should assist in the transition, which should be a gradual one. With a doctor's guidance, an insulin dependency may be reduced or completely eliminated. While type II diabetes responds most dramatically to such an approach, juvenile diabetes may improve as well, with patients needing less insulin and experiencing fewer complications.

Diet . . . Since diabetes and heart disease are so closely related, many complementary physicians recommend that diabetics follow the same type of low-fat diet used by heart patients. This diet consists of organic vegetarian foods, with lots of high-fiber vegetables eaten raw, sprouted, steamed, baked, or stir fried with little or no oil. The addition of bran and other forms of fiber will pull the extra sugar out of the system. Diabetics, as well as people prone to the disease, produce too much insulin in response to carbohydrates, so that many of the following foods should be completely omitted until insulin reactions normalize: bread, pasta, potatoes, rice, corn, parsnips, bananas, raisins and other sweet fruits and vegetables. Good protein sources include organic turkey, chicken, egg whites and tofu. The ratio of carbohydrates to proteins to fats should be around 40:30:30.

Exercise . . . An exercise regimen is crucial for burning calories and normalizing metabolism, and is especially important for overweight adults who tend to be inactive. Exercise also heightens the body's sensitivity to insulin. By lowering cholesterol, exercise lowers triglyceride levels in the blood, making cells more available for glucose assimilation. This is why the insulin requirements of diabetic athletes always drop while they are engaged in swimming, soccer and other sports. Conversely athletes notice an increase in their insulin requirements when they cease their physical activities for any extended period.

Athletes are not the only ones to benefit from exercise. Ten to 20 minutes of light exercise after each meal helps to reduce the amount of insulin necessary to keep blood sugar levels under control. A brisk walk gets the body metabolism working a little bit faster so that the absorption of food becomes more efficient. That prevents blood sugar from rising too high.

An exception to the exercise-after-meals rule is for diabetics with heart disease. In these patients, exercising after eating may precipitate an angina attack because of the transfer of blood from the intestines to the legs and other parts of the body.

Allergy Testing . . . When allergies are the root of an insulin-resistance problem, testing for food allergies can be quite helpful. To determine whether a specific food is causing hyperglycemia, a doctor can monitor a patient's blood sugar before and after that food is eaten, looking for abnormal blood sugar rises. Once allergy-provoking substances are identified and omitted, the patient with insulin resistance can often reverse his or her condition.

Eliminating allergens may also lead to weight loss. People tend to crave allergy-producing foods, but when these foods are taken out of the diet, the desire for them stops.

Nutritional Supplements . . . The most important mineral for diabetes may be vanadyl sulfate. Discovered in France in the late 1800s, vanadyl sulfate was used to control diabetes before insulin was developed. It is generally taken three times a day. Other important minerals are chromium picolinate (200-600 mcg daily), elemental magnesium (500 mg daily) and potassium, all of which help normalize glucose levels in insulin-dependent diabetics. Also, zinc is essential for normal insulin production. Using alpha-lipoic acid, the universal antioxidant, has several advantages: It neutralizes free radicals in both the watery and the fatty portions of the cells, plus it inhibits blood glucose accumulation in the blood. If supplied with other antioxidants, a typical dose consists of 250-500 mg. However, for diabetic patients, it could be in the range of 600-1800 mg.

Primagedine can improve the inflammation or degeneration of peripheral nerves (neuropathy) and can prevent retinopathy (the diabetes-linked eye disorder caused by the elevated pressure in the blood vessels of the eye). To protect against cataract formation and neuropathy, a dosage of 500-1000 mg of acetyl-L-carnitine is advised. This may also inhibit cardiomyopathy, a process that partially replaces the heart tissue with fibrous material, resulting in difficulty in the blood flow. Coenzyme Q10, apart from being a powerful antioxidant, has the ability to trigger beta-cell function and enhance glycemic control, thus lessening the chance of heart damage. The suggested dosage is 100-300 mg daily.

In weight management, conjugated linoleic acid (CLA), a naturally occurring fatty acid, can play an important role. It can help lower and maintain body fat by increasing energy expenditure. A daily dose of 3000-4000 mg is suggested. N-acetyl-cysteine has the ability to protect pancreatic beta cells against glucose toxicity. Supplementation with 600 mg of NAC could restore blood glucose levels to normal. Low levels of the master hormone DHEA is linked to insulin resistance. DHEA deficiency impacts insulin's ability to regulate blood glucose. When you restore the DHEA levels back to normal, you may bring the high glucose levels back to normal. Supplementing with 15-75 mg daily just may accomplish this. Because DHEA can change into testosterone or estrogen, men with prostate cancer and women with estrogen-dependent cancer need to get their doctor's approval first.

The antioxidant flavonoid sylimarin (extracted from the herb milk thistle) can lower glucose. A specific type of sylimarin called silibinin can inhibit kidney damage related to diabetes. Vitamin C at a dose of 1-3 g cannot only reduce oxidative stress and inhibit glycation, but it can also support the capillaries and accelerate wound healing. To maintain healthy cell membranes, it is beneficial to take essential fatty acids: 900 mg of GLA from borage oil or evening primrose oil, and 500 mg of EPA and 1300 mg of DHA from fish oil. These omega-3 and omega-6 fatty acids are in herring, mackerel, salmon, fresh tuna and walnuts, or you can obtain the same amounts by supplementing.

Vitamin E has antidiabetic effects. By enhancing insulin sensitivity, it supports the immune system against oxidative stress. A dosage of 400-1200 IU of gamma tocopherol can prevent inflammation-induced complications. A dosage of 10 mg of vitamin K can help control the glucose levels.

The extract from bilberry can reduce blood glucose levels. The recommended dosage is 100-200 mg three times a day. To help utilize glucose, 800-1600 mcg of biotin should be used. In addition, 25 g of fiber is suggested for people on diets: it makes you feel fullness, extends the mealtime and inhibits overeating. Some examples of high-fiber foods are cantaloupe, grapefruit, raisins, papaya, sweet potato, oat bran and oatmeal.

Herbs . . . Dandelion root and eyebright cleanse the liver and blood, which indirectly helps treat diabetes.

Blueberry (also known as huckleberry) leaves are known to promote insulin production. Unlike many other medicinal herbs, blueberry tea is actually pleasant tasting. If you gather the leaves yourself (they grow all over the state of Pennsylvania), it's best to pick them before the fruit appears, or after it's gone. Otherwise, the berries absorb the strength of the plant.

By increasing circulation, ginkgo biloba can alleviate symptoms associated with diabetes, such as intermittent claudication and problems with the eyes.

The herbs banaba and ampalaya have great antidiabetic effects. They support weight loss and help the body handle glucose.

Other herbs that can help diabetes and other pancreatic problems include pau d'arco, cedar berries, aloe, ginger, burdock, evening primrose, false unicorn root, onion, juniper berries, cranberry, fenugreek, goldenseal, alfalfa and kelp. These herbs are safe to take along with any preexisting medications, and are especially good to take before pharmaceuticals are prescribed.

Homeopathy . . . The remedy Mucokehl from Germany may actually reverse diabetic neuropathy. People have reported getting feeling back in their extremities, as well as eyesight improvement, with this medicine.

Chelation Therapy . . . This is helpful for its ability to reduce diabetic retinopathy and foot ulcers.

What to Avoid

Diabetics need to reduce their sugar intake and increase dietary fiber. Among its many detrimental effects, sugar works to lower chromium levels. As levels of this mineral drop, pressure in the eye increases. This can cause vision problems in diabetics.

Treatment Summary

Diabetics often do well on the same type of high-fiber, low-fat diet as heart patients are given, with a carbohydrate: protein: fat ratio of 40:30:30.

Exercise can help correct a sluggish metabolism, normalize weight and keep blood sugar under control.

It is essential to identify and omit allergy-producing foods from the diet.

Minerals that can help correct blood sugar imbalance are vanadyl sulfate, chromium picolinate, magnesium and potassium. Supplementation of carnosine, acetyl-L-carnitine, N-acetyl-cysteine, coenzyme Q10, the master hormone DHEA and vitamins C, E, and K may restore glucose to healthy levels in the blood.

The homeopathic remedy Mucokehl may help those with diabetic neuropathy to restore feeling in the extremities and improve eyesight.

Chelation therapy increases blood circulation to the microcapillaries in the eyes and extremities.

Digestive Disorders

One could call digestive disorders a virtual epidemic in this country, because they affect over two-thirds of all Americans. Dr. Kenneth Bock, of Rinebeck, New York, refers to many of his patients as the walking wounded. While these people are well enough to lead normal lives, they are not functioning at an optimal level. Their early symptoms, though minor, indicate that the digestive system is unable to fully perform its job of converting food to energy and carrying nutrients to other systems.

Left untreated, the slight discomforts of chronic indigestion gradually worsen, and the early warning signs of abdominal pain, cramps, diarrhea, bloating, gas and constipation can graduate to full-blown diseases. Crohn's disease, ulcerative colitis and irritable bowel syndrome may develop within the lower gastrointestinal tract. But bowel disorders can also help precipitate seemingly unrelated diseases, such as cancer, heart disease, arthritis and renal disorders. At this point, diseases are generally treated with expensive, toxic treatments, which ignore the root of the problem.

Correcting digestive disorders in their early stages is the best way to avoid the need for invasive, harmful therapies later on. But even when caught late, many diseases can often be stopped in their tracks when attention is paid to correcting digestive imbalances.

First, it's helpful to understand the various types of digestive disorders.

Common Digestive Problems

Acid Indigestion

The term acid indigestion refers to the failure of the body to digest food properly due to insufficient stomach acid. Burping, stomach distension, flatulence and sometimes diarrhea are indications of this condition. Low stomach acid can prevent the gastric mucosa from releasing sufficient intrinsic factor, a substance essential for the intestinal absorption of vitamin B12. This may result in pernicious anemia or in subclinical symptoms such as weakness, forgetfulness and confusion.

Acid indigestion is commonly experienced after indulging in a rich, fatty, or overabundant meal. There is just too much for the body to handle, especially if food is gulped down. As a result, large chunks of poorly masticated food must be almost entirely digested in the stomach, and there simply is not enough acid for all that work. Acid indigestion may also be the result of aging, stress, or food sensitivities.

Bad Breath

Many of us take mints or use mouthwash to freshen our breath. But this will not get rid of the problem for long, as most bad breath stems from bacterial toxins in the gut. It is important to avoid being constipated, as this causes bacterial toxins to back up through the gut and be released through the mouth.

Constipation

If you are not having at least two easy bowel movements a day you are probably constipated. Many people think it's normal to depend on laxatives to combat this problem, and, indeed, Americans spend a lot of money on laxatives. What this indicates is that, as a nation, we are not getting enough exercise, water and fiber in our diet. Our high intake of processed foods is the biggest reason for constipation. Other causes of constipation are poor food choices, overeating, eating at night, drinking with meals and high-protein diets. These habits tend to hinder the digestive process, and can create mucus in the colon.

Taking laxatives creates a dependency, and only worsens the problem, as the body forgets how to have a bowel movement on its own. Laxatives can also cause bowel inflammation and bleeding. Stress contributes to the problem by constricting colon muscles. Many people refuse to have a bowel movement away from home and need to pay more attention to their body's urges.

Long-term constipation can lead to more serious problems. Indeed, holistic doctors believe that nearly half of all diseases start in the colon. Sluggish bowels cause poisons to be absorbed into the blood, where they circulate and result in extra work for the other organs of elimination: the liver, kidneys, lungs and skin. Any manner of disease, from colds and flu to arthritis, can eventually result.

Crohn's Disease

This inflammatory disease usually affects the colon, but can be found anywhere along the digestive tract, even as far up as the esophagus. The inflammation goes deep into the tissues, and can cause structural changes. Symptoms of the disease include diarrhea, pain in the stomach, nausea, fever, chills and loss of appetite.

Diarrhea

Loose, frequent, watery stools are usually a sign of another disorder, such as food poisoning, flu, malabsorption syndrome, or a more serious illness. The stool may contain mucus, pus, blood or fat. Left untreated, diarrhea may lead to dehydration and the loss of trace minerals.

Diverticulitis

Small pockets commonly form in the colon, where food particles, bacteria and viruses get stuck. Most people have these pockets and never know it, but sometimes they become inflamed and infected, a condition known as diverticulitis. This condition is accompanied by diarrhea and gas, and can be excruciatingly painful. Many doctors recommend avoiding seeded foods, such as raspberries and strawberries, which tend to clog the pockets, but once the infection is under control, a person can once again eat these high-fiber foods.

Flatulence

Flatulence is caused by the fermentation of carbohydrates in the small intestines. This may be a sign of inadequate intestinal flora, and a signal to take good quality probiotic supplements. Flatulence is also the result of poor digestion. Chewing food properly, building the liver, pancreas and gallbladder, and water, rebalancing the enzymatic activity of the stomach, can all help to eliminate this problem.

Food Allergies

Classical allergies produce immediate symptoms. But masked, or cyclic allergies, which are more common, cause problems too, although the link may be harder to trace. This type of food allergy may be the result of eating the same foods too often, or of a system imbalanced by candida, parasites, or nonsteroidal medications. Food allergies can cause a variety of symptoms, from fatigue and bloating to skin conditions, depression and headaches. The food or foods causing the condition can be discovered through IgE antibody tests.

Gastric Reflux

A small sphincter at the base of the esophagus keeps stomach acid from splashing up as food goes down. When this does not work properly, acid from the stomach backs up into the esophagus and burns tissue to produce heartburn. A hiatal hernia may be the result of gastric reflux. Sometimes chiropractic manipulation and herbs, such as licorice and slippery elm, can help.

Irritable Bowel Syndrome

Ten to 20 percent of people suffer from irritable bowel syndrome, which is characterized by alternating constipation and diarrhea, and sometimes by abdominal pain, spasms, bloating and flatulence. When the condition is severe, there may be mucus in the stools. It may also result in poor appetite, even anorexia (the absence of appetite), and varying degrees of anxiety and depression.

As with many digestive problems, the underlying cause of irritable bowel syndrome is often food sensitivities. Often the foods responsible have a delayed effect, causing a reaction 24 to 48 hours after being eaten. The most common offenders are wheat and dairy products, which are hidden in ingredients in many foods. Other common offenders include corn, coffee, tea and citrus fruits.

Malabsorption Syndrome

Malabsorption syndrome is the failure of the body to absorb nutrients due to a digestive lapse. With this problem, after a food is eaten, the vitamins and minerals do not enter the cells, but are eliminated as waste products. The resulting lack of nutrition can be manifested in multiple symptoms, including weakness, anemia and loss of appetite, weight loss, swollen abdomen, muscle cramps and bone pain. Malabsorption syndrome can be a side effect of other diseases, such as celiac disease, cystic fibrosis and Whipple's disease. It can also be brought on by nervousness, anxiety, and fear, as well as stomach or small bowel surgery and alcohol consumption.

Peptic Ulcers

Ulcers can be acute or chronic: acute ulcers are shallow and often asymptomatic, while chronic ulcers, known as true ulcers, are deep, painful and damaging to muscles. Depending upon the part of the digestive tract affected, peptic ulcers are known either as gastric or duodenal. Both produce a gnawing pain in the upper abdomen, but the timing is often different. Distress from a gastric, or stomach, ulcer is usually experienced after a meal, while pain from a duodenal ulcer, which is located in the first part of the small intestine, is generally felt on an empty stomach. This person has pain between meals or is uncomfortably awakened in the middle of the night.

Orthodox Western medicine relates ulcers to excess stomach acid and to the presence of certain bacteria, such as Campylobacter and Helicobacter pylori. In fact, some estimates attribute the bacteria to ulcers in 80 percent of the cases. While stomach acid and bacteria can cause irritation leading to ulcers, the problem is mainly due to the susceptibility of the involved area. The epithelial lining of the stomach or duodenum is weak, and therefore vulnerable to attack.

Drugs designed to block stomach acid, such as Zantac and Tagamet, are standard treatment. By masking symptoms, these appear to initially alleviate ulcers. But since they do nothing to address the real cause of the problem, ultimately, they may cause more harm than good.

The Traditional Chinese Medicine (TCM) approach has proven helpful to some ulcer patients. In TCM, not all ulcers are similarly treated. Practitioners carefully diagnose patients, looking for imbalanced systems (meridians), and base their recommendations on these findings. Some ulcer patients need to stay away from spicy foods, for example, while others do not. Some patients benefit from certain herbal combinations, and others need acupuncture.

Ulcerative Colitis

Ulcerative colitis is a chronic, episodic, inflammatory disease of the large intestine and rectum, often caused by food allergies. Symptoms are debilitating and can include excruciating pain; stools containing blood, pus and mucus; explosive bowel movements; chronic gas; distension of the bowel; ulcers; excessive diarrhea and constipation; fever; chills; anemia; and weight loss. Complications can include peripheral arthritis, ankylosing spondylitis, kidney and liver disease and inflammation of the eyes, skin and mouth. The disease tends to come and go, and a person may be fine for months at a time. Parasites and bacteria are sometimes the cause.

Diagnosis

Minor digestive problems, with their small discomforts, tend to be ignored by orthodox medicine. As conditions become more severe, diagnoses are made through X rays, scopes and blood tests and drug therapy is generally prescribed. But medications are only quick fixes, not permanent solutions, because they only mask the underlying cause of the problem.

Since a myriad of factors can cause digestive illnesses, all possible etiologies should be investigated. Complementary physicians employ multiple measures of diagnosis, including tests for food sensitivities, parasites, candida, thyroid functioning and nutrient levels. Once the cause of the problem is identified, the individual can be appropriately treated.

Treatments

Digestive disturbances respond well to nutritional protocols that include changes in diet, supplements, herbs and detoxification. In addition, stress reduction techniques can make a profound difference. Work with a holistically oriented physician who can help you tailor a program to your individual needs.

The following recommendations are basic to overall well-being.

High-Fiber Diet

Foods that work with the body are wholesome and natural, not processed and chemically altered. Basically, this means that the healthful diet contains many complex carbohydrates, which are fiber-rich foods. We ought to follow the example of primitive cultures, which do not suffer from gastrointestinal diseases seen in the modern world, and eat five to nine servings of fruits and vegetables daily. If constipation is a problem, include fresh fruits, especially apples, figs, peaches, berries, oranges and prunes. Vegetables, raw juices and sprouts are other good choices. Eat lightly and go on a short vegetable or fruit juice fast, if possible. It is also helpful to drink a glass of warm water in the morning and take a tablespoon of olive oil before retiring at night. The rest of the diet should focus on whole grains and legumes, with small amounts of nuts and seeds. Note that, despite its name, whole wheat bread contains a lot of white flour. Consider, as better sources of fiber, brown rice, barley, millet and buckwheat. In addition to fiber, green leafy vegetables are high in magnesium, a mineral that helps the muscles of the intestines contract in a rhythmic fashion (peristalsis) to help with bowel movements.

Note that a healthy diet need not be bland. Common spices and herbs are more than flavorful; they actually aid digestion. Allspice and rosemary can relieve indigestion, basil and dill can calm an upset stomach, while cayenne and horseradish stimulate circulation and quicken digestion. Spices move foods through the system more easily with little distress to the GI tract. They also promote elimination through the increase of perspiration through the skin.

Foods with Flora

We have more bacteria in our digestive system than we have cells in our body. We may not realize it, but these good bacteria do a lot for us by allowing us to benefit from the vitamins we take in, and by acting as our first line of defense against other microbial organisms. Unfortunately modern living often destroys these friendly colonies through stress and drug use, particularly antibiotic use. It is therefore important to repopulate the digestive tract with natural flora by eating natural foods with high-quality bacteria, such as tempeh, sauerkraut and yogurt.

Food Preparation

When preparing foods, it is important to maximize digestibility without altering the integrity of the food's cellular structure. This means the avoidance of irradiated foods, foods prepared in microwaves and overcooked foods. Many foods should be juiced or eaten raw, as cooking destroys important enzymes. When cooking, steaming is generally preferable to boiling, although boiling in one inch of water is better than boiling in six inches of water, and boiling for five minutes is better than 20. If prepared foods are chosen, it is best to eat those closest to their natural state. For example, frozen peas are preferable to peas that have been boiled and canned. The type of cookware is equally important; aluminum cookware should be avoided because the aluminum gets into the food and can lead to many serious health problems.

Herbs

As we've mentioned, nature supplies us with a great variety of herbs for strengthening digestion and overcoming everyday problems. Those with digestive problems should keep the following in mind:

Aloe Vera . . . The valuable phytochemicals contained in aloe vera can help correct many chronic conditions, including indigestion, malabsorption syndrome, leaky gut syndrome, spastic colon and ulcerative colitis.

Chamomile . . . This is a gentle yet highly effective remedy for irritable bowel syndrome and other digestive disturbances accompanied by anxiety. A cup of boiled water can be poured over a heaping tablespoon of dried chamomile flowers and strained after several minutes. Taken with honey, this is a delicious, soothing tea that can be consumed throughout the day, between meals and before retiring at night.

Fennel . . . Fennel helps alleviate flatulence, cramps and indigestion. It can be taken as a tea, or the seeds can be chewed.

Ginger . . . A cup of ginger tea in the morning, with bee propolis and raw, unheated, organic honey, will invigorate the system and promote good digestion.

Nettles . . . Nettles make a good tea to take for diarrhea. Usually diarrhea causes a loss of trace elements. Nettles tea is a good source of these minerals, as well as of chlorophyll.

Oats . . . Oat tea will soothe a nervous stomach and strengthen a weak digestive system.

Origanum . . . This is known to strengthen the stomach and stop flatulence.

Licorice . . . Licorice is an herbal aid for alleviating heartburn and recovering from ulcers. In fact, this herb may be as helpful as standard medications for healing gastric and duodenal ulcers. Licorice stimulates the production of prostaglandins that promote healing to the whole gastrointestinal tract, but especially the stomach. The deglycyrrhizinated form of the extract (DGL) prevents blood pressure elevation. Taking licorice three to four times a day can provide tremendous relief.

Turmeric (Curcumalonga) . . . The Ayurvedic and Chinese plant from the ginger family has anti-inflammatory qualities, which improve inflammation in the stomach (gastritis). Turmeric also enhances bile production, which helps break down fats. In some instances, turmeric reduced the secretion of acid from the stomach.

Green Tea (Camellia Sinensis) . . . Researchers found that the polyphenols in green tea have shown great promise in preventing stomach cancer and gastritis in test tubes. Green tea might also reduce inflammation connected to Crohn's disease and ulcerative colitis. Studies show that people who drink more than 10 cups of green tea a day are less likely to develop liver disease. Green tea can be used in capsule or liquid-preparation form as well.

Herbs that stimulate liver activity also improve digestion, and include agrimony, dandelion, barberry, wild yam and milk thistle. Herbs that soothe and coat the digestive tract include mallow, chickweed, mullein and plantain. Other herbs to investigate include balmony, barberry, cayenne, gentian root, ginseng, goldenseal (on a temporary basis), coltsfoot, lobelia, wild cherry bark, skullcap, slippery elm, wormwood and angelica. When constipation is the problem, these herbs can be taken on a temporary basis: cascara sagrada bark, senna, flaxseed, bayberry root bark, goldenseal root and red raspberry leaves. Other herbs that prevent or improve digestive disorders are astragalus, Jamaica dogwood, lemon balm, peppermint, saw palmetto and yarrow. Herbs and olive oil can also be added to warm-water enemas.

Supplements

Supplements give the body extra concentrated support. It's a good idea to start slowly and build up to an optimum level, and to use supplements under the guidance of a knowledgeable health professional.

Antifungals . . . These natural alternatives to antibiotics can help get rid of parasites and yeast overgrowth. Grapefruit seed extract, pau d'arco tea, garlic, artemesia and various homeopathic remedies all have an antifungal effect. Sometimes antifungal medications, such as Nystatin or Diflucan, are prescribed by a physician. Antifungals work best when accompanied by a yeast-free diet.

Antioxidants . . . To support the digestive system, a person may need up to 800 IU of vitamin E, one to six grams of vitamin C and between 25,000 and 50,000 IU of beta-carotene. Patients with severe cases of inflammatory bowel disease may benefit from higher doses of nutrients given intravenously. Using this route, a person may be given 20,000 mg of vitamin C to start, with the amount subsequently graduated up to 50,000 mg. In addition, nutrients such as magnesium, B vitamins, glutathion and glycyrrhizin may be used.

Bioflavonoids . . . Vitamin C works even better in conjunction with bioflavonoids. Quercetin and pycnogenol are especially important because of their anti-inflammatory and immune-enhancing properties. Usually 300 mg of quercetin and 25 mg of pycnogenol, three times a day, are recommended.

Coenzyme Q1O . . . Inflammations respond well to this nutrient when 50 to 100 mg are taken two to three times daily.

Digestive Enzymes . . . Stomach or pancreatic enzymes can be useful aids to digestion.

L-Glutamine . . . L-glutamine nourishes and heals the entire lining of the upper and lower intestines, and is especially helpful for patients who are losing weight. Anywhere from 3 to 10 grams are needed. Since this is a large amount, glutamine should be taken under the guidance of a health care practitioner.

Magnesium . . . People who tend to get constipated are often deficient in this vital mineral. Using 200 to 300 mg of magnesium twice a day will not only help with the peristaltic activity of the GI tract, but will address a deficiency in a large number of individuals.

Omega-3 Fatty Acids . . . A number of studies prove that fish oils have anti-inflammatory effects. Between 1000 and 2000 mg can be taken two to three times daily with meals; take less if belching or nausea results.

Peppermint Oil . . . Clinical tests have long shown peppermint reduces colonic spasms. One capsule of enterically coated peppermint oil can be taken two to three times a day, on a temporary basis, to remove this discomfort. A handful of patients will get a burning sensation in the rectum after using peppermint oil, in which case the therapy should be discontinued. Chamomile tea can be taken instead.

Probiotics . . . Literally translated, probiotics means for life, and the word refers to products that replenish the healthy bacteria in our digestive systems. Hundreds of studies show lactobacillus acidophilus, Bifidobacterium bifidum, and fructo-oligosaccharides to promote overall good health. They are especially important to use after antibiotic therapy, vaginal yeast infections and urinary tract infections.

Psyllium Seed and Wheat Bran . . . These products are helpful for overcoming constipation when a high-fiber diet alone does not seem to make a difference. Wheat bran should be used only by people who do not have wheat allergies.

Digest RC . . . This is a natural herbal remedy that helps relieve digestive complications. It is very popular in Eastern Europe, where the dangerous health behavior of the population (poor diet, heavy drinking and smoking) significantly affects the mortality rate. Digest RC combines black radish juice (promotes bile production in the liver for fat and protein digestion) and artichoke (elevates bile levels even further, resulting in a healthier flow through the bile ducts). Peppermint is another ingredient that triggers enzyme production and the secretion function of the stomach. Charcoal (from linden bark tree) is an important component of Digest RC due to its toxin-absorbing ability. This ingredient is also used for indigestion or nervous vomiting. Cholic acid, a liver enzyme, is significant in improving digestion, as is calcium phosphate, which is capable of neutralizing stomach acid. These supportive elements taken together can increase the digestion of fats and meat protein. One or two capsules before high-fat meals is suggested.

Artichoke Leaf Extract . . . Using the large, deeply serrated leaves of the artichoke plant, we could protect the liver, enhance bile production and lower lipid levels. Artichoke has powerful compounds that show antioxidant qualities. Taking one or two 300-mg capsules with meals can be beneficial for patients with gastrointestinal problems.

GastroPro . . . Two 900-mg capsules taken daily from a formula containing polyunsaturated phosphatidylcholine (PPC) can aid in digesting fat and plays a role in inhibiting bowel strictures.

Bowel Detoxification

Getting rid of toxins is an important first step for many people with bowel disorders. Until this is done, none of the nutrients for rebuilding the system will make much difference. Detoxification can be approached in many ways. Bentonite is a clay-like substance, used in a drink that draws out toxins from the colon. Colon therapy also eliminates stored wastes and restores proper tissue and organ function. Some physicians place their patients on elimination diets, consisting of hypoallergenic foods, until a time when the body can handle certain foods again on a rotational basis. Total parenteral nutrition, or intravenous feeding, is used in extreme cases to quiet down the colon before other dietary approaches are tried. These are all excellent methods for healing an overburdened digestive tract.

Stress Reduction

The expression butterflies in my stomach reflects an example of how our thoughts and feelings affect us physically. A large bundle of nerves, known as the solar plexus, is located in the stomach area. When our nerves are stressed in any way this is often the first place to be affected. This is why we have "gut" reactions.

The best way to deal with mental and emotional problems is to address the issue at hand. When anxiety interferes with clear thinking, there are many techniques for helping us to overcome those stresses, including meditation, biofeedback, yoga, tai chi, hypnosis and breathing techniques. Remembering to take time each day for the things we enjoy such as gardening, playing a musical instrument and spending quality time with friends and family is also important for our digestive wellness and for our total well-being, as well.

What to Avoid

Poor Food Choices

Digestive disorders often result from food sensitivities; therefore, problem foods must be eliminated from the diet. People suffering from inflammatory bowel diseases usually need to stop eating wheat and certain other grains, dairy products, sugar and specific carbohydrates. Doctors who take people off foods they are sensitive to often see dramatic improvement in only a few weeks.

In addition to allergy-producing foods, there are some common rules of what not to eat for good health. In general, the substances to stay away from are: processed foods; saturated fats; artificial colorings, flavorings, and preservatives; irradiated produce and herbs; canned foods; foods grown in chemical fertilizers and those treated with pesticides or wax; and overcooked foods. When one is constipated, foods to stay away from include starchy grains, meat and dairy products.

Drugs

Antibiotic overuse is the underlying cause of many health problems that begin in the digestive system. Antibiotics do not discriminate between good and bad bacteria; rather they destroy bacteria indiscriminately and alter the flora in the gut, leading to an overgrowth of yeast. Yeast infections are believed to be contributing factors to many illnesses, including inflammatory bowel diseases. Antibiotics can also have the effect of altering bacterial structure. When this happens, good bacteria may begin to produce toxins that harm the gut. Many problems may result, including illnesses that seem to be unrelated to the digestive tract, such as chronic fatigue syndrome and fibromyalgia. Nonsteroidal anti-inflammatory medications, caffeine, nicotine and alcohol are other drugs that can wreak havoc on digestive health.

Parasites

Parasitic infections can cause chronic gastrointestinal problems that are quite common throughout the world. It is important to take as many precautions as possible against contracting these microbes, such as washing hands after using the toilet, and not ordering salad foods in restaurants. Anyone who suspects that they have this condition should see a doctor who specializes in the treatment of parasites. A testing procedure known as an endoscopy is the best method for identifying parasites that attach themselves to the intestinal wall, because these parasites are often missed in routine stool analysis.

Improper Chewing

Chewing constitutes the first stage of digestion, and sets the stage for how much nutritional benefit we receive. Unless chewing is slow and thorough, saliva will not mix sufficiently with food. Improper chewing leaves food chunks too large to pass easily through the esophagus and into the stomach for the next stage of digestion. When improperly chewed food reaches the stomach, excess stomach acid is secreted to break down oversized food particles. This subjects the inner linings of the stomach and intestinal tract to high levels of acid, which is extremely corrosive and, over time, damaging. This can aggravate digestive problems, causing everything from indigestion and heartburn to ulcers.

Drinking with Meals

Drinking with meals should be minimized or avoided, as fluid dilutes digestive juices, making the breakdown of food more difficult. Incompletely digested food causes irritation of the bowel lining and can lead to ulcerative colitis. Toxins from incompletely digested food can enter the bloodstream and activate an immune reaction. Drinking while eating also encourages gulping down food chunks that would otherwise be chewed more thoroughly. This is dangerous and can result in choking.

Eating under Stress

People tend to not chew thoroughly when nervous, anxious, or hurried. In addition, digestive enzymes are not properly secreted because stress adversely affects normal enzyme production. Up to 50 percent of the nutrients in a meal can be lost when one is eating under stress.

Eating Hard-to-Digest Foods

When foods are difficult to digest, the body oversecretes gastric juices. This highly acidic state can be internally damaging. Proteins are difficult to digest because they are made up of bonding peptide linkages, long beaded chains that must be broken down by gastric juices before they can be digested and utilized. Some peptides are more difficult to reduce than others. Those with lots of fat surrounding them, such as the peptides in meat, are difficult enough, but not nearly as bad as those in deep-fried or charcoal-broiled foods, which are held together by strong bonds of molecules that are very hard to separate.

Treatment Summary

Digestive disorders can be due to a myriad of factors. Therefore, a complete checkup is needed to uncover the cause of the problem.

Cultures that eat high-fiber foods have few digestive disorders. Spices further enhance digestion, and the addition of foods containing flora equips the gut with the microorganisms needed to ward off microbial invaders.

Foods should be eaten as close to their natural state as possible to avoid loss of vitamins and enzymes and prevent damage to the food's cellular structure.

Herbs and nutritional supplements are often used to strengthen digestion; a health professional can help tailor a program to your unique situation.

Ways of getting rid of stored-up toxins that interfere with digestion and elimination include the use of bentonite clay colon therapy elimination diets and intravenous feeding.

Since our emotions and our digestive functions are intimately related, we must address emotional issues as they arise, and engage in activities that promote relaxation.

See also: Allergies.

Dysmenorrhea

Commonly known as menstrual cramps, dysmenorrhea is part of the experience of millions of women worldwide. However, painful periods do not have to be accepted as an inescapable product of the female menstrual cycle, and can actually be prevented by adhering to several basic guidelines. First, it helps to understand the underlying causes of this common condition

Causes

Dysmenorrhea usually begins when contractions within the uterus become distorted. These contractions are governed by receptors within the uterine lining, which receive stimulation from hormonal and psychological factors. Women who have an excess of prostaglandins, which are the chemical messengers that affect the uterine receptors, are left susceptible to overstimulation and, consequently, are more likely to experience dysmenorrhea. One way in which prostaglandin production can become exaggerated is by eating foods that the body is allergic to. For instance, some women are prone to yeast reactions; hence, indulging in baked foods, breads, pastries and processed fruit juices can facilitate the onset of dysmenorrhea.

Another factor implicated in dysmenorrhea is poor nutrition. Unfortunately, most people tend to indulge in diets that lack nutritional value, and consequently hazardous toxins in the form of synthetic preservatives, additives and caffeine are able to undermine their systems' functioning. Proteins that are obtained via red meat and dairy products contain dangerous hormones that can have an adverse effect upon our bodies, as can oily and fried foods.

We have to differentiate between primary and secondary dysmenorrhea. In primary dysmenorrhea, there is no underlying cause for the painful or difficult menstruation. In secondary dysmenorrhea, very often some gynecological disease, most often endometriosis, triggers the symptoms.

Symptoms

Dysmenorrhea is usually characterized by spasmodic cramps, but achiness, sensations of heaviness in the lower abdomen and pain in the lower back or thighs can manifest as well. Additional symptoms include vomiting, nausea, loss of appetite, headaches, dizziness, anxiety, lethargy, depression and diarrhea. In most cases, dysmenorrhea occurs at the start of menstruation and persists for only a few hours, but sometimes, acute cases can manifest premenstrually and persist for days. Stress can sometimes exacerbate dysmenorrhea. Something that many women report lessens the problem is the birth of a child; periods experienced afterwards are not as problematic.

Treatments

Nutrition

Since poor eating habits can contribute to excessive production of prostaglandins, reforming the diet can have a profound effect in terms of curbing menstrual cramps. Cool, green foods are effective in abating inflammation and hot stabbing pains, while legumes, flaxseed oil, organic grains, oatmeal and steamed green vegetables can provide further relief. Deep-sea fish, such as tuna, salmon and mackerel, are also recommended.

Some nutritionists assert that menstrual cramps with emotional origins can be combated via tofu consumption. Cooking warm tofu with sweet spices, such as pumpkin pie spice or nutmeg, can be especially helpful in soothing the nerves and promoting overall relaxation.

Supplements

A deficiency of magnesium can encourage the release of prostaglandins and the occurrence of spasms; hence, daily consumption of magnesium citrate supplements can act as an effective preventative agent. Start at 300-500 mg daily, and gradually augment the dosage until bowel tolerance is attained. When DHEA is deficient, naturally rebalancing the hormone can reduce symptoms. For the headaches and blemishes that manifest prior to menstruation, evening primrose oil is a supplement that can be consumed on a daily basis.

Herbs

Popularized by the Chinese, gardenia and philodendron can be obtained with a prescription from an herbalist. The herb corn silk can be used to eliminate bloating that is induced by excessive hormones in the blood supply.

Chinese medicine describes dysmenorrhea as "blood stagnation in the lower abdomen," accompanied by "yin deficiency," "lung heat" and "liver fire." Acupuncture with Chinese herbs supports the yin, lowers the heat and eliminates the fire. Possible herbs that free the flow of the qi and the blood are aurantium fruit (zhi ke), lindera root (wu yao), cyperus tuber (xiang fu), cnidium (chuan qiong), persica seed (tao ren) and safflower (hong hua). When the application of pressure and/or warmth feels good, the following herbs are helpful: cinnamon bark (rou gui), evodia bark (wu zhu yu) and a widely used formula called warming menses formula (wen jing tang). When there is an aversion to cold and the limbs are cold, fennel seed (xiao hui xiang) and dry ginger (gan jiang) offer relief due to their "warm" properties. A popular formula, StagnationEASE (shao fu zhu yu tang), shows positive effects as well.

When one feels heat in the abdomen and has low-grade fever, coptis (huang lian) and peony bark (mu dan pi) might be the solution. heat-clearing blood-regulating decoction (quing re tiao xue tang) is a combination that can clear "damp" heat. In case of thin menses with a pale color and small volume, ginger (ren shen), astragalus (huang qi), angelica (dang gui) and rehmannia (di huang) are suggested. The chi blood tonic formula (ba zhen tang) is a time-tested solution for this type of dysmenorrhea, the so-called qi blood deficiency pattern. When the abdominal pain is accompanied by dizziness, sore back and flushed face, white peony root (bai shao) and cornus fruit (shan zu yu) work as a kidney-liver tonic. Also, the formula liver tonic (tiao gan tang, made by Life Extension,) is recommended.

Another combination, women's rhythm, can be used to ameliorate bloating. Another formula, xiao yao wan, which can be obtained at herbal pharmacies in Chinese ethnic neighborhoods, aids the digestive process, reduces menstrual pain and soothes angry emotions. Yunnan pai yao is a blend of herbs that can be employed to stabilize profuse bleeding, mitigate stabbing pains and reduce swelling.

Green tea is a way of enhancing energy by stimulating the digestive system without excessive quantities of caffeine. It creates a cooling sensation, and can help alleviate sharp, stabbing menstrual pains. A pinch of green tea should be added to a pot of boiling water and allowed to sit for five minutes. Then the tea can be sipped throughout the day.

Aloe vera can be used to treat several symptoms that commonly accompany menstrual cramps, including headaches, irritability, stabbing pains, fever, blemishes and bad breath. Furthermore, aloe vera is effective in decreasing acidic levels in the stomach and liver, and it can be a mild laxative. Aloe vera can be consumed in a juice, tea or water mixture.

Consumption of the herb dandelion can help the body eliminate impurities. Capsules or tea are available forms of this herb.

Sarsaparilla is useful in quelling hot, stabbing pains; this herb is also a diuretic.

Black cohosh is used as an alternative to estrogen replacement therapy. It is a potent agent for reducing the suffering that accompanies painful menstrual periods.

Dong quai increases the effects of ovarian and testicular hormones. It is effective in treating hot flashes, PMS and vaginal dryness, and it eliminates cramps.

Wild yam root is often used for dysmenorrhea and pelvic pain. It relaxes muscle spasm and reduces inflammation. It is good for a wide range of female disorders.

Turmeric, a tropical herb from the ginger family, may be beneficial as well.

Homeopathic Remedies

Homeopathy is an effective way of treating dysmenorrhea with no side effects, as the dilution process used in creating the remedies renders substances completely harmless. Homeopathic medicines are always keyed to very particular symptoms.

The remedy colcynthis can be used to treat acute cramps that occur suddenly during the first day of menstruation. Severe irritability and extreme anger are also part of the picture for this remedy. In addition, if the pain is substantially reduced when your knees are held firmly near your stomach, then you may wish to try colcynthis.

When the body feels more comfortable near warmth and you are suffering from spasmodic cramps and bloating, magnesia phosphorica should be administered. This potent remedy has proven effective in approximately 85 percent of the cases in which it is used.

The remedy pulsatilla should be used when cramps and the blood flow are inconsistent. Pulsatilla can be used to alleviate cutting and tearing pains in the lower back or kidney regions. Emotional signs include gentleness and weepiness. Also, the patient will have a desire to be with other people during menstruation and will prefer to be in environments with fresh air, rather than in warm stuffy rooms.

Viburnum should be employed when the menses are exceedingly late and very light. Cramps affect the sacrum and thigh regions and are accompanied by a cessation in bleeding. In addition, the patient may feel faint.

Cimifuga is for women suffering from spasmodic cramps that radiate across the thighs and pelvis, and from premenstrual headaches. As the flow of blood intensifies, pain increases as well. Emotionally, the patient may seem exceedingly nervous or depressed.

Chamomilla should be consumed when the woman is either hypersensitive or insensitive to pain. Also, she may be extremely irritable and argumentative. When menstrual bleeding increases, reliance upon coffee, stimulants and sedatives is also heightened. Furthermore, symptoms become intensified when they are accompanied by anger.

Aromatherapy

Marjoram, lavender and clary sage all possess analgesic qualities that can be used to assuage dysmenorrhea. Eighteen to 20 drops of any of these essential oils can be assimilated into a lotion or oil and massaged into the abdomen and lower back. Inhaling the cooling fragrances of rose, lavender or sandalwood can be helpful in subduing sharp, stabbing menstrual pains.

Exercise

Exercise, particularly of the type that stretches the body, can do much to minimize cramps. Relaxed swimming may be helpful. Also, a yoga class can be an invaluable aid in teaching dysmenorrhea sufferers helpful moves.

Stress Reduction

Stress can have a whole range of adverse effects upon the body, one of which is exacerbation of dysmenorrhea. Consequently, engaging in a stress reduction program can help in both the long run and the short run. Engaging in deep abdominal breathing, meditation and tai chi are some suggestions for eliminating stress and stress-induced pain. Visualization, music method therapy and the deep desire to be healed could also calm symptoms.

Other Approaches

It is no coincidence that women who have menstrual cramps also suffer from back and/or neck pain. The sexual organs—the ovaries, fallopian tubes, uterus, cervix and vagina—all need healthy nerve connections from the spine. When problems arise that irritate the nerve, it can lead to painful cramps. A chiropractor may bring relief. Spinal adjustment of the cervical vertebrae, especially the third cervical, produces positive results.

Poor elimination is frequently associated with dysmenorrhea. Hydrotherapy (colon irrigation) helps cleanse the system. Abdominal castor oil packs, when used prior to the menstrual period, assist in the cleansing of the alimentary canal. Hot Epsom Salt packs, placed over the lower abdomen, lessen menstrual pain. Sitz baths may also help in pelvic pain relief. Acupressure massage reduces the bloated feeling, as well as the sharp pain. The recommended electrotherapy form is the use of a device called the radial appliance, which balances circulation and increases relaxation. Stimulation along the spine has a calming effect. Pulses of magnetic energy around the pelvic area have a healing, rebalancing effect.

What to Avoid

Several foods encourage excessive production of prostaglandins, which interact with the uterine lining and ultimately can induce the exaggerated uterine contractions associated with menstrual cramping. Foods that should be avoided include hot spices, sugar, fried, greasy foods, alcohol and stimulating foods, such as garlic and onions. In addition, white potatoes have been implicated in the onset of dysmenorrhea.

Treatment Summary

A healthy diet can minimize the occurrence of menstrual cramps; recommended selections are cool green foods, legumes, flaxseed oil, organic grains, oatmeal, steamed vegetables, deep-sea fish and tofu.

Evening primrose oil and magnesium citrate supplements can counter the effects of dysmenorrhea.

Herbs and homeopathic remedies can alleviate uncomfortable menstrual symptoms.

Fragrant essential oils, massaged into the abdomen or lower back, can help reduce cramps.

Exercise, with an emphasis on stretching, may provide relief.

Deep abdominal breathing, meditation and tai chi are stress reducers that may help in overcoming painful periods.

Ear Infections

Ear infection is the number one reason for visits to pediatricians; by the age of three, two thirds of all youngsters have seen a doctor for this reason. This amounts to 30 million doctor visits a year, at a cost of $2.2 billion.

Several groups are at high risk for ear infections: children with allergies, children who were exposed to alcohol or tobacco smoke in the womb, children who were not breast-fed, those exposed to cow's milk within the first six months of life and those placed in day care.

The problem stems from a hypertrophy, or increase in cell size, of lymphoid tissue surrounding the eustachian tube. The eustachian tube becomes blocked, and, as a result, there is a backup of fluid. When the middle ear is affected, the condition is known as otitis media. When the external canal is involved, it is known as otitis externa. Here, boils and discharges may be present.

Treatment

Bacteria or viruses can cause ear infection. Frequently, the condition develops from the flu. Ear infection can cause temporary hearing loss. In severe cases, scar tissue can block the ear, affecting the hearing, and should be surgically removed.

Standard medical therapies for middle ear infections are antibiotics and decongestants. If several trials of these aren't effective—especially since a growing number of bacteria are becoming resistant—the next step is to place tubes in the ears. But according to research, these methods do not make a positive difference in the long run. Studies show that children receiving antibiotics are just as likely to get recurrent infections as those who do not. Some even report a greater likelihood of recurrent infections when antibiotics are given. Similarly, tubes provide relief initially, but the ear infections do not stop. All the tubes do is provide a drainage system for the pus. This is because the cause of the problem is not addressed.

Natural treatments, by contrast, go to the root of the problem, and begin with pre- and postnatal care. Simple precautions before and just after giving birth can prevent ear infections from developing. Expectant mothers should completely avoid smoking and alcohol, eat nutritious foods and take care of their mental and emotional health. After birth, breast-feeding is preferable to bottle-feeding, as many studies show that children who are breast-fed for six months or more have far fewer ear infections than their bottle-fed counterparts.

Treating Allergies

When ear infections first develop after a child is introduced to solid foods, parents should suspect allergies as the cause, according to Florida homeopathic physician Dr. Mark Frank. The first step, he says, is to discover what substance causes the allergy, and then to eliminate it. Most commonly, this is cow milk; the earlier it is given to the child, the sooner infections start. Problems may also stem from wheat, corn, soy and other foods.

To test for allergies, remove the suspected food for four days. On the fifth day, return it to the diet. If symptoms are exacerbated soon afterwards, that suggests a likely cause of allergy.

Supplements

An important step in recovery is building up the child's immune system with nutrition. If the mother is still breast-feeding, these nutrients can be taken by the mom:

Omega-3 Essential Fatty Acids . . . These play a major role in breaking up inflammatory processes. One of the best foods for this purpose is flaxseed oil. Flaxseed oil must be stored in the refrigerator, and never cooked.

Antioxidants . . . Zinc boosts the immune system, as do beta-carotene, the B-complex vitamins and vitamin C (ascorbic acid), all of which have a mild anti-inflammatory effect.

Lactobacillus, Acidophilus or Bifidus . . . When antibiotics are given to the little patient, lactobacillus, acidophilus and/or bifidus should also be administered to replace the good bacteria. Either ¼ teaspoon of powder, one teaspoon of liquid or half of the content of a capsule can be given two hours after the administration of the antibiotic, one time per day.

Homeopathy

Homeopathic remedies, which are chosen according to the patients presenting symptoms, can be highly successful in the treatment of ear pain and infections, and in the prevention of reinfection. A physician looks for the severity of pain, and whether or not there is fever, nausea, vomiting and diarrhea. In addition, the color of the ear and the presence of fluid are taken into account. These are some common remedies a homeopath might choose:

Belladonna . . . Symptoms include tearing, burning and throbbing pain in the ears, causing a child to cry out in sleep. The ear is clogged and the person hears humming noises. The ear may also be red, hot and overly sensitive to sound. The eardrum appears to bulge and the parotid glands and cervical lymph nodes may be swollen. The patient feels worse when touched, with noise, in drafts and when lying down, but better when sitting up.

Ferrum Phosphoricum . . . This is a remedy to think of if belladonna fails. Here patients are pale with flushed cheeks. They tend to be anemic and to have repeated infections in both ears. Symptoms worsen at night, when the patient is jarred, and with motion. Cold applications provide relief.

Mercurius . . . Symptoms are like those for belladonna, but are more intense in regard to redness and pulsating pain. Glands are enlarged and the throat is deep red. The pharynx is red and pus-filled and the eustachian tube is inflamed. Breath is foul, a state that worsens at night and with warmth. Sweat accompanies fever.

Chamomilla . . . This remedy helps earaches due to teething. The child is frantic, whiny, restless and inconsolable, wanting to be held and nursed constantly. One cheek is hot, while the other is pale and cool. The youngster wants, but then refuses, everything. Symptoms worsen with heat, anger, open air and at night, and get better when the child is carried and kept warm.

Pulsatilla . . . Symptoms resemble those for chamomilla. The remedy comes from the windflower and, likewise, symptoms are changeable. Infections may fluctuate between the right and left ear, discharges may alternate from yellow and green to clear. The child feels worse with heat, in the evening and after eating rich, creamy foods, and better in the open air, with motion, and with cold application. Repeated ear infections make hearing difficult.

Hepar Sulphurs Calcareum . . . This helps earaches accompanied by chills, splinter-like pains in the ear, hypersensitivity to touch and noise and a tendency to have boils in the external canal.

Kali Muriaticum . . . This remedy can be used to help the healing of the eardrums.

Arnica . . . In cases of fallopian tube placement, arnica taken three or four times a day can reduce inflammation and help the body get used to the presence of the tube.

Anas Barbariae . . . It may be given to children in cases of repeated infections.

Adjunctive Therapies

A washcloth soaked in warm water or a warm hot-water bottle placed around or on the ear often alleviates earaches. As long as no puncture wounds to the eardrum exists, drops of mullein oil with hypericum can relieve pain. Or olive oil, warmed slightly with a bit of crushed garlic (which is taken out before using the oil), can be dropped into each ear instead. This is a soothing antiviral and antibacterial remedy. The liquid extract of the antiviral echinacea combined with the antibacterial goldenseal can reduce acute infection. The daily administration of echinacea should not go beyond two weeks or the herb will lose its effectiveness.

The Chinese herbal formula called minor bupleurum is a potent agent in preventing the recurrences of ear infections; the suggested amount is 3 to 5 drops for a period of 5 days each week for one month (followed by a three-week break). This format may be repeated for six months. Chinese medicine distinguishes between types of ear infections. When sticky pus is present, due to the "heat in the lung," the suggested herb combination is magnolia flower, scutellaria flower, rhizome of anemarrhena, cimicifuga rhizome, xanthium, capejasmine fruit, ophiopogon root, white tribulus fruit, lily bulb, loquat leaf, gypsum, dahurian angelica root and licorice root. In cases of "dampness retention," the recipe is a powder of ginseng, poria, white atractylodes rhizome, pulp of lotus seed, licorice root, amomum fruit, platycodon fruit, Chinese yam, coix seed and white hyacinth bean. When a "deficiency in the kidneys" occurs, applying boiling anemarrhena, yellow corktree bark, pulp of dogwood fruit, prepared rhemannia root, poria, oriental water plaintain rhizome, moutan bark, prunella spike and Chinese yam may improve the condition. Colloidal silver may improve the symptoms of ear infection. To keep the passageway between the middle ear and the nasal cavity (the eustachian tube) open, massage the ears. Keeping the child with ear infection hydrated with spring water, soups, herbal teas and diluted fruit juices helps.

What to Avoid

Leaving a baby lying flat on his or her back to suck on a bottle is dangerous; the fluid can drain directly into the middle ear. Propping up the infant at a 30-degree angle is advisable. Exposure to cigarette smoke, pet dander and items that collect dust could be causing an allergic reaction. Avoid taking a child with an ear infection on an airplane flight. Lastly, there is a great chance for infection exposure at child-care centers, where children can pick up antibiotic-resistant strains of bacteria from each other.

Treatment Summary

Expectant mothers who engage in healthful lifestyles are less prone to have children who suffer from ear infections. Breast-feeding after birth further reduces risk of infection and enhances the child's overall well-being.

Ear infections may be the result of allergies to cow milk or other foods, such as wheat, corn and soy. These substances should be identified and eliminated from the diet.

Supplements that build the child's immune system are essential fatty acids, zinc, beta-carotene, ascorbic acid and B vitamins. A mother can take these nutrients and pass them on to her child during breast-feeding.

Several homeopathic remedies can alleviate ear infections.

Eating Disorders (Anorexia Nervosa and Bulimia)

Anorexia nervosa is a long-term refusal to eat, stemming from physical, mental and emotional factors. It's a problem seen mostly in women, particularly teenagers, who typically start out on a weight-loss program but then don't know when to stop. Bulimia, which involves periods of intense overeating, or binging, followed by vomiting or purging, is also more common in women than in men.

Unfortunately, the media has glorified an unnatural ideal of feminine thinness, adding greatly to the prevalence of these eating disorders. Couple these two conditions with a third, obesity, and distorted eating patterns become a virtual epidemic in our culture.

Causes

Research has shown that anorexia nervosa, bulimia and obesity can often be attributed to a deficiency of the mineral zinc. Evidence of the impact of zinc deficiency upon the body was discovered during the 1930s, when animals fed zinc-deficient diets developed anorexia. Further indication of the significance of zinc is provided by people who suffer from morbid obesity, a condition in which the victim's lifespan is considerably shortened and susceptibility to disease is heightened. Studies reveal an inverse relationship between the level of obesity and the level of zinc in these people's bodies. Although the zinc factor has not been identified as being either causal or an effect of obesity, it's interesting that patients on the opposite side of the spectrum—those with anorexia—have also demonstrated zinc deficiencies. Further studies of people who suffer from eating disorders have revealed that patients who do not overcome their mineral deficiencies have less of a chance of recovering from an eating disorder.

The richest supply of zinc within the female body is located within muscle tissue. Not surprisingly a common symptom of anorexia involves the deterioration of muscle mass. Anorexics who do not receive a sufficient amount of zinc in their diets actually consume their own muscle tissue to compensate for the lack. When the body begins to "scrounge" for zinc from the heart, irreversible damage can occur. When the supply of zinc within cardiac tissue is consumed, the heart, which is comprised of one percent zinc, is at risk of several disorders, including bradycardia, tachycardia and arrhythmia. Eventually, heart failure can occur, which is why anorexia nervosa should always be treated with utmost seriousness. Even the recuperation process for an anorexic person can be hazardous, since any weight gain can overburden the recovering heart.

Yet another adverse effect of zinc deficiency is loss of taste. Studies have shown that zinc-deficient individuals have difficulty synthesizing the proteins that would enable them to experience various flavors. Interestingly, eating disorder patients who are given an initial dosage of zinc supplement are often unable to taste the zinc when it is in their mouths. If you have ever consumed zinc supplements, you are probably well aware of their pungent metallic taste. An inability to experience zinc's potent flavor is a lucid indication of a zinc deficiency.

Another common contributory cause of eating disorders is stress, and stress can facilitate the onset of mineral deficiencies as well. Since women are more susceptible to stress-induced mineral deficiencies than men, they compose a greater percentage of eating disorder cases. A possible explanation for the difference is that the male prostate contains a rich supply of zinc; indeed, zinc located within the prostate is vital to the production, mobility, viability and quantity of male sperm. When a man encounters stress, zinc depletion is improbable due to the man's inordinate auxiliary supply. Women, though, are forced to withdraw quantities of zinc from surrounding tissue; hence, a deficiency is more likely to develop.

Unfortunately most victims do not realize that the cessation of eating will inevitably culminate in malnutrition. While the manifestation of a zinc deficiency remains a common occurrence among eating disorder patients, other minerals vital to the body functioning can become depleted as well. Two of these, potassium and iodine, are essential to proper thyroid maintenance. Since the thyroid is responsible for metabolism rates, any interference in its operation can actually inhibit our ability to remain thin. When a thyroid malfunction occurs, the rate at which calories are burned is dramatically decreased. So, women who think that they can prevent weight gain by throwing up their meals or going on extreme diets can end up actually compounding their problem.

Symptoms

Besides obvious weight loss and muscle deterioration, symptoms of anorexia nervosa include loss of menstruation, an extreme fear of becoming overweight and a distorted self-image; in other words, a very thin person will see herself as being overweight. Other symptoms are low energy, mood swings, long-term constipation and tooth decay. Starvation is like a drug: It causes the body to produce endorphins, which, in turn, cause the so-called starvation high. This natural high eases the symptoms, but, unfortunately, encourages dieting. The bulimic's compulsive eating binges are followed by self-induced vomiting, or the person may take laxatives or diuretics on a consistent basis. The continual cycle of bulimia will result in malnutrition and dehydration. As with the anorexic, heart functioning may become adversely affected.

The final form of eating disorder, obesity, is characterized by excessive storage of fat inside of the adipose tissue and organs of the body. Usually, the effects of obesity become quite evident on the exterior aspect of the body as well. Obesity makes exercise more difficult, which, in turn, increases the problem. The heart becomes affected here, too: It has to work harder and harder to move all that weight.

Treatment

Minerals

Since the zinc plays such a pivotal role in the mechanism of appetite, zinc supplementation is a significant part of the treatment of eating disorders. Liquid zinc is the recommended form. Supplements in the form of powders, tablets, or capsules first have to be broken down by stomach acids, and since many eating disorder patients are unable to properly digest nutrients, these are not as effective as the liquid form of the mineral.

The importance of liquid zinc is hard to overstate. Prior to the discovery of this versatile supplement, the expected recovery rate for eating disorder patients was only between 20 and 30 percent, while the current recovery rate is approximately 65 percent for bulimics and 85 percent for anorexics. Patients who have had a long history of eating disorders often report that they no longer have any desire to binge or purge after adherence to a zinc supplementation program.

A valuable benefit that liquid zinc provides is its ability to combat depression. This is important because many people with eating disorders are clinically depressed. Often, eating disorders develop as part of a response to a traumatic event, with depression being another facet of that response. For this reason—and because anorexia, in particular, can be life-threatening—eating disorder patients should be under the care of a competent medical professional. Zinc supplementation, although highly beneficial, is only part of the picture of the anorexic's or bulimic's recovery plan. Attention to the person's emotional outlook is another vital aspect.

Other important minerals for those with eating disorders can be obtained via sea vegetables, such as dulse, kelp, sea palm and nori. In addition to their valuable mineral content, sea vegetables also contain an ample quantity of other vital nutrients, including beta-carotene and vitamin B12. Since sea vegetables provide such a concentrated source of minerals, only a minimal quantity is necessary to eliminate a deficiency. In fact, mineral supplementation can be effectively achieved by adding a meager two tablespoons of a dried sea vegetable to a soup.

To re-establish healthy bacteria in the gastrointestinal tract, supplement with three capsules of lactobacillus daily. Acidophilus and bifidobacterium may be beneficial as well. Depression, typical in those with eating disorders, can be countered with amino acids such as L-tyrosine (100 mg for each 1 kilogram, or 2.2 pounds, of bodyweight, twice a day) or L-phenylalanine (500 mg taken with vitamin B6). Inositol, the simple sugar that feeds the brain, can be supplemented (2 g daily) to combat depression. In mild or moderate cases, the herb St. John's wort may be beneficial, for it also alleviates anxiety, insomnia and fatigue. (Do not take St. John's wort during pregnancy).

The essential fatty acids in evening primrose oil (two 500-mg capsules three times a day) and gamma-linoleic acid (GLA) help the body to rebalance its weight.

In cases of poor digestion, digestive aids such as betaine, pepsin, glutamic acid, apple cider vinegar, Swedish bitter, pancreatin and vegetable enzymes may be helpful. A test ordered by a naturopath or holistic doctor can show what kind of maldigestion the patient has. Afterwards, an individual therapy can be tailored to suit the digestive system's needs.

Stinging nettle juice can provide lots of nutrients to the depleted body of an anorexic or bulimic. Ginseng can boost energy. Taking 1 tbsp. (juice form) of the following herbs can stimulate the appetite: wormwood, yarrow, angelica, dong quai, centaury, milk thistle, gentian root, chamomile, peppermint, fennel, dandelion, saw palmetto, ginger, gotu kola, ginseng, lady's slipper, licorice, passion flower, skullcap, red yam and yellow dock.

During the early phases of a supplementation program, many eating-disorder patients have an intense phobia of gaining weight and are thus reluctant to eat large quantities of food. Consequently, small concentrated sources are often initially prescribed to quell their fears. Since bulimics eat in private and generally will not stop until interrupted by vomiting or another person, changing their eating habits is oftentimes difficult. Encouraging them to eat with others gives someone else some degree of control over these habits and helps the bulimic to establish a better relationship with food.

While sea vegetables remain an ideal selection, other rich mineral sources are available in the form of green foods, such as chlorella, spirulina and blue-green algae, or of grasses, such as barley greens, barley grass and alfalfa. Since many eating-disorder patients tend to suffer from dehydration, taking these remedies in a drink can be especially beneficial. The malnutrition state of anorexia and bulimia can often inhibit a patient's ability to perceive the body's need for liquid; hence, ensuring proper saturation should be an integral part of the treatment process.

Eating disorders are symptoms of unaddressed psychological or mental problems, fear, anxiety, low self-esteem and lack of self-confidence. After first dealing with the physical aspects of the disorder, psychological help and cognitive behavioral therapy should be used to support the patient in building a new mind-set. Very often, anorexics attack and punish their own body in an attempt to immunize themselves against pain and vulnerability. They deal with unmet needs by teaching themselves not to need. People with eating disorders are often trying to gain control over their weight because they feel the other aspects of their lives are out of control. Anorexics often are high achievers who try to create the "perfect" image that is often depicted in the media. An all-or-nothing attitude is common. Sometimes the anorexic tries to stop him- or herself from growing up.

Bulimia usually starts as a compulsive overeating, a craving for comfort food to fill a void or emptiness in one's life. That leads to bingeing, eating large amounts of food in short periods of time, followed by horror, guilt and hopelessness over the inability to control these desires. It is true that food can take the edge off of uncomfortable emotions, but recovery starts when one learns to face those feelings without seeking comfort in food. Healing starts with admitting the problem. The next step is to make a plan. It should be one's choice to take back the power and regain control over one's life instead of living in denial. As people with eating disorders typically have a history of setting unrealistic expectations for themselves—in effect, setting themselves up for failure—the change should be done in small steps, with victories planned one day at a time.

Prevention

Prevention of eating disorders starts with the education of youth. Young people should be taught the importance of exercise as a way of strengthening and beautifying their bodies. Food, then, can be seen as a fuel to keep us moving, feeling good and functioning at our best. Also, children should be taught exactly what constitutes a healthful diet, and how to prepare simple dishes. And they should understand how junk food could contribute to obesity and other problems.

Finally, we have to keep stressing to young people that most of the advertising and show business images they see of the female body, both on screen and in print, are thinner than most girls can hope to be while still eating healthfully. Only a small percentage of women have body types that can fit into the current idea of glamour without compromising their nutrition.

Treatment Summary

Liquid zinc greatly improves the chances of recovery from anorexia and bulimia.

Other important minerals are available in sea vegetables and green foods, such as chlorella and alfalfa.

Eating disorders must always be treated in the context of the patient's emotional state.

Good exercise and nutrition habits, as well as an understanding of our culture's distorted images, should be part of children's education.

See also: Obesity.

Endometriosis

Endometriosis is a condition in which the cells that line the interior of the uterus dislodge and grow outside the uterine cavity. The cells in their normal state build up in the uterus every month when estrogen levels are high. In this way, they assist in making the lining of the uterus suitable for pregnancy serving as a nest in which the fertilized egg will be implanted. If pregnancy does not take place, the lining breaks off when the estrogen level becomes low, and it emerges as menstrual flow. In the case of endometriosis, though, these cells can attach to a variety of areas. They may grow anywhere in the pelvis, on the fallopian tubes, ovaries, bladder, intestinal surfaces, rectum, colon, ligaments, or appendix. Endometrial tissue has even been found in more distant places within the body such as the lung or armpit.

The cells that grow outside the uterus act as if they were in the uterus; in other words, they grow during periods in which the estrogen level is high and create blood when estrogen levels are low. However, when endometrial tissue grows in areas other than the uterus, there is no exit for the blood when estrogen levels drop. Therefore, the blood will then collect in these areas, causing cystic structures, scarring and other types of damage to these organs. Over five million women in the U.S., mainly in the 20 to 40-year-old age group, are afflicted with this problem.

Causes

The causes of endometriosis are unknown at this time. However, there are theories as to why this condition develops. One possible cause may be that during menstruation the blood flows backward as opposed to outward. If that is the case, menstrual blood is able to go through the fallopian tube and gain access to the pelvic and abdominal cavity. The cells from this blood can then embed themselves outside the uterus in other tissues and organs.

Another theory is that the cells in the uterine lining migrate through lymphatic channels for implantation outside the uterine cavity. Genetic predisposition to the condition may play a part. So may a deficiency in the immune system. The theory here is that through some hormonal and chemical influence, endometrial tissue becomes activated at different times in the cycle, causing tissue to proliferate in abnormal areas. There are also studies showing that exposure to dioxin, a chemical found in pesticides and certain types of waste incineration, may be an additional cause of endometriosis. Lastly childbearing in conjunction with various methods of birth control may also be responsible.

Symptoms

There are generally two symptoms of endometriosis: pain and bleeding. Pain is the main symptom and may be either minimal or severe. It occurs because of inflammation and scarring of affected tissues. The area where the pain is felt and the degree to which it is experienced will depend on the site of the endometrial tissue and the degree to which it is implanted. The pain might occur just prior to menstruation and be attributed to menstrual cramps. However, some women experience pain during intercourse at any time during the month. It is also possible for pain to be felt during urination, due to implantation of the cells in the bladder; during bowel movements as a result of colon and rectal implants; and in the ovaries and extending to the back and buttocks, or down the legs. There may also be pelvic pain during a gynecological examination.

Bleeding problems might persist as well. There may be internal bleeding as well as bleeding from various orifices in the body (such as nosebleeds). It is important to note that recurrent bleeding at specific times of the month should lead one to suspect endometriosis.

Other symptoms may include bladder infections and fatigue.

Diagnosis

The only way to truly confirm endometriosis is through a surgical process known as laparoscopy. This procedure allows the doctor to biopsy the tissue. Sonograms and MRIs can also be helpful in diagnosing the problem, but are not completely accurate.

Treatment

The ultimate treatment for the most severe cases of endometriosis is a hysterectomy in which reproductive organs that are scarred and damaged are removed. However, this is a serious surgical procedure that should only be explored as a last result when the condition has become very serious and other approaches have failed.

One of these approaches is traditional drug therapy that generally consists of medical prescriptions for pain, and suppression of estrogen, to reduce endometrial growth. Medications given may include indomethacin, ibuprofen, Naprosyn and danazol. However, there may be adverse side effects, such as arteriosclerosis, bone loss, weight gain, edema, changes in breast size, acne, excess hair growth, hot flashes and deepening of the voice.

Hormones are another aspect of conventional therapy. They are given to simulate pregnancy in order to slow down and prohibit the progress of endometriosis. This method, too, may produce unpleasant side effects, such as depression, painful breasts, nausea, weight gain, bloating, swelling and migraine headaches.

Some newer compounds, which diminish pain and reduce the mass of endometrial tissue, may produce fewer side effects. They are called gonadotropin releasing hormone compounds and are sometimes given by injection.

Diet

Since conventional treatments for endometriosis have their drawbacks, it may be beneficial to explore natural solutions, starting with a dietary approach, to alleviate symptoms and reverse the problem. There are foods that may reduce estrogen levels, and thus diminish or slow the growth of endometriosis. A mostly vegetarian diet is recommended, with an emphasis on soy products, alfalfa spouts, flaxseeds and legumes. Another dietary strategy is to consume foods that aid in excreting estrogen from the body through the intestinal tract. A high-fiber diet works to this end; think in terms of whole grains and fresh fruits and vegetables. You want the diet to be low in fat; avoid, particularly, products high in saturated fat (such as dairy products and red meat), but make sure to get enough essential fatty acids (omega-3 and omega-6, in the form of flaxseed oil, fish oil, evening primrose oil or ground flaxseeds). Lastly, the liver may aid in lowering estrogen levels. Therefore, it is a good idea to eat foods high in the B-complex vitamins, such as whole grains and legumes, and avoid alcohol, fat and sugar, in order to promote a healthy liver.

Supplements

Vitamin and mineral supplements can also be helpful in reducing inflammation. Recommended supplements include:

Vitamin C . . . The dosage should be based on a woman's bowel tolerance; stop short of the level causing diarrhea. Combining vitamin C with 750-2000 mg of bioflavonoids rebalances estrogen levels.

Vitamin B6 . . . A dosage of 50 mg should be taken twice a day. The pyridoxal-5-phosphate form (P5P) is even better because it's easier to metabolize.

Beta-Carotene . . . A dosage of 150,000-200,000 IU decreases related cramping, fluid retention and fatigue.

Selenium . . . The recommended dosage is 400 mcg.

Vitamin E . . . The recommended dosage is 800-1200 IU.

Vitamin A . . . Supplementation of 1000-5000 IU restores vitamin A levels (low levels are typical in women with excessive menstrual bleeding).

Zinc . . . The recommended dosage is 30-50 mg per day.

Iron . . . Use in case of severe menstrual bleeding.

Calcium . . . A dosage of 1000-1500 mg daily helps to maintain muscle tone and lowers the chance of cramping. Taking 200 mg of magnesium two to three times a day helps absorb calcium.

Choline . . . The suggested dose is 1000 mg, along with 1000 mg of inositol and 300 mg of methionine.

Herbs

Herbal supplements work similarly to vitamins in that they assist in decreasing inflammation. Recommended herbs include white willow bark and a formula suggested by a Portland, Oregon, gynecologist, Dr. Tori Hudson that contains equal amounts of chasteberry, dandelion root, motherwort and prickly ash. The recommended dosage is one teaspoon taken three times daily. Milk thistle (silybum marianum), vervain (verbena officinalis) and blue flag (iris versicolor) support the liver. In cases of pelvic congestion, squaw vine (mitchella repens), red root (ceonothus americanus) and red raspberry (rubus idaeus) may be beneficial. The bereberine-containing goldenseal and dong quai have also shown the ability to relax the uterine muscles. Yellow dock can be taken in cases of iron deficiency due to heavy menstrual bleeding. White willow bark can decrease inflammation and fever caused by menstrual cramps. Echinacea is a great immune system enhancer, which is the key to recovery. Wild yam is an herb that helps rebalance the hormones. Yarrow has multiple qualities: it stops the bleeding, stimulates the liver and heals infections. To deal with estrogen excess, a lipotropic combination including milk thistle, choline, inositol, hexaniacite, methionine and dandelion might be beneficial. Phytoestrogens—the plant forms of estrogen from red clover, black cohosh and genistein—help to expel the unneeded estrogen by replacing it.

Homeopathy

Belladonna can be beneficial in cases of heavy menstrual bleeding. Calcarea phosphoricum is suggested when backache accompanies the period.

Chamomilla might bring relief when the menses contains dark blood clots. Cimicifuga racemosa can soothe unbearable pain around the hip area.

Hellerwork

Hellerwork is a body technique that helps to refine body structure through deep tissue work. It has been shown that patients with endometriosis have muscle spasms, which is one of the causes of pain. Thus, Hellerwork instructs women to relax their muscles to ease the symptoms. This therapy strives to create a healthy balance of mind and body by freeing misalignments in body structure, working to improve everyday habits that contribute to the problem and working through emotional issues that may affect a woman physically.

Oriental Medicine

Women with endometriosis may want to consider some of the natural therapies used in Traditional Chinese Medicine (TCM). One approach is to decrease the size of the endometrial mass through the use of laser acupuncture. Other TCM techniques are retention enemas or injection into the endometrial nodes with common sage root. TCM practitioners advise abstaining from sexual intercourse at the time of menstruation, as it can cause the migration of endometrial tissue into the pelvic cavity and result in an imbalance of energy. They also advocate using acupuncture to release obstructions from the liver, spleen, heart, lung and kidney in order for energy to move freely within the system.

Other Treatments

Contrast sitz baths can reduce pain by increasing circulation. Try sitting in hot water for three minutes, then in cold water for one minute. Repeat this three or four times, twice a day. Castor oil packs applied to the abdomen may also help. Practicing Kegel exercises—contracting and releasing the pelvic muscles—may ease the symptoms. Vigorous exercise that raises the heart rate is also beneficial. Lastly, avoid using tampons.

Treatment Summary

Switch to a mostly vegetarian, high-fiber, low-fat diet and be sure to consume foods high in the B-complex vitamins.

The following nutrients and herbs can help reduce inflammation: vitamin C, beta-carotene, selenium, vitamin E, white willow bark and a formula containing chasteberry, dandelion root, motherwort and prickly ash.

Hellerwork is a body technique that teaches women to relax their muscles to ease the pain caused by muscle spasms associated with endometriosis.

TCM recommends increasing pelvic flow, avoiding sexual intercourse during menstruation and using acupuncture to release obstructions.

Environmental Illness

The environment in which we live affects the way both our mind and body function. This is not a new concept. In fact, even thousands of years ago people knew that they could become ill from certain foods and products. Today as our society continues to produce more toxic chemical substances that can result in immune deficiencies and mutations, researchers and some practitioners within the medical community are beginning to give more credence to this area of study. As *Environmental Magazine* writer Alyssa Burger points out, naturalists have recently seen how chemical contamination of animals' habitats have caused mutations in certain species. That chemicals can affect humans in physically subtle, as well as overt, ways is beyond question.

Females are most likely to develop ailments related to toxic chemicals in the environment because exposure to certain toxins can create an imbalance of estrogen in a woman's body. Once in the body, many chemicals mimic estrogen, and are therefore known as xeno-estrogenic compounds (xeno meaning foreign). But males, too, can be adversely affected by xeno-estrogenic compounds. Animal studies show that a variety of male reproductive disorders, ranging from sterility to undescended testicles to odd sexual behaviors, may result from environmental factors.

Causes

From silicone breast implants; to artificial colors, flavors and preservatives in foods, drinks and drugs; to the nerve gas encountered by our Gulf War troops; to the hormones used in the dairy industry, today's society exposes us to a wide variety of chemicals that can affect our systems. Dioxins, to name one infamous group, are byproducts of the manufacture of herbicides; they increase the likelihood of cancer as well as negatively impact the endocrine system. Organochlorine pesticides, of which DDT is the most notorious example, affect fertility. Other widely used chemicals found in toiletries, spermicides, household detergents, plastics and food-can linings can affect the health of susceptible individuals as well.

Artificial colors, flavors and preservatives in foods, drinks and drugs are also potential causes of environmental illness. Tap water, foods containing additives, inorganically grown vegetables, certain meat products and hydrogenated oil all bear toxic chemicals. Fluorescent lights, perfumes and fragrances, detergents, air fresheners, disinfectants and even the products with which we furnish our homes, such as carpeting, paint and mattresses, can release chemicals at a low level. We commonly have all of those in our bedrooms, and, if they are giving off toxic fumes, this is not a good situation because the bedroom is one room in the house that really needs to be safe. Our bodies tend to detoxify at night while we are sleeping. However, if the bedroom is a toxic environment, not only can't we detoxify, but we also increase the amount of chemicals to which we are exposed, which continually weakens our systems.

In addition to chemicals, there are other environmental factors that need to be addressed. Exposure to radiation, radon, car exhaust, tobacco smoke, heavy metals and electromagnetic fields are other factors that can create immune system deficiencies.

The more poisons a person ingests or inhales, the more inclined he or she is to becoming sick. The poisons collect in body fat until capacity there is at a maximum. They then move all around the body through the circulatory system, manifesting themselves in a variety of symptoms. While anyone may become ill from environmental factors, those most at risk are people who reside or work in a sealed building that lacks windows or a good ventilation system; those who work with chemicals, computer chips, gasoline, or formaldehyde; those who are allergic or sensitive to certain foods, molds, or chemicals; those who take a variety of antibiotics; those who live near commercial properties involved in chemical manufacturing or toxic incineration; and those who are under a great deal of stress, which leads to poor eating habits.

Considering all the risk factors and the products to which we're exposed, it may seem as if everybody is fated to suffer environmental illness. That's not the case, though, because we can educate ourselves to lessen the risks and build our immune systems.

Symptoms

Different people react to environmental conditions in different ways. Symptoms can include the following: exhaustion, muscle weakness, muscle aches, joint pains, heart irregularities, asthma, increased sensitivity to odors, food allergies and intolerances, flu-like symptoms, ringing in the ears, burning in the eyes, mild or severe headaches, bloating and other intestinal problems, colon problems, sleep disorders, loss of balance, skin disorders, inability to concentrate, memory loss, anxiety and panic attacks, depression, learning disabilities, sensitivities to changes in the weather, persistent infections (especially yeast), autoimmune disorders and multiple chemical sensitivity syndrome. Allergies are known to contribute to the symptoms of ADD/ADHD, autism and chronic fatigue syndrome.

Since there are so many possible symptoms, environmental illness can be difficult to diagnose. Routine blood tests frequently yield normal results and lead doctors to believe that no problem exists. It is always a good idea for persons who suspect environmental illness to examine the following: where they feel ill (e.g., at work, at home, or in a new residence or office); whether their surroundings or lifestyle expose them to toxic substances; and whether they have recently had any new products introduced into their home or office, such as new carpeting or paint. Fortunately, there are some medical practitioners who do recognize environmental illness as a possibility when unexplained symptoms arise. Occupational and environmental physicians can order tests that examine, for example, pesticide and mineral concentrations in the blood, to help determine whether a person suffers from chemical exposure.

Treatment

While no conventional medical treatment exists for environmental illness, there are some things that people can do to minimize or reverse the damage and better protect themselves from continued exposure.

Detoxification

Two forms of detoxification have had encouraging results in the reversal of environmental illness. One is heat stress detoxification, which involves wood saunas, hot sand packing, steam baths and sweat lodges. This method requires the guidance of a trained practitioner, since it necessitates an understanding of toxins and their effects on the body. Another approach is biotoxic reduction. This is a two-week medically managed program that incorporates aerobics, sauna therapy and increasing niacin levels. Enemas and colonics provide relief to the overtaxed liver and also help to expel parasites, bacteria and yeast overgrowth. A detoxifying clay bath can help expel toxic materials from the system. Professional supervision is highly suggested. There are treatments that can be included depending upon the individual.

Diet

The foods we eat have a great impact on our system. Many of the meat products in this country contain toxins, concentrated in the tissues since animal feed is often treated with chemicals. Also, crops are treated with pesticides, which can then get into our systems, through the fruits, vegetables and grains we eat. That's why buying organically grown food, whenever possible, is recommended. Poultry that is organically fed can also be considered. Furthermore, before you drink or cook with your tap water, it should be purified.

Air and Water Purification

The indoor and outdoor air quality plays a significant role in the development of environmental illness. The filtration of indoor air in the home and workplace is important in preventing and treating multiple chemical sensitivity syndrome, which can develop because of massive exposure to highly toxic substances or ongoing exposure to low doses of toxic materials. People with MCS might need HEPA (high efficiency particulate adsorption) filtration, which filters out small particles, such as dust mites, dander, pollen, mold, fungal spores, cockroach dust and tobacco smoke. HEGA (high efficiency gas adsorption) filtration removes gases, exhaust fumes, organic hydrocarbons, pesticides, formaldehyde from materials used in home construction, paint solvents, chlorine and cleaning chemicals. Activated carbon removes low-level ozone. The perfect air purifier has a built-in ultraviolet lamp that kills bacteria and viruses through photo-oxidation; these bacteria and viruses are too small to be removed by even the finest filters. This ultraviolet light has 10,000 times more intensity than sunlight, and when it reacts with oxygen, it produces negative ions and activated oxygen, which are needed for concentration and sleep. When needed, a personal, lightweight, negative ionizer can be worn around the neck. An ionic air cleaner can also be used in the car to get rid of airborne impurities and to freshen the air. Few people are aware of the fact that they can absorb more chlorine from a shower than from drinking water. Chlorine, lead, iron oxides, bacteria, hydrogen sulfide and other inorganic contaminants can be filtered out by 99 percent using a carbon shower filter.

Supplements

There are many nutrients that can help reverse the effects of chemical exposure. Since exposure to chemicals affects people in different ways, the recommendation will vary depending upon the individual. However, some of the supplements that have proven helpful are vitamins C and E, L-glutamine, carnitine, glucosamine sulfate, magnesium and chelated manganese. In addition, antioxidants, such as green tea tincture and alpha-lipoic acid, and digestive enzymes have proven to be beneficial.

Since we are exposed to an increasing number of toxic materials every year, the liver's role as detoxifier is becoming even more important. Poor liver function can initiate allergic reactions. For instance, psoriasis could be cleared with liver supporting supplements, herbs (such as milk thistle, burdock and dandelion), N-acetyl-cysteine, taurine, SAMe, arginine and MSM.

Because of exposure to chemicals and other materials, or as a reaction to weather changes, irritant eczema may develop. (See *Skin Conditions.*) The health of the gut is also an important factor. Parasites can enter the body through the consumption of infested water or improperly cleaned food, and can lead to leaky gut syndrome. Restoring the balance of the gut flora is essential. The inhalation of molds, fungi or other irritant agents can result in sick-building syndrome, which can manifest as asthma. Outside of mild to drastic lifestyle changes, avoidance of irritants and dealing with anxiety, stress and fear, there are herbs and supplements that reduce the symptoms of asthma, such as magnesium, lobelia, lavender and tei fu lotion. (See *Allergies.*)

Reduction of Electromagnetic Pollution

In our environment, we are surrounded by electrical appliances such as computers, televisions, microwave ovens, cell phones and digital clocks that are encircled by electromagnetic fields, which are associated with the risk of cancer. Microwave ovens work by radiation, causing modification in the molecular structure of food. Cell phones work by using both continuous wave and microwave RF (radio frequency), and, according to Blake Lewitt, author of *Electromagnetic Fields,* "When it comes to cell phones, a worse frequency could not have been chosen for the human anatomy." Through their heating effect, cell phones can raise the temperature of the brain by 2 degrees Fahrenheit after only 20 minutes. The long-term exposure to these emissions causes biological damage, creating hot spots in the brain; it breaks the blood-brain barrier, allowing toxins and proteins to leak into the brain. By disrupting the brain's electrochemical communication, cell phones can cause forgetfulness and sudden confusion, and lead to Alzheimer's disease, cancer, Parkinson's disease, multiple sclerosis and accelerated aging. The exposure to cell phone transmissions triggers histamine production, resulting in an increased number of asthmatic cases.

Furthermore, bystanders can be affected by secondhand microwave and radio-frequency pollution; children, whose tissues have a greater capacity absorption, are especially at risk. Headsets and shields such as MLC-524#, developed by Steven Horvat, operate by altering the positive-negative magnetic fields and offer partial protection. Try to reduce the length of cell-phone calls, and turn the cell phone off as often as possible. It is best not to keep cell phones close to the ovaries, testicles, or heart.

What to Avoid

There is a lot that people can do to minimize the toxicity of their environment. If you suspect that you are suffering from environmental toxins, test the effect of removing suspect products containing harmful chemicals from your surroundings. Plastic-lined tin cans, as well as foods microwaved in plastic wrap, should be avoided. If you must microwave, be sure to use microwave-safe containers. Stay away from fatty animal products, as these contain toxic chemicals, including dioxin. Synthetic fragrances in personal care products, such as perfumes, aftershave, and cosmetics, can also cause harm. It's better to buy unscented products and add pure, natural fragrances. In addition, ensure that at least the bedroom is one room in your house that is free of toxins.

Harsh, fluorescent lighting that flickers 100 flashes per second can cause headaches and an inability to concentrate. These devices work based on the concept of synchronizing and controlling brain waves. In hospitals, avoiding the use of latex gloves and the sterilizer gluteraldehyde (use hydrogen peroxide instead) can save missed workdays by nurses, doctors and staff.

Don't overlook your travel habits. Did you know that car exhaust affects people inside the vehicle more than those on the outside? Always keep a window rolled down. Carbon and hepa car filters, found in newer, upscale models, may help. Finally if you're a jogger, try to follow a route that's away from heavy traffic. You don't want to undermine your health while engaged in an essentially health-enhancing activity.

Treatment Summary

Heat stress detoxification and biotoxic reduction have provided relief for people with environmental illness. Both programs require the guidance of trained practitioners.

Given that many foods contain chemicals that weaken the immune system, the following are recommended: fruits, vegetables and grains that are organically grown, organically fed poultry, purified water and avoidance of foods containing food additives or other chemical substances.

Supplemental nutrients that can help reverse the effects of chemical exposure include vitamins C and E, L-glutamine and carnitine.

Measures to remove toxic substances from your environment include avoiding foods microwaved in plastic wrap, buying unscented personal care products, using a carbon shower filter and keeping car windows open when you're on the road.

Eye Disorders

The eyes are a part of the body that can easily be taken for granted until a problem arises. The reason eye problems, in one form or another, are inevitable is that throughout the human body, new cells are continuously replacing old ones. However, this is not the way things are done in the eye. The cells of the lens of the eye with which you are born, stay with you for the duration of your life. It is also important to keep in mind that the eye is made up of 65 percent water and 35 percent protein. In fact, this represents the highest concentration of protein in the human body.

Most of the problems people have with their eyes occur gradually and generally do not produce many symptoms; therefore, without regular visits to the doctor, immediate attention and early prevention are essentially sacrificed. To further complicate the issue, conventional treatments tend to achieve only short-term solutions that can sometimes make the eyes worse. Therefore, given the discomfort eye conditions can create, in addition to the potentially serious, long-term ramifications, it is important to understand the most common disorders and their impact.

What Can Go Wrong with the Eyes

Cataracts

This is when the lens of the eye becomes fogged, due either to a decrease in the fluid surrounding the lens, poor circulation, or nutritional deficiencies. Cataracts can impair the detail of a person's vision by causing a haze and preventing light from penetrating the lens. This condition tends to get worse over time, even to the point of blindness in the most extreme cases. Cataracts can affect either one or both eyes. The link between cataracts and improper nutrition has been well documented in a plethora of clinical studies.

Diabetic Retinopathy (DR)

For adults, diabetic retinopathy is the main cause of visual problems and blindness. It affects an estimated 20 million people. To thwart this vision problem, it is essential that diabetics have the condition detected early, through a dilated eye examination, to prevent vision problems and blindness.

Note: A 2001 study concluded that the bioflavonoids quercetin, myrcetin and kaempferol inhibit diabetic cataracts.

Glaucoma

Similar to cataracts, this disorder also causes a gradual loss of sight, initially affecting a person's peripheral vision. Glaucoma usually occurs after the age of 40. However, when congenital, it can occur earlier. Twenty-five percent of Americans are afflicted with this disease, and it has led to blindness in over 60,000 of them.

The optic nerve is quite sensitive and can be affected by fluid, sunlight, infection, circulatory problems, exposure to toxins and nutritional deficiencies. In glaucoma, pressure on the eye tends to progressively increase, damaging the optic nerve. This causes gradual vision loss and, without proper care, can eventually lead to blindness. In fact, glaucoma is one of the principal causes of blindness in the U.S.

Macular Degeneration

Another primary cause of blindness is the condition that occurs when the tiny area in the center of the retina, the macula, deteriorates. The macula records images and then transmits them through the optic nerve to the brain. This condition affects primarily the elderly, as it is the leading cause of blindness in persons over age 55. It occurs for a variety of reasons, including nutritional deficiencies, circulatory trouble and atherosclerosis. Exposure to electromagnetic fields, particularly through heavy computer use, has also been implicated.

Myopia

This is the condition generally referred to as nearsightedness. Light entering the eye achieves clarity in front of the retina as opposed to on the retina, where it would normally come into focus. This results in difficulty seeing objects that are far away.

Hyperopia

The opposite of myopia is known as hyperopia or farsightedness. Here, the carrier wave of light adjusts to achieve images behind the retina. Thus, a person with hyperopia has trouble seeing objects in very close range.

Symptoms

One symptom common to all of the aforementioned disorders is vision impairment, whether it's the inability to see objects up close or far away, or the gradual loss of vision. In the case of glaucoma, there are additional symptoms, including headaches, eye pain, redness in the eyes, nausea and vomiting and an abnormally wide pupil.

Treatment

Conventional treatment for eye disorders includes surgery, drug therapy and corrective eyewear. Surgery is generally used in the case of cataracts and glaucoma. However, there is always some risk with surgery and the conditions may not be reversed. Drug therapy used for glaucoma, can produce serious side effects, such as asthma, depression, loss of libido and high cholesterol. It, too, does not guarantee a cure. In the case of corrective eyewear for both near- and farsighted individuals, the muscles in and around the eyes tend to worsen, since they begin to rely on prescriptive lenses to improve vision. As for macular degeneration, traditional medicine does not even have a way of dealing with it, viewing it as an untreatable condition.

Some natural solutions have been found not only to prevent and also improve all these disorders, but, sometimes, to correct them as well. Plus, they can provide results in a manner that is much easier on the system than conventional medical treatments. Some of these therapies are cited below:

Nutrition

Nutrition is key in dealing with eye problems not only because it can help correct a disorder, but because it will prevent future problems from occurring. Keep in mind that the eyes are dependent upon the rest of the body for nourishment. In particular, the eyes rely on the liver and kidneys, as well as on the circulatory system, to eliminate toxins from the bloodstream and to metabolize and deliver the appropriate nutrients.

The vitamins and minerals associated with eye care are vitamins E and D, for the general maintenance of healthy eyes (low blood levels of vitamin E are closely associated with increased cataract risk) vitamin A, for proper liver metabolism and digestion (vitamin A is especially important for the health of the retina); vitamin C, for ridding the bloodstream of toxins (vitamin C is highly concentrated in the aqueous humor and the corneal epithelium of the eye, and scientific literature is filled with studies showing that vitamin C gives considerable protection to the eyes; vitamin C levels exist in the lens at amounts that are 30-50 times those found in other parts of the blood); glutathione, for helping rid the eye of excess fluid (glutathione maintains the water balance in the lens); selenium, the carotenoids and niacin, for increasing circulation; all the B vitamins (specifically, riboflavin, the deficiency of which a recent epidemiological study found is linked to a decreased risk for cataracts, and which, after glutathione has fought free radicals, removes the oxidized glutathione); omega-3 and omega-6 fatty acids (found in fish oils), for decreasing inflammation; and a balance of magnesium and calcium, for proper muscle control. While these nutrients can all be taken in the form of supplements, it is important to get them from one's diet, as well. Overall, a low-fat, dairy-free, vegetarian diet is a great way to get the nutrients essential for proper eye care. In particular, carrots, green leafy vegetables (such as beet greens, spinach and broccoli) and yellow, green and orange fruits (particularly in the form of fresh organic fruit juices) are excellent sources of vitamin A. Furthermore, sulfur-rich foods, such as eggs, garlic and asparagus, increase the amounts of vitamins C and E in the body.

A noted study examined subjects to ascertain the level of activity of antioxidants in the lens and vitreous of the eye. The study determined that the decreased levels of glutathione peroxidase in diabetics were considerable. Furthermore, the diabetics' vitamin C levels were also decreased. Another study established a link between diabetes and decreased amounts of antioxidants in the body. In essence, diabetes impairs the shield of protection that antioxidants provide. To bolster that protection, diabetics need to make sure that supplementation with antioxidants is ongoing.

In fact, numerous studies show that the eyes of younger people have high levels of antioxidants, which provide protection against the above-referenced eye disorders. The eye of an older person has lower levels of these antioxidants, which serve as an invitation for free-radical damage. To help combat this problem, nutrient-enhanced eyedrop solutions are now available on the market.

Lutein and zeaxanthin are two carotenoids that exist in high concentrations in the macula, retina and crystalline lens of the eye. Studies show that both of these carotenoids protect the eye from macular degeneration and cataract formation. Good sources of lutein are dark green leafy vegetables. Good sources for zeaxanthin are yellow-colored fruits and vegetables, such as peaches and corn.

It should be noted that even the naysayers who attempt to discredit alternative medicine cannot refute the scientifically documented link between supplementation and the prevention and treatment of cataracts. The proof is incontrovertible, like the sun rising in the east. In a nutshell, free-radical damage is a major cause of cataracts.

Lastly, ginkgo is a flavonoid that inhibits free-radical damage to the eye. And for the eye to function at peak levels, it needs large amounts of the free-radical scavenger taurine, the most abundant amino acid in the retina.

Herbs

Herbs complement the nutrients a person receives from his or her diet. Specifically, herbs that allow for better circulation so that more nutrients can reach the eye are ginkgo biloba, gotu kola and hawthorn berry. The same effect can be found in the common spices marjoram, cayenne pepper, ginger and garlic.

Bilberry pine bark extract, and grape seed extract can be used to fortify the capillaries that furnish the eye with fluid and aid in the prevention of lens impairment. Recommended dosage is 120-160 mg daily.

Diagaku eye drops and shi hu are Chinese herbs useful for healing dry or inflamed eyes. For the correction of early cataracts, the Chinese herbs zhang yan, baineiting eye drops and ming mu may be beneficial.

Lycium rehmarinia is an herb that helps maintain the health of the retina.

Vision Therapy

Dr. Robert Michael Kaplan, author of *The Power Behind Your Eyes,* is a behavioral optometrist who practices vision therapy. One of the best methods, according to Kaplan, for correcting vision problems on an emotional and physical level is breath work. One technique he recommends is called the integrated breath. The method involves breathing in, breathing out and then pausing. This is performed three to five times consecutively in a slow manner to prevent hyperventilation.

Kaplan follows this foundation exercise with a procedure that he calls eye crossing. While classical vision care warns people not to cross their eyes for fear of getting stuck in this position, Kaplan believes that eye crossing, when done in a relaxed manner without straining, can increase vision fitness. The easiest way to cross the eyes is to position one of the thumbs about eight inches in front of the eyes. While focusing attention on the thumb, notice how everything behind it doubles. This is a good sign because it shows that the left and right eyes are participating equally.

Kaplan believes that the cross-eye exercise will increase one's ability to stay centered in life because when you pull the left eye and the right eyes in, you are looking closer at the self. This is also a valuable exercise for children who are developing vision, for people who experience motion sickness (see: Motion Sickness) when reading in a vehicle and for individuals who experience concentration difficulties and stress from working on computers or reading books for sustained periods.

Kaplan recommends visual hygiene practices that can easily be incorporated during the day. First, he advocates taking vision breaks while working. A person should periodically look up from the book or computer, and focus on the distance. Another tip for improved vision includes writing on an angled surface rather than a flat desk. This avoids leaning over, which strains the shoulders and back, and limits blood flow to the eyes. Additionally, good lighting is important. People should surround themselves with natural light by working near windows, skylights, or full-spectrum lighting. Lastly, it is important to take frequent body-stretching breaks every 20 minutes to an hour, to increase nerve flow from the spine, shoulders and neck. Kaplan explains that after people practice vision therapy, eyeglasses may become too strong. A vision therapy oriented practitioner can lower the prescription. In that way, eyesight can improve.

More Eye Exercises

Exercises can be helpful in preventing or correcting particular conditions. Overall, daily activity is recommended to help lower interocular pressure and increase circulation. This could even take the form of a brisk walk. Specific exercises that may be included in an individualized program include the following:

To enhance peripheral vision, imagine a clock. In visualizing the clock, rotate the eyes counterclockwise from 12 to nine and then back again. Then move the eyes in the opposite direction, from 12 to three and back. This should be done without the help of corrective eyewear, using the thumb as a guide. During the exercise, the person should be attentive to objects on the perimeter of the scope of vision. This drill can be done three times daily.

For strengthening the eye muscles, focus clearly on an object, and bring it in closer until that object becomes blurred. At this point, stop and take deep breaths until sight turns clearer. Then the object can be brought in closer again and the procedure repeated.

Another muscle-strengthening exercise involves sitting in the middle of a room and, without moving anything but the eyes, gazing up to the ceiling and then following the visual path in a straight line down to the floor. This can be repeated several times. Then the same process should be done looking from one side of the room to the other. Deep breathing should be performed during this exercise.

To release tension in the eyes, while in a comfortable position, cover the eyes with the palms of the hands. Visualize a peaceful place while performing deep breathing. One can also visualize a time in the past when one's vision was better, in order to picture the eye in its proper shape.

Massage can increase circulation to the neck and subsequently to the eyes.

Additional Therapies

Acupuncture and acupressure are sometimes used to lessen tension and improve vision. Practitioners apply pressure to specific points surrounding the eye and clear the energy paths connected to the eye, such as the stomach, urinary bladder and gallbladder meridians. Reflexology is also used for eye problems. Practitioners of this technique explain that there are reflex points in the foot—specifically located between the second and third toes—that, when massaged, can clear nerve blockages to the eyes. Biofeedback techniques can assist in regulating eye focus and muscle movement to result in improved vision. These are performed with special instruments that use sound to help teach muscle control.

What to Avoid

Particular foods and environmental factors can be harmful to the eyes, resulting in vision impairment. These include artificial sweeteners, as they contain toxic substances which can negatively affect the optic nerve; caffeine, which affects circulation; alcohol, as it can damage liver function; sugar, which may hinder enzyme function; lactose, a form of sugar found in dairy products; tobacco; steroids; the toxin mercury found in dental amalgam fillings; and exposure to direct sunlight, which can increase oxidative damage to the eyes.

Treatment Summary

Nutrients important to eye health include vitamins A, C, D and E; glutathione; selenium; the carotenoids; niacin; all the B vitamins; omega-3 and omega fatty acids, and the proper balance of magnesium and calcium.

Some herbs that help the eyes by allowing for better circulation are ginkgo biloba, gotu kola and hawthorn berry. The field of vision therapy offers exercises and lifestyle advice that can help strengthen the eyes. Daily activity is important to help lower interocular pressure and increase circulation. Also, specific vision exercises can help with particular problems.

Acupuncture, acupressure, reflexology and biofeedback are other techniques used to improve vision.

Fever

Contrary to what most of us think, a fever is really a friend in that it tells us that our body is handling an internal crisis. The hot feeling we experience is an indication that the body is working hard to burn up pathogenic microbes. High, prolonged fevers can be dangerous, however, and can result in convulsions or even death.

The definition of a fever is an abnormal rise in body temperature. Some consider a fever to be a body temperature of 100 degrees Fahrenheit or higher. Others define it simply as an increase above normal daily variations.

Fevers are caused by infectious agents, such as bacteria, viruses, and other microbes, and by noninfectious agents, such as inflammation and immune response. Exercise, anxiety, dehydration, cancer, anemia, nerve disease and drugs may also bring them on.

Treatment

Since fever is a part of the body's natural healing process, eradicating it should not necessarily be your goal. If a mild to moderate fever is part of your case of the flu or a cold, you can work with it to cleanse the body by consuming foods, particularly in juice form, that are high in chlorophyll, vitamin C and other antioxidants. Supplementation with zinc appears to reduce the duration of a fever. The herb fenugreek also seems to be able to reduce a fever. Kidney chi, the herbal diuretic used in traditional Chinese medicine, is an effective agent that relieves excess "damp-heat" conditions. It also improves symptoms brought on by any kind of infection, plus it purifies the kidneys and relieves water retention. Kidney chi's ingredients are 100-percent natural Asian dandelion, plantain seed, motherwort, Job's tears, fu ling, di fu zi, akebia, alisma, cork tree bark and chrysanthemum powder. Tinctures or teas from natural herb remedies such as catnip, elderflower, sage, yarrow, Angostura bitters, gentian, lemon balm, white willow bark, spearmint, peppermint and feverfew are also useful for reducing fever. Echinacea should be taken at the first sign of a cold, the flu or a fever. Save the aspirin or Tylenol for those times when the fever lasts for more than a day or is high.

Note: Aspirin has been associated with the serious condition known as Reye's syndrome in children and teenagers who have taken it while they had the flu or chicken pox. Consult a physician before giving aspirin to children.

Homeopathy

Homeopathic physicians key their remedies to very specific symptoms and sensations experienced by their patients. Here are some of the remedies they use when fever is a problem.

Aconitum . . . The fever appears suddenly after exposure to cold, dry winds, and rises rapidly within the first few hours, going up to 104 or 105 degrees Fahrenheit. The patient feels restless, anxious and frightened of never recovering.

Belladonna . . . If aconitum does not take effect within 12 hours, homeopathists give "the deadly nightshade," belladonna. Indications for this remedy are being flushed and congested, with dry, hot skin. Covered areas perspire, while the feet remain icy cold. There is no thirst and the tongue is bright red. Extreme sensitivity to light, noise and motion may result in a throbbing headache. This is a remedy used for fever with convulsions or hallucinations.

Ferrum Phosphoricum . . . If belladonna does not produce the desired results, this remedy is an option, as it works well in the first stages of a fever.

Bryonia . . . Think of "bry" rhyming with "dry" and you know when this remedy is recommended. Bryonia is for dry hacking coughs, and for dry parched lips accompanied by thirst. Symptoms worsen in cold, dry wind. Unlike the restless belladonna patient, the bryonia individual remains motionless to avoid achiness.

Gelsemium . . . This is a remedy often used for patients with the flu or summer colds. The yellow jasmine plant from which it is derived resembles this person's appearance: dull, droopy, drowsy and yellow. Low energy causes lethargy and a heavy sensation in the limbs. Fever is slow to start, but is long-lasting, and is accompanied by a chill and great thirst.

Baptisia . . . Onset of fever is sudden and high, and often accompanies intestinal flu. There is sudden vomiting, diarrhea, foul breath and a dull, reddish, unhappy appearance. Symptoms worsen at 11 A.M. Emotionally, the patient is fearful and frustrated.

Apis Mellifica . . . When the fever is accompanied by alternating bouts of sweating and dry body heat, this herb may do the trick.

Aromatherapy

The essential oils of aromatherapy can help lower fever and lessen congestion. Clove bud (antiseptic), bergamot (antiviral), eucalyptus (antibacterial), peppemint, sage, clary sage, basil, chamomile (anti-inflammatory), lavender and black pepper oils (toxin-expelling) all have the ability to soothe fever symptoms. These oils can be used in a warm bath or an electric burner, or added to a base oil as a body rub. Peppermint oil mixed with a carrier oil and applied to a cool, wet towel, which is then wrapped around the troubled spot, can bring down the body's temperature.

See also: Colds and Flu

Fibroids and Uterine Bleeding

One in five women over the age of 35 is afflicted with fibroids, with women of African American descent being especially prone to the problem. Fibromyoma uteri and leiomyoma uteri, the medical terminology for fibroids, are benign tumors that originate from muscle tissue and adhere to either the inner or outer uterine wall. Fibroids usually develop as a result of varying estrogen levels in the body, and provide a natural way for the body to cope with hazardous toxins. Most fibroid patients have indulged in unhealthy diets and exercise habits. The Asian medical perspective is that fibroid development can be a product of angry emotions, prolonged or dilatory menstruation, or abortion. After an abortion, cells from the terminated fetus may remain in the endometrial wall and eventually serve as the foundation for fibroid production.

Symptoms

While the presence of minute fibroids cannot be ascertained by symptomatic evidence, larger fibroids, which take time to develop, are frequently accompanied by agonizing menstruation, urinary tract infections, chronic infertility and uterine bleeding. Fibroids positioned on the inside of the uterine wall are often responsible for uterine bleeding, which commonly results in the performance of a hysterectomy. Fibroids located on the muscle wall of the uterus are not associated with uterine bleeding and are therefore seldom removed from the body.

Generally benign, fibroid tumors are growths in the muscle tissue of the uterus. Although less than one tenth of one percent of fibroids might be malignant, their accompanying uncomfortable symptoms may include heavier menses, a sense of tiredness, fullness and discomfort in the pelvic region, swollen or distended belly and inability to conceive. Pelvic distension, in addition, is felt to be unstylish these days and may result in a woman desiring a drastic surgical or nonsurgical procedure to remove her fibroids. We recommend a thorough physical examination to rule out any more severe condition masked by the sense of belly fullness (such as ovarian cancer or growths, for example), and upon the diagnosis of fibroid tumors alone, we recommend examining all options, such as diet modification, herbal supplements used under the care of a qualified medical practitioner, stress reduction and lifestyle modification.

Fibroids may have a genetic or strong dietary component, as they seem to run in some families. This may indicate a condition called estrogen dominance, where hormonal imbalance between estrogen and progesterone can lead to a variety of symptoms, such as variable length of the menstruation cycle, heavy periods and fluctuating fertility. Disruption of the endocrine system can be caused by a variety of factors, from birth control pills to after-the-fact contraceptives, such as the morning-after pill, dietary influences and estrogen-like substances that are found in city environments. All of these influences can disrupt normal bodily functioning and even thyroid function, which can lower the body's energy and decrease immune response.

Treatments

The medical establishment traditionally follows one of two approaches. The first, myomyectomy is used to eliminate small, harmless fibroids and does not alter a woman's ability to bear children. Hysterectomies are prescribed for women who have fully developed fibroids and suffer from chronic symptoms, such as heavy bleeding. A significant percentage of the hysterectomies performed are totally unnecessary and are actually quite hazardous. In addition to an abundance of physical complications, a hysterectomy can have severe psychological ramifications. What's more, out of the 750,000 hysterectomies performed each year, 2500 result in the death of the woman.

Myoma Coagulation and Other Alternatives to Hysterectomy and Reconstruction

Too often, women who have hysterectomies were not offered safer alternatives by their physicians. Unfortunately, the public is unaware of the benefits of a recently developed laser procedure known as myoma coagulation, or myelosis. Myoma coagulation originated in Europe, where fibroids are eliminated with the use of special lasers that puncture the tumor and deflate it. The operation is effective because it restricts the flow of blood to the fibroid, after which the tumor can be lanced. After the fluid drains, harmless tissue is left behind, and there is no need for extraction.

Since the uterine wall is debilitated by the procedure and unable to sustain pregnancy, likely candidates for myoma coagulation are women who are uninterested in postoperative pregnancies. In addition, the procedure can be performed only if the tumor is less than 6 inches in diameter. Fibroids that surpass the size limit can be treated with Lupron, a medication that decreases the production of estrogen in the body and causes a 30 to 50 percent reduction in the size of the tumor. The fibroid reduction lasts for only a limited amount of time, but during this period, myoma coagulation can be performed, further reducing the fibroid by up to 75 percent. When this occurs, the threat of uterine bleeding is virtually eliminated. When Lupron is used alone, without surgery, the tumors tend to return.

A new procedure is being tested in London, where MRI (magnetic resonance imaging) guides the insertion of needles into the fibroids and a laser is then used to reduce the size of the tumors. Although still testing this procedure, scientists are hopeful because it is a more precise method than laser treatment without the use of imaging.

Another new process called ex-ablate uses MRI technology for imaging and then ultrasound waves for destroying the fibroid. The affected area is brought to a higher temperature, which then shrinks the tumors. It is not known whether this procedure may cause infertility in the patient.

Uterine fibroid embolization is a procedure in which surgeons have effectively blocked blood flow to the site of the fibroid tumor. Most women who have this procedure experience a decrease in fibroid discomfort. However, since this is a new procedure, some of the drawbacks may include death from infection or embolism, infection from the procedure, infertility, sexual dysfunction, hormonal disruption, blood clot and allergic reaction to the material used to block the blood flow to the fibroid.

Radical surgical treatment such as removal of the entire uterus has been available for fibroids for a number of years, but there is an increased risk for heart disease, and an untold number of women suffer from urinary incontinence, pelvic floor prolapse and postsurgical pain as a result of the disruption of the pelvic-floor musculature. In addition, these women are relegated to a lifetime of hormonal disruption, and if they choose hormone replacement therapy, the accompanying risks for cancer.

Pharmaceutical treatments for fibroids may include birth control pills. Additionally, GnRH-agonists are thought to reduce the size of tumors by reducing estrogen production in the ovary. The tumors regrow when treatment is stopped.

Some doctors will treat the effects of estrogen dominance with an external cream from naturally occurring plant sources of progesterone, while others believe that progesterone treatment can only contribute to the causes of estrogen dominance. The antiprogesterone advocates believe that fibroids can increase during pregnancy, a period of higher progesterone production.

Nonsteroidal anti-inflammatories (NSAIDs) are also prescribed by doctors. However, there are well-documented risks associated with this option. Nonsteroidal anti-inflammatories carry the risks of additional bleeding and stroke. There are a number of natural inflammation reducers outlined in several books that discuss the overall benefits of natural Cox-2 inhibitors, such as Thomas Newmark's *Without Aspirin.*

Because the hormonal system is delicate, one should be aware of the possible consequences of playing radical experimenter with the endocrine system either by surgery or hormonal supplementation.

Dr. Allan Warshowsky says that in order to really get rid of the underlying cause of the fibroids, one must address all of the other issues in the life of the person that may be causing stress and imbalance. Dr. Christiane Northrup discusses the fact that uterine problems may be the result of stored emotions.

Nutrition, Supplements and Exercise

The development of fibroids can also be lessened by dietary modification. Women who wish to reduce the size of their fibroids or prevent their further growth should incorporate large quantities of protein into their diets. But the protein should come from healthy sources, such as vegetables and whole grains like quinoa, amaranth, millet, buckwheat, oats and brown rice. Legumes also may be beneficial in hindering the formation of fibroids. Soy products, including soy beans, tofu, soy milk, miso and tempeh, contain a good supply of isoflavones, which have been found to combat tumor growth. Soy foods are good to include in the diet, as they block stimulation of the body by "bad" estrogen-like environmental substances (xenoestrogens).

Numerous types of beans, including black beans, pinto beans, lentils, lima beans and chickpeas, are useful in preparing a variety of meals and constitute a good protein source.

A balance of natural sources of omega-3 and omega-6 essential fatty acids should be included in the dietary equation.

In addition to consuming adequate quantities of protein, it is important to drink a minimum of 2 quarts of purified water daily to promote proper functioning of the kidneys and bowels. Organs involved in the excretion process can facilitate the discharge of excess estrogen and consequently lower the potential for fibroid development. A high dietary intake of fiber can act as a deterrent to fibroid growth due to fiber's estrogen-reducing capabilities. Citrus fruits and berries, which contain ample quantities of vitamin C, can further stabilize the body's estrogen levels.

Yeast infections may encourage fibroid growth by possibly contributing to estrogen dominance. Ran Knishinshy, an herbalist, has a complete dietary program for treating yeast infections in the body.

Sometimes excessive uterine bleeding is brought on by liver poisoning and can be effectively treated by abstaining from food consumption for limited periods of time. Milk thistle, dandelion and yellow dock root can help the liver detoxify and thereby reduce the effects of overbalanced estrogen in the body. Be sure to seek medical guidance, though. When paired with an extensive hygiene regimen, temporary fasting can alleviate symptomatic bleeding in cases that do not necessitate hospitalization.

Although the medical explanation is still unclear, supplements of oil-soluble liquid chlorophyll have also demonstrated their ability to treat abnormal cases of bleeding. For maximum results, two or three capsules should be taken two to three times per day. In addition, a balanced mixture of natural organic oils, including flaxseed and borage oils, can fortify the uterus and protect it from chronic bleeding.

Women with abnormal uterine bleeding accompanied by anemia should supplement their diets with iron, but remember to seek medical supervision and adhere to recommended dosages, as excessive quantities of iron have been linked with cancer and coronary disease. Vitamin E should be taken in quantities of 400 IU daily while 1000 mg vitamin C with bioflavonoids can be taken five times per day. A recent medical investigation correlated symptoms of uterine bleeding with deficiencies of vitamin A; hence, daily consumption of vitamin A supplements is recommended. Additional supplements include 100 mg of evening primrose oil three times daily, plus silica.

The incorporation of an exercise routine into your daily routine can enhance the discharge of excess estrogen from the body, thus reducing the possibility of fibroid development. Exercise can increase regularity of menstruation by increasing ovulatory regularity and decreasing overall body weight (which can lead to hormonal imbalance). Increased weight is also linked with a higher rate of endometrial cancer.

Herbal Remedies

There are several herbal remedies that can alleviate fibroid symptoms. Fifteen drops of shepherd's purse taken three times daily can aid in controlling uterine bleeding, while the herb white ash can facilitate the reduction of fibroids. False unicorn root can be useful in treating severe bleeding when 15 drops are mixed with water and consumed on an hourly basis. The Chinese herb dong quai, which contains useful phytoestrogens and acts as a muscle relaxant, has demonstrated its ability to alleviate cramps attributed to fibroids. This herb should be consumed in quantities of 500-1000 mg per day. Han man cho, another Chinese herb that is also known as warriors grass, enhances functioning of the spleen and uterus, and can control severe bleeding. Some additional herbs commonly prescribed by holistic practitioners to treat fibroids and uterine bleeding include red raspberry, ladies' mantle, yarrow, white dead nettle, partridge berry, goldenseal, motherwort, stone root and ginger. Red clover may work in the younger years, but not during menopause. Vitex or chaste tree tincture may be helpful for long-term use. Alternating the herbs taken each month can help the patient to avoid side effects. In addition, some herbs have little-known side effects. For example, black cohosh and chamomilla used every day may cause irritability; hops may cause inability to conceive; and large doses of panax ginseng may cause tiredness.

Edgar Cayce recommended castor oil packs, and www.caycecures.com has information on how to use them effectively.

Energetic medicines relatively unknown in the U.S., such as Ayurvedic medicine, may bring some relief, as well.

Homeopathic Remedies

The homeopathic remedy aurum muriatium can aid in the reduction of fibroid size when the patient does not suffer from any adverse symptoms, such as bleeding. Hydrastinum muriaticum has demonstrated its ability to decrease the size of larger fibroids that form on the anterior uterine wall. Fibroids in this location often burden the bladder and promote frequent urination and pain.

Acupuncture

Acupuncture points that correspond to the uterus are located on the ankle. Electrical acupuncture is used to promote the elimination of fibroids; it is believed that the electrical currents create stimulation that contributes to the removal of the fibroids from their position on the uterine wall.

What to Avoid

As discussed earlier, the most nutritious sources of protein are whole grains and beans. Pesticides and growth hormones in meat also add to the hormonal challenges faced by our bodies. Meat should be avoided. If you do eat meat, limit intake to three ounces per day, a quantity that can fit in the palm of your hand. Furthermore, meat products should originate from healthy sources. Avoid consuming meat from animals that were not free-range or grass-fed. Animals injected with synthetic hormones and antibiotics are quite unhealthy for the human body.

It is also important to avoid an excessively fatty diet because fatty foods are estrogen stimulators. Furthermore, studies have correlated obesity with heightened estrogen production within the body. The liver, which aids in the elimination of excess estrogen, can be protected by avoiding fried foods, illegal drugs, coffee, alcohol and processed or refined foods. Additional foods to be avoided include diet sodas, pizza, donuts and other pastries and potato chips. In addition to being laden with growth hormones and pesticides, meat and dairy also contain arachidonic acid, which can lead to inflammation and pain.

Treatment Summary

Standard medical practices for fibroids include myomectomy, to eliminate small, harmless fibroids, and hysterectomy to remove fully developed fibroids accompanied by severe, chronic symptoms.

Myoma coagulation and reconstruction is a surgical technique in which lasers deflate tumor growth. When performed by a well-trained medical doctor, it is far safer than the standard hysterectomy.

Newer techniques, such as uterine fibroid embolization, exablation and experimental techniques with MRI guided lasers may bring safer and more effective surgeries to market that do not have the unsung but terrible side effects of the hysterectomy.

Eating wholesome proteins, and drinking four quarts of purified water daily as well as concentrating on citrus fruits and other vitamin C rich foods, can create an internal environment less conducive to the growth of fibroids.

Beans and whole grains can contribute to a better progesterone/estrogen balance within the body.

Short-term fasting and liquid chlorophyll can diminish uterine bleeding.

Vitamins E, C and A, as well as evening primrose oil and silica, offer extra protection.

Exercise lowers estrogen levels, thus lessening the chance of developing fibroids.

Herbs for strengthening the uterus include shepherd's purse, white ash, false unicorn root, dong quai and warrior grass, another Chinese herb.

Stimulating points connected to the uterus, via acupuncture, can help.

Foot and Leg Problems

People take their feet and legs for granted—until something goes wrong and suddenly their personal transport system isn't working so well. The fact is, foot and leg problems slow down large numbers of individuals each year. In general, most foot and leg problems are preventable or can be treated effectively with simple home remedies. At other times a condition may require professional guidance. Fortunately, there are a number of holistic podiatrists who can help.

Because we're so dependent on our feet and legs, it's worth becoming familiar with common conditions affecting them, and with how best to prevent and treat these.

Types of Problems

Peripheral Neuropathy

Peripheral neuropathy is characterized by a burning, pins and needles, tingling or itching sensation in the feet. This condition commonly begins as a result of either sensory dysfunction or malfunction in the motor nerves; improper functioning of these nerves can be induced by metabolic disorders, such as diabetes, and by other diseases. The peripheral nervous system contains nerves that travel from the brain and spinal cord to the rest of the body. Interestingly enough, approximately one third of HIV patients develop symptoms of peripheral neuropathy. In actuality, HIV can cause peripheral neuropathy, but it is usually a side effect of the drugs. In some instances, peripheral neuropathy may be the result of vitamin deficiencies or diabetes.

Patients with diabetes tend to suffer from extreme cases of neuropathy and often experience complete numbness in the lower extremities. When proper nerve enervation is hindered, tissues tend to break down, leaving the external aspects of the foot susceptible to abrasions, wounds and sores. In light of the fact that approximately 20,000 diabetics undergo leg amputation each year, getting treatment for these problems is essential.

Other metabolic disorders that are frequently responsible for peripheral neuropathy are thyroid hyperactivity and hypoactivity. Also, patients with kidney disease, liver disease or hepatitis A, B or C have a tendency to suffer from mild cases of numbness or pins and needles. Injury to the nerves can be induced as well by even the most moderate forms of trauma, including pounding of the feet. In addition, toxic chemicals and medications, such as pesticides, antidepressants and especially chemotherapy, have been found to induce peripheral neuropathy.

Recent advances in modern technology have enabled doctors to establish the origin of a neuropathy problem by analyzing both motor and sensory nerves. Painful nerve conduction studies that utilize needles have become virtually antiquated, as new holistic and noninvasive techniques provide doctors with computerized analysis of the foot that can trace peripheral nerves to their roots in the spinal cord. Today's instrumentation is capable of determining whether a patient's neuropathy is a result of heavy metal toxicity from mercury dental amalgam fillings or excessive exposure to lead, cadmium or arsenic. People can be exposed to these harmful elements simply by drinking unfiltered tap water. As metal accumulates within the body, the nerves in the lower extremities begin to degenerate, and peripheral neuropathy is compounded. Prolonged exposure to these types of hazards necessitates immediate attention before the damage becomes irreversible. Mercury fillings can be removed and replaced with less hazardous substances, while heavy metal accumulations can be eliminated via chelation therapy.

There are two holistic remedies that have proven to be especially effective in ameliorating neuropathies: ozone therapy and vitamin C therapy. Ozone therapy enhances the detoxification of tissue by heightening the elasticity of the red blood cells, which are then able to infiltrate small arteries and nourish the nerve cells. Vitamin C therapy can have a profound effect upon every tissue within the body. This versatile vitamin can act as a direct healing agent or as a coenzyme facilitator of essential chemical processes within the body.

Particular B vitamins have been found to help with symptoms of peripheral neuropathy. Among these vitamins are B1, B12 and folate. Also, some people have found that taking a multivitamin that includes vitamin E along with a B-complex supplement (make certain that it contains folate) helps relieve symptoms of peripheral neuropathy. Vitamin B12 can be given through shots into a muscle, a method that many believe supplies the body with more vitamin B12 than do vitamins.

Lastly, additional supplements that have shown some effect on peripheral neuropathy are magnesium, alpha-lipoic acid (also known as thioctic acid) and gamma-linolenic acid (GLA).

External Problems

People who engage in rigorous athletic activity such as long-distance running, sports or even race-walking, are often prone to exterior foot and leg injuries. Participating in an athletic activity for a lengthy period of time can be especially detrimental, while engaging in an activity after a period of abstinence can also facilitate injury.

Blisters . . . Sometimes a new pair of shoes can adversely affect the foot by causing blisters. Areas of the foot that are susceptible to abrasion or the formation of blisters should be treated with Superskin, which has proven effective in preventing external foot irritations. Superskin is a liquid that is applied by rubbing it directly into the skin. Before using this product on your entire foot, it is advisable to test a small hidden area on the skin to determine if an allergy exists.

Wounds . . . Seek medical care for serious wounds where infection could be a problem. During the initial treatment of a wound it is advisable to apply an evaporating wet dressing that will allow the cut to reach a desirable level of dryness. Once this is achieved the wound should be covered with an emollient dressing that can further aid the injury. A simple dressing that allows proper wound drainage is important. Vitamin E, aloe vera and vitamins A and D are some natural substances that can be used in such a dressing. The potent healing ability of vitamin E was demonstrated in a study of patients suffering from gangrene. Scientists concluded that even advanced forms of the condition could be treated with large dosages of vitamin E.

An internal approach to wound healing involves large intravenous supplements of vitamin C. Furthermore, intravenous ozone therapy can eliminate viruses, fungi and bacteria that may be hindering the healing process. Finally, a topical solution of ozone gas, which is comprised of an ozone/oxygen mixture encased in a balloon-like plastic container, can be applied to further cleanse the skin. Ozone has met widespread popularity in Europe, where it has proven to be quite useful in treating burn victims.

Warts . . . Warts stem from a viral infection. T-cells, part of the body's immune system, are designed to combat this type of invader. When they are unable to successfully perform their duties, the viral intruders are able to form a small tumor on the skin surface. Warts that develop on the underside of the foot are given a special designation: plantar's warts. Treatment of warts encompasses two main aspects. First, immune system functioning needs to be rejuvenated via vitamin and mineral supplementation and stress reduction. In the final analysis, a healthy immune system is the best defense against warts. Recently, doctors have used squaric acid (a very dilute solution causing an allergic skin reaction, which has been demonstrated to help dissolve warts) to ignite the immune system response. External treatment is the second approach. The external use of salicylic acid is an old treatment that is still administered. However, newer remedies, including ozone therapy and the use of liquid nitrogen, have proven more effective.

Dry Skin on the Feet and Legs . . . This condition can be caused by poor nutrition or hindered circulation. A simple homemade moisturizer can serve as an inexpensive and effective substitute for costly products. Most commercial moisturizers contain hydrogenated vegetable oil, an ingredient that can be effectively replaced with several home products. Safflower, sunflower and canola oils are all excellent moisturizers, while a mixture of vegetable oil and the oil from vitamins E, A and D capsules is another effective solution for dry skin. The latter concoction can be refrigerated to ensure its potency.

When using a homemade ointment, spread a small amount directly onto the skin and rub away any excess. For maximum results, apply the ointment right after your shower or bath while the skin is still wet. This way the moisture is locked into your skin under the coat of oil.

Calluses and Corns . . . Calluses tend to develop on the bottom of the foot, and corns form on the top, on the side or under the foot. Calluses are caused by thick accumulations of dead skin, while corns originate from calcified protrusions on the bone that either press against the skin from inside the foot or receive external pressure from a shoe, the ground or another toe. Since corns and calluses consist primarily of dead skin, they are not terribly dangerous and can be eliminated via the use of a pumice stone or other abrading apparatus. Since metal can cut through skin, resulting in infection, it is advisable to avoid any type of metal tool. In addition, before using a pumice stone or other tool, you should clean it with peroxide or alcohol in order to eliminate the possibility of bacterial or viral infection.

In most cases, the development of a corn can be averted by selecting a pair of shoes that do not squeeze or put pressure on the toes. The formation of calluses and corns underneath the foot can be prevented with shock-absorbent insoles. If this method is not successful, you may require an orthotic device that can correct any bone misalignments. Sometimes the formation of calluses or corns under the foot can be induced by a malfunction in a completely different region of the body. For example, if the spine, neck, head or pelvis are even slightly out of alignment, your gait will be adversely affected, and consequently, excess pressure will be placed upon certain areas of the foot, which may lead to the formation of a corn or callus. A meager two percent of corns or calluses necessitate professional attention. Surgery should be avoided whenever possible, as there is no guarantee that it can provide worthwhile relief. Unfortunately, many times the performance of foot surgery will leave the bottom of the foot permanently susceptible to pain.

Rashes . . . Sometimes people acquire a blistering skin rash when they come into contact with a certain kind of soap or detergent. A mixture of liquid aloe and purified water added to a bandage or gauze pad can be effective in combating this type of condition. A key element of the treatment process is allowing the solution to evaporate directly from the skin. After it dries, the concoction should be repeatedly reapplied, and eventually the irritation will disappear. It is important to continually rewet the bandage once it has dried, in order to prevent it from adhering to the wound. In certain cases of rash that necessitate it, when the acute blistering has completely vanished, intravenous vitamin C therapy can provide long-term relief, while more severe cases may necessitate ozone therapy. Ozone therapy can also be administered for psoriasis, a type of skin rash.

Athlete's Foot . . . Athlete's foot is a common, fungal skin infection that is usually a product of a weak immune system, excess acidity and warm, moist conditions. Poor T-Cell function, which can be contributory, may be corrected through stress reduction and nutritional supplements, and ozone therapy can aid the immune system further. Keeping the feet cool and dry is essential. It is important to remove sweaty socks and to avoid the use of talcum powder. The substance often contains asbestos, which can be absorbed by the lungs, leading to illness later in life.

There are several new sock materials that have proven useful in preventing the accumulation of sweat. During the winter, Thermostat and Thermax can keep the foot dry and warm, while during the summer, Coolmax can be used to keep it dry and cool.

Since athlete's foot is an acid condition, acid-forming foods, such as red meats, should be eliminated. Other foods to avoid include foods high in phosphates, such as sodas, sugary foods and fried foods. It may be beneficial to include cultured foods, such as yogurt, tofu or kefir, and to drink plenty of water to help flush out toxins.

Herbs with antifungal activity are recommended for athlete's foot. Pure aloe vera skin gel, or ointments containing cat's claw, echinacea or tea tree oil, can be applied topically. Myrrh and goldenseal powder, dusted on the foot and covered with a sock, may also help.

Another way to treat the condition is with magnets. Advocates of this method explain that magnets can be effective because they increase oxygen to the area, creating an environment that is not conducive to pathogenic microorganisms.

Fungal peeling may be due to dehydrated skin, and is a sign that essential fatty acids are low. Evening primrose oil can help here.

It is also helpful to wash the fungus under the toes with negatively charged water, to wear cotton socks and to go barefoot in a clean home when possible. To prevent susceptibility to reinfection, boosting the immune system with healthful nutrients is the best idea.

Joint Pain

Many adults develop arthritis in their lower extremities. Osteoarthritis, which develops after a long history of wear and tear on the joints, can be prevented by maintaining alignment in all parts of the body. A proper alignment regimen incorporates treatment of the upper body by a trained chiropractor or osteopath. A foot examination can also be beneficial, and in some cases, the use of orthotics may be required. Appropriately fitted orthotics can help certain people eliminate unnecessary wear and tear on their feet. Stretching exercises are important for eliminating muscle strains, while strengthening exercises can aid in balancing muscle groups and preventing joint strains. When joint aches have already manifested, consumption of several nutritional supplements, such as boron, glucosamine sulfate, boswellia, vitamin C and vitamin E, can help combat the pain. In addition, vitamin C and ozone therapy can be employed to quell the symptoms of osteoarthritis.

Many people have found relief by using glucosamine and chondroitin sulfates. Both are natural parts of healthy joint tissue. They have proven so effective and popular that they can now be purchased at neighborhood drugstores. Both supply the materials necessary for cartilage to repair and rebuild itself. They also provide protection against the enzymes responsible for attacking cartilage. However, their ability to repair is not verified merely by anecdotal evidence, but by countless studies that have proven their ability to stimulate the growth of new tissue, as well as to suppress the enzymes responsible for eroding cartilage.

A recent study analyzed the effectiveness of glucosamine and chondroitin in combating osteoarthritis of the knee. The study proved that glucosamine lived up to its reputation as a kind of panacea for the condition; it even demonstrated its ability to narrow joint space. Chondroitin demonstrated its effectiveness in dealing with problems concerning mobility. Both chondroitin and glucosamine sulfate stop and reverse—absent the side effects of traditional drugs—damage to joints. They have also proven their ability to build healthy new cartilage.

It should be noted that prevention is the best cure. To enable your joints to perform at the peak level, you should manage your weight and exercise frequently.

Rheumatoid arthritis is a condition in which one's own immune system turns against the body, leaving the bones and joints of the lower extremities susceptible to degeneration. When this form of arthritis manifests, high dosages of vitamin C can be used to restrain the immune system from causing any further damage. After the immune system has become pacified by the vitamin C, it can reinitiate functioning at a more tranquil level.

Many people develop bunions during the course of their lives. While there's a common belief that bunions are a byproduct of ill-fitting shoes, in reality they are inherited from one generation to the next. Although improper footwear can facilitate the development of a bunion problem, a genetic predisposition for bunion formation must exist regardless of your shoe selection. Young children with the genetic tendency for bunion formation can be fitted with corrective shoe inserts that are capable of eliminating the potential problem. Shoe inserts used during the early stages of development can prevent further degeneration of the bone structure and allow the bones to become realigned. Once a child has reached the age of 12, his or her foot is almost fully developed; hence, the potential for future bunion development becomes more difficult to eliminate. Although bunions usually do not appear until later in life, the use of a properly fitted orthotic during the early stage of development and throughout life can act as an effective preventive agent. In addition to being unattractive, advanced forms of bunions frequently result in the development of arthritic joints, which cannot be corrected without surgery.

Another common joint disorder that affects the foot is gout. This disease frequently manifests in the big toe joint the ankle joint, and the heel. When the kidneys are unable to assimilate the purines found in certain foods, an excessive accumulation of uric acid infiltrates the blood supply leaving the body prone to the disease. Both carnivores and vegetarians should be wary of gout, as certain foods in both of their diets contain inordinate quantities of gout-inducing purines. Some examples include meat, poultry, red wine, beer, fish, cauliflower and kidney beans.

Ingrown Toenails

Almost everyone incurs an ingrown toenail at some point in life, and this problem can be quite frustrating and painful. The best way to deal with a persistent ingrown toenail condition is to cut toenails straight across. Unfortunately people have a tendency to cut out only a small section of the nail in the corner of the foot, allowing the nail to grow directly into surrounding flesh.

To eliminate an ingrown toenail, take a small piece of cotton and roll it between your fingers. Using a toothpick, lift the ingrown nail and slip the cotton under the nail. Instead of irritating nearby skin, the nail will grow over the cotton buffer. The piece of cotton should be replaced every few days. It is important to remember that an ingrown toenail can become an expensive and agonizing problem if it does not receive adequate attention when it first develops.

Athletic Injuries

In general, if an injury does not improve significantly within 24 hours, you should seek professional help. In the meantime, here are several suggestions that can help extinguish the pain of minor internal injuries. (Broken bones, of course, always require professional care.) The first step in treating an internal injury is the application of ice. Apply ice for 10 minutes straight, and then keep the ice off for another 10 minutes to prevent the skin from becoming frozen. Ice therapy should be continued for at least the first two days after the injury occurs, or until the pain desists. Sometimes people resume activity prior to completion of the healing process, and consequently the injury becomes aggravated and swelling can once again occur. If you experience pain, it is important to apply ice, but once the pain has stopped and healing has begun, warm, wet compresses should be used for 10- to 15-minute periods on the injured region. This second form of therapy can aid circulation and enhance the healing process. So, in summary, during the initial stages of an injury, use cold therapy while sensations of sensitivity during the actual healing process should be treated with heat.

Another important element of the healing process is the performance of non-weight-bearing exercises immediately after the occurrence of the injury. It is important to engage the joints and muscles of the foot, ankle and leg in full-range-of-motion exercises. Since any initial movements may hurt at first, you should rub ice over the injured area to numb it. Once you have applied ice for several minutes, move the muscles and joints in a full range of motion. These motions will enable the body to naturally eliminate scar tissue and prevent adhesions from developing. Massage therapy can be especially beneficial for muscle, tendon, or ligament injuries in the lower extremities, while additional treatment can be obtained via ozone and vitamin C therapy.

Forty-eight hours after the occurrence of an athletic injury, moderate stretching exercises should be incorporated into the daily treatment regimen. Stretches should be executed slowly in a long, continuous and pulling manner. Each stretch should be performed for approximately 20 seconds. Never use a bouncing motion. Proper stretching can enhance circulation in the injured area, can mitigate spasms by extending the tendons and ligaments to their correct length and can prevent future spasms. After several days, you should move on to strengthening exercises. Before you initiate exercise, you should identify any weak muscles that may have actually contributed to the occurrence of the injury. Once you have done this, you can work on restoring equilibrium to all of the body muscle groups so that future injury can be averted. Professional guidance is always helpful when beginning exercises, especially when the injury is acute.

Internal Foot and Leg Problems

A heel imbalance can be induced by a variety of factors, including arthritic ankles and joints, plantar fasciitis, which is an inflammation of the muscle under the foot arch, and heel and bone spurs. People who are plagued by heel imbalances can benefit from another product, known as the Heel Hugger, a small elastic ankle brace that can stabilize both the ankle and the knee. People who incur multiple ankle sprains usually have a tendency to suffer from chronic knee ailments as well. The Heel Hugger can provide an effective means of preventing these types of injuries.

Many people mistakenly believe that heel and bone spurs are the result of too much calcium, but the opposite is true. Remember, calcium is the most plentiful mineral in the body. It comprises 1.5 to 2 percent of the total body weight. The bones have more than 99 percent of the body's calcium. When there is too little calcium, the body leaches this mineral from the bones, and then deposits it into the heel and foot. Calcium works best when it is taken together with magnesium, in a ratio of 1500 mg : 750 mg. Unless heartburn is a problem, the addition of hydrochloric acid can further enhance the effect of these nutrients. Several other nutrients and herbs have analgesic and anti-inflammatory properties; these can be used alone or in combination for the treatment of bone spurs. Vitamin C relieves swelling and works best in combination with bioflavonoids. Between 2000 and 4000 mg of vitamin C and 100 mg of bioflavonoids are needed on a daily basis. Additionally, one gram of shark cartilage daily may help alleviate inflammation and pain. Sage, rosemary and alfalfa can be made into a tea. Alfalfa is particularly good for this type of problem because it contains calcium. Bee pollen, yucca root and devil's claw may also produce excellent effects. Externally, a hot linseed or castor oil pack can be comforting. Just place the oil on a heated cloth and wrap it around the affected foot.

Foot injuries can often be traced to improper walking. The F-scan is a popular diagnostic device that can discover the presence of a foot imbalance with the use of a pressure-sensitive mat. First, a patient is instructed to walk across the mat, which registers the amount of pressure being applied by each foot. Then, the data is converted by a computer into color printouts. Analysis of these printouts by a doctor can offer an explanation as to why a patient is experiencing pain when he or she is walking.

Circulatory Problems

Varicose veins are one of the more common circulatory problems, yet most people remain unaware of the variety of alternative treatments that are available. In general, the health of our veins can be enhanced by maintaining proper weight, exercising to improve circulation and eating foods and nutritional supplements that support the liver. Much blood circulates through the liver, and if the liver becomes congested, the whole venous system can back up. This, in turn, adds pressure on the veins, damages valves and results in varicose veins. Foods that support the liver include beets, artichokes and dark-skinned fruits and berries, such as blueberries, cherries and dark-skinned grapes. Also, milk thistle and dandelion are helpful herbs for the liver. In addition, gotu kola, horse chestnut and butcher's broom help strengthen veins. Supplemental phosphorous and vitamins B and C can be beneficial for the veins in the legs and feet. People with deep varicose veins should also invest in supportive stockings.

It should be noted that some doctors suggest using blueberries during pregnancy for the prevention and treatment of varicose veins and hemorrhoids. The suggested daily amount is 1/2 to 1 cup of fresh blueberries. When supplementing, the recommended dosage is 100–500 mg per day (with 25-percent anthocyanosides). These should be taken in two or three doses.

Deep varicose veins are usually characterized by red and brownish markings, light dots and especially dark, concentrated areas above the ankle and lower leg. Severe cases are characterized by a permanent discoloration of skin. When skin discoloration is exhibited, the body is providing us with a warning that something deep within the body, such as the valves, is not functioning properly. As the veins swell, the legs and feet can become plagued by itching and, eventually, sores and open wounds known as varicose ulcers will develop.

Another common product of varicose veins, phlebitis, is characterized by inflammations within the veins and clotting of the blood. If a blood clot breaks away from the vein, a life-threatening pulmonary embolism may ensue. Obviously, discovering a varicose vein problem during its early stages and immediately instituting an appropriate treatment plan is essential in eliminating serious health risks.

Another widespread circulatory problem that frequently affects the legs and feet is intermittent claudication brought on by arteriosclerosis, or hardening of the arteries. The most effective preventive measure for this condition is regular aerobic exercise. Supplements of vitamins C and E can also be beneficial because of their ability to promote blood flow while chelation or ozone therapy can be used once the condition has already developed. Ozone therapy helps because it increases the flexibility of red blood cells, enabling them to slip through clogged arteries, while chelation therapy removes toxic byproducts from the arteries, rendering them more pliable. Both methods can provide an effective alternative to coronary bypass and leg surgery.

Proper Foot Attire

When selecting a shoe, choose a size that allows you at least half an inch from your big toe to the end of the shoe. One way of determining whether or not a shoe fits properly involves taking the insole out and placing your foot on it. By using this method, you can see if the shoe is appropriate in both the length and width. After you have made your selection, break the shoes in gradually by wearing them for short periods each day. This way you can avoid injury or irritations. As your tolerance grows, you will be able to comfortably wear the shoes for the entire day.

As for sneakers, there are a multitude of sneaker manufacturers, and each manufacturer offers an extensive selection of products; hence, consumers are under the impression that finding proper foot attire to suit a specific need, takes some time. In reality, the best type of sneaker for walking, shopping or doing housework is the running shoe. This type of shoe offers a significant degree of protection from the elements. It is comprised of highly advanced shock-absorbent materials that can shelter the entire foot, from heel to toe. Furthermore, these shoes are extremely flexible in the ball of the foot and offer stability in the rear.

Treatment Summary

Peripheral neuropathy can often be successfully countered with ozone and vitamin C. These increase the blood's elasticity and help to detoxify and nourish cells.

External wounds of the legs and feet should be properly dressed to prevent infection and speed up the healing process. An effective dressing allows the wound to drain properly. Initially, an evaporating wet dressing should be used. Next, the wound should be covered with an emollient dressing, incorporating vitamin E, aloe vera, vitamin A or vitamin D.

Wearing well-fitting shoes can usually arrest corns. Corns and calluses can also be prevented by wearing a shock-absorbent insole or an orthotic device.

For athlete's foot, ozone therapy is an effective remedy especially when used in conjunction with stress reduction, nutritional supplements and keeping the feet dry and cool.

Maintaining proper body alignment with the help of a chiropractor or osteopath can prevent joint pain. In some instances, orthotics and strengthening exercises may be necessary, as well as supplementation.

To prevent ingrown toenails, cut the nails straight across. Cotton over a toothpick can be used to lift the ingrown toenail out of the skin.

Sports injuries that do not heal within 24 hours should be handled by a medical professional. First aid involves the application of ice. Once pain subsides, apply warm, wet compresses. Non-weight-bearing exercises, stretching and massage therapy may be indicated later to restore full range of motion.

Heel imbalances may be corrected with a product known as the Heel

Hugger. Heel and bone spurs may be healed with extra calcium, magnesium and other nutrients.

Varicose veins can be treated with nutrients and supportive stockings.

A regular exercise routine, vitamins E and C and chelation or ozone therapy can help eliminate intermittent claudication.

Gallstones

Approximately 20 million Americans, most of whom are over 65, suffer from gallstones. There are a concentration of bile components, like cholesterol, biopigments and salt, all of which form little stones and block the common or cystic bile duct. As these pieces accumulate and enlarge, the gallbladder becomes inflamed, resulting in severe pain. If left untreated, the stones can cause digestive incapacity and become life threatening.

Causes

According to new research, it appears that the problem underlying gallstones is related to a deficiency in hydrochloric acid or to a food intolerance. Gallstones are also occasionally due to cysts, tumors, Crohn's disease, pancreatitis or roundworm infection. Obesity, diabetes, hypothyroidism, hyperlipidemia and crash diets with sudden weight loss can lead to increased cholesterol in the blood and the formation of gallstones. Hormone therapy, birth control pills and pregnancy may also elevate the cholesterol levels due to increased hormone estrogen levels. Even though gallstones typically are crystallized cholesterol, some blood disorders, such as sickle cell anemia, and severe liver disease can trigger the development of gallstones from the waste product bilirubin.

Symptoms

Most people with gallstones never know they have them and are able to lead normal, comfortable lives without medical intervention. Abdominal ultrasound, CT or X rays can detect the presence of stones early. When symptoms do appear, however, they can include bloating, belching and a sharp pain or spasm under the ribs or under the right shoulder blade after eating fatty foods, as well as low-grade fever, chills, nausea, vomiting and indigestion. Cholecystitis, the inflammation of the gallbladder, might occur when stones become lodged in the cystic duct, blocking the flow of the bile. A more severe blockage can take place between the liver and the intestine, causing pain and jaundice (yellowish color of the white of the eyes or of the skin). If the stones block any of these ducts for a prolonged period of time and are accompanied by persistent pain, jaundice and fever, it could lead to serious damage to the gallbladder, liver or pancreas. This can even be fatal. In this case, surgery might be the most viable option. The surgery might call for removing the gall-bladder (laparoscopic cholecystectomy). The surgeon operates while watching a monitor that is connected to a camera. People can lead quality lives without a gallbladder.

Treatment

Diet

Basically a person needs to be on a low-fat, no-sugar diet and abstain from coffee and other forms of caffeine. A vegetarian diet is generally the best one to follow, and the following foods should be included: dandelion root, beet greens and black radish greens. These foods help to increase the flow of bile, needed to break down fat.

Gallbladder Flush

Gallstones are easier to prevent than treat, but once they are there, a gall-bladder flush is sometimes effective in getting rid of the problem. According to Linda Rector Page, author of *Healthy Healing: An Alternative Healing Reference*, the flush consists of a three-day fast on olive oil and lemon juice, then six days of olive oil plus lemon, carrot, beet and cucumber juices, as well as a potassium broth containing carrots, spinach, celery and parsley. The liquids should be taken four to five times a day.

Following the flush, it is best to follow an alkaline diet with lots of sea vege-tables and concentrated green juices, such as chlorella, barley grass, spirulina and wheatgrass, to boost the liver and gallbladder.

The Chinese medicine practitioner Julia Chang suggests taking one table-spoon of gold coin grass tincture with the olive oil-lemon juice flush, as well as curcumin, to increase energy flow. If the gallstones are extremely packed, 3 teaspoons of flaxseed oil mixed with warm water may help. For those who are also constipated, an additional intestinal cleansing with bentonite clay, psyl-lium husks and lots of water may be beneficial.

Supplements

People with gallstones should check to see whether they are deficient in hydro-chloric acid. Lipotropic supplements, such as choline, omega-3 and flaxseed oil, are good to take three times a day. Other useful supplements include inositol, methionine, vitamin C and phosphatidylcholine, which is a refined form of lecithin. The amino acid taurine can help increase bile formation. Also, the plant enzymes bromelain and papain help digest protein and are anti-inflammatory. The supplementation of betaine hydrochloride, a source of hydrochloride, can help you digest proteins and fats. The typical dosage is about 325-650 mg in pill form, taken with each meal.

Herbs

Bitter herbs that normalize liver function and help to produce bile should be taken. The herb milk thistle, also known as silymarin, is one such herb. Other good herbs to take are goldenseal, cardamom and Oregon grape, which are high in the active ingredient berberine. Dandelion is also excellent for the liver and can be taken in large quantities. Additionally, turmeric is excellent for its anti-inflammatory properties. Boldo, furmitory, great celandine and artichoke leaves are all prescribed in Europe for gallbladder pain. These should be taken with medical supervision because they might cause lodging of the stones or even rupture. This is because they enhance movement of the gallbladder. Gravel root or chamomile tea will help dissolve gallstones. The Chinese herbal combination li dan xiao yan soothes acute to chronic inflammation of the gallbladder caused by stones. Its active ingredients are lysimachia (the whole plant), andrographis (the above-ground part), Japanese honeysuckle flower, chinese skullcap root, buplcurum root, yin-chen wormwood (the young shoot) and isatis root. To lessen the discomfort that may accompany this dosage, li dan pai shi may be taken. Li dan pai shi contains herba capillaris, lysimachiae weed, raical skullcap root, turmeric tuber and costus root. The classic Chinese formula lung dan xie gan wan is capable of purging the "heat" from the liver-gallbladder area, thus stimulating the stagnating liver qi. The mixture's ingredients are gentanae root, hare's ear root, raical skullcap root, gardenia fruit, alismatis stem tuber, tangkwei root and foxglove root. The herbal supplement combinations of jin dan pian, li dan pian and lungden shegon wan also support the gallbladder and liver.

What to Avoid

Certain foods aggravate gallbladder disease, the most common offenders being eggs, onions and pork. Dairy products and any other foods high in fat also tend to intensify the problem. Sugar may aggravate the gallbladder and should therefore be avoided. Note that being overweight places a person at high risk. It is advised that one lose weight gradually. Vigorous exercise, which decreases estrogen production, may lower the chances of developing gallstones. Certain prescription drugs may do so as well; check with your physician if this is a concern.

Treatment Summary

Follow a low-fat, no-sugar, no red meat, no dairy and caffeine-free diet. A nine-day liquid fast called a gallbladder flush may help dissolve gallstones.

A variety of supplements and herbs may help dissolve gallstones and support the return of health.

Headaches

Each year a large number of Americans are plagued by headaches. While sometimes the degree of severity is trivial, at other times headaches can lead to excruciating agony. There are two basic categories of headaches: tension headaches and migraines. Tension headaches are common to everyday life and are usually associated with a sensation of pressure or band-like tightness on either side of the head. Migraines, on the other hand, do not occur on a daily basis and are characterized by intense discomfort. Starting with a slight throbbing sensation, migraines can rapidly crescendo into an oppressive pounding in the head.

The number of Americans affected by migraines, according to the National Headache Foundation, has been estimated at 28 million, of which 11 million are victimized by chronic migraine. Since hormones play a decisive role in the onset of migraines, an overwhelming majority (about 20 million) of migraine sufferers are women. Clinical evidence shows that migraines are brought on by an abrupt dilation of the blood vessels, which burdens the brain with excessive amounts of pressure. This can be caused by a variety of conditions. Migraine is classified as a hereditary disease. When both parents suffer from migraines, the odds are 75 percent that the children will also be victimized by migraines.

Causes

First of all, migraines are commonly exacerbated by allergic reactions to elements in the diet or the environment. Dietary reactions include allergies to foods, artificial food additives and food combinations. Reactions to alcoholic beverages, especially red wine and beer, are quite common, as are reactions to tyramine and MSG. Tyramine is an amino acid found in cheese, yogurt, yeast extracts and smoked fish, while MSG is a flavor enhancer sometimes used in Chinese food and other products. People who are allergic to wheat, dairy products, eggs and corn may experience migraines if they indulge in these foods. Sodium nitrate, which is common in most cold cuts and frankfurters, and aspartame, an artificial sweetener that reduces the level of serotonin in the body have also been implicated in migraines. Furthermore, reactions to caffeinated products, such as coffee, soda and chocolate can trigger a migraine. Environmental reactions include reactions to hazardous fumes emitted from home furnishings, cleaning products, carpeting and other sources.

Sometimes migraines can result from cranial faults or deformities in the cranial bone structure. The position of cranial bones can be adversely altered by intense trauma to the head, such as whiplash, being hit on the head or birth trauma. According to the beliefs of Chinese medicine, a meridian imbalance, which can be diagnosed by an acupuncturist or practicing kinesiologist, can also influence the occurrence of migraines. The meridians are a system of 12 bilateral electromagnetic channels of energy within the body. When energy is entrapped within one of these channels, a meridian dysfunction occurs, and consequently a painful migraine results.

Hormones, too, can play a role in causing migraine headaches. Sixty-percent of all female migraine sufferers relate the occurrence of migraines to their menstrual cycle. Although the medical community is still uncertain as to the exact relationship between the development of migraines and the level of the hormone estrogen in the body, it is evident that this hormone somehow plays a key role in their occurrence. One hypothesis is that estrogen affects the functioning of the nervous system and the level of serotonin in the body, a substance that may facilitate the onset of migraines. Women who use birth control pills are more likely to experience acute migraines, while women who have recently experienced menopause are less susceptible to them due to the reduced quantities of estrogen in their bodies. Reliance upon hormonal replacement therapy in post-menopausal women can contribute to the reoccurrence of migraines.

A deficiency of magnesium in the blood is another predisposing factor. An insufficient intake of this vital nutrient has also been correlated with the onset of the myofacial disorder known as fibromyalgia that is characterized by migraine-like symptoms.

It is not generally acknowledged, but prescription drugs administered by medical doctors and even over-the-counter drugs can promote migraines. Simple painkillers, including mixed analgesics, acetaminophen and aspirin, which are supposed to treat headaches, can actually contribute to their onset. In fact, overuse of these products has been cited as a cause of migraines. When painkillers are used in excess, the body becomes accustomed to their presence in the bloodstream and will experience withdrawal symptoms when the supply is depleted.

Another contributing factor to migraines is a cervical subluxation in the upper portion of the neck, a condition common among people who frequently talk on the telephone. Often, people have a tendency to cradle the telephone receiver between their shoulder and neck, causing the vertebrae to assume a distorted position. People who like to read in bed are also likely candidates for cervical subluxation because the propped position of the head shifts the vertebrae and places excessive pressure upon the nerves, increasing the likelihood of a migraine.

Quite a few migraine sufferers have a habit of clenching their temporalis muscles (which are located on the side of the skull) while they are sleeping. This may be the reason they suffer from migraines. There is a small FDA-approved device that your dentist conforms to your front teeth (and that is worn while you are asleep) that is designed to combat this teeth clenching. It lessens the strong clenching of the temporal muscles (see *TMJ Disorder*) by avoiding the contact between the upper and lower rear molar and canine teeth. Tension-style migraines that are a result of teeth clenching are thus eliminated or lessened.

According to the publication *Heart Disease,* New York dentist Dr. Mark Friedman has an unusual way of dealing with migraines. Believing that migraines occur when there is inflammation above the last two upper molars that press on nerves, he invented a device that sends cold water to a piece of metal placed on the inflamed area. This cooling procedure appears to successfully soothe the pain caused by migraines.

Although stress cannot be considered a direct cause of migraines, prolonged exposure to stressful situations and anxiety can compound the symptoms.

Symptoms

Some cases of migraines are preceded by the presence of certain warning signs, including sensations of flashing lights or zigzag lines. The appearance of these ominous warning signs, called an aura, foreshadows the occurrence of a migraine. The actual headache usually occurs within 20 minutes of the warning signs on the opposite side of the head. Although the aura is usually characterized by visual stimuli, sometimes it can take the form of other sensations, such as the detection of odor, lingual difficulties, disorientation, tingling or numbness. Early detection of these warning signs can allow the victim some time to prepare for the onset of a migraine.

Unlike regular headaches, migraines are characterized by pain on only one side of the head. In addition, nausea, vomiting, fatigue, irritability, vision problems and sensitivity to light and sound commonly occur.

Treatment

Migraine sufferers are usually given nonsteroidal anti-inflammatory medication, such as ibuprofen, or special migraine medicines that can be used during acute attacks. Muscle tension headaches are commonly treated with minor analgesics and a combination of massages, hot showers and other muscle relaxation techniques.

Pressure Point Therapy

Pressure point therapy can be used to alleviate even the most intense tension headaches. There are several pressure points that promote muscle relaxation. One is the hand. By placing the thumb in the webbed area between the first and second fingers, and applying pressure in the direction of the first finger, headache pain can often be lessened.

Since most tension headaches begin in the back of the neck and the shoulders, there is a special procedure designed to manipulate the head. While sitting down and bending the head forward, position the thumbs just above the neck and below the occipital bone, approximately one and a half inches away from the midpoint of the neck. When you locate a bump, apply pressure for 10 to 15 seconds. A useful technique for treating headaches on the side of the head involves placing the finger one-and-a-half inches above the ear on the temple. When you locate a tender area, press for several seconds until the tender area disappears. Also, pressing a half-inch above the eyebrows for several seconds can further reduce headaches. There are a few reflex points below the eyebrows as well. Each point is located approximately a half-inch apart and should be pressed in an upward motion for five or ten seconds. Squeezing the bridge of the nose for five or ten seconds can also be useful. The reflex points under the cheekbones should be manipulated starting near the nose and slowly moving the index fingers a half-inch at a time toward the ears. After these points are treated, proceed to the neck and shoulder region.

Massage Therapy

Sinus headaches can be alleviated by massaging under the neck and proceeding upward through the hairline to the top of the head. Remember to squeeze the muscles located at the back of the neck and shoulders, and carefully manipulate the various acupressure points, including the bridge of the nose, below the cheekbones, under the eyebrows and under the forehead. When you are treating a migraine, you should lie down and place a cold compress over the eyes and head for a few minutes. Gently massage the temples for a few seconds, and then stretch the head back in order to release any energy blockages. This procedure alleviates migraines because it relieves tension in the muscles, increases circulation and facilitates the transport of oxygen to the brain.

Reflexology

The practice of reflexology is founded upon the principle that manipulation of the foot can aid the rest of the body. Therapy for migraines is usually initiated by creating a relaxed environment, which can include using a shallow basin of water to soften and warm the feet. There are several points on the foot that are involved in the treatment process. The big toe, reflexologists explain, corresponds to the head, while the other toes also relate to the head and to the sinus region. The ridge located under the toes relates to the neck and shoulders, and the ball of the foot corresponds to the chest and lungs.

A key factor in quelling the onset of a migraine is relaxing and comforting the body. The little notch just under the ball of the foot relates to the solar plexus, which is vital to emotional processes. Reflexologists explain that by placing the thumb on this point during inhalation and removing it during exhalation, the solar plexus is relaxed, allowing emotions to flow freely. Another activity that can aid in relaxation involves wringing the foot as if it were a washcloth. And a technique called the lung press involves pressing the ball of the foot with the right fist while supporting the foot with the left hand. The pressing motion of the fist should gradually be brought down to the heel. This technique also promotes relaxation, and should be performed three times consecutively.

During a session with a reflexologist, a wide variety of techniques are used, and both feet are treated. Sessions end with both feet being massaged, followed by a few minutes of quiet rest and a glass of water to flush out harmful deposits.

Aromatherapy

Aromatherapy, or a combination of aromatherapy and other treatment modalities, can be quite effective in subduing headaches. Lavender oil may aid in combating migraines by relaxing the neck muscles and releasing tension. This oil should be massaged into the back of the neck and temples prior to pressure point therapy. One or two drops of peppermint oil can be applied as a massage oil, like lavender oil, added to drinking water or inhaled from your palm or a tissue.

Herbal Remedies

Aloe vera is especially beneficial in alleviating headaches induced by pollution or acidic foods. The herb feverfew may be used to combat migraines.

Lungtanxieganwan is used in Traditional Chinese Medicine to ameliorate headaches brought on by anger or constipation. The herb xiao yao wan treats headaches prompted by allergies, premenstrual syndrome and hypoglycemia. Valerian is of use for headaches characterized by nervousness and insomnia, and can also treat migraines and dizziness that are associated with air travel.

Allergy Control

Since migraines induced by allergic food reactions may take hours to fully develop, patients often need to keep a journal, listing all of the foods they have consumed in order to effectively expose the culprit. In ascertaining the presence of a possible food allergy, patients can place a sample of the suspect food under their tongue. If there is truly an allergic reaction, muscles that were once strong will be weakened by the food, and there will be variations in the intensity and frequency of the pulse. Future migraines can be prevented by eliminating the allergy-inducing food from the diet.

The frequency of migraines caused by environmental allergic reactions can be reduced by keeping household plants. Plants have the ability to assimilate various toxins that are found in our homes. For instance, spider plants demonstrate the capacity to absorb formaldehyde, which is commonly discharged by plywood, synthetic carpet, particle board and new upholstery while chrysanthemums can aid in absorbing fumes released by glue, varnish and lacquer. Alternatively, one can attain a similar effect by drinking an herbal tea that contains chrysanthemums.

Craniosacral Therapy

Although an examination of the skull for cranial faults is considerably more difficult than detecting a food allergy, proper diagnosis, followed by corrective measures, can help prevent future migraines. Cranial faults often escape detection due to the subtle motions of the cranial bones. Many people who suffer from migraines with cranial origins have internally rotated frontal bones. This condition frequently results in the occurrence of a migraine accompanied by eye pain. What craniosacral therapists do is manipulate bones to relieve pain. Treatment with this modality consists of pressure, applied at varying levels, to different parts of the head.

Other Modes of Treatment

Migraines induced by hormonal imbalances can be combated with supplements such as vitamin B6 and evening primrose oil that stabilize hormonal levels. Migraines characterized by a meridian imbalance can be treated by either an acupuncturist, who will rely upon the use of needles, or a kinesiologist, who will manipulate the meridians using a finger. Either type of practitioner can be effective in restoring the balance of energy. The treatment of migraines caused by upper cervical subluxation should be performed by a competent chiropractor, who can adjust the region and eliminate the subluxation. As we have mentioned, some cases of migraines are induced by excessive reliance upon medication. People who suffer from this category of migraine should, while under the supervision of a holistically oriented physician, halt consumption of these products. Gradually, the body will lose its dependence upon the medication and can readjust to normalized conditions.

Migraines induced by a magnesium deficiency can be remedied with a combination treatment of magnesium supplements and malic acid. There have been a large number of studies detailing the relationship between magnesium and migraines. According to one study, two double-blind trials found that supplementing with oral magnesium may not only reduce or eliminate migraine episodes, but also may reduce the incidence of these attacks. The report stated that oral supplementation with magnesium could be recommended for most patients with migraine. Also, lowered serum and intracellular levels of magnesium have been found in migraine sufferers.

Another report showed that 90 percent of juveniles who suffered from migraines and had decreased magnesium levels were returned to normal when treated with oral magnesium picolinate. This study seemed to imply that low brain magnesium levels are responsible for migraines. Since the necessary dosages vary from one individual to the next, a physician should be consulted before beginning magnesium supplementation.

By now, it should be apparent that a central theme of this book—and a central theme to any health program worth its salt—is prevention. When it comes to migraines, vitamin B2 (riboflavin) is a key player in preventing migraines. One Belgian study hypothesized that because the brains of migraine sufferers had reduced mitochondrial phosphorylation, riboflavin could be used because of its potential to increase mitochondrial energy efficiency and would result in a prophylactic effect. During the study, an oral dose of 400 mg of riboflavin was given to the study's participants for a minimum of three months. The findings supported the conclusion that high dosages of riboflavin may be an inexpensive, effective remedy for migraines.

As in the case of vitamin B12, researchers believe that some migraines may be caused by mitochondrial dysfunction. An indispensable part of the mitochondrial electron transport chain is CoQ10, which seems to play an important prophylactic role in preventing migraine. One clinical study showed that after three months of receiving a daily amount of 150 mg of CoQ10, there was a significant decrease in the average number of days that the patients had migraines. The report did not note any side effects.

Butterbur root appears to prevent migraines from occurring. This is because it acts as an antispasmodic on the vascular walls. One double-blind test demonstrated that butterbur was 77 percent effective as a preventer of migraines. The suggested daily dose is 50 mg two times per day.

Glucosamine is an anticoagulant that, in some instances, stops migraines from occurring. The suggested minimum daily dose is 1500 mg.

Picamilon, a compound that is similar to a vitamin, easily penetrates the blood-brain barrier to enhance brain circulation. Picamilon has been shown to significantly decrease headaches on one side of the head.

Stress-related migraines can be treated with the herb feverfew (also known as featherfew and bachelor's buttons), which acts as a sedative and can be consumed as either a tea or in capsules. Feverfew is an herb with a long history of treating the same types of ailments that are treated by aspirin, among them headache. Feverfew's prowess at successfully treating migraines has become legendary. As with Dr. Friedman's device above, feverfew attacks inflammation, relieving a principal cause of migraines. Specifically, feverfew attacks two substances known as inflammatories, serotonin and prostaglandins. By inhibiting these, feverfew helps avert spasms of the blood vessels that can lead to headaches. The recommended dosage is one cup of tea per day or one or two capsules of the freeze-dried extract version. Meditation, progressive muscle relaxation, yoga and moderate exercise, such as swimming and walking, can be employed to further reduce stress and improve the emotional state.

Additional Supplements

When the herb feverfew is accompanied by 250 to 500 mg of magnesium and 125 mg of ginkgo biloba on a daily basis, the symptoms of migraines can be drastically reduced. This combination of supplements has met remarkable success in the treatment of people who regularly suffer from migraines, and can serve as an effective substitute for conventional treatments. Supplements of niacin have a tendency to create a flushing sensation in the head, which in turn eliminates excess blood and quells the onset of migraines. Finally recent studies have shown that daily supplementation of 1000 to 2000 mg of omega-3 fatty acids, found in fish oil, and riboflavin (see above) can decrease the frequency and severity of migraines.

What to Avoid

Although some causes of migraines are beyond our control, others, such as food allergies, can be effectively combated by avoiding certain products. Clinical research has correlated the consumption of red wine and other alcoholic beverages with the occurrence of migraines in certain people, while other research has implicated chocolate as a contributing factor. Monosodium glutamate is another frequent cause of migraines. While Chinese food is infamous for its use of MSG, surprisingly, a variety of other foods, including salad dressing, sauces, frozen and prepared foods and soups, incorporate MSG. Caffeine and artificial sweeteners, such as aspartame, have also been found to promote migraines. Studies have revealed that foods containing quantities of the mineral copper, such as wheat germ, shellfish and nuts, can act as migraine-inducing agents. Citrus fruits should also be avoided, due to their tendency to increase intestinal absorption of copper. Many people who suffer from allergy-induced migraines have cited reactions to dairy products, particularly various types of cheese, as the root of their problems. Cheese, smoked fish, yogurt and yeast extracts contain an ingredient known as tyramine, which has been known to increase susceptibility to migraines. Sodium nitrate, common in cold cuts and frankfurters, is yet another cause.

In addition to abstaining from foods that provoke allergies, it is important to avoid missing meals and to avoid excessive exposure to stress, as these are two factors that contribute to the onset of headaches.

Treatment Summary

Pressure point therapy is useful in treating tension headaches. A qualified massage therapist can promote recovery from sinus headaches, migraines and tension headaches.

Pressure applied to specific areas on the feet can be effective in the alleviation of headaches, even migraines.

Several essential oils work to release tension, thereby alleviating headaches. Migraines are often reactions to allergy-producing foods. Tests for food allergies will let you know which foods to eliminate.

Cranial faults in frontal head bones can cause migraines accompanied by eye pain. A craniosacral therapist can manipulate these bones to promote wellness.

Supplements that can support the body in overcoming headaches include vitamin B6 and evening primrose oil.

The herb feverfew, magnesium and ginkgo biloba work to reduce migraine symptoms.

Niacin, as well as omega-3 fatty acids and riboflavin, arc othcr anti-migraine nutrients.

Heart Disease

Up until recently, heart disease killed more Americans than any other ailment. (Cancer replaced it, moving heart disease to second place.) Each year approximately $50 billion is spent attempting to combat it. Approximately 61 million Americans have heart disease, and more than 2,600 Americans die from it each day. There are a wide variety of factors that contribute to heart damage. Anything that serves to damage the inner lining of the blood vessels and impedes the transportation of oxygen and nutrients to the heart can be defined as a risk factor. During the initial phases of heart disease, destructive agents ranging from tobacco, artificial food additives and gasoline fumes, to sustained high blood pressure may contribute to hardening of the arteries, commonly known as arteriosclerosis. As time progresses, the accumulation of calcium joint deposits, scar tissue, fat and cholesterol in the arteries leads to the formation of atherosclerotic lesions and eventual arterial blockage. The blockage of arteries going to the brain often results in a stroke, while blockage relating to the heart can cause heart attacks.

Types of Heart Conditions

Arteriosclerosis is the most common type of heart disease in the U.S. It is characterized by a slow, progressive thickening and hardening of the arterial walls, and loss of elasticity due to excessive calcium buildup along the vessel linings. Diet is a big factor in this process, as it is the buildup of cholesterol and fats on the inner walls of coronary arteries that narrows these arteries, impedes the circulation and can eventually cause heart attacks.

Angina pectoris is a spasm of the heart muscle that occurs when clogged arteries do not permit adequate oxygen flow to the area. This creates a situation analogous to that of a person exercising beyond their oxygen capacity. The angina pectoris patient will experience pains in the chest or deferred pains to the shoulder, wrist or jaw. Most of the time, the problem stems from a blockage of blood flow caused by atherosclerosis (a kind of arteriosclerosis).

Congestive heart failure is another condition that can result from the progressive thickening and hardening of the arteries. It occurs when inefficient functioning of the tissues creates an imbalance in the amount of blood being pumped in and out of the heart. In this situation, the narrowing of the vessels causes the blood inflow to exceed the outflow, which can eventually overwhelm the heart and result in hazardous fluid backup, fill the lungs, legs and other organs.

Congenital heart disease is caused by a persistence in the fetal connections between the arterial and venous circulations. Under normal circumstances these connections are terminated at birth, but in babies who suffer from congenital heart disease, these connections continue to exist. A prime example of this is the presence of ductus arteriosus, which attaches the pulmonary artery and the aorta. In addition, congenital defects involve the partitions between the cardiac cavities and the vessels surrounding them. In newborn "blue babies," who suffer from a condition known as cyanosis, the pulmonary artery is excessively narrowed, and the ventricles are connected by abnormal openings, resulting in insufficient oxygen intake and a bluish skin tone. Modern technology has helped improve the outlook for infants suffering from this problem.

Rheumatic heart disease, associated with rheumatic fever, is characterized by damage to the entire cardiac region. It was once the leading form of heart disease among children and adolescents, but is now quite uncommon due to the widespread use of antibiotics.

Myocarditis, which is common in older adults, can be described as a degeneration or inflammation of the heart. It often results in dilation, which is the enlargement of the heart muscle due to weakness or hypertrophy, which is the overgrowth of the muscle tissue.

Cardiac arrhythmia refers to the abnormal beating of the upper (atrial) or lower (ventricular) chambers of the heart. These palpitations, which may be experienced as pounding or thumping in the chest and the sensation of having missed a beat, generally indicate that the heart needs nutrients, and that it is overworked and tired. The condition is related to poor intestinal function, associated with gas and fermentation in the stomach and allergy. Caffeine may be a precipitating factor.

A major factor associated with various forms of heart disease is high blood pressure, or hypertension. Hypertension is commonly caused by poor dietary habits, including excessive intake of sugar, caffeine, alcohol or salt; lack of exercise; high stress; or being overweight. Over time, subclinical hypothyroidism can also make a patient prone to hypertension, a fact that the medical profession often misses.

Heart disease is sometimes associated more with men than with women. But women at menopause and beyond should be aware that as estrogen levels drop so, too, does estrogen's protective effect on the cardiovascular system.

Medical data shows that twice as many women die from heart disease than from all forms of cancer combined. In short, risk factors associated with the onset of heart disease should be of concern to everyone.

Symptoms

During the initial phases of heart disease, there are no clear indications that the disease is present, since the illness develops quite gradually and can take years before it assumes its deadly status. Symptoms of heart disease usually become evident only after the arteries become severely blocked, as is the case with arteriosclerosis. This disease is sometimes called "the silent killer" because its victims are often unaware of its presence until the first heart attack.

Some early warning signs that may indicate arteriosclerosis include leg cramps during walking, changes in skin tone and temperature, chest pain, shortness of breath, headaches, fatigue, dizziness and memory defects. People who suffer from congestive heart failure may also experience shortness of breath, accumulation of water in the lungs and swelling of the ankles, while angina pectoris patients will encounter pains in the chest and other body parts. The deferment of pain to other parts of the body associated with angina may bewilder people, but it is important to acknowledge the cardiac origin of these sensations.

Factors that damage the arteries are high-normal levels of glucose, insulin, iron, homocysteine and fibrinogen, and any level of C-reactive protein above the optimal level. (See *Stroke.*) Of these, homocysteine, a naturally occurring amino acid in the body, is especially dangerous. Numerous studies over the past 10 years have demonstrated that with only a slight elevation in the blood level of homocysteine, a person's chances of suffering from heart disease are increased. This is so *even in the absence of any of the other risk factors.* Fibrinogen, a blood protein that plays a critical role in normal and abnormal clot formation, contributes to the buildup of plaque and may assist in blocking the arteries after an unstable atherosclerotic plaque bursts. If fibrinogen increases above normal levels, there is a possibility of a blood clot. If fibrinogen levels fall below normal, the threat of a hemorrhage looms. Excessive glucose levels could speed up the glycation process that is responsible for arterial stiffening, while excessive insulin inflicts direct damage to the endothelium.

Treatment

Finding a qualified professional advisor is crucial in preventing and treating heart disease. Your doctor should be personally interested in your situation, and should possess extensive knowledge of your family history of heart disease, blood pressure, cholesterol level, stress level and weight. Only after taking these factors into consideration can a proper cardiovascular health program be administered.

Traditional Approach: High Blood Pressure Medication

People who suffer from high blood pressure have traditionally been treated with medication. But pharmaceutical propaganda notwithstanding, there is one problem with this approach. Studies indicate that prolonged dependence on prescription high blood pressure medication can cause adverse side effects and can actually compound heart disease. Should people, then, discontinue medication use? Not without a physician's guidance. It is recommended that patients do not discontinue use on their own without first consulting their doctor, because this can lead to a dangerous elevation of blood pressure and eventual stroke. Before discontinuing your consumption of prescription drugs you should work with your physician on discovering a method that will allow your body to cope naturally with high blood pressure. Changes in lifestyle and diet will be key in this process and understand that the process may take some time, and that your dependence on the pharmaceuticals may continue for several more years, or even the rest of your life.

The First Linchpin of a Natural Approach: Nutrition

Dean Ornish's classic study, in which heart disease patients were placed on strict vegetarian diets and were instructed to follow aerobic exercise and relaxation programs, have provided clear evidence that heart disease can be effectively treated and even reversed. Many nutritionists feel that the reduction of dietary fat intake is vital to preventing heart disease, especially angina. The intake of fatty foods, which on average comprises 40 percent of an American's diet, should be reduced to, at most, 20 percent. In fact, some health practitioners feel that fat intake should be as low as 10 percent.

While saturated fats are the worst culprits, too many unsaturated fats have also proven to have potentially harmful effects on the body. People who consume a large amount of unsaturated vegetable oils will experience a fall in blood sugar level when the body becomes tired. When this occurs, the adrenaline level rises and the unsaturated fats that the body has stored are drawn out, causing the lining of the blood vessels to become polluted.

People should try to consume a diet of vegetarian whole foods. Complex carbohydrates—fruits, vegetables, beans, and whole grains—are the basis of such a diet. Plant pigments known as flavonoids, which can be found in vegetables, fruits and some beans and grains, provide healthy protection against heart disease that cannot be provided in other forms. However, since studies show that up to 75 percent of the population release too much insulin in response to carbohydrates in the diet, the type and amount of carbohydrate foods may need individual monitoring.

Many Americans were brought up with the notion that only animal products could supply the necessary amounts of protein. But this assumption is false, as research has demonstrated that grains and legumes, such as rice and beans, can provide a healthy source of protein without harmful fats. Clinical studies have shown that increased intake of fish can be useful in combating heart disease and some forms of cancer. Fish oils from sardines, mackerel, salmon and cod contain the valuable omega-3 and omega-6 fatty acids. Consumption of tofu, which is low in fat and high in fiber is yet another way to promote the development of a healthy heart and prevent cancer.

Plenty of pure water will help to normalize blood pressure and end angina pain, according to Dr. Batmanghelidj, author of *Your Body's Many Cries for Water*. As we grow older, we tend to lose our perception of thirst and tend to drink too little water. As a result, our cells become dehydrated, and a process of reverse osmosis occurs. This means that to maintain vital cell function, the body filters water into the cells from outside of them. The result of this transfer of water is increased blood pressure.

Dr. Batmanghelidj warns that angina can be set off by too little water. So, to regulate blood pressure and put an end to angina pain, he recommends drinking half of one's body weight in ounces. In other words, a person weighing 150 pounds needs to consume 75 ounces of water daily, which represents more than nine glasses.

Supplements

The consumption of certain dietary supplements can assist in the maintenance of a healthy heart and reduce dependence on prescription medication. Antioxidants, in particular, such as vitamins C and E, can shelter the arteries and heart from free radical damage by protecting the tissues that line the artery walls.

Vitamin C . . . Vitamin C supplementation should be an integral part of everyone's life, as it works to prevent cancer, heart disease and other serious disorders. This vitamin should be consumed in quantities of 500 to 1000 mg three to five times per day because of its tendency to be excreted from the body.

Vitamin E . . . Vitamin E can be especially useful in preventing blood clots because it reduces the adhesive qualities of clot-inducing platelets. Thus, E helps prevent strokes and heart attacks. It has been estimated that if everybody supplemented their diet with 200 to 800 IU of vitamin E per day, the incidence of stroke in our country could be reduced by up to 20 percent. By having E reduce the occurrence in blood clotting and oxidation in the arteries, these vessels are able to heal and recover briskly, guaranteeing the clear passage of oxygen through the arteries and into the tissue. Vitamins C and E work even better with the addition of beta-carotene and selenium.

Vitamin K2 . . . A recent study in the *Journal of Nutrition* reported that increasing vitamin K2 (menaquinone) reduced the risk of coronary heart disease.

Bioflavonoids . . . Studies show that bioflavonoids protect against cardiovascular disease and heart attacks. The bioflavonoid quercetin is particularly important in this regard. Good food sources of these substances include the white membrane in oranges and grapefruits, as well as grapes, plums, apricots, cherries, currants and blackberries. Between 100 and 300 mg should be taken daily.

Coenzyme Q1O . . . Coenzyme Q10 is a heart-helping nutrient in that it assists the cell mitochondria—the main source of cell energy—in the burning of fats and reduces high blood pressure and arrhythmias. This substance serves as an antioxidant by preventing oxidative damage and hardening of the arteries. Coenzyme Q10 is especially important for angina and congestive heart failure patients. The recommended dosage for people with less severe heart ailments is 50 to 200 mg per day, while people with more serious conditions may require 400 mg.

Essential Fatty Acids . . . We need to include the essential fatty acids (omega-3 and omega-6) in our diet to minimize heart disease and other ailments. Good sources of omega-3 fatty acids are fish, fish oil supplements and flaxseed oil. Omega-6 fatty acids are found in evening primrose, borage seed or black currant seed oils. The two complement each other and both should be taken daily. Generally, 3000 mg of omega-3 and 2000 mg of omega-6 should be divided into three doses.

Folic Acid and Vitamin B12 . . . These nutrients assist in the reduction of blood levels of homocysteine, a substance linked to heart disorders. Furthermore, a 14-year-long study reported in *JAMA* proved that females who took the highest amounts of folic acid had 47 percent less coronary heart disease than women who ingested the least quantities of folic acid. Astonishingly, for each additional 200 mcg of folic acid, there was an 11 percent decrease in the risk of coronary heart disease. The scientific literature indicates that amounts of 400-2000 mcg of folic acid are optimal to reduce the risk of heart disease.

Also worth noting is the connection between vitamin B6 and heart disease. In one study involving over 80,000 females, the females who took the highest amounts of vitamin B6 had a 51 percent less occurrence of coronary heart disease than those who took the least amount. Amazingly, for each additional 2 mg of B6, the risk for coronary heart disease dropped by 10 percent. The suggested daily dose of vitamin B6 to combat heart disease is 10-100 mg.

A study conducted in Poland showed that supplementation with folic acid (500 mcg daily), vitamin B6 (300 mg daily) and vitamin B12 (1000 mcg weekly) reduced the level of homocysteine in the blood by half (from 20 to 10 micromoles/liter). An added benefit of vitamin B6 supplementation was that it reduced thrombin, a blood-clotting enzyme.

However, taking folic acid with vitamins B6 and B12 produced even more favorable results. Studies have shown that supplementing with a combination of these three supplements not only reduced homocysteine levels, but also cleaned out arterial plaque.

There is only one way to learn your homocysteine levels: by taking a homocysteine blood test. When the homocysteine level is above 7, you would be advised to supplement with the aforementioned combination of folic acid and vitamins B6 and B12.

Note: By reducing the consumption of meat and other methionine-rich foods, you will lower your homocysteine levels.

L-Arginine . . . The amino acid L-arginine facilitates the body's production of nitric oxide, which has an anti-angina and antistress effect upon the arteries in that it enables the muscles in the arterial walls to relax. Supplements of L-arginine can also prevent platelet-induced arterial spasm by hampering the buildup of plaque on the arterial walls. Supplementation is generally at a level of 2 or 3 grains of L-arginine per day.

L-Carnitine . . . The burning of fat within the cell's energy makers, the mitochondria, is enhanced by the amino acid L-carnitine, whose presence is required to lure the fat into the cell. Once inside the mitochondria, the fat is burned for energy that our bodies use. L-carnitine enables the body to recover quickly from fatigue, and when combined with supplementation of vitamin E, this nutrient is a capable combatant of heart disease. Taking 500 mg twice a day on an empty stomach is recommended.

Lecithin . . . Derived from soy, lecithin supplies the body with inositol, choline and phosphatidyl choline, three nutrients that aid in the maintenance of healthy arteries and the emulsification of fat. Lecithin can reduce plaque in the arteries, lower blood pressure and ameliorate angina pectoris. Lecithin granules are like finely chopped nuts, and can be sprinkled on cereals. Liquid lecithin can be blended into healthful beverages.

Magnesium . . . Approximately 80 percent of the American population is magnesium-deficient. Magnesium, which should be consumed in quantities of 600-1000 mg daily, is an advantageous nutrient because it enhances circulation by permitting the muscles in the arterial walls to rest. It is useful in ameliorating many forms of heart disease, including hypertension and arrhythmias.

About 100-200 mg should be taken in the morning on an empty stomach; the remainder is best absorbed before bedtime.

Niacin . . . Clinical studies have indicated that niacin (use the non-flush version), also known as vitamin B3, can help prevent heart attack and heart disease fatality. In addition, evidence suggests that it can be an effective combatant against cancer. Note: Niacin should only be taken under medical supervision because of its tendency to hamper liver function.

Selenium . . . A lack of this important trace mineral has been associated with hypertension. Generally, 200 mcg daily is recommended.

Taurine . . . Supplementation of taurine, an amino acid that acts as an antioxidant, can help fortify cardiac contractions and consequently enhance the outflow of blood from the heart. The consumption of 500 mg of taurine twice a day can be a key factor in avoiding congestive heart failure and arteriosclerosis.

Acidophilus and Fructo-Oligosaccharides . . . Both products increase helpful intestinal bacteria and thus eliminate the harmful germs. As a result, heart palpitations due to intestinal problems diminish, and heart strength increases.

Calcium and Potassium . . . These are important since low levels of calcium and potassium may also result in heart palpitations.

Maxepa/EFA . . . Individuals who do not consume adequate quantities of fish should be pleased to learn that the heart disease-deterrent essential fatty acids found in fish oil can be provided with the supplement Maxepa.

Some additional supplements to consider are the vitamin B complex, choline, inositol, niacinamide, phosphorous, GLA, cod liver oil, brewer's yeast and wheat germ. Also, for people who are deficient in thyroid hormone, supplements of thyroid extract are important because, among other things, they reduce the risk of heart attack. The natural form is better than the synthetic.

Herbal Treatments

Herbs are a source of nutrition that can assist in treating and preventing heart disease. Among the many choices available, garlic shines as a cardiovascular disease preventive: It contributes to the lowering of cholesterol levels and elevated blood pressure, and helps prevent blood clots in the arterial walls when taken along with vitamin E. It also helps stimulate and revitalize the heart muscle and strengthen the peripheral circulation, as well as circulation within the heart. Eating a crushed garlic clove, once in the morning and once at night, has a revitalizing effect on the heart. For those sensitive to the social implications of eating raw garlic, 500 mg of deodorized garlic can be taken twice a day. Two other cooking spices that help to counteract atherosclerosis are ginger and turmeric (the yellow spice used in curry powder).

Cayenne, which contains the active ingredient capsaicin, has multiple functions, including the abilities to lower blood pressure and cholesterol levels and prevent heart attacks and strokes. Studies find that using the entire herb is more effective than using capsaicin alone.

Hawthorn berry is versatile, with the ability to improve arrhythmias, angina, blood pressure and arterial hardening. In addition, the daily consumption of hawthorn berry can enhance circulation and treat valvular insufficiency, irregular pulse and abnormal acid levels in the blood. The herb is used widely in Europe for early stage congestive heart failure, as it has been found superior to medications for slowing down the condition. The recommended dosage is generally 160 mg, divided into two doses a day, although people with more challenging conditions may need up to 160 mg three times daily.

Bugleweed can help alleviate heart palpitations and high blood pressure. Lily of the valley is also effective against palpitations.

Ginkgo biloba aids small blood vessel circulation.

Mistletoe can relieve heart strain, stimulate circulation, and lower blood pressure. Fifteen drops of the extract or three cups of the tea can be taken three times a day. Remember not to misuse this particular herb by exceeding the recommended dosage, and do not eat the mistletoe berries.

Motherwort can be used to secure cardiac electrical rhythm, but be sure to seek medical supervision when taking this herb. It can be added to warm water (10 to 20 drops) and consumed as a tea.

Tansy is another herb for heart palpitations and can also be ingested as a tea. It can be taken three to four times a day, an hour before meals and just before sleep.

Wild yam enhances the body's production of DHEA, a hormone needed to prevent the onset of heart disease.

Alfalfa, which is especially useful in preventing arteriosclerosis and calcium deposits, should be consumed in the seed form, either mixed in salads or by taking six teaspoons per day.

Arjuna is an Ayurvedic herb for improving circulation to the heart and normalizing high blood pressure. It also helps to reverse soft tissue damage to internal organs and muscles.

Indian snakeroot, also known as Rauwolfia, possesses hypotensive properties, according to clinical studies from the U.S., Britain and India. The plant grows wild in India and Africa, and has been used for centuries to treat various conditions affecting the nervous system, including anxiety, fear, snakebite and abdominal pain. Rauwolfia is used in hypotensive medications and is found most effective for mild conditions when the whole herb is taken, and when it is used over an extended period of time.

Black cohosh is an American herb that has the ability to help lower blood pressure and act as a sedative by inhibiting vasomotor centers in the central nervous system.

Some additional herbs that can be used to alleviate and prevent heart disease are bilberry, valerian root, kelp and butcher's broom.

Chelation Therapy

Many health practitioners agree that chelation therapy is the most effective way of treating heart disease because of its ability to fully reverse all the disorders associated with the arteries and cardiac region. This form of therapy provides an attractive alternative to bypass surgery, which treats only a limited portion of the body's arteries and blood vessels. One of the major advantages of chelation therapy is its ability to improve the functioning of the brain by ameliorating the symptomatic dizziness and the mental degradation associated with artery blockage in the upper body. The average patient will experience significant results after 30 exposures to the therapy. After the initial treatments, maintenance treatments are usually needed once a month or every other month to preserve the benefits the patient receives.

Chelation therapy consists of the usage of an IV apparatus and a chemical known as EDTA. During the procedure, the patient is seated in a comfortable chair and a bottle containing the EDTA is situated several feet above the head of the patient. The EDTA solution slowly flows from the bottle through the IV, and finally into the patient's veins, where it filtrates into the blood and circulates around the fluid spaces that surround the cells. The entire procedure usually lasts for approximately three hours.

What chelation therapy does is cleanse the body by removing potentially harmful substances, such as lead, uranium and nickel. The EDTA is also able to combine calcium with calcium deposits in the arterial walls, which the kidneys then discharge out of the body. Furthermore, the EDTA promotes softening of the arteries by eliminating the buildup of scar tissue within them.

People in their 40's are prime candidates for chelation therapy, since most people in this age group will experience some amount of arteriosclerosis as a result of excessive cholesterol intake and the buildup of calcium, scar tissue and fat within the arteries. Chelation can successfully eliminate these risk factors and can turn back the clock for many potential heart disease victims. It is an excellent idea to initiate therapy during the early stages of heart disease, as studies have indicated that the reduction of arterial calcium accumulation between the ages of 40 and 60 can be vital to curbing the development of arteriosclerosis.

Chelation therapy has also achieved widespread success in the treatment of people who already suffer from an advanced form of heart disease, such as angina or intermittent claudication. Treatment of these patients frequently results in the complete disappearance of the symptoms that have plagued them. In numerous cases, people with angina who were unable to participate in relatively simple activities experienced remarkable improvement in their abilities. People in their 70's and 80's sometimes require a number of treatment sessions beyond the average 30 because of the accumulation of pollutants that have attached to their arterial walls over the years, but their systems can even eventually be cleaned out as well.

Overall, when chelation is combined with an extensive regimen of aerobic exercise, correct dietary intake, proper supplementation and stress reduction, this therapy can provide an extremely effective means of averting heart disease or dealing with a condition that already exists.

Exercise

Any exercise program should be initially supervised and okayed by a medical doctor to ensure that medical problems do not worsen with activity. Many people benefit from an exercise routine that burns 2000 calories a week. Three kinds of exercises therapeutic for the heart are lifting of light weights, yoga and aerobics:

Light Weight Exercises . . . Lifting light weights benefits the heart when exercises are directed at expanding the chest area. This allows the heart more room to breathe. These three exercises are particularly helpful.

1. Lie down on a bench with two- to three-pound dumbbells and perform lateral flies. As you inhale, stretch both arms to the side. Hold the breath in as you bring the dumbbells back overhead. This exercise opens the rib cage and gets more oxygen and energy into the chest area.
2. Lie down on a bench and bring the dumbbells straight back overhead while breathing in deeply. Bring them back down to the front while breathing out.
3. Squat down to perform a deep knee bend while holding a light (20-pound) barbell or broomstick across the shoulders. Breathe in deeply as you bend. Hold the breath, and then blow it out audibly as you rise.

Yoga . . . The best yoga exercise for opening up the chest area is the cobra posture. In this exercise you lie on the floor with your stomach to the ground and your feet together. Slowly arch the body up towards the ceiling, beginning with the eyes, head and neck. Take care not to overarch the neck. The palms of the hands can touch the floor in a push-up position, or the hands can rest alongside the body with the palms facing up. This second option will give less of a stretch but necessitate more work for the head, neck and chest.

Breathe in deeply as you lift. Once in position, breathe lightly in and out. After holding the posture for several seconds, gradually come back down, chest first and head last. Generally, the cobra is performed three times. During the first round, the arms are stretched out alongside the body. During the second two rounds, the palms are down on the floor. The body is raised higher with each successive round.

Aerobic Exercise . . . Walking is an aerobic exercise that is beneficial to the heart and highly recommended by physicians, as it is something almost anyone can do. Other types of aerobic exercise are jogging, running, water-walking, swimming and bicycling. Choose an exercise or exercises that you enjoy doing, so that you will be more likely to continue with your routine. Remember, though, to get medical clearance before you begin any new activity.

The Power of the Mind

Although physical factors such as diet and exercise play a big part in preventing or combating coronary disease, it is crucial not to overlook the spiritual health of the mind in relation to the body's ability to heal itself. People should try to let their minds as well as their bodies relax by engaging in cardiovascular exercise, deep breathing, biofeedback, yoga and massage therapy. A mixture of aromatic oils, such as ylang ylang, lavender, peppermint or marjoram, combined with massage oil, can enhance a massage by calming the body and lowering the blood pressure.

A positive relationship and understanding with one's soul can enable the body to combat disease more effectively, as a healthy soul is able to influence an effective bodily response. People who have undergone traumatic experiences, such as divorce or the death of a loved one, will often suffer from symptoms of heart disease because they have lost touch with the desire to remain healthy. These people need to reconnect with their souls, regain confidence in themselves and work on effectively expressing their emotions.

Many times people inappropriately internalize the stress in their lives, converting it to self-destructive habits, such as overeating, alcoholism or recreational drug use. Prolonged exposure to stress can actually induce red blood cell clotting by increasing the adhesive qualities of the platelets. Increased clotting contributes to the accumulation of atherosclerotic plaque, arterial blockage and, eventually, heart attack. When people are able to relax, their blood pressure decreases, halting the buildup of waste along the walls of the arteries.

Improvement in a patient's mental health can have a profound effect upon the functioning of the immune system, as well. When we feel loved, favorable hormones are produced by the endocrine system, enabling the muscles to relax and oxygen to flow more freely. In short, paying kind attention to one's own emotional state and making positive changes in attitude when necessary, can be a rewarding complement to the physical treatment of coronary disease.

Lancet described type D behavior as a risk to having heart disease. Withholding and denying emotions by, say, declining to cry when crying is appropriate—for instance, upon learning of the death of a loved one—and not being socially connected (two traits of a person with a type D personality) seem to contribute to heart disease and stroke.

Another study involving 2800 men and women over 55 years of age demonstrated how even slight depression is able to increase cardiac mortality by 60 percent. However, a significant depression could triple the rate of cardiac-related deaths.

According to a 2002 study from Duke University, men who had cardiovascular disease and who went through four months of stress management (1½ hours weekly) significantly reduced their cardiovascular events.

What to Avoid

An overly sedentary lifestyle and obesity are to be avoided, as these factors can contribute to high blood pressure. In addition, it is important to eliminate our dietary intake of animal protein, saturated fats and saturated oils, salt, fried foods, caffeine, tobacco, alcohol and heavy starches, because these foods contribute to the deposit of pollutants within the walls of the arteries. The presence of hydrogenated vegetable oil or vegetable shortening on a product's ingredients list should serve as a reminder to stay away from that product. Avoid margarine at all costs. At one time, people believed that polyunsaturated oil assisted in the reduction of cholesterol levels, but we now realize that the high trans-fatty acid content in margarine only promotes heart disease. Unfiltered tap water can be a problem; it can eventually lead to coronary damage due to pollutants in the water supply. While sufficient amounts of pure water protect the heart, other beverages are not good substitutes, particularly caffeine and alcohol, which are dehydrating.

Finally, let go of stress in any way that you can. Stress reduction is not a frill. As discussed earlier, the reduction of stress in one's life decreases the risk of heart disease and heart attack by eliminating unnecessary free radical damage to the tissues and by relaxing the walls of the arteries.

Treatment Summary

There is clear evidence that heart disease can be effectively treated and reversed through a low-fat diet program.

Drink sufficient amounts of pure water.

Supplements and herbs can be taken to combat many forms of heart disease. Antioxidants, in particular, are vital.

Chelation therapy can reverse disorders of the arteries and cardiac region.

Light weight exercises, yoga and aerobics are excellent forms of exercise that can benefit people at risk or who are suffering from heart disease.

Spiritual, emotional and mental health play a role in the body's ability to heal itself.

Heat Exhaustion and Heatstroke

Heat exhaustion and heatstroke (also known as sunstroke or heat hyperpyrexia) come from an overexposure to the sun or high temperature. While most people are careful not to overdo it, there are times when they may not be mindful of the power of the sun, such as when they are vacationing in a tropical country where they are not used to the weather.

Symptoms

Heat exhaustion is characterized by weakness, dizziness, nausea and muscle cramping from a loss of fluid and salt, while heatstroke is more severe. When the temperature of the body exceeds 104 degrees Fahrenheit, or when the victim has suffered a seizure or is in a coma, it means that heat exhaustion has turned into a stroke. Heatstroke is a medical emergency and a far graver condition than heat exhaustion. In fact, its mortality rate ranges from 40 to 80 percent. It affects every organ in the body except the pancreas. It threatens a person—if not quickly reversed—with cardiovascular failure, permanent brain damage and death.

Note: To distinguish between heat exhaustion and heatstroke, ascertain the victim's state of mind. Oftentimes the victim will have an altered mental status.

Treatment

First Aid

A commonsense first-aid approach would be to get the person out of the sun, and to provide rest, fluid replacement and cooling. Cooling can be accomplished by applying ice packs and wrapping the person in a cool, wet sheet. When the condition is severe, the individual should be rushed to a medical facility as soon as possible. This applies especially to the person who is in shock, as evidenced by shivering, incoherence and confusion. Fluids containing electrolytes are also important. These drinks supply the person with calcium, potassium and magnesium, minerals that must be replaced as they drain out of the body quickly during heat exhaustion and heatstroke. Foods high in these nutrients include dark leafy greens, nuts, seeds, whole grains, sea vegetables, blackstrap molasses and bananas. Mail companies sell these drinks, but their effect can also be obtained from a solution that incorporates lemon juice, lime juice, green drinks, mineral water or salt water.

Vitamins

The role of antioxidants in combating free-radical damage to the skin should not be overlooked. Antioxidants can be taken orally or used topically on the skin. Foremost among these antioxidants are vitamins A, C and E. When the skin is protected, it can protect you from heat exhaustion and heatstroke.

Herbs

Second- or third-degree burns occurring with either condition can be minimized with the help of pure aloe vera. The gel, placed directly on the skin, will hydrate the skin immediately. Taken internally as a juice or gel, aloe vera further will promote healing by providing the body with a multitude of electrolytes.

The following herbs have long been in use to reduce fever or lower the body's temperature:

Chinese Skullcap . . . Reduces the temperature by dilating the blood vessels close to the skin's surface.

Elder Flower with Peppermint Leaf . . . Treats fever.

Subprostrata . . . Dilates the blood vessels, thus reducing the body's temperature.

Willow Bark . . . A staple of Native American medicine to treat fever.

Note: Cayenne pepper has capsaicin, which may lower the body temperature by stimulating the sweat glands.

Homeopathy

The main homeopathic remedy for sunstroke is belladonna. Homeopathic practitioners use it when symptoms include a throbbing and pulsating headache. The face is flushed and hot, and the extremities are cold. The pupils may be dilated, and the person feels worse when touched or laying down flat. Persons treated with belladonna usually do not feel thirsty.

Glonoinum (nitroglycerin) is used if the individual has a fever and is flushed and sweaty. The sufferer may complain of having a hot face but cold extremities.

What to Avoid

The worst thing to give a person felled by heat is alcohol. Some people are under the impression that alcohol will revive the person, when in actuality it only dehydrates the tissues further.

Treatment Summary

A person suffering from heatstroke or exhaustion should be given immediate first aid in the form of rest, fluid replacement and cooling. The condition may be a medical emergency that requires hospitalization.

Aloe vera can be applied topically or taken internally.

Belladonna is a homeopathic remedy for sunstroke.

Hemorrhoids

Hemorrhoids, also known as piles, are swollen blood vessels that cause the mucous membranes of the lower rectum or anus to protrude. When the projection is above the inside opening of the anus, it is referred to as an internal hemorrhoid. This tends to be painful and causes bleeding with bowel movements. Hemorrhoids that appear outside the anal opening are called external hemorrhoids; these do not usually cause bleeding, but may cause discomfort.

Generally, hemorrhoids affect people with sedentary lifestyles, as well as people who eat too many dairy products and constipating protein and starch. The problem may also be due to diarrhea and the overuse of laxatives, poor circulation, putrefaction of old waste matter and straining to defecate. Pregnant women are especially susceptible, and are advised to avoid constipating foods for this reason.

Treatment

Diet and Lifestyle

Although we tend to think of hemorrhoids as a local problem, the condition is generally due to a systemic imbalance. As mentioned above, straining to have a bowel movement places pressure on the blood vessels and is a primary cause of the problem. This can be avoided by eating a high-fiber diet, getting sufficient exercise and drinking eight to 10 glasses of water daily, all of which encourage softer, bulkier stools that pass more easily. Magnesium aids peristalsis and can be very helpful. Vitamin C loosens stools, making bowel movements easier. Additionally, taking bioflavonoid supplements, such as those derived from rutin (600-4000 mg per day) has been shown to significantly reduce swelling, bleeding, itching and other hemorrhoid symptoms.

Similarly, the product Daflon, which contains the food-derived flavonoid diosmin, reduced symptoms in the majority of hemorrhoid-inflicted pregnant women who used it in trials in dosages of 1000-3000 mg per day.

Herbs

Some simple herbs may have a healing effect. Aloe vera juice, for one, is a gentle laxative that increases circulation and soothes the alimentary canal. A person can begin with one teaspoonful of the gel and work up to one table-spoonful or more, if needed. A Chinese herbal formula called Fargelin may remedy the condition quickly by improving circulation to the area. Slippery elm and marshmallow also soothe an irritated digestive tract. Either one can be used to relieve constipation. They should not be used, however, if there is diarrhea or mucus in the stool. Additionally, butcher's broom and horse chest-nut are useful for this problem, especially when there is pain and numbness in the feet and legs. A pint of blueberries every day can also help.

Psyllium, which is high in fiber, has also been shown to have benefits in re-lieving constipation. It is effective in the amount of 7 g, taken three times daily. Otherwise, 2 tablespoons of psyllium seeds or 1 teaspoon of psyllium husks can be mixed with juice and taken two or three times per day. However, it is crucial to consume adequate liquids when taking psyllium. *Caution: Do not* take psyl-lium if you already take the prescription drug nitrofurantoin or digitalis.

The use of horse chestnut extract has also been reported to reduce hemor-rhoid symptoms. Choose either an extract that is standardized for a 16 to 21 percent aescin content or an isolated aescin preparation, so that you will be getting 90-150 mg of aescin per day.

Combining external treatments with internal ones speeds up the recovery process. Witch hazel is an astringent herb that may be topically applied in an ointment base three or four times a day. Botanicals can also be made into a poultice by grinding up herbs, placing them inside a cloth and applying them to the skin. This helps to break up congestion, lessen inflammation and re-move toxins. Suggested botanicals for such a compress include lemon juice and vitamin E, as well as witch hazel.

Herbs and oils added to bath water can provide further relief to an irritated system and improve circulation. Cyprus oil is a venous tonic that is used in the treatment of hemorrhoids. Five drops of the essential oil can be added to the bath. Alternatively, a therapeutic bath can be made by covering three handfuls of chamomile and one handful of witch hazel, nettle, echinacea or calendula with boiled water. The herbs should be covered and allowed to steep for about an hour. The herbs should then be strained and the liquid poured into a tub-ful of water.

Finally, adding a quarter of a cup of Epsom salts to four inches of bathwater will reduce all swelling.

Treatment Summary

A high-fiber diet, exercise and eight 10-ounce glasses of water daily allow for elimination without straining. Magnesium, vitamin C, the product Daflon and bioflavonoids may also be helpful.

Numerous herbs can be taken internally, applied externally, or used in a bath to soothe and heal hemorrhoids.

Hepatitis

Hepatitis is a viral infection that damages the liver. There are three types of hepatitis, called A, B and C, for which the virus has been identified. Hepatitis A is usually spread by food or water contaminated with feces; hepatitis B and C are spread via tainted blood products used in transfusions, unsterile needles or sexually. Hepatitis A has a slow onset and most people fully recover, while hepatitis B and C begin and progress rapidly. Hepatitis B and C can lead to prolonged illness, including cirrhosis of the liver and death. Not only is hepatitis C a serious international public health problem, but it is also currently the most common reason for liver transplants in the United States.

Having a weakened liver makes one more susceptible to hepatitis. Factors that may contribute to weakening of the liver are other viruses, such as cytomegalovirus and Epstein-Barr virus. Degenerative substances that harm the liver include toxic chemicals in the environment, as well as alcohol and drugs that cause liver cells to die. Liver-harming medications can include tranquilizers, chemotherapeutic agents, antibiotics and anesthetics.

Symptoms of hepatitis include mild or severe fatigue, upper respiratory problems, nausea, vomiting, multiple joint aches or tenderness, muscle aches, headaches, loss of appetite, fever, jaundice, low blood sugar, anxiety, depression, nervousness and visual changes.

In cases of accidental exposure to hepatitis B (such as through a needle or other contact with infected blood, serum, semen, or vaginal or other body fluids), hepatitis B immunoglobulin (HBIG) should be given within two days to two weeks, to prevent infection, along with the vaccination series for hepatitis B, if no immunity has been established.

If diagnosed, you must reduce the risk of passing the virus by taking proper precautions. Remind your doctor, dentist and other practitioners that you are a carrier. Cover all cuts and open sores with bandages. Wipe a blood spill promptly, then clean the area with a 1:10 ratio of bleach to water. Do not share razors, needles, syringes, nail files, clippers, scissors, toothbrushes, or any other object that may have come into contact with your blood or body fluids. Dispose of personal items such as tissues, menstrual pads, tampons and bandages in a plastic bag. Use condoms, and alert those with whom you have sexual contact as to your condition. If you are pregnant, tell your doctor; a child born to an infected mother should be vaccinated within 12 hours of birth.

Treatment

Conventional medicine has approved the use of interferon alpha and lamivudine for the treatment of chronic hepatitis B. However, in a large percentage of interferon alpha patients, the drug poses toxicity problems, which manifest in a number of ways, ranging from flu-like symptoms to depression. Pegylated interferon is now being used before interferon for the treatment of hepatitis C because it has the benefits of easier administration and fewer side effects.

Lamivudine, which is also prescribed to HIV patients, and is well tolerated, helps suppress the virus' replication, and delays disease progression. But since treatment with one agent is associated with a viral strain's developing resistance to that agent, combination therapies are likely to be the wave of the future.

A hopeful new therapy, for both its therapeutic value and benefits on immune response, is thymosin alpha-1. This therapy augments the functioning of the T-cells, triggers maturation of lymphocytes and encourages reconstitution of immune defects. It has an outstanding safety record and may be taken safely with other therapies. Unfortunately, although thymosin alpha-1 is available in over 20 different countries, it has yet to gain approval by the FDA. Depending on the results of currently ongoing trials, we could see the introduction of thymosin alpha-1 as a therapy in the United States very shortly.

Nutrition

Recovery from hepatitis depends largely on restoring the integrity of the liver. Many holistic approaches therefore focus on liver detoxification and strengthening. A whole foods vegetarian diet prevents the liver from being overworked. Such a diet also contains phytochemicals, plant chemicals that help prevent acute damage or even protect a person from developing problems in the first place.

A good daily drink for liver cleansing consists of lemon juice or cider vinegar in water with a teaspoon of honey and royal jelly. A mid-morning snack of apple, carrot or cranberry juice, or a vegetable juice with green powder, will further purify the liver. Roasted dandelion, peppermint, pau d'arco and Japanese green teas are also good for this purpose. Try 10 eight-ounce glasses of fresh, organic dark green and yellow vegetable juices daily and add one ounce of aloe to five of the glasses.

Supplements

The supplementation of antioxidants is critical to minimizing the oxidative stress of hepatitis. Oxidative stress is believed to be the cause of the tumors that appear after years of chronic liver inflammation. Reports have shown nutritional antioxidants to be both therapeutic and preventative agents, reducing both inflammation and damage to tissues.

In a randomized, double-blind study, vitamin E was shown to be highly successful in combination with conventional hepatitis treatments due to its powerful antioxidant properties. Other important supplements to consider include quercetin, vitamin C (taken intravenously and orally), essential fatty acids, B-complex vitamins (especially B12) and selenium. Selenium has been proven to have a protective role against hepatitis B, and viral hepatitis patients should take 200-400 mcg of selenium daily to ward off liver cancer. Zinc, a companion trace mineral, may also be of benefit.

New information shows that glutathione is necessary for maintaining the liver's redox state and is essential to the liver's performance. Glutathione levels in the body may be enhanced by taking 600 mg of N-acetyl-cysteine (NAC) once a day, 20-30 g of whey protein once a day, 250 mg of alpha-lipoic acid twice a day and 500-1000 mg of L-glutamine once a day. If administered intravenously, alanyl glutamine or free glutamine may be used at the same dose.

S-adenosylmethionine (SAMe) is vital for liver function and regeneration. It is also an effective antidepressant. A dosage of 200 mg of SAMe may be taken three times daily.

Polyunsaturated phosphatidylcholine (PPC), sold under the name Gastro-Pro in the United States but available only as a drug in Europe, may be taken in divided doses totaling 1800-2700 mg daily. PPC protects cell membranes and helps regenerate liver cells. It works very effectively in conjunction with vitamin E and milk thistle.

Herbs

The best herbal support is derived from silymarin, a milk thistle extract. The key ingredient in this herbal aid, silibinin, accelerates the rate at which protein is synthesized in the liver, so that cells are regenerated faster. A member of the daisy family, milk thistle is widely used in India, where hepatits is seen in epidemic proportions.

Curcumin, an ingredient in turmeric, has anti-inflammatory properties.

Astralagus stops free radical damage and aids detoxification processes.

The Japanese frequently eat burdock root, a bitter herb known for its ability to cleanse the liver.

The Chinese herb phyllanthus and the ganoderma mushroom have been shown to act against hepatitis B.

Dandelion root is used for hepatitis and jaundice because it stimulates the liver and gallbladder. When large quantities are taken, patients are sometimes cured in a short period of time.

Red clover fights free radicals, attacking liver cells and helps the system to detoxify.

Evening primrose oil will also benefit the liver and spleen and is especially good together with echinacea. The oil contains prostaglandins, which help reduce inflammation.

Another valuable herb for the treatment of hepatitis is Oregon grape root. This herb contains berberine, a substance that aids in liver metabolism. Interestingly enough, similar species of the herb grow throughout the world and are used by separate cultures for blood and liver cleansing; while Native Americans have long valued Oregon grape root, Chinese and Indian cultures have their own species of the plant.

Barberry is yet another herb useful for this condition, especially when combined with goldenseal and lobelia. However, as barberry is quite bitter, only small quantities can be tolerated.

Alfalfa is important because it relieves liver inflammation. Additionally, alfalfa is a good source of vitamin K, which helps prevent bleeding.

Jamaicans have long used Jamaica weed, a form of phyllanthus, in the treatment of hepatitis. This plant contains ingredients that can kill the hepatitis B virus in vivo, something that is difficult to accomplish using allopathic medicine.

Many liver disorders accompany candida problems. In these instances, pau d'arco or garlic should be taken for its antifungal effects and for immune support.

Other herbs that improve liver function include aloe vera, buckthorn, wild yam, wood betony and yellow dock.

Ozone Therapy

All forms of hepatitis have shown improvement with intravenous ozone, and hepatitis can sometimes be fully eliminated after several sessions. The modality appears to increase immune system activity, enabling the body's own defenses to wipe out aggressive viral organisms.

What to Avoid

Steer clear of all foods that stress the liver in order to avoid toxicity. This includes food additives, preservatives and artificial sweeteners. Sugar can promote liver inflammation and free radical damage. Instead, eat organic foods.

Alcohol kills liver cells and leads to cirrhosis. Many drugs can aggravate the problem, as well. Even certain herbs can be toxic to the liver in high amounts. Avoid germander, comfrey, ginbu-1, skullcap, mistletoe, pennyroyal and chaparral leaf. While 500 mg of licorice root extract taken three times a day may be beneficial, take it only under a medical worker's close supervision to ensure that no unwanted increase in blood pressure occurs.

Do not load the body with excess iron, which is toxic to the liver. However, since anemia is often a result of hepatitis treatment, it is important to work closely with your physician in order to maintain proper levels. Be careful not to eat spoiled or moldy peanuts, which can contain a toxin associated with the acceleration of hepatoma. Fresh peanuts do not contain this toxin.

Corticosteroids, while useful against other forms of hepatitis, can be dangerous when used in cases of viral hepatitis.

Treatment

Organic, chemical-free foods that replenish the liver are detoxifying and strengthening. These include many plant foods, as well as vitamins C, B and E, selenium, SAMe, the product GastroPro and glutathione.

Numerous herbs strengthen the liver. The most noteworthy is the milk thistle extract, silymarin, which can actually reverse liver damage.

Ozone therapy can sometimes reverse hepatitis in a matter of a few sessions.

Excess iron, moldy peanuts and corticosteroids should be avoided.

Once infected, a person must take care not to transmit viral hepatitis to others.

Herpes

One aspect of the aftermath of the sexual revolution was an epidemic of herpes outbreaks. While much feared in the 1970s, this contagious condition was overshadowed by the advent of AIDS in the early 1980s. Today, though less publicized than AIDS, herpes is far more prevalent, affecting, in one form or another, 80 percent of the American population. Over half the population gets cold sores from time to time, the result of herpes simplex virus 1 (HSV1). Others become afflicted with shingles, a herpes zoster infection, years after they get chicken pox. Additionally, people get Epstein-Barr, the form of herpes that causes mononucleosis. Still others break out in genital herpes, an infection caused by herpes simplex virus 2 (HSV2).

Causes

Herpes is a contagious virus that lives in nerve cells. Periodic attacks occur whenever the immune system is below par. Any kind of emotional, mental or physical stress can lower the body's defense system and create the perfect climate for an outbreak. Common physical stressors include illness, menstrual periods, vaginal yeast infections, too much sunlight or friction (which breaks down skin cells), allergies and certain foods. Prescription drugs that lower immunity can cause an attack. Examples of such medications include antibiotics, steroids and antidepressants. Also, genital herpes can be sexually transmitted, and pregnant women can transmit the virus to their unborn children via blood or through direct contact with infected tissue during delivery.

Symptoms

Genital herpes causes surface sores on the skin and lining of the genital area. In men, penile blisters may appear on the tip of the foreskin and turn into surface sores for several days before healing. In women, sores can appear on the cervix, vagina or perineum. These sores may be accompanied by a discharge or vaginal blisters. There is often a burning sensation, especially at the onset of an outbreak. Other symptoms may include urinary problems, fever and lymphatic swelling. Intercourse is painful and should be avoided during an outbreak to prevent sexual transmission. HSV2 occurs intermittently and usually lasts from five to seven days.

Oral herpes attacks the skin and mucous membranes on the face, particularly around the mouth and nose. These cold sores tend to appear as pearl-like blisters. Although they are short-term, they can be irritating and painful.

Herpes zoster, the result of the varicella zoster virus (VZV), may cause agonizing blisters on one side of the body, usually on the chest or abdomen. Pain is usually felt before effects are seen. Symptoms may last from a few days to several weeks.

Treatment

While there are no cures for herpes, drugs are commonly given to lessen symptoms. The most famous of these is acyclovir, also known as Zovirax, which supposedly reduces the rate of growth of the herpes virus. Others include famciclovir, vaalacyclovir and penciclovir. Herpes medications have many potential side effects, including dizziness, headaches, diarrhea, nausea, vomiting, general weakness, fatigue, ill health, sore throat, fever, insomnia, swelling, tenderness and bleeding of the gums. In addition, acyclovir ointment can cause allergic skin reactions. While acyclovir stops DNA replication of the virus nearly 100 percent of the time, it also halts the patient's DNA synthesis 1 percent. Furthermore, the widespread use of acyclovir promotes the development of drug-resistant strains of the virus.

Natural remedies, which are kinder to the system, are effective in shortening the length of the outbreaks and in diminishing their frequency. These are some to know about:

Nutrition and Lifestyle

When herpes strikes, it's always a good idea to rest and eat lightly. Short fruit fasts, with plenty of pure water and cleansing herbal teas, can be helpful. Good herbs to include are sage, rosemary, cayenne, echinacea, goldenseal, chaparral, red clover, astragalus and burdock root.

Beneficial bacteria, such as those found in yogurt and in supplements of lactobacillicus and acidophilus, support the digestive processes necessary for the maintenance of the immune system.

Other nutrients that directly enhance the immune system include garlic, quercetin, zinc gluconate, buffered vitamin C, vitamin E and beta-carotene or vitamin A. Bee propolis is anti-inflammatory and high in B vitamins, which combat stress. Also good are bee pollen, blue-green algae and pycnogenol.

The over-the-counter drug Tagamet, or generic cimetidine, has demonstrated immune-enhancing powers. It has proven effective in preventing and shortening durations of herpes outbreaks. The suggested dosage of cimetidine is 200 mg three times a day and 400 mg at night, as soon as early indications of an outbreak emerge. Refer to the package insert for specific dosage information and possible drug interactions.

At the start of each day, DHEA may be taken in a 15-75-mg dose. A blood test should be taken after three to six weeks of DHEA therapy to monitor that desired levels are being reached (350-430 mcg/dL for women and 400-560 mcg/dL for men). DHEA will increase testosterone in the body, so women with estrogen-dependent cancers and men with prostate cancer are not advised to use this treatment. In addition, the possibility of having these cancers should be ruled out before its use. Essential fatty acids (EFAs) assist in the elimination of saturated and partially hydrogenated fats, providing relief for many herpes sufferers. EFAs also promote the stability of cell membranes, which makes cells less prone to allowing the herpes virus to enter.

Garlic reveals its antiviral properties when taken in amounts of 1000 mg twice per day during an outbreak.

One to three 300-mg capsules of lactoferrin should be taken, especially in the early stages of infection.

There is controversy surrounding the use of L-lysine as a herpes-outbreak therapy. However, many researchers comment on its effectiveness. Those who suffer from frequent outbreaks should take L-lysine in the amount of 1000-1500 mg per day. Foods that naturally contain lysine include yogurt, cheese, fish, potatoes, eggs and brewer's yeast. During outbreaks, it is recommended that patients increase lysine consumption and reduce their intake of arginine (found in walnuts, peanuts and seeds).

Olive leaf extract (500 mg) should be taken three times a day, at mealtimes, during outbreaks.

Probiotics, such as lactobacillus plantarum, are not only effective for healthy digestion, but also for ulcerations of the mouth when taken three times a day.

Homeopathy

Homeopathy will build the immune system, not merely suppress symptoms. The following remedies are used to treat herpes homeopathically. Note that you shouldn't touch the formulas directly; that may disturb their vibration. Rather, they should be placed under the tongue until dissolved. Also, coffee, mint, camphor and chamomile must be avoided, as they act to cancel the effects of the remedies. It is also important to note symptoms. As they change, so, too, must the homeopathic remedy.

For cold sores:

Natrum Muriaticum . . . When sores are on the lips, especially in the middle of the lips, the 30c potency should be taken twice a day.

Phosphorus . . . Cold sores that manifest above the lips, accompanied by itching, cutting and sharp pain, need the 30c potency twice a day.

Petroleum . . . For cold sores that erupt in patches, and become crusty and loose around the lips and mouth, petroleum is indicated. A 9c potency is needed three times a day.

Apis . . . Apis helps cold sores around the mouth and lips that are accompanied by stinging, and painful blisters that itch and burn. A 6c potency is needed three to four times daily.

For female genital herpes:

Natrum Muriaticum . . . This remedy is indicated when the herpetic lesions are pearl-like blisters and the genital area feels puffy, hot and very dry. A 6c potency may be beneficial when taken four times a day.

Dulcamara . . . Women who tend to get a herpes outbreak in clusters on the vulva or on the hair follicles around the labia and vulva every time they catch a cold or get their period, are given dulcamara in a 12c potency, two to three times a day.

Petroleum . . . This may help if herpes eruptions form in patches and the sores become deep red and feel tender and moist. Outbreaks usually occur during menstrual periods, and most often affect the perineum, anus, labia or vulva. A 9c potency should be taken three times a day.

For shingles:

Arsenicum Album . . . This remedy benefits most cases of shingles, especially when the individual feels worse in the cold and after midnight, and better with warmth. If taken at the onset of an attack, it is best taken in a 30c potency twice a day for two to three days. After the first three days, arsenicum album is indicated if there is a burning sensation in the areas that were affected by the zoster eruptions (typically the chest and abdomen). At this point 12c, taken two to three times a day, is best. This remedy is excellent for getting rid of the burning sensation that is often present.

Hypericum Perforatum . . . Hypericum is a remedy for any kind of nerve pain. It is indicated whenever there is intense neuritis and neuralgia, with burning, tingling and numbness along the course of the affected nerves. Hypericum perforatum should be taken in a 30c potency, two to three times a day.

Essential Oils

In France, essential oils are well respected for their medicinal properties and used in place of antibiotics to combat various inflammatory ailments, including cold and canker sores. Aromatherapist Valerie Cooksley, author of *Aromatherapy: A Lifetime Guide to Healing with Essential Oils*, suggests this mouthwash recipe: Mix 5 drops of peppermint, bergamot or tea tree oil with raw honey. Then add this to a strong sage or rosemary tea. Rinsing with the formula several times a day, balances the pH of the mouth and helps to heal infections. Daily use may even prevent outbursts from arising.

Cooksley recommends dabbing a Q-tip with myrrh oil and then applying it directly onto cold and canker sores to relieve pain. Another aromatherapist, Sharon Olson, dabs a cotton swab with diluted tea tree oil and places that on the cold sore to kill the virus. She follows this up with soothing lavender oil and aloe vera gel. A beneficial byproduct of the therapy, she explains, is its ability to lift the spirits and clear the mind.

Ozone

Intravenous infusion for four weeks along with IV drops of vitamin C, water-soluble vitamin A and glutathione helps fight herpes.

What to Avoid

Stay away from anything that upsets the nervous system, such as caffeine, alcohol and hard-to-digest meats. Foods high in the amino acid arginine, such as chocolate, peanut butter, nuts and onions, are also associated with higher incidences of outbreaks.

Toothbrushes should be changed frequently, and completely dried before reuse to prevent reinfection. Soaking toothbrushes in baking soda or hydrogen peroxide also fights germs. Since stress promotes outbreaks, it is important to make time for activities that alleviate tension. Possibilities include biofeedback, yoga, meditation, deep breathing and exercise.

Treatment Summary

Antiviral drugs are routinely given to herpes sufferers to alleviate symptoms, but these have many potential side effects.

During a herpes outbreak, one should rest, avoid stress and eat light, cleansing foods. There are many beneficial herbs that can be taken as teas. A variety of nutrients directly support the immune system. Homeopathy offers several remedies for combating herpes. Further, the product Tagamet, DHEA, L-lysine, lactoferrin, olive leaf extract, EFAs, garlic and probiotics also have positive effects.

Essential oils can be used internally or externally in place of antibiotics to stimulate the immune system and relieve inflammation and pain.

See also: Cold and Canker Sores.

High Cholesterol Level

Most Americans, including doctors, are victims of a mass campaign against a substance produced by our own bodies. Cholesterol is a steroid that is essential for the maintenance of the body's cells. It is not necessarily the monster we have been led to believe that it is. It helps the liver digest fats and works with protein and lecithin to transport fats through our blood. Not only that, but cholesterol helps manufacture important male and female sex hormones. In addition, cholesterol helps keep skin moist. Cholesterol is so important that if not enough comes from food, the liver manufactures it. It is so essential that, unless it is oxidized, it is produced daily to build the membranes of new cells that must be formed in place of dead and dying cells.

Most of us think of cholesterol as a type of fat, but, as mentioned above, it is really a special kind of alcohol, called a steroid alcohol or sterol. Normally, most cholesterol is found in cells, and only a small amount is found in the blood. Doctors do not worry about cholesterol in the cells, but when levels in the blood get high, the substance can clog arteries and put a strain on the heart.

A serum cholesterol level that is between 125 and 200 mg per 100 ml of blood is generally a safe one, in my opinion. Opinions on this differ widely, though; some experts say that a 175 mg cholesterol level is high; others place the acceptability cutoff as high as 275. You should discuss this issue with your own practitioner.

Actually, the cholesterol number alone is not enough to say that a potentially dangerous situation exists. It is also important to test triglyceride and lipoprotein levels (as part of a regular SMA-24 blood test). An elevated triglyceride level indicates a poorly functioning liver or pancreas. This is dangerous because triglycerides are blood fats and may play a part in clogging the arteries with harmful plaque. Lipoproteins are compounds composed of fat and protein, and of particular interest to the health-conscious are high-density lipoproteins (HDLs) and low-density lipoproteins (LDLs). HDLs are low in cholesterol and high in phospholipids, and are considered the "good guys" by heart specialists because they lessen the chance of heart disease. Having too many LDLS, on the other hand, are what doctors worry about. LDLs contain high levels of cholesterol and have a tendency to stick to the walls of arteries and build up as plaque. Too many LDLs, therefore, increase the risk of atherosclerosis, a condition in which the arterial walls are damaged by cholesterol and result in normal blood flow being blocked. An important factor to consider when testing cholesterol is the ratio of HDL versus the total serum cholesterol level. Ratios of 4:1 or better (i.e., the first number is lower than the four) are desirable.

Treatment

Dependence on cholesterol-lowering medications is unnecessary and unsafe. Plus, many have toxic side effects. Unless a person suffers from a rare genetic disorder called hypercholesterolemia, where high blood cholesterol levels begin at birth, there are safer, more natural ways to keep cholesterol levels down.

Eating less cholesterol-containing food would seem to be a good approach, and indeed the goal of lowering high dietary cholesterol intake has received much publicity in recent years. The problem is that cutting out eggs, steak and diary products does not necessarily correct high blood cholesterol. While cutting down on fatty foods is an excellent suggestion for most Americans who eat far more fat than they need, this approach alone may not be sufficient for lowering cholesterol because cholesterol is produced by the body. The body may respond to a sharp reduction in cholesterol by manufacturing more on its own. The body can make as much as 1500 mg of cholesterol a day, more than six times the amount normally eaten!

It is interesting to note that certain ethnic groups, such as the Masai tribes of Africa and the Eskimos, have high-cholesterol diets and yet have low levels of serum cholesterol and few incidences of heart disease. So, factors other than cholesterol intake must obviously come into play. Some of these factors are genetics, nutritional status, stress, exercise, age and blood triglyceride levels.

Diet

Instead of cutting out cholesterol-rich foods completely, a better approach might be to add more fiber. Roughage increases the speed at which the body eliminates cholesterol. Pectin, found in apples, is especially good for this. Also, eating old-fashioned hot grain cereal, such as rolled oats, oat bran, barley or buckwheat, is helpful in this regard. Adding pectin-rich apples to the cereal doubles the benefit. It is especially important to have 4-6 g of soluble fiber such as pectin, guar gum or psyllium before eating any meal high in fat.

Caution: Do not take psyllium if you already take the prescription drug nitro-furantoin or digitalis.

Chitosan is a fiber made from material in shellfish. It has proven effective in improving bowel functioning and reducing the body's cholesterol levels through elimination. As with other fibers, however, trace-mineral absorption will be reduced along with fat. Therefore, take trace minerals at a time other than when fiber is consumed. Three to six 500-mg capsules of chitosan may be taken along with 1000 mg of asorbic acid before a meal high in fat.

Another interesting finding is that a small amount of polyunsaturated fat may lower serum cholesterol levels by 5 to 10 percent. Linoleic acid, found in cold-pressed oils, fish (not shellfish), nuts, seeds and nut butters, is especially good.

Policosanol, a supplement that comes from natural sugar cane, contains octa-cosanol, an alcohol found in the waxlike coating of fruits and leaves. Studies show that policosanol: normalizes cholesterol as well as or better than do drugs; hinders arterial lesions from developing; prevents LDL-cholesterol oxidation, which destroys blood vessels; and inhibits clot formation and abnormal platelet aggregation. Millions of people across the globe use policosanol. The suggested dose is one tablet twice per day with meals, both morning and evening.

Artichoke leaf extract has impressive cholesterol-lowering advantages. In a number of studies, artichoke leaf extract has been shown to actually restrict cholesterol synthesis, an effect that persists for hours following initial exposure. As a supplement, 300 mg of artichoke leaf extract can be taken three times a day.

The benefits of garlic are undeniable. Studies have shown that liquid garlic extract inspires cholesterol reduction and protects the arterial lining from damage caused by oxidation. But most importantly, garlic prevents thrombosis, the cause of arterial blood clots and the main reason for strokes and heart attacks. In supplement form, garlic is beneficial for this condition in doses of 900-8000 mg per day.

Incorporate curcumin, otherwise known as turmeric root, into your diet. This ancient spice has been proven to cause significant cholesterol drops in a mere matter of days. Like garlic, turmeric also helps to inhibit the formation of abnormal blood clots. To receive its full benefits, take 900-1800 mg of curcumin daily.

Another ancient remedy that has recently been revived in the West is gugulipid. Gugulipid is derived from the resin of a certain type of north Indian tree. It should be taken in 140-mg doses once or twice per day.

Green tea will also lower undesirable forms of cholesterol. Drink one to three cups of green or black tea, or take one 350-mg capsule of 95-percent green tea every day.

Fish oil can reduce triglycerides by more than a third, on average, and is especially beneficial when taken in conjunction with garlic. If the fish oil causes stomach upset, perilla oil may be substituted. Perilla oil is a relatively new essential fatty acid source and is much easier on the gastrointestinal tract. Fish oil is preferable, however, if triglyceride levels are especially high.

Foods high in vitamin B6 (pyridoxine) are helpful. As this water-soluble vitamin tends to get lost in cooking, it is best to include plenty of raw fruits and vegetables in the diet. Leafy green vegetables are especially high in B6.

Lecithin-rich soy products, such as tofu and tempeh, are also important. Numerous studies have shown that soy protein plays a beneficial role in cardiovascular health. The phytochemicals in soy appear responsible not only for reduced incidences of heart disease, but for fewer cancers as well. Taking 5-6 g (about 2 teaspoons) of soy powder or a 135-mg capsule of 40-percent soy extract twice daily may be helpful.

Supplements

Many people are deficient in vitamins and minerals that keep cholesterol levels under control. Niacin (vitamin B3) is important for cholesterol control and can be found in a variety of foods, including leafy greens, wheat germ, beans, peas, salmon and tuna. It can also be taken as a supplement, though most individuals cannot handle the 1000 to 3000-mg dose needed for cholesterol-level suppression. Niacin helps to lower triglycerides as well as cholesterol and to raise beneficial HDL levels. Note that niacin should be used cautiously by those with a history of gout, liver dysfunction or diabetes. In high levels, niacin can cause liver toxicity. People with hepatitis should not take niacin. When taking niacin in dosages exceeding 1000 mg per day, liver enzymes should be monitored every six months. The effects of niacin are enhanced by vitamin C. Flush-free niacin (to prevent a reddened face) should be used.

One of vitamin C's many wonders is that it helps to lower cholesterol; anywhere from 1000 to 10,000 mg are needed each day (requirements increase in colder months and during periods of illness and stress). Vitamin C is best used in combination with bioflavonoids, especially rutin and quercetin. When combined with lecithin, it helps to dissolve arterial plaque. (Encapsulated liquid lecithin should have a phospholipid-choline content of at least 35 percent, and should deliver a minimum potency of 51.5-percent phosphatides. Granulated lecithin should be labeled 25-percent phosphatidyl choline, and should not have soy flower added to it.)

Vitamin E (400-800 IU daily) should not be overlooked. Vitamin E slows aging, and it is a known protector against several dozens of diseases. It will also improve circulation to the heart.

Vitamins B6 and methionine balance triglyceride levels, and ultimately help to normalize cholesterol.

Studies reveal the best cholesterol-lowering minerals to be chromium, calcium, magnesium, zinc and selenium. Selenium may be taken in the amount of 200-600 mcg per day.

Warning: monitor the use of supplements to reduce cholesterol. Have a cholestorol blood test 45 to 60 days after beginning the regimen. If supplements fail, drugs may be considered.

Herbs

Ginger and cayenne decrease liver production of cholesterol and triglycerides, according to studies. In addition, plenty of garlic should be eaten, as it lowers cholesterol and thins the blood, lessening the chances of dangerous blood clots. Raw garlic is most effective, but even cooked, this herb has a therapeutic effect. Deodorized capsules and pills are least effective, though, because it is the allicin, the smelly part of the garlic, that makes it useful. The ganoderma mushroom helps reduce cholesterol, triglycerides and total number of fats in the bloodstream.

Exercise

Exercise seems to help raise HDL and lower LDL levels, although it may take several months before there is a noticeable change.

What to Avoid

Many people replace cholesterol-rich foods with artificial ones—fake eggs, margarine, imitation bacon, nondairy cream, etc. But there is no evidence supporting that these fake foods prevent heart trouble, and they are associated with a higher incidence of cancer.

Foods containing refined sugars lead to an unhealthy buildup of fats in the liver and tissues. They also lower the level of healthy HDLs and increase the unwanted LDLs. Refined foods should be replaced with complex carbohydrates—fruits, vegetables and whole grains. Note that alcohol is high in refined sugar and should be avoided.

Many medications, including steroids and contraceptives, can increase cholesterol and triglyceride levels and destroy the nutrients needed for maintaining normal levels. In fact, studies reveal that people on steroid medications have a 50 percent increase in blood cholesterol levels. Excessive amounts of protein and cooked foods can also destroy cholesterol-controlling nutrients. Another factor that tends to raise cholesterol levels is stress, which is one of the reasons that stress avoidance—or management—is so important.

Treatment Summary

Cholesterol-lowering medications are unsafe and unnecessary except for people suffering from the rare disorder hypercholesterolemia.

Soluble fiber, especially pectin, helps to eliminate excess cholesterol from the body. Chitosan may be taken. Small amounts of polyunsaturated fats may lower cholesterol levels as well.

Exercise raises good cholesterol (HDL) and lowers bad cholesterol (LDL), over time.

Supplements that keep cholesterol under control include policosanol, niacin, vitamin C, bioflavonoids, liquid lecithin, vitamin E and the B vitamins, as well as chromium, magnesium, zinc and selenium.

Ginger, garlic, curcumin, gugulipid, artichoke extract, green tea, soy protein and the ganoderma mushroom lower cholesterol and tryglycerides.

See also: Heart Disease.

Hypoglycemia

Hypoglycemia is a defect in the carbohydrate metabolism whereby blood glucose reaches lower than normal levels. As glucose is a particularly important metabolic fuel for the brain, lowered glucose can result in a host of central nervous system disorders. The main cause of low blood sugar is a diet high in refined carbohydrates. Unfortunately, the average American diet, which is rich in processed foods, sugar, soda and coffee, is practically a prescription for hypoglycemia. These foods require little digestion and get absorbed too rapidly into the bloodstream. As a result, the blood sugar level becomes unstable. With sugary food consumption, the level shoots up and too much insulin is secreted by the pancreas. The blood sugar level then drops. At this point, people tend to reach for more refined carbohydrates and the cycle continues.

Symptoms

Hypoglycemia causes sustained stress, which can result in a variety of symptoms, including weakness, headaches, visual disturbances, food and chemical allergies, chronic fatigue, emotional problems such as anxiety and mood swings, confusion, chronic yeast infections and even asthma. Often, people don't realize that low blood sugar underlies their symptomalogy. Nor do medical professionals realize that hypoglycemia is the problem in many cases. For many people, this ignorance has sad consequences. Hypoglycemic individuals have been institutionalized because they were thought to be emotionally imbalanced and incapable of making rational decisions. Complicating the issue is the fact that tests rarely detect hypoglycemia. If a diabetic undergoes a five-hour glucose tolerance test, the condition shows up. Otherwise, it usually goes undetected.

Treatment

Naturopathic Viewpoint

Naturopaths view hypoglycemia as a disease of civilization. The overburdening of the system that culminates in hypoglycemia stems from the kinds of diets most people eat and the high stresses they endure. According to Dr. Paul Epstein, a naturopathic physician practicing in Norwalk, Connecticut, alleviating the problem usually involves attention to diet, supplementation and emotional support. He advocates making the following changes in order to banish this problem.

Analyze Your Current Diet ... To find out what foods may be causing the problem, a naturopath often takes a complete patient history and uses the information to make the patient aware of what is being eaten that is causing distress. Troublesome foods are then eliminated and replaced by those that provide the body with optimal support.

Avoid Simple Sugars ... Simple sugars must be avoided at all costs since they cause the pancreas to overproduce insulin. They also lack B vitamins and other essential nutrients found in complex carbohydrates that are needed to metabolize sugar into energy.

Simple sugars come in a variety of forms: sugar, fructose, glucose, corn sweeteners, corn syrup, fruit sugar, table sugar and brown sugar. They are found in alcoholic beverages and are hidden in many canned, packaged and frozen foods as well.

In cases of hypoglycemic attack, it may be necessary to immediately take a substance containing simple sugars, such as fruit juice. Couple the sugar with a source of protein—a slice of cheese, for example—to slow down the system's absorption of the glucose and avoid rapid changes in levels.

Eat a Diet High in Complex Carbohydrates ... For years, hypoglycemics have been told to eat high-protein diets when abundant complex carbohydrates are what they really need. If a person with low blood sugar eats a piece of fruit to overcome fatigue, 30 minutes later the fruit is digested. As a result, glucose enters the blood, raises the blood sugar level and restores energy. If that same person eats a lean steak instead, he or she has to wait six to seven hours for the meat to leave the stomach. It takes even longer for the amino acids derived from the meat to be translated into usable energy. Carbohydrates deliver required energy rapidly and efficiently while protein not only takes longer to get energy to the cells but even depletes the body in the process because it takes a lot of energy to create energy from protein.

Eat Vegetable Protein ... As protein sources, vegetable foods are generally preferable to animal-derived foods. Foods such as nuts, seeds, grains and Jerusalem artichokes provide time-released energy.

Add Fiber-Rich Foods . . . People with sluggish digestion or constipation may benefit from additional dietary fiber. This can help slow down the absorption of glucose into the intestinal capillaries. Slower absorption allows a more gradual release of insulin and a faster normalization of blood sugar levels after meals.

Avoid Caffeine and Nicotine . . . Caffeine and nicotine overstimulate the adrenal glands. When these substances, other stressors and a generally poor diet are combined, the adrenals can enter into a state of emergency. They become depleted of important vitamins such as B-complex vitamins and vitamin C.

Use Herbs Known to Rebalance the Blood Sugar . . . Herbs associated with balanced blood sugar include black cohosh, panax and Siberian ginseng, dandelion, gentian, ginger, cinnamon, uva ursi, licorice root and huckleberry leaves. Goldenseal is helpful but should only be used for short periods to prevent the depletion of B vitamins. Astragalus, by contrast, is a tonic herb that can be safely used on a daily basis. It boosts energy by providing adrenal and immune support, and can be taken as an extract or made into a soup by boiling the root.

Pay Attention to When You Eat . . . When you eat is just as important as what you eat. The hypoglycemic person generally needs to eat frequent, small meals to provide the body with a steady supply of food that is easily and slowly converted to glucose.

Supplement the Diet . . . Dietary changes alone may be sufficient to overcome hypoglycemia. Still, you may want to reinforce an improved diet with supplementation. First, consider supplements that support the regulation of blood sugar. These include adrenal extracts, glucose tolerance factor, zinc and chromium, nutrients that allow insulin to do its job more effectively. In addition, B vitamins supply crucial enzyme cofactors essential for carbohydrate metabolism. L-carnitine, L-glutamine and vitamin B6 also help lessen cravings for sugar. Vitamin E increases energy naturally, so a person doesn't feel the need for an artificial jolt from caffeine or sugar.

When deprived of glucose, brain cells may die. Research suggests that vitamin B6 protects against neurological damage due to hypoglycemia. Take 25-50 mg of vitamin B6 every day.

To avoid deficiency, consume 200 mcg of chromium daily. Chromium enables the liver to release sugar to the body. Chromium occurs naturally in foods such as whole grains, molasses and brewer's yeast.

The amino acid cysteine is an effective treatment for hypoglycemia because it assists in the neutralization of insulin overload in the blood, especially when taken with vitamin C and vitamin B1. New users should begin in the first week with daily doses of 500 mg of cysteine along with 1500 mg of vitamin C as well as 250 mg of vitamin B1. In the second week, take these same dosages twice per day. In the third week, begin taking these doses three times daily.

Consider adding glutamine powder to a protein drink every day or taking several 500-mg glutamine tablets along with your regular supplements. This amino acid is the primary agent in rebuilding glucose, which contributes to energy production.

There is some evidence to suggest d-manno-heptulose, a sugar extract taken from avocados, inhibits excess insulin secretion and the resulting hypoglycemia. Take d-manno-heptulose just after meals. The recommended dose is 100 to 200 mg, but will vary from person to person.

Supply Liver Support . . . The liver stores glucose as glycogen and breaks it down in the process called gluconeogenesis. Certain botanicals, such as dandelion root, Siberian ginseng and beet leaf, aid in this process. Celandine, methionine and choline are substances that work to maximize liver efficiency. Lipotropic factors also help control blood sugar by boosting liver function. These are especially helpful for people who have flatulence, hemorrhoids, difficulty digesting fats, light-colored stools or elevated fat levels.

Supply Adrenal Support . . . A person who is highly stressed or suffering from allergies, chronic inflammations, fatigue or nervous and emotional disorders should consider supplements that support the adrenal glands. The number one adrenal strengthener is pantothenic acid. Other beneficial supplements include freeze-dried adrenal gland extract, Siberian ginseng root, vitamin C and zinc. Royal jelly also provides excellent nourishment for the adrenals.

Supply Pancreatic Support . . . Digestive aids that support the pancreas might be indicated when there is impaired digestion.

Get Emotional Support . . . Knowing what to eat and what not to eat is one thing. Using this knowledge is another. Naturopaths often offer their patients support as they alter lifelong habits and struggle with issues at the core of their resistance to change.

The American Academy of Family Physicians has stated that 80 percent of all visits to family physicians are due to stress-related complaints. Stress is a critically important factor to address when hypoglycemia is the problem. According to Dr. Epstein, one doesn't treat hypoglycemia—one treats a person who has hypoglycemia.

What to Avoid

People with hypoglycemia need to avoid simple sugars, processed foods, concentrated foods, alcohol, nicotine, high-protein diets, caffeine and stress.

These stimuli are known to precipitate attacks. Aspartame, the chemical used in artificial sweeteners, should be eliminated as well.

Treatment Summary

While dietary needs may differ from person to person, a general rule of thumb is to avoid all simple sugars and to eat complex carbohydrates, vegetable proteins and fiber-rich foods.

Eating frequent, small meals is a good idea, as it slowly converts food to glucose.

Eliminate caffeine and nicotine.

Herbs that help to normalize blood sugar levels include black cohosh, ginseng and dandelion, among others.

Supplements that provide overall support may be beneficial, as well as those that benefit specific organs, including the liver, adrenal glands and pancreas. Take B6, chromium, cysteine, vitamin B1, vitamin C and glutamine daily. The consumption of avocado sugar just after meals may be beneficial.

Hypoglycemia patients often need emotional support to encourage the development of new habits.

Hypothyroidism

The thyroid gland makes hormones that control metabolism. Hypothyroidism occurs when too few hormones are produced due to decreased thyroid gland activity. The condition often goes undetected; estimates, though, put the number of people affected as high as 40 percent of the U.S. adult population.

Symptoms are numerous and can include chronic fatigue, feeling cold all of the time, inability to lose weight and skin conditions such as acne and eczema. In addition, there can be psychological components of the condition, particularly chronic depression, anxiety and panic as well as poor concentration and poor short-term memory. Sexual complications may include a low sex drive, impotence and infertility (especially low sperm count). Chronic constipation, hair loss, heart palpitations, brittle nails, muscle weakness and muscle and joint pain are additional symptoms. Women often experience menstrual problems, such as excessive bleeding, painful or irregular periods, scanty flow, cessation of menstruation, premenstrual syndrome and very late or very early onset of menses.

Also, an increase in age-related and immunodeficiency disease such as arthritis, cancer and heart disease, is associated with populations that are low in thyroid hormone.

When thyroid hormone levels are low, the body doesn't produce enough heat, so the extremities tend to be cold. Cold fingers, cold toes and a cold tip of the nose are common indicators that not enough heat is being produced. In general, being colder than other people can be an indicator that one's thyroid output is insufficient.

Treatment

Conventional treatment for hypothyroidism is often clouded by misdiagnosis and by incomplete testing. Because there are such a great variety of symptoms, other diseases are often blamed, and the condition goes undiagnosed. For example, hypercholesterolemia, or too much cholesterol in the blood, is often diagnosed in place of hypothyroidism. Treatment with restrictive diet or cholesterol-lowering medication often causes liver irritability and does nothing to address the underlying thyroid malfunctions.

Another problem is that T4 or thyroxin hormone levels are commonly used as the sole diagnosis for hypothyroidism. But levels of two other hormones—T3 and thyroid-stimulating hormone, or TSH—should also be tested. Furthermore, the TSH reference range that many labs consider normal is 0.2-5.5 mU/L, with numbers greater than 5.5 commonly considered indicative of thyroid deficiency. However, new studies show that TSH readings as low as 1.9 are even a warning sign for abnormal thyroid activity. In such cases, there may be an autoimmune attack on the thyroid, which can result in significant thyroid impairment. Furthermore, in individuals with TSH values exceeding 2.0, studies show an increased risk of the patient's developing hypothyroid disease within the next two decades. In individuals with TSH concentrations above 4.0, there is a greater risk of heart disease. Finally, research confirms that thyroid deficiencies can be the cause of excess cholesterol production.

Hypothyroidism may be caused by poor general nutrition, especially too little high-quality protein. Water fluoridation is also thought to be a potential thyroid suppressant. Huge quantities of foods in the cabbage family can suppress thyroid function as well, but this is extremely rare. Thyroid antibody levels should also be tested to rule out autoimmune thyroid conditions.

Standard treatment for hypothyroidism consists of prescription synthetic thyroid hormone. Synthroid, one of the most widely used drugs in the United States for this condition, has been under attack by the FDA in recent years for problems with stability, purity and potency. Other synthetic drugs for thyroid disorders, such as levothroxine, have also been questioned for their effectiveness. Thyroxine, another traditional treatment, was recently shown to be of no benefit to its users in a study that compared it to placebo. The side effects and interactions of such treatments are similar to the symptoms of hyperthyroidism, which include fever, sweating, nausea, heart failure, menstrual problems, hair loss, headache, tremors and inability to sleep. Synthetic hormone treatments are also associated with a multitude of drug interactions, including with anticoagulants, beta-blockers and estrogens.

Natural thyroid hormone is much more effective, but it has become increasingly difficult to obtain. The vast majority of glandular products are derived from bovine (beef) sources. The exception is pancreatic extracts that are usually derived from pork.

Smart consumers who purchase glandular products would be best served by buying them from respectable companies. Glandulars that are improperly processed fall far short of the desired results. If the glandulars are not suitably prepared, natural lipids, vitamins, minerals, enzymes and hormone precursors are destroyed. Natural glandulars, such as Armour Thyroid, contain thyroid from the glands of pigs.

Physicians who question the purity or consistency of natural thyroid extracts should contact the not-for-profit Broda O. Barnes Research Foundation (*www.brodabarnes.org*). Dr. Barnes spent over half a century on research, treatment and teaching in the field of thyroid and other endocrine problems.

It is important to take vitamin A, vitamin C, vitamin-B complex, vitamin B12 and vitamin E for this condition. Coenzyme Q10 taken in a dosage of 100-250 mg per day is also beneficial. Be sure to take adequate amounts of the minerals magnesium, manganese, zinc and selenium. Selenium should be taken in the amount of 200-600 mcg daily. Selenium assists in the removal of toxins from the body, and deficiency in this mineral is toxic to the thyroid.

Patients may be started on the lowest possible dosage of thyroid hormone and gradually built up. Improvements should be noticeable after 30 days, with full effects occurring after 90. This medication is usually taken for life.

Absorption of thyroid medication is limited by a number of factors, such as the taking of certain calcium supplements, antacids containing aluminum hydroxide, iron sulfate, Dilantin and Tegretol.

Hypothyroidism can also be caused by an underlying autoimmune disorder. For treatment of this type of thyroid malfunction, it is best to initially treat the underlying disorder. For example, iodine deficiency demonstrates the importance of the intake of the proper amounts of iodine for the thyroid to function properly. Not enough of iodine, which is found in seafood and seaweed, in the diet, can actually cause hypothyroidism. However if the underlying autoimmune disorder is the cause of hypothyroidism, iodine will be an ineffective treatment, and may actually cause increased irritation.

Deficiency of the amino acid tyrosine (a precursor of thyroxine) also causes hypothyroidism. A dose of one gram per day for adults is advised.

Some naturopathic physicians find a formula called Energetics to be helpful in normalizing thyroid function. The formula consists of many of the supplements listed above, such as tyrosine, organic iodine (in the form of thyroxin-3), vitamin B2, niacinamide, zinc, chromium and liver concentrate. Depending on the patient's requirements, this formula is given from one to three times daily in one or two tablets each time.

DHEA, which aids in the body's metabolic functioning, may also be taken. While a dosage of 25 mg taken one to three times per day is suggested, it is important to have the blood tested to ensure you are reaching optimal levels.

Melatonin should be taken on a daily basis at bedtime in a dose of from 300 mcg to 6 mg.

Aerobic exercise may provide additional support. A regular routine, centered on long walks or intense activity like jogging or bike riding, in which one burns 2000 calories, is recommended.

Treatment Summary

The conventional approach to hypothyroidism usually consists of giving a synthetic thyroid hormone.

Natural thyroid hormone is more effective than the synthetic type, but more difficult to obtain. The formula Energetics may be helpful. Under proper circumstances, vitamin A, vitamin C, vitamin-B complex, vitamin B12, vitamin E, coenzyme Q10, magnesium, manganese, zinc, selenium, iodine, the amino acid tyrosine, DHEA and melatonin may be beneficial.

Aerobic exercise may help to correct a low-thyroid condition.

Infertility

Infertility is a widespread problem today. In the U.S., it affects approximately 17 percent of all couples that are of childbearing age, which translates to about five million Americans. There are many factors—physical, emotional and environmental—that contribute to infertility.

To understand infertility, it helps to understand the conditions necessary for a couple to be able to have a baby. First, the man has to be able to produce healthy sperm. Second, eggs need to be produced from the woman's ovaries. Third, the woman's fallopian tubes have to be clear and open in order to allow the sperm to reach the egg while it is in the fallopian tubes, and to allow for easy passage of the egg to the uterus. Fourth, the lining of the uterus needs to be suitable for the fertilized egg to be implanted. Finally, once the egg is implanted, a woman must create the necessary hormones in order to sustain the fertilized egg. Obviously, there are many things that can go awry along the way.

Causes

First, we must examine the possibility of male infertility. While infertility is often attributed to the woman, it is actually male infertility that is the problem 40 percent of the time. Male infertility may be due to low sperm count, decreased sperm motility or aberrant sperm morphology. There are several reasons these happen. Low sperm count may be due to undescended testicles that were not repaired, trauma to the testicles, large amounts of exposure to X rays, the taking of certain drugs or an infection after puberty that was accompanied by high fever. More often, it is a reversible condition—such as poor diet, overuse of saunas, ultra-vigorous exercise, lack of exercise, drinking, smoking, obesity, chronic infection, the wearing of tight slacks or underwear, or poor general health—that contributes to the impaired sperm production. Optimal scrotal temperature falls between 94 and 96 degrees Fahrenheit. Temperatures exceeding 96 degrees halt or inhibit sperm production. Therefore, in many men, a reduction in scrotal temperature will often result in fertility.

Low sperm motility makes it difficult for the sperm to travel from the vagina and up through the fallopian tubes to fertilize the ovum. Decreased sperm motility may be related to any of the factors listed above. Alternatively, it may be the result of an enlarged prostate gland or male hormone imbalance. There might also be a blockage of the vessels traveled by the sperm, which can be caused by varicosity, inflammation or infection.

A topic of some debate in Europe is the effect of birth control pills and estrogen-like chemicals on male infertility. These chemicals are not biodegradable by stomach acids and get into the environment—the soil and water—through urine. Thus, they get into the food chain, and in that way they can affect males and females alike.

The second condition necessary for conception is ovulation. A woman's inability to ovulate is most commonly due to some kind of hormone imbalance. The menstrual cycle is regulated by the adrenal, pituitary and thyroid glands. Problems with the functioning of any of these may cause a failure to ovulate.

Birth control pills and other sources of estrogen are sometimes the cause of hormonal imbalances. Fertility specialists report that women who have taken birth control pills for an extended period of time have difficulty reestablishing their monthly cycles. This may be due to oral contraceptives causing pituitary hormone deficiency as well as their precipitating a deficiency of B vitamins, both of which contribute to hormone balance. Further, an inordinate amount of weight loss or gain, excessive stress, poor diet, sleep deficiency and thyroid problems may disturb normal endocrine function. (According to Dr. Dahlia Abraham, a complementary physician from New York City, a woman can determine whether she has a problem with hypothyroidism by taking her temperature. On the third, fourth and fifth day of a woman's cycle, she should place a thermometer under her armpit first thing in the morning. If the mean average on those days is below 97.5 degrees Fahrenheit, then she is most likely hypothyroid.)

In addition to hormone imbalances, there are other potential causes of ovarian failure. Zinc deficiency, abnormal body fat distribution, obesity or being underweight may also result in abnormal ovarian dysfunction.

Third, if it is found that a woman is able to ovulate regularly and successfully, another potential cause of infertility problems that can be explored is blockage of the fallopian tubes. A sloppy abortion may lead to blocked fallopian tubes. Further, chlamydia (which may be promoted through the use of birth control pills), use of IUDs, and use of certain drugs may cause this problem, as these factors can result in pelvic inflammatory disease and subsequent scarring, which may hinder the ability of the ovum to get though the tube and into the uterus. Narrowing or blocking of passages may also be due to inherited difficulties; a disease such as salpingitis, tuberculosis or endometriosis, or by other infections of the womb.

If the cervix is infected, excess mucus from the infection or inflammation can force the sperm out. There may be polyps preventing sperm from entering the uterus.

Malposition of the uterus or uterine fibroids may also make labor difficult or lead to sterility. These problems should be resolved prior to conception. Fibroids are usually related to hormonal imbalance, specifically an excess of estrogen. Although there are no herbal remedies for malposition of the uterus, gynecologic manipulation by a specially trained chiropractor or osteopath may help, along with pelvic and breathing exercises.

The fourth condition that must be met is the lining of the uterus must be able to nurture the fertilized egg. Endometriosis may deter this from happening as cells that normally build up in the uterus each month in preparation for pregnancy can actually grow outside the uterus, resulting in fertility problems. Nutritional insufficiency may also affect the ability of the uterus to sustain the embryo. In these cases, conception may actually transpire but the ovum may not have the appropriate nutrients to develop. This results in unrecognized spontaneous abortions, which may lead to a label of infertility.

Other possible causes of infertility are low plasma copper concentrations, abnormalities of the reproductive system, heavy metal toxicity, genetic damage from electromagnetic radiation, lack of knowledge about the fertility cycle and antibodies that may be produced by either party that can destroy the man's sperm.

Symptoms

The obvious symptom of infertility is the inability to conceive after an appropriate length of time trying, generally considered to be a year. However, what is not always acknowledged by society is the emotional aspect of the problem. Couples can experience anguish, mourning, loss of self-esteem and marred self-image. Infertility can also result in difficulty between partners, as it is so often related to sexual issues. Communication problems between the partners can be exacerbated as they grapple with infertility. In as many as a quarter of all women who struggle with infertility, nonphysical or emotional problems are to blame. This is why it is extremely important to pay close attention to diet and to eliminate fatigue when attempting to conceive.

Treatment

Treatment for infertility ranges from drugs to surgery to in vitro fertilization, the method in which the man's sperm is used to fertilize his female partner's egg outside of her uterus. The embryo is then implanted inside the womb for her to carry to term. This may cost approximately $10,000 per cycle.

Modern assisted reproductive technology (ART) also offers the ability to fertilize donor eggs and then implant the eggs in the infertile woman. Thus, a woman is able to bear a child that is not genetically related to her. This method is generally even more costly, as it could run up to $15,000.

When a uterus suffers from such abnormalities that it cannot sustain a pregnancy, a fertilized egg may even be implanted into the womb of a "surrogate" mother, who then carries the baby to term. However the development of a child within a woman's womb is a very personal process. Over time, it may grow difficult for the surrogate mother to part with the infant, regardless of whether the child genetically is hers or not.

For women with problems ovulating, clomiphene may be prescribed. Clomiphene causes ovulation in about 75 percent of women, but only 40 to 50 percent actually become pregnant. Prolonged use of the drug has been linked to ovarian cancer. It often causes undesirable side effects such as headaches, vision problems, nausea, breast tenderness, hot flashes and swelling of the abdomen. Five percent of the women who use clomiphene end up conceiving multiple children at the same time, primarily twins. Five percent of users also develop ovarian hyperstimulation syndrome, in which the ovaries enlarge and fluid shifts from the bloodstream into the abdominal cavity.

If treatment with clomiphene is unsuccessful, gonadotropin is used. This hormone, derived from postmenopausal women, is extremely expensive and has very severe side effects. Gonadotropin is injected into the muscle, simulating maturation of ovarian follicles. While 95 percent of women using this treatment ovulate, only 50 to 75 percent become pregnant, with a very high incidence of multiple births.

Therefore, it is important to know that there may be alternative natural solutions that can be tried prior to (or in conjunction with) using other conventional methods of treatment. Some natural approaches are outlined below, although couples should of course work with a holistically oriented health practitioner to get individualized guidance.

Learn How to Identify When Ovulation Begins

Women are most fertile at certain times of the month, and it is important to know how to pinpoint these times. Establish when you are ovulating by using a sensitive thermometer and keeping a chart. Take your temperature just before getting out of bed in the morning. Before ovulation, your waking tempcrature should be slightly below normal, between 97 and 97.8 degrees Fahrenheit. But in the second half of the cycle, two weeks prior to menstruation, your temperature will increase slightly, by .5 to 1 degree. This indicates ovulation. Vaginal discharge during this period is usually clear in color and slippery in texture, permitting the sperm to penetrate the cervix.

Select Healthy Lifestyle Choices

First, it is important to provide the body with proper nutrients by eating a well-balanced, healthy diet. Therefore, it is suggested that fat and food additives, such as nitrates, nitrites and MSG be avoided. Fasting for a few days may even provide assistance in the case of fallopian tube blockage. It is further recommended that the following substances be avoided completely as they inhibit fertility in both men and women: tobacco or nicotine products, caffeine, alcohol, heavy metals, environmental hazards (e.g., pesticides and herbicides) and drugs such as marijuana and cocaine. Additionally, relaxation techniques have been proven to enhance fertility by increasing vigor and reducing stress, anxiety, depression and fatigue. Lastly, one or both partners may be anxious about becoming pregnant, and a lot of tension can build up around this issue. It is important to address this through some type of emotional or spiritual work. Support, whether it comes from an individual counselor or a group, can make a big difference in one's outlook.

Supplements

While a good diet will benefit the system and positively impact chances for becoming pregnant, the addition of specific nutrients can further enhance the male and female reproductive systems. Talk to a nutritionally oriented health practitioner. In general, the following are some of the more important nutrients to consider.

Especially important for men:

Zinc . . . Studies show that consuming 25 to 50 mg of zinc a day has a positive impact in helping men overcome impotence. In addition to supplementation, foods containing zinc should be eaten; these include nuts, seeds, whole grains and brewer's yeast.

Vitamin E . . . This nutrient may improve the sperm's impregnating ability. Food sources rich in vitamin E are wheat germ, whole grains and uncooked nuts.

L-Carnitine . . . Infertility due to low sperm motility may be due to insufficient carnitine levels. Carnitine is generally recognized as being important for the heart muscle, as indeed it is. But studies have also shown that 3000 mg of oral L-carnitine, taken daily for four months, will increase spermatozoa motility, as well.

Reishi (Ganodenna) Extract . . . Recent studies of infertile men with chronic genital inflammation secondary to infection by the human papilloma virus (HPV) find reishi extract effective for overcoming the condition. Taking the extract significantly reduces inflammation of the skin in these patients and improves sperm parameters.

Other nutrients helpful to men are selenium and vitamin D.
Especially important for women:

Vitamin B6 . . . This vitamin is particularly important for women as it can help adjust progesterone and estrogen levels. The recommended dosage of B6 is generally from 100 to 300 mg per day. Good food sources of B6 include eggs, rice, soybeans, oats and whole wheat products.

Other vitamins that have been proven to help increase fertility in women are: iron (35 mg); folic acid (one mg three times daily), to help normalize blood chemistry; vitamin B12, to help normalize reproductive function; colloidal silver, to help cleanse the system when chlamydia is causing infertility; and bioflavonoids (found in broccoli, green peppers, parsley and citrus fruits), to help develop a healthy uterine lining.

Important for both men and women:

Vitamin C . . . This nutrient is beneficial to both men and women as it has the ability to dispose of toxic metals from the body that can interfere with pregnancy. Generally, the recommended dosage is 100-200 mg daily. Food sources of vitamin C include broccoli, cantaloupe and any type of berry.

Oriental Naturopathic Medicine

This type of Eastern approach to infertility strives to create an overall healthy environment within the woman that allows for proper digestion, menstruation and hormonal balance. It also focuses on raising the man's sperm count and sperm motility. One aspect of Oriental treatment involves increasing pelvic blood flow to correct fallopian tube obstruction and/or problems with ovulation. This method encompasses the use of laser acupuncture, retention enemas and injection of common sage root into the endometrial nodes.

Vitex agnus castus, while not containing hormones in itself, helps to correct deficiency of either estrogen or progesterone.

Chamaelirium luteum, especially popular in Britain, is well known for its effects on female infertility. It helps to prevent miscarriage, uterine hemorrhage, over-relaxation and prolapse of the uterus.

Unicorn root, commonly used for infertility and impotence, is also beneficial for miscarriages caused by a lack of strength. It may be used safely throughout pregnancy.

Oriental naturopathic medicine advocates practicing good sexual hygiene to reverse endometriosis and enhance fertility. Practitioners suggest that couples avoid intercourse at the time of menstruation, saying that it can result in an imbalance of energy and cause the migration of endometrial tissue into the pelvic cavity.

The use of acupuncture is another Eastern approach in treating infertility. The idea is to release obstructions from the liver, spleen, heart, lung and kidney in order for energy to move freely within the system. This can potentially impact fertility by overcoming possible hormonal, psychological and emotional factors that are connected to those organs.

Herbs to tone renal/adrenal function are part of the Oriental approach, since reproduction is considered related to the kidney. Recommended herbs include wormwood, which is actually a European herb that can be consumed along with the Chinese herbs daughter seed and fructose litchi (a red berry); dong quai, which can be taken as a tea or in capsule form; kelp, which is rich in iodine and thus beneficial for hypothyroidism; and ginseng, as it contains a lot of zinc, which may help strengthen the male reproductive system.

Western Naturopathic Medicine

According to Dr. John Pizzorno, naturopath and midwife, one type of treatment that may counter infertility is a hydrotherapy procedure used to ease pelvic inflammatory infection. Essentially, this procedure uses sitz baths and has a woman submerge herself in a tub of hot water for five minutes with her extremities outside the tub. The water level should extend to her umbilicus. She should then alternate to a bucket of cold water for one minute (here the water level should be just underneath the umbilicus, so there is less cold water than hot water). This procedure should be done three to four times daily. After a period of participating in this regimen, she should start getting a discharge that may indicate that the body is emitting scar tissue and toxic material from the ovaries and fallopian tubes. However, it is recommended that women avoid unprotected sex for several months during this treatment. The reason is that prior to completion of the treatment, there may be partial blockages, which could result in problem pregnancies should conception occur during this time.

Herbs

Lastly, there are some herbal supplements that have been known to increase fertility and, therefore, should be kept in mind. Fennel and anise have both been known to promote menstruation and facilitate birth. Red raspberry leaf tea contains a lot of iron, as well as other nutrients, making it beneficial to the reproductive system overall. Ginkgo biloba improves circulation, and therefore may help to overcome impotence.

Treatment Summary

Male infertility should be considered. Sometimes a simple change in scrotal temperature can eliminate male infertility.

Many modern treatments for female infertility used in the West are incredibly expensive. Some methods have legal and ethical consequences that need to be considered by all parties involved. Many have alarming side effects.

Learn to identify when ovulation begins. This can be done by observing: (1) an increase in temperature approximately two weeks prior to menstruation in addition to (2) a change in the color and texture of vaginal discharge to more of a clear, slippery substance.

Because proper nutrients and optimal chemical balance offer the best chance of becoming pregnant, it is important to make healthy lifestyle choices. A well-balanced diet, relaxation techniques and avoidance of bad habits or substances known to inhibit fertility should be considered.

Vitamin and mineral intake can make a difference. Specific recommendations for men are zinc, selenium and vitamins E, D and C. Particular suggestions for women include vitamins C, B6 and B12, in addition to iron, folic acid, colloidal silver and bioflavonoids. It is worth talking to a nutritionally oriented health practitioner, because each individual's system and situation are unique.

Oriental naturopathic medicine uses acupuncture and herbs in treating infertility.

A hydrotherapy procedure can be used to ease pelvic inflammatory infection. It prescribes that a woman alternate between a tub of hot and cold water to help the body emit scar tissue and toxic material from the ovaries and fallopian tubes.

Learning Disorders

Teachers from past decades may recall the occasional hyperactive student. This is in dramatic contrast to today's world, where between 3 to 9 percent of children are classified as having some type of behavioral or learning disability. In the United States alone, over 6 million youngsters are currently diagnosed with one of the most common of these, attention deficit hyperactivity disorder (ADHD). ADHD has been called attention deficit disorder (ADD), hyper-kinetic syndrome and even minimal brain syndrome. Many adults, too, are being told that their learning suffers because of this condition.

Though prescriptions for drugs such as Ritalin and Strattera have escalated in recent years, Nancy O'Dell, Ph.D., and Patricia Cook, Ph.D., offer a unique program, developed in the early 1970s by professor Miriam Bender, as a sub-stitute for the traditional pharmaceutical treatments. In an interview with the author of this book, they claim that during the past 30 years, their treatment has benefited countless patients. Their techniques are detailed in their book, *Stopping ADHD*.

Professor Bender hypothesized that a developmental delay in a reflex was the cause of ADHD. In essence, the theory claims that reflexes are founda-tional. If there are problems with the foundation, then there will be problems with everything that is built on that foundation. Bender believed the key was the symmetric tonic neck reflex (STNR), which sends signals to the neck and arms that they should work opposite of the legs: if the arms bend, the legs should want to be straight, and vice versa. Babies depend on this precise reflex to lift themselves off of their bellies as they learn the skills that will enable them to crawl. If the baby does not crawl properly for a minimum of six months, the STNR will stay at an immature level. When it remains at this under-developed level, symptoms develop that could be improperly diagnosed as ADHD. Hence, when a child has trouble sitting still in a chair, paying atten-tion, obeying directions or writing, she is quickly labeled as having ADHD and summarily given prescription drugs.

Many children diagnosed with ADHD share common characteristics with children considered to be gifted. Often, intelligent children, because they display these characteristics, are sent to a specialist in ADHD. This misdiagnosis can start a domino effect that takes the child through a battery of unnecessary drugs, doctor visits, psychological problems, and so on. According to Drs. O'Dell and Cook, in at least 75 percent of cases, STNR is a chief contributing factor for the ADHD symptoms and affects a minimum of 10 percent of the population. Because of sudden infant death syndrome (SIDS), more and more babies are placed on their backs while sleeping to decrease the odds of being victimized by SIDS. This has resulted in an increase of persons with immature STNRs, because not being placed on their stomachs prevents them from crawling (try crawling on your back!).

Still, others might ask, why the sudden epidemic? Is our modern world, with its exposure to too many chemical pollutants, causing brain disturbances that make learning difficult? Or are medical advances enabling us to better detect a condition that was there all along? Since the diagnosis is subjectively based, perhaps the condition is not real at all, but only a fabrication.

Medical practitioners differ widely in their beliefs. At one extreme, ADHD is said to be a bona fide medical condition that needs pharmaceutical control. At the other end of the spectrum, doctors believe ADHD to be nonexistent. Many of these physicians express alarm at the growing population of medicated children, especially since a diagnosis is based on observations of behavior and not measured through neurological tests. Thus, any child who exhibits noncompliant behavior may be diagnosed with a learning disorder.

According to Nina Anderson, author of *ADHD: The Natural Approach*, in many cases children are being labeled with a disorder such as hyperactivity when, in fact, they may simply be normal kids who are particularly bright and require a more active social and educational experience as an outlet for their intelligence. Even the question-and-answer forms used for diagnosing ADHD are strikingly similar to those used to identify children as gifted and talented.

So, is ADHD a disability or merely a difference? Many members of the medical field take a middle ground. They believe that learning disorders such as ADHD do exist, but that they should be viewed in a broader context. They see these disorders not just as psychological or behavioral disturbances, but as nutritional, biochemical and medical issues as well.

Above all else, it is important to obtain a proper diagnosis. ADHD is not recognized as a biological medical condition, but purely as a set of symptoms. It is marked by an inability to pay attention, complete tasks or concentrate, and is sometimes accompanied by hyperactivity. Some observable signs include motor problems (such as excessive fidgeting, constant leg and hand movements, and abnormal motor skills), attention problems (including procrastination and extreme disorganization), mood disorders (such as bursts of anger, extreme hopelessness, frequent interruptions and low self-esteem) and addictions and alienation (such as trouble maintaining relationships).

The American Psychiatric Association has declared that between 3 and 7 percent of the childhood population has this disability, with three boys having ADHD for every one girl. According to studies, up to 6 percent of adults could be considered to have ADHD, as well. ADHD is now classified into three types: inattentive, hyperactive-compulsive and combined. ADHD should be diagnosed by someone with adequate training in behavioral science, and is best diagnosed using a team approach. Diagnosis should be based on a detailed medical history, as well as on observations. A person needs to have experienced the disorder in a persistent and disabling manner for six months prior to the age of seven in order to qualify as having ADHD. Many are wrongly diagnosed without this information.

Many other conditions may be mistaken for ADHD. Survivors of sexual or physical abuse may exhibit symptoms similar to ADHD, but these are actually the result of post-traumatic stress syndrome. Individuals with bipolar disorder are also likely to be misdiagnosed with ADHD. However, bipolar-disorder sufferers exhibit both hypersexuality and conflicts with parents with greater intensity than do those with ADHD. Misdiagnosis can come at a harsh price: Stimulant medications such as Adderall are contraindicated in people with psychotic or schizophrenic tendencies, for instance, because they exacerbate symptoms. Many individuals who were wrongly prescribed stimulant ADHD medications saw their symptoms deteriorate into dangerous, often deadly, psychotic episodes.

Children often take ADHD medications every day for years and years. But there are side effects to long-term drug use. Furthermore, drugs only mask symptoms and do not get at the underlying pathology, if there is one. Therefore, it's preferable to get at the source of learning disabilities and try to correct the fundamental problem.

Causes

Learning disabilities may be a consequence of several factors, toxicity and nutritional deficiencies being just two of these. With the increasing amounts of pesticides, processed foods and environmental toxins to contend with, our bodies—and more specifically, our brains—are being deprived of important nutrients. When this happens, normal brain chemistry is impaired such that this organ will send irregular signals to the rest of the body, subsequently resulting in abnormal mental, emotional and behavioral patterns.

Food allergies may be responsible for some learning problems, as they allow inflammatory compounds to permeate the bloodstream and affect normal brain function. Additionally, hypothyroidism may be an underlying factor, since an underactive thyroid may cause the brain to operate incorrectly.

Chronic exposure to mercury, a known neurotoxin, may also be to blame for the explosion in learning disabilities since World War II, when amalgam dental fillings became popular. It is biologically possible that ADHD and developmental disorders such as autism, speech and language delay are all due to such exposure. Amalgam fillings, therefore, should not be used. Also, great care should be taken in the removal of such fillings.

A similar link may exist between these disorders and exposure to thimerosal (a topic that has generated headlines across the nation recently), a mercury-containing compound that has been used since the 1930s in vaccines routinely administered to children. In 1999, the U.S. Public Health Service and the American Academy of Pediatrics recommended removal of thimerosal from children's vaccines. As change happens slowly, however, an unknown number of vials are still believed to be in circulation. If vaccines must be used, take care to ensure that they do not contain thimerosal.

Elevated mercury levels have also been found in people who consume a great deal of fish. While fish may have other nutritional benefits, eating more than two fish meals per week is ill advised.

Studies show that mothers who are cocaine users have a greater likelihood of giving birth to children with ADHD. Prenatal exposure to cocaine seems to give rise to disruption of the brain systems charged with regulating arousal and attention span.

New research pinpointing some of the biochemical and genetic changes evident in people with ADHD is emerging. One theory that is gaining support is that certain people do not produce enough dopamine and other neurotransmitters in response to stimuli ordinarily found pleasurable, such as love, reproduction and eating. These individuals may instead seek other avenues to get their needed "rush," such as compulsively eating junk food or sugar, taking drugs or engaging in risk-taking behavior. Defects in dopamine-receptor genes may be to blame.

It is important to take strength in the fact that nutritional and lifestyle strategies will increase neurotransmitter levels naturally. Through behavior modification, increased exercise, changes in diet, supplementation and the creation of a chemical-free environment, parents can find an effective approach to treating ADHD.

Treatment

Cocaine, which is one of the most reinforcing and addicting of the abused drugs, has pharmacological actions that are very similar to those of methylphenidate (Ritalin), which is now the most commonly prescribed psychotropic medicine for children in the U.S.

—Research Report, *Archives of General Psychiatry* (1995)

Conventional treatment relies on drugs to attempt to control behavior. Ritalin, or methylphenidate, is the most well-known ADHD drug. It was originally developed for narcolepsy patients. Now Ritalin can also be found in Adderall, which is the most widely prescribed drug for people with ADHD. Adderall is a combination of four different amphetamine salts and stays in the body longer than Ritalin alone, so the user experiences fewer highs and lows. Other stimulants that are prescribed for ADHD include Dexedrine (dextro-amphetamine), Desoxyn (methamphetamine) and Cylert (pemoline).

The amphetamines prescribed for ADHD are classified by the Drug Enforcement Agency as Schedule II stimulants. In the same category as "uppers" and "speed," methylphenidate is categorized as a stimulant because it has the effect of increasing alertness and physical activity. It makes dopamine more available in the brain, and works by suppressing all spontaneous behavior. As a Schedule II drug, it is characterized by the DEA as "having a high abuse potential with severe psychic or physical dependence liability."

One of the most worrisome side effects of treating ADHD with stimulant medication is the possibility of addiction. The stimulants prescribed for ADHD are chemically similar to illegal street drugs such as dextroamphetamine ("dexies"), methamphetamine ("crystal meth") and especially cocaine. In fact, Ritalin provides the same four-hour high as cocaine. The only difference is that it takes four times longer to leave the system.

Studies also indicate that the use of stimulant drugs for the treatment of ADHD may prime the brain for later cocaine use. This means that cocaine has a stronger effect than it would otherwise have had. The abuse of methylphenidate itself is also on the rise. Unlike substances such as alcohol and illegal drugs, it is easier for young people to obtain. Tablets are often crushed and snorted like cocaine. Ironically, adults are often imprisoned for making and taking the same sort of drugs that are regularly administered to children.

With or without medication, studies show that people with ADHD are more likely in general to fall prey to addictive behaviors, such as smoking and drinking. This factor should be considered before the administration of stimulants for ADHD.

The long-term use of stimulant drugs, including amphetamines, is known to have serious side effects. Since stimulants decrease appetite, one side effect is growth suppression. Adderall's package insert warns, "Patients who are not growing or gaining weight as expected should have their treatment interrupted." Stimulants also cause cardiovascular problems such as increased blood pressure, as well as liver damage.

Severe neurological side effects have also been demonstrated. Studies show that children as young as 10 years have developed bipolar disorder as a direct result of being on ADHD stimulants. Neurotransmitter problems also develop and manifest in symptoms such as social withdrawal, sleeping disorders, facial tics, depression, passivity, anxiety, tiredness, depression, meaningless repetitious or obsessive-compulsive behavior, headaches, zombie-like behavior and meaningless compulsive activity. This inspires an endless cycle in which, to counteract the emotional disturbances the child has developed as a result of the prescription medicine, the child is prescribed more antidepressants, mood medications or sedatives, each of which has their own side effects.

Aside from the deaths due to overdoses or drug interactions, many instances of sudden death due to cardiac arrest have been reported in children who took the prescribed dosages of stimulant ADHD medications. Many of these children had latent, undetected structural cardiac abnormalities that could not be detected by the simple blood test and heart monitoring that is routinely done.

Adderall and other stimulant ADHD medications also have serious drug interactions with certain antidepressants. Stimulant use with tricyclic antidepressants results in an alarming and sustained increase of amphetamine in the brain and can cause heart failure. Taken with MAO-inhibiting antidepressants, they have toxic, potentially fatal neurological effects.

Furthermore, is it unclear whether the long-term benefits of using these drugs, if any, come close to outweighing the risks. While stimulants may show short-term effectiveness in controlling overactive, impulsive, inattentive or aggressive behavior, studies conducted over the past 40 years show that children who took stimulant ADHD medication ultimately "achieved" (earned a high school diploma, stayed out of prison, and so on) no better than their nonmedicated counterparts.

A variety of nonstimulant drugs is also becoming available for ADHD. These include atomoxetine (which has enjoyed a good safety record), gabapentin (which is an anticonvulsant that has been used in adults with bipolar disorder), bupropion (which has been safe in the treatment of adolescent children with depression), modafinil (which induces wakefulness without being a stimulant) and tomoxetine (which has traditionally been used as an antidepressant). These appear to be well tolerated for the most part.

Behavioral Techniques

People with ADHD need established routines in their lives in order to function. Parents should clearly articulate to their children what the appropriate times are for bed, play, eating, school and doing homework. Parents are responsible for consistently making sure that this schedule is adhered to and amended as necessary. This also fosters healthy communication between parents and children, which furthers the healing process. In addition, older children will benefit by using a planner. Its consistent use will make their lives more manageable, even into adulthood.

Encourage your child to look you in the eyes during oral communication. Make sure that what is being said is being acknowledged with authenticity.

Avoid bombarding your child with too much information at once. Too much overstimulation confuses ADHD sufferers, causing eventual shutdown.

Incorporate meditation into your child's lifestyle. Meditation is a proven means of increasing the ability to pay attention. One simple technique is to use a metronome and allow the child to tap in time with the tone.

Massages are helpful in that they relieve stress, which contributes to ADHD. More important, they help lower blood viscosity. With respect to ADHD adults especially, this minimizes hypercoagulation, a disorder that leads to low oxygen and death in tissues. Hypercoagulation has not only been linked to cognitive disorders such as ADHD, but to lowered immune function, heart disease and cancer. Turmeric, ginkgo and ginger may also be used to help control this disorder.

Studies have shown that exercise, through the release of dopamine to the brain, is effective in controlling the symptoms of learning disorders. Vigorous exercise should be performed for one half hour three to four times a week. Additionally, one half hour of moderate activity most days of the week is also recommended.

Biofeedback electroencephalograph (EEG) training, proven extremely effective in the treatment of alcoholism, can also empower children with ADHD to end their dependence on stimulant medications. Biofeedback teaches children to enter a peaceful alpha brainwave state and utilize other neurological pathways in order to control impulses, increase attention and process information better. Between 20 and 40 sessions are usually required.

Supplements

It is crucial to nourish the brain with the types of nutrients it needs to function properly. This is especially important in a child's first three years of life, when 90 percent of brain development occurs. Children who do not get enough essential nutrients suffer in terms of intellectual capacity and attention span. Sadly, a survey of over 3000 children in the United States by the Department of Agriculture showed that less than 1 percent received daily requirements under the five food groups, and 16 percent met none of these requirements at all.

Studies link deficiencies of essential fatty acids (EFAs) to ADHD. Deep-sea, cold-water fish such as salmon, tuna and herring all contain docosahexaenoic acid (DHA), which is the most important EFA for supporting the brain. Children should take 1000 mg of fish oil daily, while adults may take 1000-2000 mg a day.

Magnesium and selenium are two vital minerals that everyone needs but that we don't all get enough of. In fact, low magnesium levels are related to cases of hyperexcitability and inattention. The recommended daily dosage is 200-500 mg of magnesium and 100-200 mcg of selenium. Calcium supplements are also of benefit.

Zinc is another key nutrient, since an insufficient amount of this mineral in the body may impede enzyme function and subsequently hinder normal brain function. As a supplement, 20-40 mg a day is suggested.

Sulfur amino acids are also significant, as they help in eliminating toxins from the body. Children will also respond to vitamin B1 and vitamin B6. B vitamins are extremely important because they help synthesize neurotransmitters and help brain enzymes to use carbohydrates for energy. Vitamin C should also be taken to help maintain neurotransmitters.

Choline, which facilitates the return of acetylcholine to the brain, can be taken in amounts of 1000-6000 mg daily. However, since the choline powders available for children have an undesirable flavor, the best way to get enough choline is through DMAE. DMAE furthers the synthesis of acetylcholine. Children should begin at a low dose of 50 mg taken twice a day on an empty stomach. Over time, if there are no side effects, they may build up to 250 mg per day. At higher doses, side effects include muscle tightness, headaches and insomnia. The same approach should be taken for adults, who may take twice the amount recommended for children.

Phospholipids, such as phosphatidylserine, are vital to functioning of the neurons and to brain metabolism. Children with neuronal dysfunction may take 100 mg of phosphatidylserine daily, while adults may take 100-400 mg a day.

Amino acid deficiency is prevalent among children with ADHD. Children can take 250-500 mg of L-glutamine and $\frac{1}{8}$ teaspoon of gamma-aminobutyric acid (GABA) daily. Adults may take 1 g or more of L-glutamine and up to $\frac{1}{4}$ teaspoon of GABA each day. It is also important to eat adequate protein.

Theanine can help calm the nervous system without acting as a sedative. Children may take up to 200 mg daily, while adults should take 300-400 mg daily.

Stress-reducing herbs such as valerian and lemon balm are beneficial, as stress is a contributor to ADHD. Ginkgo and ginseng improve blood flow to the brain. Spirulina is a detoxifying algae that may help take aluminum and other toxins out of the body. One study showed an 81 percent improvement in test scores when children took 1 gram of spirulina each day for half a year.

Since high levels of thyroid hormone may contribute to ADHD, the possibility of an imbalance should be explored in both children and adults with ADHD. Hormone-lowering drugs, supplementation and dietary changes may help.

While inappropriate for children, DHEA may be supplemented by adults, since it is a neurosteroid that is associated with ADHD. Adults must have a blood test first in order to have the proper dosages prescribed and to ensure that hormone-related cancers are not present.

Dr. Alan Cohen has found that many people have responded to the correct diet and supplement program. Do remember, though, that while these nutrients can all be taken as supplements, diet is of prime importance. An organic diet, free from all additives and preservatives, is recommended so that exposure to toxins is limited and the amount of nutrients the body receives will be maximized.

Clean Schools, Clean Diet

Dr. Doris Rapp is a board-certified environmental medicine specialist, pediatric allergist, and author of many books, including *Is This Your Child's World?* Dr. Rapp emphasizes the connections between chemical sensitivities, poor nutrition, food allergies and alterations in behavior: "The tendency is to place children with learning and developmental problems into special classrooms with special education teachers. But maybe stopping the dyed sugary cereal for breakfast would eliminate the problem. I had one child whose IQ was verified at 57. After discovering her sensitivities and making the appropriate changes, her IQ zoomed to 125. This switch is from retarded to superior. How many other children are getting D's and F's, when they can be getting A's and B's?"

Dr. Rapp adds that medical science has now documented the fact that children's brains can actually be altered by exposure to certain chemical odors. These odors can interfere with the blood flow to the brain, which, in turn, can alter functioning in particular parts of the brain. She explains that if the speech area is affected, the child may stutter, speak too fast or not be able to remember words. If the frontal lobe is affected, the child may suddenly bite or hit, or become irritable, withdrawn, moody or depressed. Dr. Rapp mentions that in the past, psychologists often blamed parents for problems that actually stemmed from an environmental illness.

Rapp cites the experience of the Ontario school system, after psychologists there noted that standard treatments for learning problems were not taking effect. The schools called in environmental physicians, such as herself and Drs. Lyndon Smith, Alex Schauss and Marshall Mandell. All basically gave the same advice: Improve the children's nutrition and keep classrooms free of chemicals.

These suggestions worked. Better nutrition and clean classrooms not only increased academic performance and attendance, but some children who were being taught at home were able to return to school. As Dr. Rapp points out, there's no good reason that we in the U.S. can't follow Ontario's lead.

What to Avoid

Dr. Cohen suggests that heavy metals, such as antimony, aluminum, arsenic, lead and cadmium, should be avoided, since a percentage of autistic children have been found to have high concentrations of these substances in their bodies. Avoid pollutants, including PCBs. Incorporate the use of air and water filters in your everyday life.

Many children with learning disorders seem to have a gluten and casein sensitivity. Casein is a protein found in milk, therefore dairy products may have to be removed from the diet. Gluten is found in grains, and therefore wheat, spelt, oats, barley and rye may also be problematic.

Further, since many children with learning disabilities have compromised immune systems, indicating an overgrowth of candida yeast that allows for increased production of toxins, they should be placed on a yeast- and mold-free diet.

While food allergies are individual in nature, there are certain common food allergens that parents may want to keep in mind. These are corn, soy, eggs, tomatoes, yeast and peanuts. Allergy testing and an elimination diet may be helpful. Keep in mind that the foods that have been the most genetically altered are most likely to be allergenic.

Avoid food coloring and other additives, such as preservatives, bleaches and artificial flavorings, as studies have shown these are responsible for sleep problems, irritability and restlessness. Again, an organic diet of fresh, whole foods is best.

Most importantly, sugar intake must be reduced in the ADHD child. Studies show that sugar causes all of the problems of ADHD, including aggression, inattention and hyperactivity. ADHD children have also been shown to have abnormal rhythms with regard to cortisol, the stress hormone, something that is usually experienced by individuals with difficulty breaking down carbohydrates. Instead, when given sugar, ADHD sufferers release a mere half of certain adrenal hormones (such as epinephrine), which counterbalance drops in glucose due to high insulin. ADHD children have been observed to overcompensate by becoming hyperactive after eating sugar in order to produce these hormones. This finding is reinforced by strong recent evidence showing how medications that enhance the function of these hormones improve symptoms.

Treatment Summary

ADHD is a learning disability that has been woefully overdiagnosed, and has created a great deal of wealth for the major drug companies. A proper diagnosis by an expert in behavioral science—or, preferably, by a team of experts—is essential. The conventional stimulants prescribed for ADHD are associated with a laundry list of drug interactions, contraindications, horrific side effects and unknown long-term effects.

The incorporation of a structured daily routine, exercise, massage, biofeedback training, and other behavioral and lifestyle modifications can significantly relieve ADHD symptoms and facilitate the removal of stimulant medications.

Nutrients that can enhance brain function include EFAs, magnesium, selenium, zinc, sulfur, amino acids, vitamin B1, vitamin B6, vitamin C, calcium, choline, DMAE, phospholipids and L-glutamine. Spirulina, theanine and herbs such as ginkgo and ginseng can be of benefit.

An additive-free, organic diet low in sugar maximizes learning potential.

Evaluating the diet for possible allergens, and then eliminating them, can be helpful.

Keeping school and home environments free of harmful chemicals can enhance learning.

Lupus

Lupus erythematosus is an autoimmune disorder in which the body attacks its own connective tissue or collagen. For most sufferers (overwhelmingly women between the ages of 20 and 40), lupus is a mild disease affecting only a few organs. But for others, it can be serious and life-threatening. People of African, Native American and Asian ancestry develop the disease more frequently than those of European background. Lupus is believed to result from a combination of genetic and environmental factors, but the exact cause of the disease is not known.

Symptoms can include achy joints, fever, nausea, dizziness, vertigo, prolonged or extreme fatigue, arthritis, a rash that goes across the bridge of the nose and cheeks, kidney problems (including renal failure), pleurisy (chest pain), sun and light sensitivity, hair loss, Raynaud's phenomenon (fingers turning white or blue in the cold), seizures, anger and depression, mouth or nose ulcers, nail fungus, headaches and anemia. These indications can be made worse by infections, antibiotics, extreme stress, hormones (especially estrogen) and certain drugs.

The quality of life for many lupus patients has increased dramatically in recent years as newer and safer drugs have become available.

Treatment

Lupus is often treated with steroids, such as prednisone and corticosteroid compounds. Taken long-term, these can cause great damage to the liver, eyes and other organs, as well as weakening of the bones. This is one of the reasons that alternative approaches to the condition are worth looking into.

The supplementation of antioxidants will help minimize free-radical damage caused by exposure to toxins in the environment.

Omega-3 essential fatty acids from fish will alleviate many symptoms resulting from inflammation, and may prove more beneficial than prescription medications.

Taking a formula that includes copper, calcium, vitamin D3, magnesium and folate can minimize bone loss. Vitamin K may also be taken, but not by individuals who use anticoagulant drugs.

Glucosamine and chondroitin can be taken to minimize the pain associated with arthritis due to lupus. To help alleviate chronic aches, DL-phenylalanine powder or L-tyrosine powder may also be taken.

Herbs

Herbs that promote detoxification may be of benefit to lupus sufferers. Pau d'arco, a blood cleanser and aloe vera juice or gel, which neutralizes and flushes toxins from the body, can both help in this regard. Cat's claw, flaxseed oil and omega-3 fatty acids can reduce inflammation. Other helpful nutrients include black walnut, which is anti-inflammatory and antiparasitic, and gotu kola, which nourishes the nervous system.

DHEA

Dehydroepiandrosterone (DHEA) is a hormone produced by the adrenal glands. Many diseases, including lupus, are associated with low levels of this hormone. In studies, women with lupus were given high levels of supplemental DHEA, and some dramatic improvements were seen. In women, 15-25 mg per day is recommended, while men may take 50 mg per day. Before beginning DHEA therapy, however, you must see your doctor to establish baseline values and to rule out the possibility of hormone-related cancers.

Acupuncture

An acupuncturist will take into account the whole range of symptoms each individual manifests, and tailor treatment accordingly. In general, acupuncture increases circulation of blood and what the Chinese refer to as qi, or vital energy, which in turn decreases pain.

Exercise

A regular exercise program helps to keep mobility in the joints, build endurance and to detoxify the body.

Flushes

Enemas and colonics are of great importance in cleansing the body, which is necessary for the alleviation of lupus symptoms. Massage further stimulates detoxification. Colloids, which are metals (such as silver) suspended in solution, are designed to bypass the intestines and enter directly into the cells.

These have detoxifying, antifungal and antibacterial effects, and help to clear arthritic symptoms.

Healthy maintenance of the gastrointestinal tract is the best way to improve immunity, as roughly 80 percent of immune function takes place there. Therefore, a probiotic formula should be taken to supply the area with beneficial bacteria. People with chronic disease states should take a probiotic formula containing FOS, which is a nutrient for intestinal flora. To support the liver, milk thistle should also be taken.

SAMe also protects the liver, and acts as an antidepressant, as well. In divided doses, 1200-1600 mg of SAMe may be taken daily.

Aromatherapy

Aromatic oils have a positive effect on the emotions as well as the body. Joint pain can be alleviated with pine, cedar and other tree oils. A technique aromatherapists recommend for relaxation is placing a drop of chamomile, lavender, lilac or neroli on the palms, rubbing them together, cupping the hands around the nose and breathing in. It is important to use natural oils of a pure quality, and to dilute these before applying directly to the skin.

Physical and emotional stress should be avoided as much as possible to prevent flare-ups. L-theanine tablets in the amount of 100 mg may be taken up to four times a day in order to improve mood, boost concentration and aid relaxation.

What to Avoid

Lupus symptoms vary widely and can be adversely affected by stress and lifestyle. Working at a job one dislikes, for instance, can exacerbate symptoms. Environmental toxins should be eliminated to the greatest extent possible. Foods that stress the system include the obvious villains: processed foods, sugar, caffeine and carbonated beverages. There are also less obvious triggers, healthy foods that set off an allergic inflammatory response. People commonly have problems with peanuts, soy, wheat, corn, milk and acid-producing foods such as meat, dairy products and oranges. Problem-causing foods can be individually identified through allergy testing.

Treatment Summary

Lupus is conventionally treated with steroid drugs, which can damage organs and bones. Herbs are a natural treatment that can benefit lupus sufferers as they cleanse the blood, flush toxins from the body and reduce inflammation.

Studies reveal that DHEA supplementation yields improvement in the condition.

Acupuncture can decrease pain associated with lupus.

A regular exercise program, massage therapy, enemas and colonics flush the system of toxins and help to remove arthritic symptoms.

The essential oils used in aromatherapy can alleviate joint pain and create a feeling of relaxation.

Lyme Disease

Lyme disease is an acute inflammatory condition that can cause joint pain and heart and nervous system symptoms. Its name comes from the place where it was discovered in 1975: Lyme, Connecticut. Although Lyme disease occurs in other parts of the U.S., as well as in other countries, the highest concentration of Lyme disease is in the northeastern United States. Lyme disease is sometimes referred to as "the Great Imposter" because it is frequently misdiagnosed as another disease.

Causes

The spirochete that causes Lyme disease was not identified until 1982. The spirochete, borrelia spirochete (later named after researcher Willy Burgdorfer, Ph.D.), is a type of bacterium in the same family as the one that causes syphilis. This spirochete is transmitted through the bite of a deer tick. Not all deer ticks are infected, but a good percentage are. Note that deer ticks do not reside just on deer; various animals can pick them up. In fact, it is not at all uncommon for people to get deer ticks from their pets after the pets have been running around in the woods or even on a lawn that has trees and bushes.

Some may see Lyme as just a simple infection. However, it is much more than that. It is a complicated disease that may involve other coinfections, especially of the parasitic pathogens Babesia and Ehrlichia.

Symptoms

Some people manifest the classical identifying sign of an inflamed, slightly raised bull's-eye rash. The rash is usually painless, but can be stinging, and often occurs from several days to weeks after the tick bite. It may manifest in an area other than where the original bite happened.

Many other symptoms can be present. Some of these are unexplained fevers, sweats, chills, flushing, weight loss or gain, fatigue and tiredness. Neurological signs include muscle cramps, twitching, headaches, neck creaks and cracks, neck stiffness, tingling, numbness and facial paralysis, such as in Bell's palsy. Mood swings, irritability and depression, as well as memory problems, can occur too.

Signs are not necessarily persistent; they tend to come and go, so that a person with Lyme disease may feel severe symptoms for a week and only mild effects for several months.

Studies involving animals that were infected with Lyme disease show that in less than one week after the infection, the lyme spirochete could be inside tendons, muscles, tissue, the heart and the brain.

The Importance of Tick Removal

Once a person is bitten by a tick, the longer it remains, the more of a chance there is of infection. Usually, a tick must feed for 24 hours before it will transmit infection. Most people will therefore reduce their major problems if the tick is spotted fairly soon and removed.

The way to dislodge a tick is with tweezers, never with fingers. (If tweezers are unavailable, protect the fingers with a paper towel.) Grab the insect close to the head, and pull it straight out. The tick should then be cellophane-taped to a card for identification purposes, so that a doctor or health department can see whether or not this was a deer tick.

If some tea tree oil is available, before attempting to remove the tick place the oil on a piece of cotton and then onto the head of the tick. This will help kill the tick within minutes, making it even easier to yank out and further minimizing the amount of harmful bacteria absorbed into the system.

Diagnosis

According to Dr. Michael Schachter, of Suffern, New York, Lyme disease cannot be diagnosed by one single antibody test alone, since tests give false negatives 30 percent of the time. There are also about 10 percent false positive readings, where the patient does not have the disease even though the blood test says he does. For this reason it is best to make a diagnosis based on a combination of laboratory tests and manifesting symptoms.

New York City's Dr. Martin Feldman says that although the antibody test is the most common diagnostic tool used today, there is also a PCR enzyme test, which is superior for identifying spirochetes. Even better is electrical acupuncture, which can tap into the spirochete's energy fields right away. The device used can also test a person's reaction to different therapies, and, ultimately help test the individual's return to wellness.

Dr. Feldman adds that people can be infected by Lyme disease to different degrees, depending on the state of their immune systems. In order to see whether or not the body has the ability to effectively fight off the spirochete, Feldman begins his diagnosis by taking a complete profile of the person's immune system status. Some signs of lowered immunity include frequent or lingering colds; recurrent infections; sinus problems; digestive disorders; skin problems; PMS; candida overgrowth; parasitic, viral, or fungal infections; allergies; and chemical sensitivities.

Treatment

Antibiotic therapy is the primary treatment given for Lyme disease. Basically, four groups of antibiotics are used. These include those in the penicillin family, the tetracycline family, the cephalosporin family and the macrolide family.

There is a controversy within the medical establishment regarding the best way to utilize antibiotic therapy in treating Lyme disease. Many doctors treat the condition with short courses of antibiotics. These physicians argue that you can get rid of the disease after a one- or two-week course. Others say that the Lyme disease organisms can hide in the tissues for long periods of time, and that short courses of antibiotics frequently do not get to them. They feel that large closes of medicine over long periods of time, generally from four to six weeks, may be needed.

The way antibiotics are administered depends on various factors. In milder cases, in the newly infected, and as a prophylaxis (for people who have just gotten a tick bite and think they might be getting Lyme disease), it is sometimes recommended that people take oral antibiotics for a period of time. In more severe circumstances, or in cases that do not respond to oral treatment, antibiotics may be given intravenously.

Some holistic practitioners do agree that antibiotics can be an important therapy when taken at the early stages of the disease. However, that treatment alone is not enough. At a minimum, anyone on antibiotics, particularly on long courses, should be taking yogurt or an acidophilus supplement to prevent the overgrowth of yeast. Additionally, many other measures for destroying the spirochete and enhancing the immune system should be taken.

Diet

Organically grown foods should be eaten in their natural form whenever possible, with an emphasis on fruits and vegetables. Nuts and seeds, as well as whole grains, should be used. When a person eats meat, organically raised animals should be the source, to avoid weakening from chemical contamination.

Supplements

Dr. Schachter feels that large amounts of the amino acid glutamine should be fed to the immune system so that it can quickly overcome any infection, including Lyme disease. Although glutamine is naturally made by the body, insufficient amounts are produced during times of stress. When an infection is present, the body will resort to breaking down muscles to get more of this vital substance, resulting in a wasting away of the body. Glutamine is even more important when antibiotics are taken because large doses of antibiotics can cause yeast overgrowth, damage to the intestinal lining, leaky gut syndrome and poor absorption of nutrients, all conditions that glutamine can help repair. Additionally, glutamine is an essential part of the glutathione molecule, a major antioxidant produced by the body. The best way to take glutamine is as a teaspoon of powder, somewhere in the range of 5 g three times a day, or a teaspoonful three times a day. Higher doses may be needed for some Lyme disease patients.

Sometimes, vitamins and minerals need to be injected into the patient. This is because the Lyme spirochete, and other bacteria, viruses and fungi in the person's system weaken the intestinal tract so that oral supplements are not fully absorbed. Injectable nutrients bypass the gastrointestinal system, and at the same time, help to heal the digestive tract, so that oral nutrients can have a greater effect. Some nutrients a doctor may administer in this fashion are vitamin C, B vitamins, particularly B6 and B12 and the minerals chromium, magnesium, calcium, zinc, manganese, copper, molybdenum, selenium and glutathione.

The joints can be nourished with calcium, magnesium (when the source of your discomfort is primarily muscle pain, extra magnesium—in a dosage of 30-420 mg per day—and malic acid may provide comfort), manganese, copper and vitamins A and D, as well as glucosamine sulfate and chondroitin. Other basic nutrients for immune repair are bioflavonoids, gamma linoleic acid, essential fatty acids, zinc and selenium.

Furthermore, fatty acids, such as borage and fish oils, help to reduce the inflammation that is often associated with Lyme disease. When energy levels are low, carnitine and alpha-lipoic acid, renowned as energy boosters, may provide a lift.

Bio-oxidative Therapies

Bio-oxidative therapies can restore health, even after other methods have failed. Some patients benefit from a very low concentration of intravenous hydrogen peroxide. Others do well on ozone therapy, where a portion of the patient's blood is mixed with ozone and then injected back into the body. Studies show that ozone therapy stimulates cytokines, chemicals in the white blood cells that help the immune system kill off offending organisms.

What to Avoid

It is important for Lyme disease patients to avoid products that weaken immunity, whenever possible. The list of these is long, and includes sugar, alcohol, caffeine, tobacco smoke, white flour products, hydrogenated fats, chemicals added to foods, fluoridated and chlorinated water, aluminum cook ware and certain medications. Some people have impaired immune systems because of their mercury amalgam dental fillings, and may benefit from their removal, with the addition of a chelating agent that helps to remove mercury from the body. It may seem troublesome to avoid all these substances, but optimizing the condition of the immune system is vital in fighting an illness like Lyme disease.

Preventing tick bites is obviously a good idea for everyone. High-risk activities include walking in the woods or on the beach near tall grassy areas and gardening. Woodpiles tend to attract mice, and therefore Lyme problems. Bird feeders attract animals, too, when the seeds spill over. Dogs and horses may carry ticks and get Lyme disease themselves. When entering high-risk areas, cover the body completely, wearing long pants, a long-sleeved shirt and a hat, and check for ticks afterwards. Ticks show up better on light-colored clothing. Be sure to shower thoroughly, while inspecting the body for ticks. Ticks usually crawl around for at least a few hours before biting, so you have some time before the tick might attack.

Treatment Summary

Cover up to avoid ticks in high-risk areas; if you find a tick on your body or your pet's, remove it promptly to avoid infection.

Antibiotics are the primary method of treatment, although there is controversy regarding how long a course is needed.

Foods selected should be chemical-free to support immune health.

A variety of supplements are helpful in combating Lyme disease, with glutamine being particularly noteworthy.

Bio-oxidative therapies can aid in treating this condition.

Lymphedema

More people are familiar with edema than lymphedema. Lymphedema affects approximately 3 million people in the U.S. and 120 million throughout the world. In edema, an excessive amount of fluid has accumulated in the tissues and the organs, causing swelling. However, lymphedema, as the same suggests, involves swelling of the skin and subcutaneous tissue because of a blockage (for example, from surgery, scarring or chronic edema) of the lymphatic vessels or lymph nodes, resulting in an accumulation of large amounts of lymph fluid in the affected region. This abnormal swelling can occur in an arm or leg (sometimes in both legs), and very occasionally in other parts of the body, such as the head or intestines. Though lymphedema can be congenital, it is usually the result of surgery, especially of lymph node surgery designed to treat breast cancer. Besides swelling, the symptoms include skin thickening, leaking of lymphatic fluid when the skin is cut or broken, and bursting pain, in which the skin feels like it is about to explode.

An estimated 1 percent of the U.S. population has lymphedema, which results from not having enough vessels to carry the lymph. Most cases in the U.S. are the direct result of trauma associated with surgical and radiation treatments for breast cancer. Other causes include parasites, automobile accidents and other physical injury. Also, some 2 million people worldwide are born with inadequate lymph circulation.

The most frequent complication associated with lymphedema is cellulitis, or streptococcal infection of the skin and subcutaneous tissue. Patients will run a high fever; the arm or leg will turn red. Other complications include leaking of lymph fluid, known medically as lymphorrhea; some people leak fluid all the time. Rarely, patients develop malignant tumors in the swollen arm or leg, so-called lymph angiosarcoma.

Lymphedema should be treated immediately, as it can be life-threatening. Early indications include tight jewelry, and skin that does not lose its indentation after being squeezed for several seconds.

Treatments

Manual Lymphatic Drainage

This simple method employs light, slow, rhythmic movements to stimulate lymphatic flow. It can be used as a preventive measure following a mastectomy, before lymphedema occurs. When used after breast removal surgery, studies show that it can reduce scarring, increase arm mobility and alleviate pain and uncomfortable sensitivity.

Complete decongestive physiotherapy (CDP) is a treatment that has been used quite effectively in Europe and has now gained acceptance in the U.S. This therapy is aimed at reducing an affected part of the body (such as an arm or leg) to its regular size. CDP has four steps:

1. Manual lymph drainage (MLD), done by a specialist.
2. Bandaging the swollen body part after the MLD session.
3. Exercise to promote an outflow of lymph fluid from the affected body part.
4. Extreme care of the skin.

Diet

An abundance of fresh, organic, live foods, such as sprouts, salads and fresh juices, aid detoxification and promote good health. The best foods to eat are complex carbohydrates; animal protein and sodium should be avoided. Green juices, such as wheatgrass, celery and parsley, contain chlorophyll, which purifies the blood and lymph. Green juices are too strong to be taken alone, however, and should be diluted with other juices and pure water.

Herbs

The following herbs are known for their anti-edema qualities: hyssop, rosemary, black licorice root, astragalus and dandelion root. Alfalfa, corn silk, juniper berries, lobelia and pau d'arco are also helpful. Garlic is valuable for its antimicrobial and antibiotic properties.

Supplements

Certain nutrients help to cleanse the lymphatic system and move materials through. These include vitamins B1, C and E as well as L-taurine, potassium and raw kidney extract.

Magnets

When properly applied to the affected region, magnets stimulate lymphatic flow. The negative pole is the correct pole to be used.

Respiration

Breathing deeply is the most cost-effective way to activate stagnant lymph fluid. One technique, recommended by California lymph specialist Dr. William Martin, is the following: Breathe deeply in through the nose and out through the mouth, in cycles of three. With each exhalation, push the air out strongly. The third time, before exhaling, hold the breath for as long as possible. While the breath is being held, imagine where the healing breath should go, and mentally direct it to that part of the body.

This exercise opens up the lymphatic ducts and speeds lymphatic flow. It also releases pain, because pain can come from a lack of oxygen at the cellular level. A word of caution: Never hold in air to the point of stress. And stop to rest if this causes dizziness.

Other ways to improve respiration include light bouncing on a small trampoline, while breathing deeply, as well as bio-oxidative therapies, which employ ozone or oxygen. Aerobic exercises prompt lymphatic drainage, and sweating removes toxins from tissues.

Minimizing Symptoms

Patients already affected can take many steps to minimize their problems. Here are some important ones to follow:

Heat should be avoided, as it causes the body to produce more lymphatic fluid. This means no hot showers, hot tubs or saunas, and wearing long sleeves and hats to avoid sun exposure.

To minimize the chance of skin cuts, gloves should be worn when gardening. Electric razors, rather than manual ones, provide less of a chance of cutting the skin.

Patients are urged to avoid strenuous exercise and the lifting of heavy objects.

Women who wear a breast prosthesis should find the lightest one possible, and bra straps should be padded. Whenever possible, bras should not be worn as they restrict lymphatic flow.

Skin and nail care should be meticulous to avoid infections, and patients should avoid going to manicurists who use their instruments on other patrons.

Patients must avoid injections to affected areas or to the arm nearest where the breast cancer was. They must avoid having a doctor take blood or blood pressure readings from that arm. Nor should they receive chemotherapy in that arm.

Mosquito bites can lead to serious infections and must be avoided.

Maintaining a normal weight minimizes symptomatology.

If airplane travel is necessary, the arm or leg should be wrapped and elevated before take off. Preparation for travel includes taking extra garlic and other natural antibacterials.

What to Avoid

The most detrimental foods contain salt, sugar and caffeine. It is also important to stay away from processed foods and artificial chemicals.

Treatment Summary

Stimulating lymph flow through manual lymphatic drainage, especially after a mastectomy, can prevent the occurrence of lymphedema.

Healing foods promote cleansing and include live green foods and complex carbohydrates. Caffeine, sugar and salt must be avoided.

Beneficial herbs have anti-inflammatory, antimicrobial and antibiotic properties.

Nutrients that promote further detoxification include vitamins B1, C and E, L-taurine, potassium and raw kidney extract.

The negative pole of a magnet placed over the affected region will speed up healing.

Deep breathing accompanied by visualization is a powerful way to promote healing.

Menopause

Menopause can be defined as the conclusion of the female reproductive phase of life. In most women, the onset of menopause occurs between the ages of 45 and 50, but it has been known to occur anywhere from age 40 to 60. In addition, menopause can be provoked at an earlier time due to uterine or ovarian surgery, or certain types of illnesses. Menopause is characterized by the decreased functioning of the ovaries, which results in reduced quantities of the hormone estrogen in the body. Not just a discrete event, menopause is actually a process, one that lasts several years or even a decade.

Although menopause is an experience common to women all around the world, those in Asian countries tend to adapt more easily to the hormonal changes involved, due to their willingness to accept the aging process as a natural transition. In Asian countries, age is associated with wisdom and respect; hence, women in these countries do not dread this stage of life. In the United States and other Western nations, advanced age is feared profoundly by women, due to cultural conditioning. This negative outlook is often correlated with the acquisition of acute menopausal symptoms. Women who are about to experience menopause, or who have already, should reexamine their attitudes and try to eliminate any preconceived ideas regarding aging. It should also be noted that acute symptoms are frequently avoided by Asian women because their diets contain ample quantities of soy products, which are high in phytoestrogens and phytoesterols. In addition, Asian women benefit from the widespread use of medicinal herbs.

As the information above indicates, menopause has traditionally been defined as a female condition. However, men have a similar condition, called andropause, but commonly referred to as male menopause, which is caused by hypogonadism, or low testosterone levels. Strictly speaking, andropause is defined as the "natural cessation of the sexual function in older men." In lay language, it means the lessening of sexual desire in men because of decreasing hormone levels.

What Women Experience

The menopausal process usually begins with variations in the menstrual cycle. The time between cycles often becomes irregular, and sometimes periods are skipped. Although menopause is usually accompanied by reduced menstrual flow, some women report heavy, irregular bleeding. Hot flashes are another common experience, while some women may experience dry skin, irritability, vaginal dryness, night sweats, urinary tract infections, mood swings, fatigue and sleep disturbances. It should be kept in mind that some women have no troublesome symptomatology at all. It is also important to mention that menopause is characterized by diminished estrogen production by the ovaries, and when this occurs, the manufacturing process is transferred to the adrenal glands. Consequently, women with healthy adrenal glands are less susceptible to experiencing acute symptoms.

A common misconception is that women will lose their sex drive once they have experienced menopause. In fact, only a small percentage lose their ability to become aroused, and these cases can be effectively treated. Actually, many women report heightened sexuality because the risk of pregnancy is absent. Another assumption whose time has gone is the belief that, after the change of life, life will no longer be enjoyable. Many women fear that their later years will be characterized by intense psychological problems. This is untrue, as women who have reached 50 years of age are not at any increased risk of clinical depression. Although some women may experience mood swings due to decreased levels of estrogen, serotonin and endorphins, these levels can effectively be corrected by natural means, and thus, symptomatic mood swings can be eliminated.

What Men Experience

The beginning of male menopause typically occurs as men enter their 40s. As men reach their 40s, most will begin experiencing physical and emotional changes. The exercise routine that formerly held their bodies together is now inadequate. Fat has slowly appeared in places where muscle used to be. Sexual activity and interest wane. Many men find their enthusiasm for living has decreased along with their sexual desire. Reports indicate that approximately 25 million men in the U.S. between 40 and 55 years of age suffer from andropause. Oftentimes, when men have low levels of testosterone, it has a domino effect on mood, mental skills, memory and sexual desire.

Testosterone is the hormone responsible for regulating the structure of proteins in the body. It governs the development of the genitals (penis and testicles). The testicles account for about 7-10 mg of the testosterone produced each day. When the testicles do not produce their normal level of testosterone, the body changes. In the cause-and-effect relationship, the low testosterone levels are the cause, and the effect is a man with a body that is falling apart, ravaged by clogged arteries, varicose veins, hemorrhoids, high blood pressure and elevated cholesterol.

Treatment for Women

The medical establishment has traditionally approached menopause as a disease, and, in that paradigm, offered hormone replacement as a "cure." In reality, menopause is not a disease; it is a natural transitional period that can be coped with using natural techniques. Unfortunately, hormone replacement therapy has become commonplace in our nation over the past few years. Although most doctors insist that replacement therapy involves the use of natural hormones, the fact is that the hormones being used are not manufactured by our own bodies, nor are they derived from natural plant sources, such as soy products or yams. Premarin, a popular hormone replacement product, is obtained from the urine of pregnant horses. Currently, 10 million women are being administered this product in capsules or in patches. Clinical studies have confirmed that the administration of synthetic hormones to patients can increase the risk of breast cancer by up to 33 percent. Furthermore, hormone replacement has been linked to upper body obesity and insulin resistance, a condition commonly associated with low blood sugar levels, elevated blood pressure and excessive insulin levels.

Treatment for Men

There are many ways men can combat the ravages of andropause. Eating a well-balanced diet with an emphasis on organically grown fruits and vegetables is a good way to escape the effects of chemicals that negatively impact the endocrine system. Men should supplement their diets with the full gamut of antioxidants. In order to counteract the physical impact of andropause on the body, men should undertake a regular exercise routine. Numerous studies have documented that high-intensity exercise helps men keep their testosterone levels elevated. Encouragingly, the exercise program works in both older and younger men.

Many men have pleasantly discovered that natural plant extracts can improve their sex drive, as well as their performance. The following is recommended for men who desire to have similar results: 5 mg of zinc, 550 mg of chrysin, 125 mg of nettle, 20 mg of ginger root extract, 400 mg of muira puama, 125 mg of maca (Peruvian ginseng) and 5 mg of black piperine (from black pepper).

Nutrition and Supplements

Fortunately, synthetic hormone replacement can be averted in favor of natural treatments that have no harmful side effects. Studies have shown that plant estrogens, such as those found in soy products, are quite helpful in combating symptoms. And soy products (for example, tofu, tempeh, soybeans) hamper the proliferation of cancerous cells. Oats, cashews, almonds, alfalfa, apples and flaxseeds also contain natural sources of estrogen enhancement, although in more modest amounts. Women who incorporate these natural estrogen-containing foods into their diets can experience remarkable relief from hot flashes. In addition, sufficient intake of magnesium, found in soy products, whole grains and beans, is important in curbing hot flashes. Increased dietary intake of fiber and reduced quantities of animal products can limit irritability, while sunflower seeds, walnuts, hazelnuts, cabbage, asparagus, broccoli, oats and barley can serve as additional combatants of menopausal symptoms.

A multivitamin/mineral supplement that has more magnesium than calcium and adequate quantities of B vitamins and vitamin C can enhance adrenal functioning and alleviate emotional disturbances. Supplements of vitamin E are recommended, too. This useful vitamin promotes the production of the brain hormones FSH and LH, which act as vital agents in the prevention of hot flashes. In addition, vitamin E reduces vaginal dryness and hot flashes. Natural sources of vitamin E, including the various mixed tocopherols, are more efficient than artificial versions. The mineral zinc is useful as well.

Supplements of the vitamin B complex are especially important during the menopausal years and can be extracted naturally from whole grains and green vegetables. Three to four mg of vitamin B5 and 150 mg of B6 should be consumed on a daily basis, while prescriptions of folic acid can serve as natural hormone replacements. Adequate quantities of essential fatty acids should also be consumed because they act as natural hormone supplements, prevent cancer and can alleviate the symptoms of aging. Essential fatty acids are also crucial in preventing dryness of the vaginal region. People on low-fat diets often suffer from deficiencies of essential fatty acids and, consequently, need to incorporate certain foods into their diets to correct the problem. Omega-6 fatty acids can be obtained from pumpkin, sesame, safflower and flaxseed oils, while omega-3 fatty acids are sufficiently supplied in diets that contain fish, fish oil capsules and flaxseed oil.

Vitamin D, which can be supplemented in quantities of 400 to 600 IU per day, is also absorbed directly from sunlight, or extracted from salmon oil. This is an important vitamin for menopausal women, especially those who live in polluted regions. Calcium supplements can prevent or curb osteoporosis and can be particularly beneficial when supplementation is initiated considerably before menopause. While many women have difficulty assimilating dairy products, calcium citrate, amino acid chelate and calcium carbonate offer alternative sources of calcium that can be easily digested. Regardless of which source you select, remember that the body requires 1300 mg of calcium on a daily basis, and even more if you have difficulty assimilating it. An analysis of an individual's calcium absorption can be performed prior to supplementation. Gamma linoleic acid, which is available as evening primrose oil, borage oil and black currant seed oil should be supplemented by menopausal women in quantities of 200 mg per day. Boron is yet another valuable source of both female and male hormones and can be effectively supplemented.

There are several other natural products that can stimulate the production of hormones during the menopausal years. Natural DHEA, commonly obtained from yam extract, can invigorate the body. Progesterone cream or serum guards against fibrocystic conditions and breast cancer, improves the effectiveness of thyroid hormones and prevents osteoporosis by replacing depleted calcium. Progesterone should be administered three to four weeks out of every month. Wild yam cream, which is an over-the-counter product, and oral progesterone supplements, can provide effective natural hormone replacement. Estriol is a beneficial hormone that has demonstrated its ability to hinder the development of breast tumors in animals and is currently being prescribed as an alternative to synthetic hormones by some gynecologists. Finally, Estrogen, a formula comprised of 80 percent estriol and 20 percent estrone and estradiol, can prevent the onset of breast cancer, osteoporosis, and cardiovascular disorders without any harmful side effects.

Certain soy products have high amounts of isoflavones (see *Osteoporosis*). Isoflavone is a phytoestrogen, also known as a plant estrogen. In the body, plant estrogens perform like a weaker version of estrogen. It is important to note that the key to maximizing the effectiveness of soy products is to consume large amounts of them over a protracted period of time. Taking them in this manner affords them the best opportunity to combat osteoporosis and help relieve the menopausal symptoms such as vaginal dryness and hot flashes. Several studies have documented soy's effectiveness in significantly reducing the occurrence of hot flushes. A double-blind, placebo-controlled study showed that women who received 60 g of soy protein isolate per day lessened their hot-flash episodes by 45 percent. Another study showed that there was a significant decrease in the occurrence of hot flushes after a six-week period among women who had taken 400 mg of soy extract and 50 mg of isoflavone daily.

Herbal Treatments

In addition to dietary modifications and natural supplements, there are numerous herbs that can enhance a woman's ability to cope with menopause if she is having problems. First of all, the herb chaste berry, commonly marketed under the name Vitex, can augment the progesterone level in the body and, consequently, eliminate many of the symptoms associated with menopause, including vaginal dryness, hot flashes and mood swings. Chaste berry can be obtained in capsules, teas and in dry or liquid extracts. Note that the medicinal capabilities of this herb, which affect the pituitary gland and hypothalamus, can take a considerable amount of time to show up. Usually, at least one or two complete cycles are required before the effects become apparent, and six months of use may be needed for sustained improvement.

Herbs that serve as natural sources of phytoestrogens and progesterone include wild yam (used as a progesterone-producing herb to alleviate hot flashes), alfalfa, sarsaparilla and blessed thistle. To assist with proper functioning of the nervous system, consider skullcap, motherwort (to relieve vaginal dryness), valerian root (to promote sleep and relieve anxiety), passionflower, ginseng, fresh oat and blue vervain. Black cohosh is a panacea-type herbal remedy that is used to treat "female problems" such as PMS, menstrual cramps, morning sickness and menopausal symptoms. Studies have credited it with helping relieve menopausal symptoms in a high percentage of menopausal women.

Dong quai, one of the most significant Chinese herbs, has proven effective in providing relief from the symptoms of menopause. It should be taken for eight to 12 weeks, or for three menstrual cycles. At the end of this period, many women have found a perceptible decrease in the negative effects of hormone imbalances. Asian healers have used dong quai for centuries to balance female hormones and to avoid the problems associated with menopause.

To treat the depression that can accompany menopause and andropause, many advocate the use of St. John's wort, an extract of the flower Hypericum perforatum. For hundreds of years, St. John's wort has been used to treat mild to moderate depression. In short, the effectiveness of St. John's wort is incontrovertible.

Homeopathic Remedies

There are several homeopathic remedies that can be effective in treating flooding in younger women. (Flooding is the condition in which menstrual bleeding stops for a period of time and then resumes profusely.) The remedy China is used by homeopaths in remedying heavy bleeding with dark, clotted blood. To treat the painful discharge of heavy, bright red, clotted blood, sabina can be used. Sabina can also be used to alleviate feelings of irritability. Secale is helpful in reducing heavy and persistent bleeding of almost black colored blood, while the remedy phosphorous can control frequent bleeding of bright red blood without any clots. Additional symptoms that can be treated with phosphorous include multiple fears, non-severe depression, chilliness and memory loss.

Homeopathic remedies can be useful in lessening the vaginal dryness and thinning that frequently accompany menopause. Sepia should be used when the vagina is itchy and dry. When vaginal dryness interferes with sexual intercourse, natmur is the remedy that should be administered. In addition, natmur can be used to control burning vaginal secretions, loss of pubic hair, depression and irritability that intensifies with consolation. These symptoms often become compounded in the later part of the morning. When dryness and headaches occur simultaneously, the herb bryonia can act as a healing agent. The homeopathic remedy nitric acid is used to treat cases of severe vaginal dryness in which extreme desiccation of the mucosa results in splinter-like sensations in the vaginal region.

Aromatherapy

Aromatherapy is an approach to menopausal symptoms that incorporates both the mind and the body. Menopausal women may want to try the application of fennel, clary sage and cyprus in a lotion or body oil two or three times a day. Inhaling peppermint or basil oil on a tissue numerous times a day is recommended by aromatherapists for hot flashes. Remember, though, not to use excessive quantities of essential oils and to avoid direct skin contact. In addition, essential oils should constitute only 3 percent of lotions or body oils. People interested in aromatherapy should seek professional supervision when they begin treatment in order to prevent harmful side effects and ensure that high-quality oils are being used. Also, professional aromatherapists can create specific oils tailored to the individual needs of their clients.

Exercise

Research demonstrates that exercise can diminish the occurrence of hot flashes in menopausal women. In order to completely reap time benefits of physical fitness, regular exercise should be initiated significantly before the onset of menopause, although any time is a good time to begin—with medical guidance.

Exercise can also be a good counter to menopausal depression and mood swings because it enhances the production of endorphins and serotonin in the brain. And considering the disease-preventive benefits of exercise, everyone should partake, at some level. Beneficial forms of exercise include biking, running, swimming, walking and dancing. Discover what you enjoy, and then keep at it. Crosstraining can also be advantageous, but be sure to perform different exercises on different days of the week in order to avoid overexerting any one part of the body.

Ayurvedic Medicine

Ayurvedic, which translated means "the science of life," has had a widespread following in India for 4000 years. The key to Ayurveda lies in the belief that balance can have a profound influence upon a person's health. Practitioners of Ayurveda examine the patients' psychological and physical health, and then custom-design a proper diet and exercise program based upon their evaluation. To alleviate menopausal symptoms, this form of therapy uses herbal phytoprogesterones and phytoestrogens.

What to Avoid

Although all women will experience menopause, some will be victimized by adverse symptoms more than others. Remember that the severity of symptoms may be dependent upon one's willingness to accept the aging process and the person's ability to adapt to the tremendous hormonal changes that occur. Adaptation includes taking some preventive measures, specifically avoiding several foods that have a tendency to compound symptoms. Clinical research has revealed that excessive intake of sugar, caffeine and alcohol can modify the blood sugar levels of the body, leading to, or compounding, psychological disturbances. Furthermore, it should be noted that studies have correlated alcohol, meat and cigarettes with premature menopause.

Treatment Summary

Beneficial plant estrogens are found in soy products, and, to a lesser extent, in other foods, such as oats, cashews, almonds, alfalfa, apples and flaxseeds.

Some important nutrients for the menopausal years are the B-complex vitamins, vitamins C, D and E, magnesium, calcium and zinc.

Herbs that may be helpful are chaste berry, dong quai and wild yam, among others.

Homeopathic remedies can help balance menstrual flow if flooding is a problem. Other homeopathic remedies are used to alleviate vaginal dryness.

Aromatherapy can be a helpful modality for menopausal women.

Exercise alleviates hot flashes and depression.

Ayurvedic medicine uses plants with progesterone and estrogen to alleviate menopausal symptoms.

Motion Sickness

Motion sickness is usually attributed to an inner ear problem, but the condition may also stem from a poor diet or allergies.

Treatment

Chewing ginger may help prevent nausea, including motion sickness and sea sickness. According to scientific studies, ginger is more effective than Dramamine, a common over-the-counter motion sickness drug, and, unlike pharmaceuticals, it does not cause drowsiness. The key to ginger's effectiveness appears to stem from the oils it contains (gingerols and shogaols). These oils calm the intestinal tract and subtly depress the central nervous system. Some of the most potent forms of ginger are the powdered, capsule form, the tea form (from sliced ginger root) and the candy form. Ginger should be taken on an empty stomach.

To help prevent jet lag and motion sickness during air travel, taking 1-3 mg of melatonin during the trip may be effective.

Pyridoxine (vitamin B6) is a water-soluble B-complex vitamin that enables over 70 different enzymes to function properly. Vitamin B6 can dilate blood vessels, and, thus, effectively treats motion sickness.

Using a finger to apply pressure (via acupressure) on the Neiguan or Pericardium-6 acupuncture point (which is above the wrist of the inner arm) has proven effective against motion sickness. Furthermore, many have been aided by applying pressure to Small Intestine 17, located underneath the earlobes, in the grooves behind the jawbone. This spot is connected to the ear's balancing mechanism.

Homeopathic Remedies

Tobaccum is a remedy recommened by homeopathic practitioners for helping dispel motion sickness, especially sea sickness, characterized by a sink-ing feeling in the stomach and nausea. As its name implies, tobaccum is made from tobacco. Cocculus can help motion sickness when there is nausea at the smell of food. The person for whom this is prescribed feels worse when looking at something moving and better when focusing on a still horizon. Arnica can be taken to overcome the achiness and jet lag that follows a long flight. Homeopathic borax is specifically suggested for nausea that is caused by downward motions, as when an airplane is landing. When motion sickness is coupled with headache, nausea and ringing in the ears, nux vomica can provide relief. Petroleum combats dizziness and the nausea one feels when riding in a car or boat. Lastly, when motion sickness is the result of reading you've done in an automobile, sepia is recommended.

Multiple Sclerosis

Multiple sclerosis is an autoimmune disease in which the myelin sheath, a fatty protective coating around nerve cells, is destroyed by the body's own defense system. The disease presents a wide variety of symptoms, which range in severity and can come and go. MS symptoms include weakness of an arm or leg, unexplained tingling or funny sensations in various places in the body, double vision, loss of vision, problems with speech or walking, increased urinary frequency, incontinence and memory impairment.

Allopathic medicine is uncertain as to the exact cause(s) of MS, but environmental, dietary and even viral factors are implicated. For some reason, people who live further from the equator have a higher incidence of the disease. Some theories attribute this difference to degrees of sunlight. Others connect it to diet, as people in northern regions tend to eat greater amounts of saturated fat.

Treatment

Because MS is an autoimmune disease, most neurologists believe that shutting down immune function is the best treatment approach. In the process, though, harmful steroids, such as Prednisone and Solu-Medrol, and even chemotherapeutic agents, may be used. Recent studies show that beta interferon injections decrease the frequency of flair-ups (which are called exacerbations), but these injections can also produce flu-like symptoms, including severe body aches, high fever and debilitating weakness.

Conventional medicine tends to neglect low-tech approaches, which can be highly successful. Changes in diet, the use of nutritional supplements and reduction of environmental toxins can all have a positive impact on MS patients.

Diet

A neurologist by the name of Dr. Swank has been studying dietary factors related to MS and publishing his results in peer-reviewed medical journals since the 1950s. His long-range studies show that strict adherence to a low-fat diet, consisting of no more than 20 grams of fat per day, produce the best results. Saturated fats, including those found in red meat, dark meat and palm and coconut oils should be eliminated or eaten rarely. This approach can improve disease management and greatly increase life expectancy, even in severe cases. More specific dietary recommendations are found in Dr. Swank's book, *The Multiple Sclerosis Diet Book.*

Supplements

Taken daily, these important nutrients have a variety of benefits. They can enhance neuron functioning, prevent free radical damage, improve circulation and increase oxygen:

Garlic—1000-2000 mg
L-cysteine—500 mg
Inositol—1000 mg
Choline—1000 mg
Vitamin C—1000 mg six times daily
Vitamin E—600 IU
Sodium selenite—200 mcg
Coenzyme Q10—up to 200 mg
Niacin—200-500 mg three times daily
Vitamin B12—1000 mcg
Vitamin B6—100-500 mg
DMG—100-400 mg

According to some studies, evening primrose oil (1500 mg) and fish oil supplements may noticeably lessen the harshness and duration of MS attacks.

In some instances, DMG contributes to a remyelinization of the sheath protecting the spinal column. Garlic is beneficial for its high sulfur content. And borage, black currant seed and evening primrose oil are valuable for their gamma linolenic acid. Studies indicate use of this substance is related to decreased severity of symptoms.

A 2004 seminal study reported in *Neurology* found that supplementation with vitamin D was linked to a 40-percent reduction in the risk of MS. The women in the study supplemented with multinutrient supplements that contained vitamin D (400 IUs daily).

Since people in the north get less sunlight, and therefore less vitamin D, it may help to take more of this vitamin. In fact, one study showed that up to 5000 units of vitamin D, taken in combination with 16 mg per kilogram of body weight of calcium, and 10 mg per kilogram of body weight of magnesium cut MS exacerbations in half. Since vitamin D can be toxic in such high doses, this plan should be followed under a physician's guidance.

Curcumin has shown potential as a treatment for multiple sclerosis.

One study detailed the effects of ginkgo (240 mg daily) on patients suffering from a mild form of MS. The group that supplemented with ginkgo, as opposed to the placebo group, demonstrated major improvements on a cognitive-function test. The group receiving the placebo did worse than before. Scientific literature has shown a scant few drugs capable of improving cognitive function. Future studies may prove ginkgo to be a valuable ally in the war against MS.

Magnets

Magnets can help to heal damaged muscle and nerve tissue. Wearing magnets or sleeping on a magnetic bed can thus play a role in the management of MS symptoms.

Biological Dentistry

Toxic vapors from mercury amalgam fillings, or bacteria lodged in the gums and teeth, can cause any number of debilitating symptoms seemingly unrelated to the mouth—even central nervous system damage. Anyone with MS should work with a biological dentist to remove toxic fillings and make other dental and periodontal corrections for improved overall health.

Treatment Summary

Studies show that adherence to a low-fat diet can result in improvement of MS and greatly increase life expectancy.

Nutrients taken supplementally can enhance neuron functioning, prevent, free radical damage, improve circulation and increase oxygen.

Use of magnets can help to heal damaged in tissue and nerve tissue.

Since toxic vapors from mercury amalgam fillings can aggravate a host of problems in the body related to MS, it is suggested that a biological dentist be consulted for removal of these fillings.

Obesity

Obesity refers to an abnormal increase in body fat, and is usually, but not necessarily, synonymous with being overweight. The distinction is most clearly seen in athletes, when muscular, 300-pound football players are not obese until they stop working out; then, muscle turns to fat. Conversely, a person whose weight falls within an acceptable range on a chart can actually have too much body fat. An impedance test is useful in determining whether one is overfat. Another alternative is to use the body mass index (BMI), which is determined by the body weight (in kilograms) divided by the height (in meters squared). A person with a BMI of 25-29.9 is considered overweight; a person with a BMI over 30 is classified as obese.

In the U.S., people often are overfat. This is largely due to the massive consumption of high-fat and sugary foods in the typical American diet. Children become addicted to this way of eating and grow into overweight adults who are prone to a variety of diseases, including gastrointestinal and cardiovascular disorders, cancer, diabetes and atherosclerosis. But even health-conscious individuals who restrict their fat and sugar intake are becoming heavier, according to government statistics. Dr. Alan Cohen, medical director of the Health and Rehabilitation Center in Danbury, Connecticut, explains that people are eating less fat and replacing it with more carbohydrates. Yet, 75 percent of the population is carbohydrate intolerant. This means that these individuals convert carbohydrates very quickly into high doses of sugar, which, in turn, stimulates the pancreas to produce insulin. When there is a high level of insulin, or hyperinsulinemia, sugar is converted into body fat, making weight loss difficult. To determine if one is hyperinsulinemic, one should get the fasting insulin levels from a blood test. Whether one is carbohydrate sensitive can be determined by a health care practitioner who performs a complete physical in conjunction with a complete health and family history. A family background of heart disease, diabetes and obesity, as well as high levels of cholesterol and triglycerides, are signs of hyperinsulinism and carbohydrate sensitivity.

Additionally, many overfat people have subclinical hypothyroidism, which is the type that does not necessarily show up on blood tests. The thyroid gland sets the rate at which we burn calories. Basic metabolic rate (BMR) is determined when one is idle. The calculated average ratio is 1680 kcal per 70 kg (154 lbs) for a man, and 1173 kcal per 58 kg, (127.5 lbs) for a woman. When the thyroid slows down, our metabolism becomes sluggish, meaning that we burn calories less efficiently. To learn whether or not subclinical hypothyroidism exists, people can take their temperature by placing a thermometer under the arm for 10 minutes before getting out of bed in the morning. Five readings yielding an average of at least 97.8 degrees indicates normalcy; an average below that may indicate hypothyroidism. Besides a low body temperature and weight gain, other signs of subclinical hypothyroidism are cold hands and feet, memory and concentration problems, dry skin, constipation, PMS and other menstrual problems, and hair thinning or loss.

Treatment

Obtaining and maintaining a normal level of body fat depends on lifelong habits that encompass a healthy way of eating and exercising. The traditional weight loss tactic of dieting, by contrast, implies a temporary restriction of food intake or calories, not permanent change, and is thus doomed to failure from the beginning. Diets create a rebound effect whereby the person not only gains back lost weight, but adds additional pounds. Repeated attempts result in a yo-yo syndrome, with the person continually losing and gaining weight. This is not only bad for self-esteem; it slows down metabolism, making it more difficult to lose weight with each subsequent try.

Most people blame failure on their lack of willpower, but they need not be so hard on themselves. The reason diets do not work can be explained by considering the way our ancestors lived in prehistoric times. For much of the time that humans have been around, there was no steady source of food. Sometimes there was plenty to eat, and at other times there was nothing. In order to survive, people's bodies had to adjust to these conditions of feast or famine. When food was scarce, metabolism would slow down to preserve energy; when there was plenty of food, it would speed up. Whether food was scarce or plentiful, women had more fat than men because they needed it for carrying babies and breastfeeding.

Dieting places the body in the famine or starvation mode, which is why metabolism slows down when people go on strict diets. When they begin to give in to their cravings, their metabolism speeds up; when one is young, this is called the rebound effect. Up until the age of 30, the body can adapt to metabolic changes brought on by dieting and then quitting, but after that it becomes less flexible. With added age, metabolism slows down and stays down. To make matters worse, the weight lost is often muscle, but the weight gained tends to be more fat than lean body mass. Fat burns fewer calories than lean tissue, with the result being that the next time around in the yo-yo diet cycle, the pounds will be more difficult to shed.

Many people mistakenly believe that a high-protein diet is a good way to lose weight. While such a diet may have dramatic effects at first, it can produce unwanted consequences over time, such as irritability, agitation, sluggishness and even damage to the kidneys and liver. Additionally, animal protein foods are usually marbled with saturated fat that clog the arteries.

Proper Eating

The best diet to follow is one that teaches proper eating as a way of life. It is generally higher in complex carbohydrates and lower in protein and fat. The ratios of calories from carbohydrates, protein and fat should be approximately 60:20:20. But for people with a carbohydrate intolerance, the proportion should be more like 40:30:30. As mentioned earlier, this will keep insulin levels down and burn more body fat. People with carbohydrate sensitivities should avoid bread, pasta, potatoes, rice, corn, bananas and raisins, getting their carbohydrates instead from other sources.

Good fruits to include are apples and blueberries because of their gel-forming fibers. Oat bran, barley and carrots can also be considered, as well as water-soluble fibers that restrain carbohydrate absorption. As these foods travel through the intestines, they provide a sense of fullness, which signals the brain to turn off its hunger appetite. Additionally, sea vegetables, such as kelp, nourish the thyroid, which in turn keeps the metabolism running smoothly. Drinking plenty of pure water is important, as well. Dieters should be wary of the no-fat craze, as avoiding fats completely can be dangerous. Each cell in our body is lined with cholesterol or fat. Plus, the fat-soluble vitamins A and E can only be absorbed when fat is present. These antioxidants work to prevent a variety of diseases, including cancer, heart disease and immune disorders. A distinction needs to be made between good and bad fats. Good sources are found in fish, avocados, nuts and nut butters and olive oil. Recent studies show that *when* we eat might be as important as *what* we eat. It is better to have a substantial breakfast, plus to eat all other meals before 6:30 P.M., since that is when the metabolic rate is high enough to use calories as energy instead of turning them into fat.

Glycemic Index

We can measure the insulin-elevating power of different foods with two index numbers. The glycemic index shows the speed of blood sugar reaction to carbohydrates. The glycemic load demonstrates the impact of the ingested carbohydrates. The use of these numbers is not entirely beneficial for obese people because their insulin level is already high, which inhibits weight loss. But the numbers can be used to control insulin levels.

Supplements

Nutrients have many important functions for the individual working to lose weight healthfully. Some help to eliminate cravings by balancing blood sugar, while others burn calories quickly by speeding up the metabolism. Here are some important ones to consider:

Chromium Picolinate . . . Chromium helps stabilize blood sugar levels, so that there is less of a craving for sweets. It also helps to increase lean body mass and boost energy. Furthermore, chromium reduces insulin resistance, which in turn decreases the storage of adipose (fatty) tissue and increases its metabolism. Between 200-400 mcg of the chelated form is preferred, as it is more easily absorbed into the intestinal tract. It is suggested that a person take vitamin E with chromium, as well as 30 mg of niacin with each 200-mcg chromium capsule.

Magesium . . . Magnesium deficiency is linked to insulin resistance and high blood sugar levels. For people going on a calorie-restricted diet, supplementation of 300-500 mg of magnesium is recommended.

Essential Fatty Acids and Gamma Linoleic Acid . . . The body needs two types of essential fatty acids: omega-3 and omega-6. Omega-3's are found in flaxseed oil, which should be cold-pressed, organic and stored in a cold place in a dark container, as essential fatty acids are light-sensitive. This oil can be used on salads and should never be cooked. If a product tastes bad, it may be rancid and should be discarded. Omega-3's contribute to weight loss by helping the kidneys get rid of excess water.

The body needs to balance omega-3 fatty acids with omega-6 fatty acids. Gamma linoleic acid contains omega-6 and can be found in evening primrose, borage or black currant seed oil. Five hundred milligrams of evening primrose oil taken in the morning may help reduce appetite.

L-Carnitine . . . A dosage of 500-1000 mg helps take fatty acids inside cells, where energy-producing mitochondria burn them up.

Lecithin . . . Lecithin helps emulsify fat, and one tablespoon is best taken in the morning with breakfast.

Potassium . . . About 300 mg daily taken in divided doses will increase energy and muscle strength.

Psyllium Husk . . . A tablespoon, once or twice daily, along with 8 to 16 ounces of water, provides extra fiber for better digestion.

Additional Supplements . . . Research has shown that daily supplementation of ascorbic acid (vitamin C) can have a positive effect for obese people who are attempting to lose weight. Other supplements to know about are hydroxy citric acid (HCA), spirulina, yerba mate and kola nut, which have been found to speed up metabolism. Supplementing a normal diet with gel-forming fibers such as guar gum produces a feeling of fullness that can make adhering to a diet easier. In addition, fiber can improve metabolism.

Hormone Rebalancing

DHEA . . . The precursor of hormones such as testosterone and estrogen can interfere with weight loss. DHEA levels decline with age. To restore the levels to those of one's youth, supplement with 50 mg for men and 15-50 mg for women. This can boost the insulin growth factor, IGF-1, resulting in weight loss. DHEA rebalancing can also cause thyroid hormone levels to drop. *Note:* DHEA supplementation is not recommended for people with hormone-related cancers.

Testosterone and Estrogen in Men . . . Obesity in men is associated with low testosterone levels and high estrogen levels (see *Menopause*). The decreased level of free testosterone in men is caused by an excess of aromatase enzymes in the fat cells or in dietary fat. The fat tissue, especially in the abdomen, actually "aromatizes" testosterone and its precursors into estrogen. The production of aromatase enzymes could get out of control if the body is low in zinc, which is a natural aromatase inhibitor. (Supplementation of 30-90 mg of zinc could be helpful.) If liver function is hampered by aging, alcohol or certain drugs, the liver cannot properly eliminate surplus estrogen, making the hormonal imbalance even worse. Men with central or visceral obesity (pot belly) are at risk of developing type II diabetes or cardiovascular disease, accompanied by impotency.

Sometimes, even though testosterone is replaced, there is still a problem with testosterone's bioavailability, which causes a loss of libido. Concentrated nettle root is capable of binding with sex hormone binding globulin (SHBG) in place of testosterone. This is a way that testosterone can reach the cell receptor sites and stimulate the libido, resulting in sexual arousal. Additionally, nettle may prevent benign prostatic hyperplasia (enlargement of the prostate gland) by inhibiting dihydrotestosterone (DHT), a metabolite of testosterone. DHT can stimulate prostate growth. Another quality nettle has is that it blocks enzymes—such as 5 alpha reductase, which can trigger prostate enlargement, excess facial hair and hair loss at the top of the head.

Insulin . . . As the cells become resistant to the hormone insulin, the body cannot release fat from storage and the person cannot lose weight. Excess insulin in the bloodstream can also contribute to weight gain by depleting glucose in the blood, a process called reactive hypoglycemia. The symptoms are a constant craving for sugar. Eating does not bring satisfaction because insulin continues to feed off the glucose. The presence of too much insulin in the blood also blocks the release of growth hormone by the pituitary gland. Decreased levels of growth hormone result in less lean muscle and more stored fat. The development of hypertension is associated with excess insulin, as are damage to the kidneys and to the vascular system. To determine if you have a high insulin level in the blood, you have to check your fasting insulin levels.

The consumption of water-soluble fibers, which have a high viscosity (gelling capability), can decrease blood sugar–insulin levels and cholesterol levels, thus promoting weight loss. Fiber should be taken before each meal with 8 to 16 ounces of water.

CLA, or conjugated linoleic acid, is a fatty acid component of beef and milk, and is a powerful agent due to its many benefits for obese people. CLA can work as an antidiabetic drug, elevating insulin sensitivity. It is preventive and a partial treatment for cancer; it suppresses arachidonic acid, which can induce inflammation. It also promotes fat loss by inhibiting fat cells. The suggested dose is 3000-4000 mg a day. CLA could be combined with guarana, a caffeine-containing herb that is stronger than coffee and tea, and that has a uniquely slow release. (Guarana, unlike coffee, has a cooling effect and is used as a rejuvenating health tonic.) Guarana triggers a decrease in the number of fat cells by promoting the release of stored fat and then helping to turn the fat cells into energy. The end result is a higher metabolic rate. With CLA, guarana is successful in getting rid of extra fat.

Thyroid Hormone. . . Hypothyroidism's major characteristic is weight gain. It could be caused by selenium or zinc deficiency, stress, overconsumption of refined carbohydrates, excessive fasting or coffee consumption, food allergies, abuse of antibiotics, intestinal microflora imbalance, or metal or chemical toxicity from dental amalgam fillings, secondhand smoke or organic compounds (such as the softeners in plastics and food wrap, an overtaxed liver or antidepressants). After determining if a low level of the thyroid hormone exists, traditional medicine uses thyroxine to make up for the missing amount of hormone the thyroid gland cannot produce. Alternative medicine suggests detoxification, stress management, a better diet and infusions of the herb bladderwrack to rebalance thyroid function. Holistic medicine offers a natural form of thyroid hormone replacement. Acupuncture combined with Chinese herbal preparations can also be beneficial.

Exercise

Eating right without exercise offers little hope for success in fighting fat. Exercise has to be part of any body-reshaping effort, and for best results, a combination of aerobic and anaerobic exercises should be performed. Aerobics burn body fat and lower the body's setpoint, or weight-regulating mechanism, making weight loss easier. Anaerobics help to build lean body mass.

A person's setpoint will work against a weight-loss effort, which is why exercise has to be brought to bear in that effort. If you are used to being 150 pounds, for example, and then drop to 145, the brain creates signals in the form of hunger until your original weight is restored. But if you exercise and make intelligent food choices when you are hungry this will help the body get comfortable with a lower setpoint.

The type of exercise you do is not as important as consistency. The idea is to enjoy the exercise enough to make it part of a routine. A half hour of walking each day is a beneficial exercise that most anyone can engage in. The pace should be comfortable, not too hard. But dancing, swimming and even gardening are other good choices.

One word of caution: Before beginning an exercise program, it is important to get a complete physical from a doctor to rule out any underlying cardiac or pulmonary problems that may preclude exertion.

Breathing Exercises

When Pam Grout, author of *Jump Start Your Metabolism with the Power of Breath*, began doing breathing exercises for energy, she found, to her surprise, that she was able to lose 10 pounds without trying. Grout subsequently learned that shallow breathing accompanies being overweight, and that deep diaphragmatic breathing improves metabolism, and, secondarily appearance. Proper breathing contributes to weight loss because it sends more oxygen to the cells, which then allows cells to rapidly burn up and eliminate wastes. When we clean out the cells with each breath, fats do not get the chance to deposit themselves there. We have a lot more energy and far better health.

These are some of the breathing exercises Grout recommends:

Lie on the floor, relaxed, with hands down at the sides and palms up. Place a slightly heavy book on your stomach. With each inhalation, allow the book to raise up as high as possible, without straining. Bring the book back down with each exhalation. This is a good exercise for learning to pay attention to breathing.

Inhale through your nose to a comfortable count. Hold the breath for four times as long as the inhalation. This allows the body's cells to get lots of oxygen. Then exhale for twice as long as you breathed in. The ratio, then, is 1:4:2. So, if you count to five to inhale, you hold the air in to a count of 20, and then you exhale through your mouth to a count of 10. As you exhale, your tummy flattens and you get all the carbon dioxide out. For optimal benefit, this exercise should be performed for 10 rounds, three times a day.

Stress Management

Cortisol, the adrenal gland's hormone, when induced by stress reacts like insulin, delaying the release of fat. We can see the importance of natural stress management, accomplished with meditation and yoga. Cognitive therapy is also vital. We have to be able to let go of "comfort" addictions. People who end up being obese often use food as a tranquilizer to give themselves a temporary high. We should dare to face and address the real issues of our life that may be suppressed. But first we must give up the excuses. Also, finding joy in life and having a sense of humor can contribute to healing. Laughter is a powerful factor in overcoming autoimmune diseases.

Colon Cleansing

Sometimes people overeat because they are not absorbing nutrients. The brain does not perceive nutrients in the blood and therefore does not signal the body to stop craving food. By restoring intestinal health through colon cleansing, more nutrients are absorbed and a person tends to eat less.

What to Avoid

As mentioned earlier, dieting is ineffective and sometimes dangerous. Healthful eating should be a way of life, which means the elimination of processed foods, bad fats and certain carbohydrates, if an intolerance to them exists. Additionally a lack of exercise, a clogged colon and shallow breathing are counterproductive.

Substitutes for fattening foods are particularly harmful. First, they are based on the assumption that a person is not willing to change his or her eating habits, thereby reinforcing unhealthy food selections. Second, they introduce harmful chemicals into the system. Be particularly wary of artificial sweeteners. Aspartame, for one, is used in popular sugar substitutes and in many diet foods. While no detrimental effects have been proven in controlled studies, there have been reports of neurological reactions, such as hallucinations, dizziness and even epilepsy. And studies on rats have linked the product to brain tumors.

A new artificial food posing a potential challenge to consumer health is the fake fat Olestra. This product has a vacuum effect on the fat-soluble vitamins A, D, E and K and on the carotinoids. These vital nutrients are dissolved into the Olestra and passed out of the system before they can be utilized. As a result, the body is deprived of important protection against cancer and other illnesses.

Treatment Summary

Dieting has been the traditional approach to obesity. However, done in conventional fashion, this implies a temporary restriction of food intake or calories—not permanent change. The best approaches are ones that strive to reverse the condition long-term.

Learning proper nutrition and eating habits is essential. A healthy diet is high in carbohydrates and lower in protein and fat.

Nutritional supplements that help eliminate cravings and burn calories include chromium picolinate, essential fatty acids, gamma linoleic acid and others.

Exercise is an essential complement to a healthy diet. Consistency of routine is more important than the type of exercise.

Breathing exercises will teach proper breathing, which will improve metabolism and contribute to weight loss.

Colon cleansing restores colon health so that more nutrients can be absorbed, lessening the tendency to overeat.

Osteoporosis

Twenty-eight million Americans have osteoporosis, which is responsible for 1.5 million fractures each year, at a cost of $10-15 billion in medical expenses. Another 18 million Americans suffer from low bone mass, which increases their chances of eventually contracting the disease. Alarmingly, half of all women over 50 will have a fracture related to osteoporosis. Fractures—which usually occur in the hip, spine or wrist—are an omen for osteoporosis. With osteoporosis, the bones become porous, thereby increasing the occurrences of fracture. Women account for 80 percent of all cases of osteoporosis, with postmenopausal women being at the highest risk. Women who have recently experienced menopause often endure heightened bone loss and the cessation of bone growth as a result of the hormonal changes that have taken place.

The onset of osteoporosis is characterized by a sustained loss in calcium, a process that occurs at a rate of 1 to 2 percent per year in women in their mid-30s and increases to 4 to 5 percent during the postmenopausal years. Some people with osteoporosis suffer from defective calcium assimilation due to a deficiency of silica or phosphorous, while others may have a malfunctioning of the thyroid and parathyroid glands, which are responsible for calcium metabolism. The parathyroid glands control the level of calcium in the blood by secreting hormones that can balance the level when a shortage arises. During a calcium shortage, excess calcium, which is stored in the bones, joints and soft tissue, is discharged into the bloodstream, resulting in the reduction of bone mass. Acid blood, a condition induced by the consumption of acidic foods, excessive quantities of animal protein, stress and the accumulation of hazardous waste products within the body, fosters osteoporosis because the parathyroid glands are forced to balance the pH level of the blood by releasing excess calcium from the bones.

There are several risk factors for the condition, including a family history of the disease and excessive dietary intake of meat, caffeine, sugar, refined carbohydrates, or phosphates contained in soda and processed foods. Frequent consumption of alcoholic beverages, cigarette smoking and a sedentary lifestyle are additional contributory causes. Furthermore, evidence has shown that women of Northern European ethnic origin and women with small frames are at an increased risk of osteoporosis.

Contrary to what we've been told, large quantities of calcium-rich dairy products in the diet can actually contribute to the condition's onset. Researchers who travel to China often anticipate a high incidence of osteoporosis because of the country's lack of dairy intake, but to their surprise, there are actually few cases of skeletal disorders. Interestingly enough, in the U.S. and other Western nations, where abundant dairy intake is common, there is a higher rate of osteoporosis.

Symptoms

People who suffer from osteoporosis often experience pain in the lower back and the occurrence of sudden fractures due to fragile bone mass. Loss in height and skeletal deformity are other symptoms. Some early indications of calcium deficiency are gum disease and loose teeth, insomnia, back pain, height loss and cramps in the legs at night.

Treatment

The conventional medical approach to osteoporosis involves the introduction of synthetic estrogen into the body. Unfortunately, estrogen replacement therapy has been linked to an increased risk of heart attack, stroke, and uterine and breast cancer. Obviously, alternative approaches to the condition are worth examining.

Nutrition

A low dietary intake of animal products and a high intake of plant foods facilitate the growth and repair of the bones. Green leafy vegetables provide abundant sources of vitamin K, beta-carotene, vitamin C, fiber, calcium and magnesium, all of which promote the development of a healthy skeletal structure. Vitamin K is responsible for the formation of osteocalcin, the essential calcium building matrix protein involved in bone mineralization. Calcium is vital because it is a key nutrient in maintaining bone density. Over 99 percent of the calcium found in the body is in the bones and teeth. The blood contains the other 1 percent. Calcium sources include broccoli, milk, nuts and seeds. The Chinese, who have a low incidence of osteoporosis, frequently consume calcium-rich sesame seeds and cook with sesame oil. Lastly, isoflavones, found mainly in soy products, affect the body much like estrogen. Isoflavones increase bone density and retard bone loss in menopausal women.

Supplements

Women over the age of 25 require 500-1000 mg of calcium per day in addition to their dietary intake, a quantity that can be obtained in supplements of calcium citrate with magnesium. Women over the age of 40 should take 1500-2000 mg per day, while estrogen replacement patients require 1200-1500 mg. Other important supplements include magnesium citrate, vitamin C, beta-carotene, selenium, boron (5 mg), strontium, folic acid, silica (100 mg), copper, zinc and manganese (25 mg). Also important are vitamin D, which is necessary in absorbing calcium (the National Osteoporosis Foundation suggests taking 1200 mg of calcium and approximately 400 IU of vitamin D) and vitamin K, which could improve bone density, thereby lessening the risk of bone fractures (but those on blood-thinning medications such as warfarin must not take vitamin K). A balanced multivitamin/mineral supplement can supply most of these nutrients, but it is advisable to supplement the zinc separately in order to avoid decreased nutrient absorption.

Another cause of osteoporosis is a deficiency in essential fatty acids (for example, gamma linoleic acid and eicosapentaenoic acid). Reports show that supplementing with essential fatty acids stabilizes or increases bone mass. Essential fatty acids also increase calcium absorption.

A hormonal supplement that can be of value is DHEA; a substance that is depleted during the later years of life and that is useful in the treatment of chronic aging symptoms.

Herbs

The herb horsetail can be a valuable source of calcium, while nettles and dandelion can supply vitamin D.

An alternative to the use of synthetic hormones is the consumption of natural ones. Natural progesterone, which can be obtained from the herb wild yam, is preferable to synthetic estrogen because it promotes the development of healthy bones without harmful side effects. And while estrogen can only eliminate calcium loss, progesterone can actually replace depleted calcium in the bones. This useful substitute can be purchased in pill form or in a cream. For maximum benefit, half a teaspoon of the cream should be massaged into the skin twice a day over soft tissue and the spinal region for a period of two weeks out of every month.

Homeopathy

Homeopathy can serve as a valuable complement to diet and exercise in the prevention and treatment of osteoporosis. Calcarea phosphorica can be relied upon for extended periods of time for the treatment of soft, weak, curved or brittle bones. Corticoid helps alleviate the symptoms of post-traumatic osteoporosis and can be especially useful for older people who have recently fractured a hip. Parathyroids can aid in the treatment of pains in the long bones, ankles, knees and hips and can be beneficial to people who experience pain while walking.

Homeopathic remedies should be administered at a potency of 200c for acute pain, while people with chronic symptoms should begin treatment with 12c to 30c. Recommended dosages should be administered in groups of three to four pellets placed under the tongue and should be consumed on an empty stomach. It is advisable not to eat 15 minutes before or after taking homeopathic medication.

Exercise

Healthy bones, to some degree, are an indication of healthy living. Thus, regular exercising is the most significant step one can take to improve the strength of the bones. The performance of weight-bearing aerobic exercise and weight lifting can be a crucial factor in avoiding osteoporosis. And even after a patient has been diagnosed with the disorder, these forms of exercise can be beneficial. Of course it is important to obtain medical supervision at this time in order to design a program that will not result in injury.

Ideally, women should initiate an exercise program long before menopause to prevent osteoporosis. Aerobic exercise can be advantageous because it allows the muscles to engage in a continuous, rhythmic workout. Weight-bearing aerobic exercise, such as jogging, dancing, stair climbing and brisk walking, promotes mechanical stress in the skeletal system, contributing to the placement of calcium within the bones.

Although non-weight-bearing aerobic exercise, such as biking rowing and swimming, does not contribute to the strengthening of the bones as much as its counterpart, it does enhance flexibility and can be especially beneficial to women susceptible to arthritis. People involved in aerobic programs should exercise for 15 to 30 minutes, two or three times per week. A full day of rest between workouts is required to allow adequate time for the muscles to recuperate.

A warm-up and cool-down routine should become an integral part of the workout. Warm-ups, which are frequently confused with stretches, are relatively simple movements that enable the body to produce heat by enhancing the circulation of blood through the muscles. The performance of a warm-up routine prevents unnecessary injury to the muscles. The legs can be properly warmed up by lying on the floor and rotating them in a bicycle fashion or by walking in place, while the arms and upper body muscles are engaged in a full range of motion exercises. After the conclusion of your exercise routine your body should be quite flexible and you can proceed to the stretching segment of your workout. Remember that stretches should resemble long, continuous pulls and that bouncing will only tighten the muscles and can cause injury.

According to Ann Berwick, a practicing aromatherapist, the incorporation of warming and stimulating massage oils, such as rosemary, ginger, sage, blackberry and eucalyptus, into the warm-up routine can help improve its effectiveness. During the cool-down portion of your workout, a mixture of juniper, rosemary and lemon can help eliminate waste products and treat stiffness.

Yoga is an effective method of evading osteoporosis because it contributes to the development of healthy bones, corrects posture and allows the muscles to remain firm and limber. In addition, participants will benefit from improved coordination and balance. By strengthening the arms, yoga helps prevent fractures of the wrist, upper arm and forearm, which are common to women who fall with outstretched arms. Furthermore, improved strength and flexibility of the muscles can aid in the aversion of fractures by absorbing the shock of a fall and a correct posture lessens the possibility of spinal fractures. Older women often become involved in yoga in the hopes of avoiding getting dowager's hump. This condition, characterized by the slumping of the shoulders and caving in of the chest, significantly limits the movement of the body and puts extraordinary pressure on the spine, which can result in compression fractures of the spinal column. Improvement in balance and coordination can prevent fractures by reducing the chance of falling and improving response time.

There are several fundamental yoga poses that are effective in combating osteoporosis. In Downward Facing Dog, an exercise that aids in the fortification of bones in the arms and wrists, the body is positioned in a standing position with the hands on the ground, forming a triangular shape under the torso. There are actually three parts of this triangle. The first part consists of the area from the hands to the hips and the second is formed from the hips to the heels, while the final part is comprised of the space on the floor between the hands and feet. When this yoga position is properly performed the burden of body weight is placed upon the arms, and consequently, bone mass in the upper extremities is strengthened.

The Warrior Pose, which helps increase muscle strength, balance and flexibility, involves standing with the legs three to four feet apart (depending on one's height) and rotating one leg slightly inward and the other outward. Meanwhile, the arms can be positioned either out to the side or above the head. This exercise strengthens the hip muscles, which is crucial to preventing osteoporotic hip fractures.

The Cobra improves posture and increases flexibility and strength of the paraspinals, which are the muscles in the rear portion of the spinal cord. This yoga position is performed by laying facedown on the floor and using the back muscles to lift the head and chest away from the floor.

Women who already suffer from osteoporosis should be wary of forward-bending exercises, since they have a tendency to overexert the back and cause compression fractures. In addition, it is advisable to seek professional assistance (i.e., at a certified instructional facility) while participating in yoga to ensure that proper technique is practiced and potential injury averted. Ideally, again, women interested in yoga should begin participating considerably before the onset of menopause in order to prevent unnecessary pain and suffering later in life. When performed correctly, yoga can indeed effectively enhance the skeletal system and serve as an early deterrent to osteoporosis.

Women susceptible to slouching can improve their posture by practicing a relatively simple exercise. Fold a blanket to the size of a box of roses and then lay down with your head and spine centered on it. Your arms can either be placed at your sides with palms facing upward or can be held in the air creating a V-shape, while your shoulders should remain on the ground on either side of the supportive blanket. When the body is slouched, the intercostals, which are the muscles between the ribs, are constricted, causing a reduction in lung capacity and compression of nearby organs. By breathing deeply in the position described above, the intercostals are able to expand and potential organ compression can be averted.

Acupuncture

Chinese women have an exceptionally low incidence of osteoporosis, and when someone does acquire the disease in China, it is effectively treated with acupuncture. This method of treatment utilizes an electrical impulse along the spinal cord, which causes the reproductive cells, known as bone stem cells, to multiply and fortify the bone structure. When combined with the supplementation of calcium and weight-bearing exercise, this type of acupuncture can be an effective means of combating osteoporosis. In addition, studies have indicated that the performance of peripheral electrical stimulation in the legs can also aid in the strengthening of bone mass.

A practitioner of Traditional Chinese Medicine (TCM) treats osteoporosis with the hybrid treatments of acupuncture and herbs. In TCM, the kidneys oversee the bones and store the qi (energy) for the bone and marrow. When the marrow of the bone is not nourished, osteoporosis results. TCM states that this happens because the yin energy is exhausted from the kidneys. Hence, acupuncturists attempt to treat osteoporosis by energizing the kidneys with a technique that stimulates qi points that are associated with the kidneys.

What to Avoid

People can prevent osteoporosis by avoiding excessive intake of sugar, white flour, caffeine, carbonated sodas, meat, salt and alcohol. Prolonged consumption of these substances promotes the depletion of calcium from the bones and diminishes calcium production. Clinical studies have demonstrated a positive correlation between caffeine and alcohol intake and the occurrence of fractures in women. However, consumers of tea have less to worry about than coffee drinkers because tea contains a moderate level of caffeine relative to coffee.

Medical evidence has also established a direct link between the smoking of tobacco products and decreasing bone mass. Female smokers have lesser amounts of estrogen and often experience menopause earlier. Note that heavy reliance upon cow's milk and other dairy products will not ameliorate the symptoms of osteoporosis, as evidence has demonstrated that cultures that do not eat these products have lower incidences of the disease. Furthermore, dietary intake of protein-rich fish, eggs and chicken should be limited, because these foods contain inordinate amounts of the amino acid methionine. Methionine is transformed by the body into homocysteine, a chemical known to encourage the development of osteoporosis and arteriosclerosis (see *Heart Disease* and *Stroke*). Finally, people who are involved in homeopathic treatment should avoid coffee and aromatic substances, such as perfumes and breath mints, as these can hinder the effectiveness of the treatment. In addition, avoid excessive handling of the pills because residue from perfumes or other aromatic substances can debilitate the potency of the medication.

Treatment Summary

A low dietary intake of animal products and a high intake of plant foods, especially green leafy vegetables, facilitate growth and repair of bones.

Vitamins and minerals important to bone health include calcium, magnesium, vitamins D, K and C, beta-carotene, zinc and others.

The hormonal supplement DHEA may be helpful.

Some herbs that can help supply the body with substances necessary to keep the bones strong are horsetail, nettles, dandelion and wild yam, from which natural progesterone is obtained.

Homeopathy can serve as a complement to a bone-building diet and exercise program.

Weight-bearing aerobic exercise and weightlifting can be crucial in avoiding or alleviating osteoporosis.

Yoga is beneficial in combating skeletal problems.

Acupuncture offers a method that can treat osteoporosis by sending an electrical impulse along the spinal cord that fortifies bones.

Parasites

Many people have parasites and don't know it. Neither do their doctors. Often, when doctors are prescribing treatments for urinary tract infection, chronic fatigue, pelvic inflammatory disease, vaginitis, candida and other diseases, they are oblivious to the actual cause of their patients' ailments—parasites. If you have a condition that has not benefited from medical care, you should consider the possibility that your condition is a product of parasites. Recent estimates have indicated that seven million people suffer from parasites in our country alone.

Invasive parasites can be broken down into two categories: worms and protozoa. Worms, such as hookworms, pinworms, roundworms and tapeworms, are able to infiltrate the body and subsist on undigested food that accumulates on the intestinal walls. These intruders especially enjoy refined carbohydrates and sugar, which become lodged in the lower intestinal region as a result of decreased nutrient absorption. Insufficient pancreatic production of digestive enzymes or enzyme malfunction are often responsible for this maldigestion and the accrual of leftovers within the intestines.

While the presence of worms in the system can have many adverse effects, most people with parasites are affected by the second group, protozoa. The simple single-cell structure of protozoa facilitates infinite reproduction and enables the organism to defeat the body's complex defense system. Protozoa can thrive for prolonged periods inside the cells of the body creating a potentially difficult situation for our immune systems, which are unable to formulate a suitable response.

Causes

Although we in the U.S. are widely known for our general adherence to sanitation and health laws, parasites continue to pester many Americans for several reasons. First, parasite infestation is commonly caused by eating in restaurants where employees do not properly cleanse their hands before preparing food. In addition, if you or a sexual partner have traveled to a foreign country that does not adhere to strict sanitation laws, the risk of contracting a parasitic infection is increased. Another risk factor for parasite infection is drinking from an infested water supply that is commonplace in many cities and suburbs abroad and even domestically. The consumption of raw fruits and vegetables and undercooked meat and fish can promote parasite infection, as can working in a hospital, day care center, garden or sanitation facility. Evidence has linked the use of antibiotics and immunosuppressive medications to infection because of their tendency to alter the intestinal system and create a climate conducive to parasite development. Parasites do not usually survive in a healthy host; therefore, the presence of parasites within a human implies that he or she may suffer from a defect in the elimination process, an unhealthy diet or poor health habits. Public tap water is also a source of parasites. Finally, the escalating frequency of parasitic infection within our nation can be partially attributed to the increasing importation of foreign delicacies, such as sushi.

The detection of parasites in the body cannot always be effectively achieved by examining stool samples, since parasites fasten themselves to the mucosal surfaces of the intestines and thus are able to avoid the stream of waste exiting the body. Intestinal biopsy can also produce misleading results because, often, an uninfected area is extracted and studied.

A more accurate method of ascertaining whether parasites are present is a rectal swab examination. This test, which was designed by Dr. Herman Bueno, utilizes fluorescent stains in the identification of protozoan parasites.

Symptoms

The invasion of the human body by parasites can cause a wide variety of chronic symptoms, which, if left untreated, may expedite the onset of other serious disorders. The presence of parasites can have an adverse effect upon the intestinal system, causing flatulence, abdominal bloating and pain, foul-smelling stool, heartburn, constipation, anal itching, vomiting, bloody or mucousy stool and diarrhea. Psychologically, parasites can promote mood swings, varying degrees of depression, nightmares, irritability, spaceiness and hyperactivity. Parasites can also drain the body's energy resulting in chronic fatigue. Additional symptoms include fever, night sweats, weight loss, loss of appetite, rashes, hives, abnormal itching, arthritis, allergy, Crohn's disease, colitis, food allergies, anemia and insomnia. In women, parasites can promote the development of cervicitis, pelvic inflammatory disease and vaginitis and can contribute to a decreased libido.

Parasites can deplete the body of nutrients such as potassium, calcium, magnesium and vitamins A, B6 and B12, and overwhelm the immune system, which can lead to severe illness. The symptoms can last for as long as the life span of the particular parasite that is causing the harm.

The varied assortment of symptoms associated with parasitic disease is attributable to the ability of the parasite to interfere with a variety of essential bodily functions. For example, research has demonstrated that parasites are capable of manufacturing enzymes that can corrode the intestinal walls and allow toxins to infiltrate other parts of the body. Also, parasites can effectively disorient the immune system, creating a situation in which our own immuno-suppressive agents attack healthy tissue and thus induce autoimmune disorders.

Treatment

Herbs

The use of herbs in treating patients with parasitic infections is often more effective than prescription medications, such as Flagyl, because herbs can be safely consumed for extended periods of time, while prolonged dependence on drugs can lead to harmful side effects. Although most medical textbooks state that the treatment of chronic protozoal infection should last only 5 to 14 days, this is proven untrue by recent research, which has demonstrated that successful therapy usually takes several weeks, or even months.

The daily consumption of raw garlic or odorless supplements can eliminate most strains of parasites, including hookworms, tapeworms and giardia, and can effectively combat fungi, bacteria and viruses, as well. Garlic can also be administered in colonics and in juices. (Add the juice of three cloves of garlic to 4 ounces of vegetable juice and drink every two hours.) Garlic has allicin, which has demonstrated its ability to successfully fight entamoeba histolytica and giardia lambia. It is antiviral, antibacterial and antifungal. It can also be used against pinworms and roundworms.

Goldenseal, which contains an active ingredient known as berberine, is another herb with antiparasitic potential, and can be especially useful in defeating bacteria, fungi and parasites, particularly giardia parasites. Goldenseal has been used for ages against any infection involving the mucous membranes of the body. Unfortunately, goldenseal, unlike garlic, cannot be relied upon for more than a month at a time.

Several drops of green black walnut tincture, Western wormweed, cloves, capsicum, quassi chips, mullein leaf, cascara sagrada aged bark, thyme sweet Annie, cinchana and elecampane root added to purified water can effectively cause parasites to be exuded from various parts of the body. This concoction should be consumed when you first awaken and again at the end of the day.

Chaparral is yet another herb with antibiotic, parasiticidal properties. A small quantity of citrus seed extract can also be an effective means of expelling parasites from the body.

Black walnut is an effective herb against ringworm and athlete's foot, and for healing cracks in the hands and the feet. The juice of the unripe hulls of black walnuts is used for parasites and fungal infections. The herb wormwood has been used for ages to fight parasites. Wormwood tea is frequently used to fight pinworms and roundworms, though it is renowned for its effectiveness against giardia. Wormwood comes in tea, liquid extract and capsule form. Note: Stay away from the pure oil. It is poisonous.

American wormseed is different from wormwood. It is a traditional herbal remedy used in the tropics to eliminate roundworms, hookworms and tapeworms. It is often used with children.

Pumpkin seeds are used especially when tapeworms and roundworms are present. Theses seeds help immobilize and eliminate worms and other parasites in the intestines. For the seeds to be most effective, one must consume large amounts of them—up to 25 ounces for adults. Most people squash them and mix them with a juice.

Grapefruit seed extract is a powerful ally in the war against parasites. Grapefruit seed extract is usually considered to be nontoxic, as the tissues do not absorb it. This permits it to be used for several months. It is most often used against giardia and candida yeast, which can take a long time to eliminate.

In addition, there are several traditional Chinese herbs that have proven their ability to combat parasitic infection. The herb baibu can eliminate pinworms from the body when it is added to a cloth containing alcohol and worn while sleeping. When ku shen is assimilated into a tea, it can aid in the purification of the lower intestinal and urogenital regions. Lei wan is yet another versatile Chinese herb that can be helpful in defeating a wide variety of parasites. A knowledgeable herbologist can guide you further.

Nutrition and Supplements

The consumption of raw garlic, onions, horseradish and raw pumpkin seeds can help prevent the contraction of parasitic infections. In addition, supplements of magnesium, vitamin B12, capsicum and calcium can aid the body in its battle with parasites. Oil of oregano has proven its effectiveness in battling parasites. One study reported in *Phytotherapy Research* focused on oregano's ability to treat gastrointestinal parasites in 14 adults. The results were startling. After only six weeks, Entamoeba hartmanni completely disappeared in four cases, Blastocystis hominis completely disappeared in eight cases, and the gastrointestinal system was better in seven of the 11 patients who had B. hominis.

Certain foods can actually heighten the possibility of parasitic infection, so avoid excessive dietary intake of these products (see "What to Avoid," below).

Other Treatment Modalities

The weekly performance of colonics can aid in the prevention and treatment of parasitic infections because the cleansing of the bowels eliminates a potential breeding ground for microorganisms. Furthermore, colon therapy contributes to the fortification of the digestive system.

Detoxifying is a natural approach that cleanses the body of parasites that are in the stools or entrenched in the intestinal walls. Natural supplements include psyllium husks, citrus pectin, activated charcoal, bentonite clay, papaya extract, pumpkin seeds and flaxseeds.

Some additional forms of therapy include hydrogen peroxide therapy ozone therapy and the application of tea tree oil, acidophilus, probiotic homeopathic 59 and colloidal silver.

What to Avoid

Being careful about what you eat is always a good idea. To minimize risk of parasitic infection, beware of crustaceans, such as crabs, lobster and shrimp and avoid consumption of pork, pork products, raw beef and sushi. If you do eat meat, when preparing the raw meat, be sure to separate your meat cutting board from your vegetable cutting board, because during the handling of raw foods millions of parasites can easily be transferred from surface to surface. In addition, avoid intake of coffee, sugar, alcohol, milk and dairy products, as evidence has shown that they can contribute to the debilitation of the immune system, and consequently facilitate the influx of parasites. Although fruit, honey and tofu have significant nutritional value, people with parasitic infections should abstain from these products in order to allow time for the body to effectively combat the parasites.

Unfortunately, restaurants usually lack ideal sanitary conditions, or even the conditions of your home kitchen, so you should try to limit your consumption of meals at outside establishments. Salads and other raw foods can be especially dangerous because they're not exposed to the parasite-killing heat of cooking and, often, food preparers do not properly wash their hands after they leave the bathroom.

When cleaning utensils, the use of a food-grade hydrogen peroxide can aid in the prevention of infection. Many times people will only wipe fruits and vegetables with a cloth before they eat them, but this is an ineffective means of ridding them of parasites. So it is important to wash these foods in a solution of food-grade hydrogen peroxide.

Although urban and suburban water supplies are treated with chlorine, parasites frequently survive nevertheless, so beware of consumption of unfiltered tap water. And even though pets may be fun to sleep with, they can carry parasites and transfer them to their owners. Also, be sure to remove parasitic worms on a regular basis, try not to walk barefoot when around animals and avoid letting pets lick your face or eat from your plate. Remember not to leave the bathroom without properly washing your hands. Finally, if you are experiencing any type of elimination difficulties, be sure to correct the problem before the onset of putrefaction, a condition that is ideal for the breeding of parasites.

Treatment Summary

Herbs can be more effective than prescription medication in treating parasitic infections because they may be safely consumed for extended periods of time. Garlic is particularly recommended.

Supplements useful against parasitic infections include magnesium, vitamin B12, capsicum and calcium.

Colonics can aid in the prevention and treatment of parasitic infection.

To minimize risk, beware of shellfish, pork, raw beef and sushi.

Beware of raw food, such as salad, when eating out.

Unfiltered tap water can present a hazard.

Parkinson's Disease

Parkinson's disease, first described by James Parkinson in 1817, is a degenerative central nervous system disorder, the result of damage to brain cells. Statistics from the National Parkinson Foundation show that there are about 1.2 million people with Parkinson's disease in the US and Canada. Although the disease is usually associated with aging, young people may become affected due to encephalitis, carbon monoxide, heavy metal poisoning or drug use.

Symptoms

For centuries, physicians have noted the first signs of Parkinson's: a small tremor in the hands or a slight dragging of one foot. Symptoms grow more pronounced when the person is stressed or fatigued. Over time, voluntary movements become increasingly difficult. Walking becomes stiffer and slower. This is followed by speech difficulties and visual problems. Then the face becomes expressionless due to increased muscular rigidity. Since the person cannot control his or her facial muscles, there is often drooling. There may also be numbing of the hands and feet. Thinking processes remain normal, but they are stuck inside a debilitated body. For this reason, as symptoms worsen, a great depression may set in and lead to a shortened life span.

While quite a bit has been ascertained about the symptoms of Parkinson's, relatively little has been learned about its cause and cure. Even today, doctors cannot recognize the beginning stages of Parkinson's. As for all diseases, a proper diagnosis is crucial with Parkinson's. Distressingly, one postmortem study showed that 25 percent of persons who had been examined and determined to have Parkinson's did not, in fact, have Parkinson's!

Yet, don't be dismayed. Quite a bit of information is known about the disease, as well as about why it develops. Also, much is known about the conventional and alternative treatments for the disease that can ease the symptoms. These treatments have been known to halt Parkinson's progress.

While there has been no definitive cause stated for the disease, it is believed

Parkinson's is caused, in part, by a shortage of dopamine. In fact, the symptoms of the disease are attributed to a loss of cells in the substantia nigra region of the brain. These cells are responsible for producing dopamine. Dopamine is a neurotransmitter, a chemical messenger between nerve cells in the brains of mammals. The parts of the brain damaged by this insufficiency of dopamine are the parts that help regulate the nervous system and the body. One might say, "Well, let's monitor the loss of dopamine. As soon as it begins, we'll know that there is a possibility Parkinson's will ensue." The only problem with this logic is that the loss of dopamine is not noticed until about 80 percent of the amount found in the brain is lost. Perhaps, one aspect of earlier detection of the disease is the earlier detection of the decline of brain dopamine levels.

Epidemiology shows that men have a higher probability of developing Parkinson's than women. Caucasians appear to be afflicted more than any other race. For some unknown reason, the disease afflicts identical twins more frequently than the general population.

Another very credible theory is that Parkinson's has environmental causes. A recent study in the journal *Nature Neuroscience* showed that rotenone, a pesticide, caused Parkinson's symptoms when given to rats. The study indicated that the pesticide might have caused the mitochondria to make free radicals, which then led to the Parkinson's disease.

Treatment

Drugs are usually given in an attempt to correct imbalances of brain chemicals, such as dopamine and acetylcholine, but these often have unpleasant side effects. In order to relieve tremors, treatments have also been given to destroy parts of the brain. For example, the nerve to the area may be cut, or alcohol may be injected into certain areas.

In the natural arena, major lifestyle changes must be addressed. Parkinson's patients do require a great deal of therapy, but major improvements are possible through natural means.

Nutrition

A fresh, live-foods diet is essential to the healing process. The diet should incorporate mostly alkaline foods, with green drinks, such as chlorella, spirulina, barley grass or wheatgrass, once or twice a day. Also good are vegetables such as red beets, carrots, spinach, green beans and red onions. Make sure all fruits and vegetables are organic, which means they were grown without chemical toxins. For similar reasons, those afflicted with the disease should consume only bottled or filtered water. Studies have also shown a link between sugar and fat consumption and the chance of developing Parkinson's. In addition, microwaving food is taboo.

Antioxidants are critical for overcoming oxidative damage to the brain and for slowing down progression of the disease. Some of the best antioxidants for this purpose contain compounds known as PCO's, found in extracts of grape seed and white pine bark. About 100 mg three times daily are generally recommended. Vitamin C is another important antioxidant for this condition that helps to flush toxins from the system. In addition, the brain nutrient phosphatidylserine should not be overlooked. Also, when a person is depressed, the amino acid DLPA has been found to work well.

Herbs that work with Parkinson's patients include hawthorn extract and ginkgo biloba. Over time, these can improve circulation, minimize leg cramp and tremors, and increase a feeling of well-being. Nervines, such as skullcap, valerian, hops and lady's slipper, can help to rebuild the nervous system.

Tyrosine and phenylalanine are amino acid precursors to dopamine, and are found in both protein foods and supplements.

Studies indicate that to properly treat Parkinson's, oxidative stress must be reduced. Chelation therapy plays an important role in eliminating iron as well as other toxins from the brain. These toxins infuse the brain with free radicals. Some think that chelation can occur only through chelation therapy. However, antioxidants can also play the role of chelators. The C and E vitamins, bioflavonoids, polyphenols (from black and green teas), grape seed extract (specifically, the proanthocyandins) and tocotrienols from curcumin also serve as chelators.

Glutathione is another important warrior in the battle against Parkinson's. It is not easily found in foods, though sulfur-rich foods remain the primary source. However, far and away the best way to obtain glutathione remains supplementation, orally or intravenously. An indirect way of elevating the body's glutathione levels is supplementing with N-acetyl-cysteine or L-cysteine.

Recent reports indicate that an up-and-coming substance in the battle against Parkinson's is coenzyme Q10. These studies show that orally consuming CoQ10 can impede the march of Parkinson's. Though other research has proven CoQ10 effective in treating Huntington's disease and other neurological abnormalities, these are the first studies demonstrating its efficacy in combating a major neurodegenerative disease. One particular study demonstrated that coenzyme Q10 supplementation at a dosage of 1200 mg per day reduced mental and physical problems 44 percent more than the placebo.

Melatonin may prove effective in treating Parkinson's. Based on a study with rats, researchers concluded that melatonin could be helpful in treating Parkinson's and other neurodegenerative disorders caused by free-radical damage.

Exercise

Exercises involving weight training have been linked to increasing testosterone levels, which in turn, elevate dopamine levels. Hence, exercising is crucial in fighting Parkinson's.

Aromatherapy

Massage with fragrant essential oils will not cure Parkinson's disease, but can have beneficial effects. Clary sage, marjoram and lavender are recommended. Anxiety, lack of energy, muscular pain, stiffness of gait and sleeping problems are all aspects of Parkinson's that may be alleviated by aromatherapy.

What to Avoid

Older adults commonly develop drug-induced Parkinson's disease after having been prescribed antipsychotic drugs, such as Haldol, Thorazine, Mellaril and Stelazine. These antipsychotics are used to sedate nursing home patients with dementia and chronic anxiety, two nonpsychotic disorders. When these drugs are discontinued, most newly diagnosed Parkinson's patients return to normal.

Studies show that toxic pesticides routinely used in agriculture and lawn care are linked to Parkinson's disease. People tend to discount low levels of exposure, but in children, the elderly and people already ill, even small amounts can be damaging, leading to any number of problems, including nervous disorders and cancers.

Heavy metals harm the central nervous system. Therefore, avoid aluminum cookware, remove amalgam dental fillings and stay away from cigarette smoking, as cigarette papers contain cadmium. Hair analysis can be performed to see if high levels of these and other metals need to be chelated out of the body.

Treatment Summary

Drugs are conventionally given to correct chemical imbalances, but they often have unpleasant side effects.

Destruction of parts of the brain is sometimes attempted to stop tremors. A nerve may be cut or alcohol may be injected into a motor area.

Maximizing nutrition, emphasizing a live-foods diet, with alkaline foods and green juices, is beneficial.

Antioxidant nutrients are extremely important for Parkinson's patients. In particular, they may benefit from L-carnitine (500 mg two times per day), phosphatidyl choline (500 mg two times per day), L-glutathione (1000 mg), L-cysteine (500 mg), ginkgo (125 mg), DHEA (25 mg), melatonin (5 mg),

CoQ1O (200 mg), L-phenylalanine (500 mg), L-taurine (500 mg), chelation therapy, vitamin C and glutathione therapy, choline (1000 mg), inositol (1000 mg), B-complex (50 mg three times per day), PCO's, vitamin C and phosphatidylserine.

The amino acid DLPA works to counter depression.

Herbs can improve circulation, minimizing cramps and tremors. Hawthorn extract and ginkgo biloba are noteworthy in this regard. Soothing, nervine herbs include skullcap, valerian and hops.

Aromatherapy may alleviate Parkinson's symptoms. Additionally, antioxidants also help: L-glutathione (1000 mg), vitamin C (5000-10,000 mg), NAC (1500 mg), alpha lipoic acid (500 mg), quercetin (700 mg), pycnogenol (200 mg).

Periodontal Disease

Normal healthy gums are pink and do not bleed, but this is rarely seen. In fact, 90 percent of Americans suffer from gum conditions, the most common ones being gingivitis and periodontitis. Unfortunately, most periodontal disease goes largely unnoticed, as it progresses slowly and silently over a period of years. That's why it's vital to understand what gum disease is, how it develops, and how to prevent and treat it.

Types of Periodontal Disease

Gingivitis

Gingivitis is an infection of the gums usually associated with poor dental hygiene and the accumulation of bacterial plaque on the teeth. Food debris, bacteria and the normal turnover of skin cells create sticky deposits that accumulate along the gum line and around the necks of the teeth, leaving a thin, white coating. If not removed, this bacterial plaque will harden within 72 hours to form calculus or tartar, material that cannot be brushed off. This makes it difficult to remove bacteria, which is the cause of swollen, infected and bleeding gums. As the gum continues to swell, pockets form near the teeth. Eventually, calculus lodges within these pockets, setting up an environment that contributes to the development of gingivitis.

Gingivitis may be triggered by a variety of factors. These can include ill-fitting fillings, birth control pills, constant breathing through the mouth, certain illnesses, such as diabetes mellitus and leukemia, and vitamin deficiencies. In addition, bacterial formations in the mouth are often the result of too many of the soft, sticky foods that are common to American diets. Vitamin C and niacin deficiencies can also result in gingivitis.

Researchers have long been baffled by the link between gingivitis and heart disease. People with gum disease—in which the gums bleed—have a 25-percent increased risk for heart disease, as compared with individuals who have healthy gums. However, the cause-and-effect link has never been firmly established.

Now, according to a 2000 study, those who have gum disease are apt to have elevated blood levels of fibrinogen (clotting factor) and C-reactive protein (CRP). (See *Stroke*.)

Periodontitis

While gingivitis is reversible, the patient who ignores the problem may advance to periodontitis, a more severe, degenerative condition causing irreversible bone loss. According to the American Academy of Periodontology, 32 million Americans are currently suffering from this silent, progressive condition. In people over the age of 35 periodontitis is the leading cause of tooth loss.

If a patient with gingivitis does not regularly disturb bacterial formations, the bacterial colonies will get denser, resulting in less oxygen available to support typical healthy and gingivitis-related bacteria. Now anaerobic bacteria begin to accumulate. These are highly pathogenic, and the result is degeneration of the underlying tissues and bone resorption.

There are several reasons people develop periodontitis. First, smoking can be implicated, as well as chewing tobacco. In addition, ill-fitting bridges, fillings and crowns (caps) harbor and encourage the proliferation of harmful bacteria. Poor dental hygiene obviously promotes periodontitis. And a significant contributing factor to the onset of periodontitis is diet. Research has shown that periodontitis was not nearly as prevalent in primitive civilizations as it is today. Without a doubt, this is due in large part to the dominance of refined foods, such as white flour and white sugar, in modern diets. Also, today, people live longer and teeth are subject to longer exposure to a wider variety of organisms. It is therefore especially important to develop good gum care habits early and to carry them throughout life.

Symptoms

Since gum disease progresses silently, some people will notice no symptoms at all. Others will be aware of subtle changes that occur in stages. As mentioned earlier, when a person is healthy, the gums are light pink, very firm and do not bleed. As plaque accumulates, the teeth will appear to have a white coating at the gum line and within five days gingivitis will manifest. During this preliminary stage of gum disease, the gums will bleed more often, especially in the morning when a person is brushing, flossing or eating something hard. In addition, the gums will exhibit moderate inflammation. This inflammation can be characterized by swelling, redness, heat, loss of function and sensitivity. Sometimes a peculiar taste and odor will develop in the mouth.

As periodontal disease becomes more chronic, a bluish or purplish tint can appear. If the disease is not treated in its initial stages, the gums can start to recede. At this time, bleeding can worsen. Sometimes, however, bleeding stops. Pockets develop and deepen in size to about the 4- to 6-mm range, and slight bone loss is exhibited. As periodontitis progresses, pockets deepen further, measuring 6 to 8 mm, or more. Continual bone loss will cause spaces in between the teeth to develop, and eventually, permanent tooth loss will result.

Treatment

There are two basic treatments traditionally used for periodontal disease. One is surgery. During surgery, part of the gum is cut away, and some bone may be reshaped. The focus of surgery today is regeneration of tissue.

The second approach is antibacterial therapy. This involves long-term behavioral change with careful adherence to a rigorous self-cleaning program that can significantly improve gum health. Many patients using this approach report gratifying gradual success. First, they notice that the gums no longer bleed when they brush or floss. After some more time, the gums stop receding and become firmer. As this occurs, loose teeth become more secure, and the bacterial infection within the gum line subsides. Consequently, inflammation resolves, pain is alleviated and the infection in the mouth is finally controlled.

Of course, prevention is the best approach to gum disease, and there is a lot that people can do in this vein, namely brushing, flossing, irrigating and receiving dental cleanings on a regular basis. Many dentists believe that preventive dentistry can quell harmful bacteria during the preliminary stages of a gum problem, but that in serious cases, it becomes more difficult to eliminate the bacteria because toxins become lodged below the surface of the gums. Pockets in excess of 10 mm deep should be treated with a special applicator device designed to cleanse deep pockets. Now accessible to the general public, this type of applicator utilizes a safe, low-pressure stream, and can be used to bathe the pocket with an antiseptic solution containing hydrogen peroxide or table salt.

There are several natural rinses that are recommended for gum infections due to their ability to eliminate the bacteria responsible for periodontal infections. One such remedy is an herbal rinse containing calendula, which is a mixture of marigolds, goldenseal and myrrh brewed into a tea. When preparing calendula, dilute the herbs with an amount of water that suits your personal tolerance. After the ingredients are brewed into a tea, the tea should be strained. Then use the liquid to irrigate the gum line, while the remaining granules can be applied during brushing. Other herbal rinses that have proven effective in treating gum disease are made from propolis, echinacea, garlic and tea tree oil.

Baking soda may be the best combatant of shallow infections. It can also aid in neutralizing the acids emitted by infectious bacteria. Baking soda can be mixed with water, or if the infection is especially bad, hydrogen peroxide. This is also a great trick for stain removal. By adhering to a strict irrigation, brushing and flossing routine, you can alleviate surface infections and quell some of the painful symptoms of periodontitis. However, you should not become overconfident, as infections hidden deep within pockets in the gum line can continue to proliferate and ravage the underlying gum structure. Most dentists will attest to the fact that surface precautions cannot reach beyond a 4-mm threshold. It is therefore advisable to work in conjunction with your holistic dentist and dental hygienist. Then, and only then, can periodontitis be controlled.

Nutrition

Proper dietary intake is crucial in preventing gingivitis and periodontitis. Fresh fruits and vegetables, whole grains, and fiber should be mainstays of the menu, according to biologic dental practitioners. Raw fruits and vegetables are especially beneficial because of their ability to enhance enzyme functioning. People who are able to assimilate dairy products should continue to do so, many practitioners advise, because dairy products can provide the body with an abundant quantity of calcium. Fermented dairy products, such as yogurt, are best, since they help maintain intestinal health. Cow's milk is also recommended; however, people who are intolerant of it should supplant cow's milk with goat's milk. If you are completely intolerant of dairy products, you can obtain an ample amount of calcium from green leafy vegetables, especially kale or dandelion greens, collard greens or turnip greens. Not only is the calcium in these last suggestions easier to assimilate than that in dairy products, but these vegetables also contain several other useful nutrients, including beta-carotene, vitamin A, vitamin C, vitamin E, enzymes and minerals.

Supplements

Sometimes proper nutrition cannot be completely obtained through our diets. If a person with periodontitis is not receiving a satisfactory quantity of calcium from his or her food intake, supplementing with calcium is a good idea. Periodontitis is frequently accompanied by blood sugar problems like hypoglycemia or diabetes, which make it more difficult for the person to effectively combat infections. Often these particular people, especially those who suffer from low blood sugar levels, will benefit by supplementing their diets with zinc, manganese and magnesium. Magnesium and calcium are both crucial to the bones that provide the foundation for the teeth. Manganese also serves to maintain the ligaments that surround the teeth, but is a nutrient often neglected by both conventional and holistic dentists. Chromium fortification should also be part of the treatment regimen, as almost 90 percent of Americans are deficient in this mineral. Chromium aids in transporting insulin into the cell mitochondria, where it is consumed and converted into energy. The micronutrients vanadium and boron are needed for proper bone structure, and silicon and zinc are important as well. Essential fatty acids are beneficial because they facilitate the transportation of calcium and magnesium through the cell membrane.

Coenzyme Q10 is a nutrient that has been used by the Japanese to treat disease in which the patient suffers from severe inflammation, strange tastes, abscesses, pus accumulations within the gum pockets and significant pain and halitosis (bad breath). CoQ10 begins its work in the mitochondria. Since CoQ10 is fat soluble, it penetrates the cell membrane, acting as the messenger link between the various enzymes in the electron transport chain. Optimal levels of CoQ10 must be present in the cell membrane for energy to be produced. No other substance can substitute for CoQ10.

In addition to energy production, CoQ10 plays a vital role as an antioxidant at the cellular level, having the ability to neutralize the effect of free radicals, which damage cell membranes and lead to disease states and aging. As early as the 1970s, researchers found that gum tissue in people with periodontal disease was often deficient in CoQ10. Subsequent studies have shown deterioration of the gums to be halted and healing to occur, sometimes within days, at dosages of 50-75 mg a day.

The homeopathic remedy cali corbonicum can be used to treat cases of periodontitis in which a person is plagued by purulent pockets without abscesses, as well as excessive saliva, halitosis, strange tastes, digestive pain and a pale or coated tongue. Calcarea fluorica is prescribed by homeopaths for patients with loose teeth, digestive problems, dry tongue and a painful burning sensation, while staphysagria can aid in combating cases characterized by black stained teeth, bleeding, bone loss, tooth decay and pain.

Homeopathy also offers preventive treatment for gum disorders with the idea that discouraging the initial accumulation of debris on the teeth can avert gingivitis and periodontitis. One remedy that can be used to prevent calculus accumulation is fragaria, which should be consumed at 6c potency twice daily. This treatment aids in dissolving existing accretions, so when the dentist scales your teeth, the process is easier.

What to Avoid

Although sometimes a genetic predisposition to gum disease exists, most cases can be averted by incorporating several simple precautions into our daily routines, and by avoiding certain activities.

Since nutrition can play such an important role in gum disease, it is obviously important to eat correctly. Try to avoid refined carbohydrates, alcohol and caffeine whenever possible. Soda should also be avoided—especially dark soda—because it will encourage the loss of calcium. Also, smoking can facilitate the onset of periodontitis. Remember that refined sugars should be eliminated, as sugar hampers several vital immune system functions, including white blood cell migration and phagocytosis, which is the ability of white blood cells to eliminate bacteria, viruses and other infectious intruders. Plus sugar can contribute to the gradual depletion of minerals needed for healthy bones and teeth. Most Americans could also benefit from avoiding excessive phosphorus consumption. Although most of us eat calcium-rich foods, only a limited quantity of this essential nutrient is actually absorbed by the body due to the fact that phosphorus, which is in red meat, soda and fast foods, can force calcium out of the body. In an attempt to replace the nutrient, the body takes calcium from bones and deposits it as tartar on teeth and in arteries. The ideal diet has a phosphorus to calcium ratio of approximately 4:10.

Treatment Summary

Surgery may be needed in some cases of gum disease.

Proper dental hygiene is vital, both to prevent periodontal conditions and to treat them.

Noninvasive approaches to gum disease include massaging the gums to dislodge and eliminate infectious debris, natural rinses to help get rid of harmful bacteria and baking soda to combat shallow infections.

A fruit and vegetable-rich diet, with whole grains and fermented dairy products, promotes gum health.

Calcium, magnesium, zinc, manganese, chromium and vitamin C are some of the nutritional supplements a person may need to combat periodontal disease.

When combined with a good diet and regular cleanings, homeopathic remedies can help reduce gum conditions.

Phobias

Phobias are overwhelming, irrational fears of specific objects or situations. People feel intense discomfort, sometimes to the point of panic, when faced with the feared object. The usual way of dealing with this problem is to avoid the stimuli entirely, which can create varying degrees of hardship.

Types of Phobias

There are three types of phobias, the first and most common being simple phobias, which affect about 10 percent of men and women, in equal proportion. Typical simple phobias are fear of animals, heights, medical procedures, needles, elevators, water and air travel.

The second category is social phobias, which involve the fear of being embarrassed or humiliated in public. Number one on the list here is the fear of public speaking. In fact, surveys show this to be more frightening to many people than the thought of death. Other social phobias include fear of being in restaurants and other public places, using public toilets, blushing in public, dating and meeting new people. With a social phobia, a person feels self-conscious about being judged to the point of not being able to function around others.

About one in 20 people are affected by the third and most severe type of phobia, agoraphobia (literally, "fear of the marketplace"). Individuals with this condition avoid public places for fear of having a panic attack. Usually, the condition begins after such an attack occurs spontaneously. Then, the person avoids going to places where he or she might be embarrassed should another attack occur. Or the person may fear being unable to escape if he must. The panic a person feels is tantamount to a severe stress reaction. Symptoms include heart palpitations, rapid heartbeat, chest pain and shortness of breath, which can leave the person thinking that he or she is having a heart attack. There may also be dizziness, nausea, sweat, a choking sensation and chills. Feelings of unreality and loss of control take over and the individual feels detached, as if dying. In milder cases of agoraphobia, people tend to avoid closed places, like grocery stores, bridges, tunnels and subways. They may go to places close to home with a person they consider safe. In the worst-case scenario, individuals remain homebound. Some will not even go from one room to another in their own home.

Causes

Phobias usually begin after the brain associates some object or situation with a frightening or traumatic event. Sometimes the connection is clear. A person who almost drowns as a child develops a water phobia, for example. But at other times the relationship is far less obvious. Elaine Magidson, of Creative Counseling in New York, tells of a client who had a phobia of butterflies. Although the woman lived in the city and was not likely to see any, she was obsessed with the possibility, and it was making her day-to-day life difficult. Special counseling techniques helped her to recall a traumatic incident in her life that took place when she was just three years old. At that time, her mother was having a nervous breakdown and being placed in a straitjacket by men about to take her away. As she watched, screaming and crying, a butterfly flew past. From that moment on, all the horror of the event became subconsciously associated with these insects.

Sometimes phobias are simply the result of people being afraid of something early in life and then spending their whole lives avoiding it. A fear of dogs may cause a child to stay away from them. This becomes a pattern, and the person still avoids them years later. Because it occurs for so long, the person's fear of dogs turns into a phobia.

Of course, parental conditioning can contribute to this. Another way a phobia might form is through modeling. A child watches a phobic parent and begins to copy his or her behavior. Some believe a genetic tendency is involved as well. Research with identical twins shows, in fact, that agoraphobia has a genetic component.

Another factor contributing to agoraphobia is upbringing, where a child has overprotective, perfectionistic or hypercritical parents. Or their parents have continually given them the message that life is a dangerous place. As a result, the child becomes sensitive and frightened of the world.

Nutritional imbalances may play a role. Too much sugar, caffeine or alcohol can cause physiological imbalances that increase stress and cause hypoglycemia, hypothyroidism and nutritional deficiencies, making agoraphobia more likely to be manifested in susceptible individuals. Certain foods and food additives can cause allergic reactions that increase susceptibility to the disorder as well. Unless these stresses are addressed, they can build up in the system until one day some incident triggers a full-fledged panic attack.

Treatment

The traditional psychological approach to phobias involves imagery and real-life desensitization. Imagery begins with placing the person in a state of deep relaxation. He or she may be asked to visualize a peaceful scene, like a beach or a mountaintop. Progression relaxation techniques may be used. Then, gradually, the person goes from imagining that safest space to ones that are more difficult, involving the feared object or experience. Someone with a phobia about elevators may go from the peaceful beach scene to a relatively unthreatening elevator scene, such as seeing himself with someone he trusts pressing a button outside the elevator door. A session or two later, he may feel comfortable enough to watch the door open. Then he sees himself going into the elevator with that person and so on, until he finally envisions himself going up and down many floors alone. This is followed by real-life desensitization, where small steps to overcoming a phobia are actually taken. People become accustomed to each small success before moving ahead. But the road is not always direct. Generally, people make progress and then fall back a few steps before moving forward again.

While this commonly accepted method works for many people, it has its problems. It involves a lot of time, which means a long-term commitment to the process. This is often difficult for phobic individuals, who may not have the time or not want to make it because discomfort is involved.

Also, anxiety-reducing medicines are commonly prescribed. While these may be helpful at low dosages when a person is first beginning desensitization, the disadvantage is that the person may only feel better while on the medication. After it is stopped, the phobia may still exist.

Natural therapies, used alone or with traditional modalities, may be effective in treating phobias and other anxiety disorders.

Inositol

Inositol is derived primarily from cereals and legumes. Inositol can influence biological activities in the body. It has been proven effective in treating panic attacks and obsessive-compulsive disorder. In one study, patients received 12 g of inositol each day for four weeks. During the next four weeks, they received a placebo. Their panic attacks decreased twice as much when they received the inositol as when they were on the placebo. The researchers found inositol to be safe and potentially therapeutic in the treatment of panic disorder.

In a double-blind, placebo-controlled study, inositol was given to OCD patients at a dose of 18 g a day. Improvements were noted after six weeks. These improvements were similar to those experienced with the orthodox drugs Prozac and Luvox.

L-Theanine

Theanine is an amino acid that is derived almost entirely from green tea. Its strength is that it easily crosses the blood-brain barrier and alters the biochemistry, thereby increasing concentration and the ability to focus one's thoughts. Volunteers were given oral doses of theanine at 50-200 mg. Forty minutes afterwards, a measuring of their brain alpha waves showed that the theanine had a relaxing effect, without causing drowsiness, in the subjects.

Adapton

Adapton is a substance obtained from a species of deep sea fish called garum armoricum. It is widely used in Europe and Japan to treat stress, anxiety and depression. It helps regulate the nervous system, thus allowing a person to better cope with mental and physical stress. Adapton also improves concentration, mood and sleep.

Lifestyle Changes

Meditation quiets and clears the mind. The results of clinical studies show that meditation causes metabolism rates and blood pressure to drop.

There is mounting evidence that regular exercise is effective in treating mild to moderate depression. A recent study concluded that there is plenty of evidence supporting the use of exercise in the treatment of clinical depression, and that aerobic and resistance exercise enhances mood states. There is no precise explanation for why exercise helps decrease depression and improve other psychiatric disorders. However, the improvements may very well be the result of the brain's release of endorphins. Endorphins calm and soothe.

Neurolinguistic Programming

Newer techniques take a quicker, more direct approach. Neurolinguistic programming, like the traditional approach, does use relaxation, but it uses several short-cut techniques that can be quite effective. Instead of involving the person in progressive relaxation techniques each time, where each muscle is tensed and then relaxed, the person gives himself a cue to get into that same calm state. The cue could be visual, auditory or kinesthetic, and might involve gazing at a candle, squeezing the elbow or saving something nice for yourself. This technique, called anchoring, saves a lot of time by creating a relaxed state immediately.

After anchoring, the next step in the "fast phobia cure" is called double-stepped association, and gets the person to step away from a scene while imagining it. It is as if the individual is watching an actor in a movie. This makes the phobia less personal and therefore less frightening.

Other interesting techniques are used to take power away from negative emotions. For example, when people are upset about something, they tend to remember it in vivid colors. Having people see the experience in black and white it lessens the intensity of feeling.

The philosophy behind these methods is that a person becomes conditioned to a phobic response very quickly, and can become unconditioned just as fast.

Educational Kinesiology

This technique is used alongside neurolinguistic programming, and involves exercises that promote better mind/body balance. These exercises distribute energy throughout the brain in such a way as to promote greater relaxation and reduce stress. For example, the brain stem becomes active under duress. When that energy is transferred to the cerebral area, more rational thought processes take over, and a lot of discomfort disappears.

A simple way to do this is to place the fingers on the middle of the eyebrows, and move them about one inch up into a soft space in the forehead. Pressing into the area for several seconds when one is anxious immediately promotes relaxation by transferring energy from the brain stem to the cerebrum.

Acupressure

There is an acupressure technique used against anxiety or nervousness. Apply slight pressure to the indentation in the center of our breastbone, known as the sternum. Holding four fingers over the area opens up breathing and releases tension.

To relieve irritability or an agitated feeling, rub the top of your shoulder and notice where it feels tightest. This will probably be close to your neck. Hold this point and breathe slowly and deeply.

Acupressure can be done on oneself, or a friend or family member can help. The idea is that the application of pressure relieves tension, as well as alleviating pain and increasing circulation.

Affirmations

Affirmations are based on the principle that our thoughts and words create our experiences. Taking a situation that ordinarily frightens us and using thoughts and words to affirm the type of situation we want for ourselves make a world of difference. An agoraphobic who has difficulty traveling might say, "I travel with ease and feel relaxed." Initially, we do not believe what we are telling ourselves. Otherwise, we would not need to be making affirmations.

But affirmations do make a difference over time. Positive thoughts and words impact our subconscious mind, enabling us to create new patterns of behavior.

Counseling

Building self-esteem and improving communication skills are essential elements in recovery. Phobias serve to protect the person in some way, and once they are eliminated the person needs support.

Affirmations can be used in conjunction with counseling, as in journal writing. One journal-writing exercise has a person divide a page in two and write on one side, "I accept myself no matter what." On the other side, all the objections to that thought can be recorded. Sometimes, by writing down negative thoughts, their positive thoughts can be explored.

Nutritional Support

Research shows certain nutrients have a positive effect on brain chemistry. Some nutrients that work to reduce anxiety are the B-complex vitamins, calcium, magnesium and GABA. Also of value in this regard are the amino acid L-tryptophane, the omega-3 fatty acids and inositol.

Herbs

Herbal agents that calm the nerves are known as nervines. A common one that is easy to find is valerian. Valerian is a tonic for the nerves that is best taken when an anxiety attack is imminent. It is especially recommended for nervous problems that are due to emotional stress or pain. While small amounts of valerian are helpful, large doses should be avoided as they can bring on depression. Lady's slipper is an eastern woodlands plant that has traditionally been used by Native Americans as a nervous system soother. People sometimes make a flower essence of it, leaving this rare species intact in the ground. Lady's slipper is often combined with other nervines, such as hops, skullcap, chamomile, passionflower or celery. Hops will calm a nervous stomach and, when placed beneath a pillow, it is said to promote sleep in an insomniac. Skullcap is a remedy for overcoming sleep disorders and agitation. Chamomile and passionflower help nervous conditions in people of all ages. Celery is yet another tonic for nervousness.

In Ayurvedic medicine, the herb that specifically alleviates anxiety attacks is called Ashwagandha. Much scientific research from India confirms that Ashwagandha calms because it is actually a nutrient for the brain and nerves.

Recently, the South Pacific herb kava kava was approved in Germany for its antianxiety effects. The plant is a species of pepper that aboriginal people have taken for over a millennium for relaxation purposes. Kava kava has become popular recently, but some cautions should be taken. First, it works synergistically with alcohol, so the two should not be used together. Second, due to its potency, a person can become impaired to the point of not being alert enough to perform such tasks as driving or operating machinery. And third, a pigment in the plant can build up in the body, causing an itchy, scaly skin condition. Fortunately, the problem will go away once kava kava is discontinued. However, this is nature's warning to use the herb sparingly.

What to Avoid

Alcohol, caffeine, sugar and nicotine cause chemical imbalances in the brain. Many people rely on these substances to avoid anxiety, not knowing that they actually cause it.

Treatment Summary

Imagery and desensitization are the traditional method of treatment for phobias. While this works for many people, it usually involves a long-term commitment and sometimes involves medications. However, there are some newer techniques that take a quicker, more direct approach.

Neurolinguistic programming is a newer method that involves short-cut psychological approaches to decondition the person from their phobic responses.

Educational kinesiology is used in addition to neurolinguistic programming and involves exercise that promotes better mind/body balance.

Acupressure can be used as a tool against phobic responses.

The use of affirmations is based on the principle that positive thoughts and words impact the subconscious mind, facilitating creation of a new pattern of behavior.

Antianxiety nutrients include the B-complex vitamins, calcium, magnesium, GABA and L-tryptophane.

Valerian and several other herbs have an antianxiety effect.

Pregnancy-Related Problems

Pregnancy is a time of promise, joy and vitality. But there can be physical problems associated with it too. Morning sickness, breast tenderness, fatigue and constipation are some of the many complaints commonly associated with term pregnancy. Further, after childbirth many women experience depression due, in part, to hormonal shifts in the body. Women should be aware that there are many natural, safe ways to alleviate pregnancy-related discomforts. Discuss these with your doctor or midwife, with the understanding that each pregnancy is different.

Common Pregnancy Discomforts and Their Management

Morning Sickness

Hormonal shifts during the first trimester decrease the secretion of hydrochloric acid in the stomach. This can lead to poor functioning of muscles that move food along the digestive tract, which in turn can lead to the nausea and vomiting in early pregnancy, known as morning sickness. The best way to alleviate morning sickness is to get plenty of rest and to eat several small, easily digested meals, since nausea typically starts on an empty stomach. Crackers should be kept by the bed and eaten before getting out of bed in the morning. Protein snacks eaten before going to bed or upon awakening at night also help.

Here are some additional ideas: Cucumber may relieve congestion quickly. A good preventive treatment consists of a teaspoon of lemon juice or apple cider vinegar mixed with a teaspoon of honey in a cup of vanilla water. This can be taken before breakfast or ahead of each meal if nausea continues past morning. Vitamins that can help with this problem include 50 mg of vitamin B6 and vitamin K. The latter is often low during pregnancy. Good sources of K include green leafy vegetables as well as cauliflower, broccoli, and cabbage.

An injection of this vitamin can help stop intractable vomiting. Acidophilus may help by balancing the intestinal pH. Ginger is great for nausea. Wild yam is an herb that can help stop nausea. While it does not contain hormones itself, it works by helping the body to balance its own progesterone levels. Other herbs to consider include fennel, peppermint and cardamon in warm milk. Catnip tea is another gentle remedy. A very dilute amount of peppermint oil can be rubbed onto the stomach or inhaled to relieve nausea and vomiting.

Constipation

This problem may also be the result of hormonal shifts that slow food transit through the gut. This can be corrected by increasing fluid consumption to at least eight to 12 glasses of water daily, as well as by adding more fiber from whole grains, bran, and fresh fruits and vegetables. In severe cases, whole psyllium seeds often help. One teaspoon of seeds is placed in a cup of water, and after drinking this, it is important to drink an additional cup of water. Castor oil and other irritating laxatives, including herbs such as cascara sagrada and senna, should be avoided. Anything causing peristalsis may bring unwanted contractions. In addition, doctors frequently prescribe iron to pregnant women to combat anemia. Iron can exacerbate constipation. Homeopathic remedies for constipation include nux vomica, sepia, bryonia and lycopodium.

Diarrhea

Diarrhea can be helped by following the BRAT diet—bananas, rice, apples and toast. Additionally, four capsules of charcoal, taken one to three hours apart, binds toxins in the bowels. However, charcoal should not be taken for more than three days, as it also binds up nutrients. Homeopathic remedies for diarrhea include podophyllum peltatum, sulfur, thuja occidentalis, veratrum album and cinchona officinalis.

Flatulence

As with other bowel problems, this occurs because the gastrointestinal tract is not moving as well as it should. Also the baby's head sometimes presses on this area. It may help to avoid carbonated drinks and to chew food well.

Sugar Imbalances

Symptoms of sugar imbalance during pregnancy can include exhaustion accompanied by puffiness, especially in the hands or feet. Gestational diabetes can develop at this time. Although it ends when pregnancy does, if left untreated, this type of diabetes can cause problems for the baby and complicate delivery. Sugar should be immunized or avoided completely; chromium picolinate lessens cravings for it and keeps blood sugar balanced. Dandelion tea or tincture (30-60 drops, three times a day) can also help.

Breast Tenderness

Breast tenderness occurs in the first trimester as the body prepares for breast-feeding, and lasts for only a few weeks. Hot compresses, hot showers and well-fitting bras without underwires can alleviate sensitivity.

Exhaustion

Fatigue is a common problem, especially during the first trimester, due to hormonal changes and the needs of the fetus. Anemia may be a factor and is often prevented by eating lots of green, leafy vegetables. Herbs, such as yellow dock, nettles and dandelion, can be taken as a tea or tincture to counter tiredness from anemia.

Heartburn

Frequent small meals are preferable to three big ones. And as is true for everyone, lying down after eating should be avoided, as this causes stomach acids to wash back up into the throat. A good herb for heartburn is slippery elm. One teaspoon of the powder can be added to water or juice, or lozenges can be taken throughout the day. Papaya enzymes are another handy item to have available. Also, two to three drops of diluted peppermint oil, placed on the back of the tongue, may relieve this problem.

Episiotomy Problems

Approximately 80 percent of women in the United States undergo this surgical procedure during childbirth to enlarge the vagina during delivery. The operation is often improperly performed, leading to problems later on when the cervix begins to push through the vagina and it appears as if the uterus is being forced out. Doctors often mistakenly diagnose this as a prolapsed uterus and recommend a hysterectomy. Tragically, 100,000 to 200,000 women are misdiagnosed with this condition each year. Corrective surgery, recently developed by gynecologist Dr. Vicki Hufnagel, easily ameliorates the problems. Repairing the vagina is a simple procedure that can be performed in 45 minutes in a doctor's office, allowing patients to go home the same day.

Treatment

Diet

Certain conditions during pregnancy—such as, anemia, hypoglycemia and diabetes—necessitate special diets and close supervision by a physician, but there are some general rules of thumb that benefit most women. These include eating a wide assortment of whole organic foods, such as grains, legumes, vegetables, fruits, nuts and seeds; eating only when hungry and; eating small, frequent meals instead of a few larger ones. Pregnant women need lots of extra protein, which vegetarians can get through extra soy products, including soy milk, tofu, tempeh, beans, nuts, seeds and fish. Plenty of pure water is needed but should be taken before and between meals. Drinking during meals dilutes stomach enzymes, making digestion more difficult. Cravings should be responded to with the most wholesome foods possible. Finally, calcium-depleting foods, such as coffee, chocolate and sodium, should be avoided.

Supplements

Folic acid is especially important during pregnancy for preventing neural tube defects. Neural tube defects such as spina bifida and anencephaly affect 1 in 1000 newborn children in the U.S. If there were a 1 in 1000 chance that you would be struck by lightning, you probably would not go outside. Reports in the 1980s touted the benefits of supplemental folic acid before a woman became pregnant. Such use, the reports stated, can considerably reduce the chances of neural tube defects. The amazing aspect of this finding is that this is true even though women who give birth to an affected child demonstrate no signs of a deficiency in folic acid.

Interestingly enough, in the United Kingdom, neural tube defects occur at a greater rate than in the United States. UK doctors recommended that women supplement with 4000 mcg of folic acid daily when trying to become pregnant. They also recommended that the women eat flour and grain products fortified with folic acid. The 4000-mcg dose of folic acid recommended by the doctors prevented 83 percent of neural tube defects! Women who supplemented with the standard 400-mcg dose of multivitamins showed only a 36-percent reduction. In addition, to combat pernicious anemia, a minimum of 1000 mcg of vitamin B12 should be consumed each day.

Recently, research has been directed at investigating how nutrition affects developing brain tumors in young children. Brain tumors are the foremost cause of death from cancer in children. Researchers have linked the incidence of brain tumors in children to the mother's diet. One researcher concluded that pregnant mothers who consumed high amounts of vegetables along with vitamin and mineral supplements substantially lessened the risk of their offspring developing tumors. To further divide the results of this study, the pregnant mothers who had eaten the most vegetables, fruits and fruit juices, vitamin A, vitamin C and folate had the greatest amount of protection for their unborn child. Since heating food destroys this fragile nutrient, it is important to take it in supplement form.

The National Cancer Institute reported that pregnant women who supplemented with folate and vitamins A, C and E reduced by half the likelihood of their children developing a brain tumor before the age of five. As in the aforementioned study, the risk reduction was related to how long and how much the women supplemented.

Women with diabetes have an increased chance of their offspring having birth defects. In general, studies have shown that multivitamins reduce the risk of birth defects. However, a 2003 study seemed to suggest that multivitamins could additionally reduce the likelihood of the children of diabetic women having birth defects.

Other important nutrients during pregnancy include a multivitamin/mineral supplement, vitamin C, vitamin B12, vitamin E and acidophilus. A doctor's guidance is needed when taking supplements during pregnancy.

Iron has traditionally been stressed for good health. But too much iron can be dangerous, and extra iron should not be taken unless tests indicate a need for it.

Calcium during pregnancy is extremely important. Note that the best source of calcium is whole foods, especially green leafy vegetables. However, if a supplement is desired in addition, calcium citrate is easiest on the stomach; other forms sometimes cause digestive upsets or constipation. A lack of sufficient calcium during pregnancy is linked to muscle cramps, backache, high blood pressure, osteoporosis, tooth problems and preeclampsia (a serious condition of pregnancy that is accompanied by high blood pressure, protein in the urine and swelling of the hands, feet and face). The only cure is to deliver the child. The manner in which calcium is assimilated is determined by a combination of factors: vitamin C availability, stress, exercise, vitamin A and vitamin D.

For women with postpartum depression, research has shown that vitamin B6 can help reestablish hormonal balance by raising serotonin levels. Patients given B6 for 28 days after delivery did not have a recurrence of postpartum depression.

Herbs

There are many herbs that can aid in relieving the discomforts associated with pregnancy. Raspberry leaf is a tonic that helps relieve almost any complaint and can be taken as a tea freely throughout pregnancy. Raspberry tea contains fragrine, an alkaloid that tones the pelvic muscles, including the uterus. The magical qualities of raspberry tea are attributed to its healthy amounts of vitamin C, as well as the amounts of vitamin E, calcium and iron it contains. The tea can be combined with peppermint for morning sickness.

To soothe cramps during pregnancy, women can try black haw or cramp bark. Ginger is one of the best natural remedies for preventing nausea, especially when accompanied by a diet of small, frequent meals, as well as fresh air and plenty of rest. Black cohosh is an old-time woman's remedy that grows in the deep, dark forests of eastern America. It was used by pregnant Native American women to ease childbirth and diminish labor pains. When taken in the last two or three weeks of pregnancy, black cohosh helps ripen the cervix and bring down the fetus. Sometimes the herb is taken together with blue cohosh.

In general, herbs to avoid are bitter (such as goldenseal and pennyroyal), those with antihistamine properties (such as ma huang and osha root) and diuretics (including buchu, horsetail and juniper berries).

Exercise

Most pregnant women benefit from a mild to moderate exercise program. The best level of exercise depends on how active a woman was before pregnancy, but most women can increase their endurance and should be encouraged to start at a comfortable level and build up. The exceptions are women whose doctors advise against an exercise program due to specific health concerns, such as pregnancy-induced hypertension, premature rupture of membranes, incompetent cervix, persistent second- and third-trimester bleeding and premature labor in a prior pregnancy or current one. Get your practitioner's go-ahead before embarking on a pregnancy exercise program.

In general, though, 60 minutes of aerobic exercise, approximately three times a week, is a good goal to work toward, although shorter workouts can be beneficial as well. Non-weight-bearing activities, such as cycling and swimming, are best, as they minimize the risk of injury and allow activity levels to remain closer to pre-pregnancy levels. Stretches that open up the pelvic area are also recommended.

Some precautions include not standing for prolonged periods and avoiding high-intensity exercises and risks of falling. The woman should not push to the point of breathlessness, and try not to raise her body temperature. After the first trimester, exercising in the faceup position limits blood supply to the baby and should be avoided as well.

Alexander Technique

Teachers of the Alexander technique seek to restore the freedom of movement so necessary for women dealing with the added demands of pregnancy.

Learning to bend, breathe and even rest properly can decrease pain and tension and ease delivery. Changes can extend beyond pregnancy and enhance stamina and overall functioning after birth.

During a session, the pregnant woman takes an active role in therapy, while the teacher acts as a guide. A woman may learn to squat in preparation for delivery or learn how to pick something up without stressing her back. Many of these movements are ones we naturally make as children but lose as adults. In addition, the teacher has one important hands-on role. Touching the clients stimulates the nervous system to respond in new, more beneficial, ways. After a lesson, people find that their movements are freer, and they report feeling lighter.

Massage

Maternity massage promotes relaxation, which is of significant value to an expectant mother and her unborn child. It also helps to stimulate lymphatic drainage of toxins and can alleviate muscle spasms, back pain, cramps, swelling in the legs, varicose veins, hemorrhoids and fluid retention. In addition, massage can promote hormonal balance and a strong immune system, as well as decrease irritability, mood swings and overheating. The therapist who understands pregnancy massage knows how to adjust pressure and focus to each stage. During the first trimester, touch must be gentle. For example, mild pressure to the bridge of the nose and forehead, and under the eyebrows and cheekbones, can unblock sinuses. In the second trimester, massage can be more rigorous and used to stimulate circulation, increase flexibility and reduce pain and spasm. Specific focus on the chest may alleviate breathing problems. In the third trimester, work is concentrated on the lower hips and sacrum to reduce back pain.

Just before delivery, a woman may be taught how to relax muscles in the perineum, the area between the vagina and rectum that needs to loosen up during childbirth. By enlarging this area, the need for an episiotomy may be eliminated. The technique involves self-massage: With clean hands and warm vitamin E or vegetable oil, the mother places thumbs or index fingers an inch to an inch and a half inside the vagina. Firm, gentle pressure is applied downward and outward until the stretch results in a burning sensation. This is held for a few minutes. The exercise is repeated once or twice a day.

During labor, applying pressure to certain acupressure points can reduce pain and anxiety, and even speed up labor. One technique involves walking the thumbs up from the sacrum to the top of the spine, holding each point for several seconds. Another is to press thumbs along the outline of the shoulder blades. A reflex point for quickening labor is located on the inside of the legs, approximately three inches above the ankle. Another is just below the anklebone on the inside (uterus point) and outside (ovary point) of the foot. These areas are pressed for approximately ten seconds.

During the postpartum period, massage can stimulate milk flow and help the uterus return to its normal size. Massaging the abdomen in a circular fashion helps to expel blood as the uterus contracts, and circling the breasts with light oil, followed by placing a flat hand on the nipple, and moving outward and upward, helps milk glands to flow.

While massage is useful for enhancing overall health during and after pregnancy and for treating a variety of conditions, there are times when it should not be used. Contraindications include vaginal bleeding, fever, abdominal pain, edema, severe headaches, blurry vision, excess protein, diabetes, high blood pressure, heart disease and phlebitis.

Aromatherapy

Using essential oils, either alone or in conjunction with massage, works on both physical and emotional levels. Aromatherapists suggest for that common bane of pregnancy, hemorrhoids, five drops of cyprus oil added to a bath. For sinus problems, try eucalyptus added to a cold air humidifier or a pan of hot water. Varicose veins may improve with cyprus and lemon oil added to a body lotion and applied to the veins in the morning and evening. Postpartum depression blues may be lifted by jasmine and clary sage added to the bath.

Only pure oils should be used, and many good ones are available from health food stores. While most are safe to try, some women experience allergic reactions to certain oils and may benefit from the guidance of an aromatherapist.

Homeopathic Remedies for Postpartum Depression

Postpartum depression, generally blamed on hormonal shifts, may also be due, in part, to overwhelming major lifestyle changes that a woman is experiencing. All of a sudden, the woman may have gone from being the center of attention to the caretaker of a helpless new individual. She may have had no experience in this new role. And even if she already has a child, each new one brings a big change in family dynamics, and in the mother's responsibilities. Also, fatigue can be a factor in postpartum depression, which can range from "the blues" to a serious, life-threatening condition.

Women experiencing depression should be under medical care. And ideally, although this is far from always the case in our society, all new mothers should be the beneficiaries of a familial and neighborhood support system.

Part of a woman's medical support system may be a homeopathic physician. Homeopathy is different from all the other forms of medicine. One homeopathic dose of medicine deals with all of the patient's symptoms. The one dose has been known to last for months. Classical homeopathy offers a wide range of remedies for postpartum depression, and a homeopathic physician can provide individualized guidance on which is appropriate for a particular woman's symptoms. The remedies include sepia, natmur, ignatia, arnica, pulsatilla, cimicifuga, kalicarbonicum, phosphoric acid, cocculus and aurum metallicum.

Another (nonhomeopathic) treatment for postpartum depression is natural progesterone. It's generally started about a month after delivery. And nutrient supplementation, undertaken with the guidance of a physician knowledgeable in this area, can make a difference.

What to Avoid

When a woman is pregnant, special care should be taken to avoid exposure to toxic ingredients found in such items as chemical hair dyes, household cleaners, paint and paint fumes, thinners, solvents, benzene, dry cleaning fluid, wood preservatives and pesticides. Radiation from X-rays and other sources is to be avoided, especially during the first trimester. It should go without saying that cigarettes, alcohol and recreational drugs are to be avoided, as well.

Toxic surroundings are also harmful. Negative people and aggravating situations cause stress. It is best to spend as much time as possible with loved ones and to fill surroundings with beauty.

Treatment Summary

Eating a wide assortment of organic foods, eating only when hungry, and eating small frequent meals, with extra protein, are some general rules of thumb for a pregnancy diet.

It's preferable to drink water between meals rather than during them.

Folic acid and other supplements, as prescribed by one's doctor, are important.

Raspberry leaf tea, and other herbal remedies can help women feel better during pregnancy.

A pregnancy exercise program will generally be based on how active the individual was prior to pregnancy, as well as any specific conditions that may emerge during pregnancy. However, aerobics tend to be the best form of activity during this time.

The Alexander technique is a method designed to restore the freedom of movement necessary for women dealing with the added demands of pregnancy.

Certain massage therapies are beneficial during and after pregnancy. Aromatherapy can alleviate specific conditions.

Homeopathic remedies and natural progesterone are two approaches to postpartum depression. Also, nutrient supplementation can relieve this problem.

Premenstrual Syndrome

Though first described in the medical literature in 1931, premenstrual syndrome (PMS) for years was not recognized by the medical establishment as an actual clinical condition. Women suffering from PMS (which refers to symptoms that occur between ovulation and the beginning of menstruation) were told that their symptoms were imaginary, and were sometimes diagnosed with psychological disorders. Between the 1920s and the 1950s, women with this problem could even find themselves institutionalized and administered shock therapy, while more recent treatments have included Valium and Prozac. Fortunately, the medical community has since acknowledged PMS as a true medical condition, and more effective remedies are currently available to alleviate its symptoms. Yet, many doctors still do not believe that there is such a condition as PMS. As a result, they fail to recognize and treat it. Of the 482 women who called the National Association for Premenstrual Syndrome (NAPS) helpline in the year 2000, 42 percent stated that their doctors were either unsympathetic or did not know much about PMS.

The occurrence of PMS has more than doubled in the past 50 years. This is probably due to the acceptance of its legitimacy as a condition. Though it is hard to believe, researchers now recognize over 150 different PMS-related symptoms that women complain about in the week or two before their period. It is hard to find a common denominator for all of these complaints, making it impossible to find a single treatment that will serve as a panacea. The one drug that most fits this bill is progesterone. Consequently, it has been the most commonly prescribed drug for PMS. Unfortunately, recent indications conclude that it is ineffective in treating PMS.

Symptoms

Premenstrual syndrome is characterized by a wide range of symptoms with different women experiencing the problem in different ways. Common symptoms are bloating, headaches, cramps, swelling, fluid retention and lower back pain. Others are breast tenderness, sugar cravings and acne, as well as depression, insomnia, anxiety, mood swings, irritability, withdrawal and forgetfulness. While the diagnosis of most other diseases involves the recognition of specific symptoms, ascertaining the presence of PMS is most dependent upon the time frame within which symptoms manifest.

Treatment

The usual medical approach to PMS involves administration of prescription drugs. As is always the case, though, prolonged dependence upon prescription drugs can have adverse side effects. Some doctors, with the idea that PMS is due to an imbalance of the hormones progesterone and estrogen, prescribe progesterone supplements. Although this treatment may adjust the hormonal levels of the body, it does not address the true origin of the problem. Progesterone's side effects include changing the length of the menstrual cycle.

Alternative practitioners provide another perspective on remedying the imbalance. They explain that excessive quantities of estrogen in the body may be a product of liver malfunction, a condition that can be effectively treated by limiting the intake of estrogen-rich foods in the diet and by improving the woman's exercise habits.

Diet and Supplements

A healthy diet is essential in both preventing and combating PMS. Women who suffer from PMS should consume foods high in fiber and complex carbohydrates, and should have snacks in between their meals in order to stabilize blood sugar levels and ameliorate symptoms. Indeed, the majority of women do not understand the benefits of fiber in dealing with PMS. Only recently has it been proven that fiber increases the intestinal clearance of estrogen. Excess estrogen is believed to contribute to developing PMS symptoms. An increase of fiber, especially in the two weeks before the period, may assist in lessening the PMS symptoms. Cool green foods, such as salads, can also be beneficial.

The diet should be as pure as possible. Contaminants found in pesticides, artificial food additives, drugs and environmental chemicals can raise the body's estrogen level, creating a deficiency of progesterone and provoking PMS. Thus, food should be organically grown and unprocessed, whenever this is possible.

According to a study in *Obstetrics & Gynecology*, women who adopt a low fat, vegetarian diet considerably reduce pain related to PMS. This diet also eased water retention and concentration problems, increased energy levels and lowered cholesterol levels.

Excessive estrogen within the body can also result from a surplus of animal fats in the diet or a deficiency of essential nutrients, such as the vitamin B complex, vitamin C and vitamin E, which are essential for the proper disposal of unnecessary hormones.

During severe bouts of PMS a good diet may have to be supplemented with additional nutrients. Vitamin B6, also known as pyridoxine, serves as a natural muscle relaxant and can reduce cramps associated with PMS. This versatile vitamin also acts as a diuretic, relieving swelling, fluid retention and breast tenderness. Vitamin B6 should be consumed on a daily basis in quantities of 200 to 400 mg and can be supplemented throughout the month. This may be part of a B-complex supplement. Remember not to exceed the suggested dosage of B6, as excessive intake of this vitamin can cause neuropathy, or inflammation of the nerves.

Magnesium, which soothes the nervous system, alleviating anxiety, irritability, nervousness, insomnia and fluid depression, can be quite advantageous when added to one's daily dietary intake in quantities of 500-1000 mg. The antispasmodic qualities of magnesium can reduce cramps and lower back pain associated with the menstrual cycle, and can also help eliminate sugar cravings. PMS appears to be related to a magnesium deficiency. Supplements of vitamin E in a dosage of 200-600 IU can aid in the reduction of breast tenderness and are beneficial in treating cramps and fibrocystic breasts, which have a tendency to enlarge prior to menstruation. The mineral zinc in the amount of 30-69 mg can be useful in minimizing depression and irritability.

Another supplement to know about is gamma linoleic acid (GLA), a precursor of prostaglandin-El, which is vital in coordinating neurological and hormonal functioning. This hormonelike substance can aid in the treatment of cramps, sugar cravings, muscle spasms, mood swings, depression, irritability and breast tenderness. Common sources of GLA include evening primrose oil and black currant oil. Also, borage oil, which is actually 24 percent GLA, can provide a concentrated source of the substance in a single capsule and is an effective substitute for six evening primrose oil capsules. One 1000 mg pill of borage oil, which will supplement the body with 240 mg of GLA, should be consumed daily.

A daily intake of 1000 mg of essential fatty acids, which can be obtained from fish and flaxseed oil, aids in the production of prostaglandin-E3, a hormonelike substance that can reduce breast tenderness. Although the essential fatty acid content of flaxseed oil is sacrificed during cooking, an ample supply can be obtained when the oil is used in salad dressings or on top of heated foods. Flaxseed oil contains lignans, which have both estrogenic and antiestrogenic activity. Lignans help reduce hot flashes, cycle changes and ovarian dysfunction.

Natural sources of progesterone, such as Mexican yams, can prevent various forms of cancer, fibrocystic breast disease and can also stabilize hormonal imbalances.

Isoflavones are substances useful in alleviating the mood swings of PMS. These are forms of phytoestrogen obtained from soybeans and other legumes that can help correct hormonal imbalances by joining in the competition for estrogen receptor sites. When the isoflavones occupy these receptor sites, inactive estrogen is displaced and eventually eliminated by the liver and colon. Organic sources of isoflavones, which include soybeans, peanuts, lentils, green peas, split peas and beans, have demonstrated the same beneficial qualities as prescription hormonal supplements without the adverse side effects.

Exercise

As with so many conditions, exercise will make a positive difference with PMS. Research has shown that regular participation in aerobic exercise can prevent negative mood swings, alleviate cramps, reduce fluid retention and limit sugar cravings. For maximum results, exercise should be performed three or four times per week.

Women who exercised moderately for a full cycle had decreases in their retention of fluid, breast symptoms and premenstrual depression. It is speculated that endorphin, the neurotransmitter, is linked to both exercise and mood symptoms. Furthermore, many believe that endorphin withdrawal leads to PMS symptoms.

Chinese Herbal Remedies

From the wide array of Chinese herbs, lungtanxieganwan has demonstrated its capacity to reduce angry emotions associated with PMS. Another Chinese herb, xiao yao wan, aids in the treatment of depression, indigestion, bloating and poor circulation. The herbal formula called Women's Harmony can also be used to improve circulatory functioning.

Herbs

Chasteberry has been proven effective in treating PMS. One study demonstrated how women with a severe form of PMS, premenstrual dysphoric disorder, responded as well to chasteberry as to the very much prescribed antidepressant Zoloft.

Cramp bark extract has been extremely effective in relaxing the uterine muscles. Because it is an antispasmodic, it has been used for centuries to ease cramps and spasms. Herbalists frequently prescribe it for treating menstrual cramps.

Some promising results have been attained using ginkgo to combat PMS. In

one study, 165 women were given 160 mg of ginkgo extract or placebo each day from the sixteenth day of one menstrual cycle to the fifth day of the next. Fluid retention and symptoms of breast tenderness improved as a result.

St. John's wort has been used for over 2000 years as a medicinal herb. Women have found relief from PMS, specifically cramping, when taking this ingredient.

Dong quai is a staple in Traditional Chinese Medicine (TCM) and is often prescribed for PMS. It helps ease hot flashes, painful menstruation and uterine cramps related to the menstrual cycle or menopause. *Caution:* Dong quai contains phytoestrogens, making it a powerful hormone balancer; hence, it should not be taken by pregnant women.

Teas

Tea has the distinctive amino acid theanine, which can lessen the effects of PMS. Theanine easily crosses the blood-brain barrier and makes delicate biochemical alterations. Unlike tranquilizers, this amino acid does not induce drowsiness, nor does it interfere with the ability to think. One report demonstrated that rats' memory and learning ability were improved by theanine.

Theanine works by closing off the anxious mode, thereby boosting the ability to concentrate and focus. In addition, theanine counteracts the hyper effect brought about by caffeine. Green tea contains a much higher quantity of theanine than other teas.

To help ease PMS symptoms, the recommended dosage is 100-200 mg of theanine.

Note: According to research at the University of Saskatchewan, an herbal combination of borage oil, flax oil, vitamin E, bioflavonoids, cramp bark extract and chasteberry fruit extract was clinically effective for women with PMS. The study, conducted over three months, showed a 67-percent decrease in 15 of the most common PMS symptoms. The study is published in the September 2001 *Journal of Obstetrics and Gynaecology of Canada.*

Homeopathic Remedies

Several homeopathic remedies have proven their effectiveness in countering PMS, but it is important to remember that only one product should be used at a time. If the remedy you have chosen does not alleviate your symptoms, homeopaths advise discontinuing its use and trying another.

The remedy lachasis can be used to combat a wide variety of symptoms, including ovarian pain, breast tenderness and headaches. Laccaninum can be used to treat swollen breasts, while bovista eases gastrointestinal symptoms, such as diarrhea. Pulsatilla is prescribed to help alleviate the emotional state in which women become forlorn and seek consolation, and natmur is used to combat the kind of melancholy and depression that tend to intensify with consolation. Additional symptoms that can be treated with natmur include headaches and cravings for salty foods. Intense depression, severe discouragement and indifference, and a sensation that the uterus has become congested and will soon drop through the vagina are a few of the symptoms that homeopathic practitioners treat with sepia. Finally, folliculinum, a relatively recent French innovation, is reported to soothe symptoms of PMS when administered on the seventh day of the menstrual cycle in a 30 to 200c potency.

Reflexology

The ancient practice of reflexology is founded on the concept that the foot contains reflex areas that correspond to various other parts of the body. By manipulating specific parts of the foot, reflexologists seek to enhance the performance of the corresponding organs and glands. Women who have used reflexology to treat PMS often praise its benefits. The pampered treatment, soft music and dimmed lights that often accompany reflexology treatments provide additional comforts and can promote the relief of stress.

According to reflexologist Laura Norman, the best way to understand the locations of reflex points is to visualize the human body superimposed on a foot. Accordingly, the toes correspond to the uppermost region of the body, including the eyes, nose, mouth, ears and brain, while the ball of the toes corresponds with the chest region—the heart, lungs and bronchial tubes. The center of the foot represents the internal organs, while the heel and ankle area is associated with the pelvic area and reproductive organs. The uterus, which is symbolized on the foot by a diagonal line midway between the heel and anklebone, can be treated by using the reflexology technique of the thumb walking around the inside area of the ankle. Rotating the thumb in a circular motion and finger walking near the uterus point can aid in alleviating PMS.

A reflexologist can guide you on the manipulation of other reproductive reflex points. Beyond this, massaging the remaining parts of the foot can be beneficial in treating PMS because all of the systems of the body interact on a daily basis. Overall relaxation can be enhanced by running the thumbs across the bottom of the feet. While reflexology is most useful in alleviating PMS when it is practiced three or four days before menstruation starts, it can be used during and after menstruation, as well.

Acupuncture

TCM recognizes groups of signs and symptoms as indicative of disharmony. In TCM, the basic imbalance that causes PMS is liver qi (energy) stagnation. The liver in TCM is responsible for the easy flow of qi and mirrors the rise and fall of hormones in the endocrine system.

Pressure Point Therapy

Another way of coping with PMS involves the manipulation of the body's natural pressure points. Positioning your hand three inches below the hip bone on the side of your leg, use your fingers to locate a tender spot. When you discover a suitable area you can initiate massage therapy. If the pressure point that you have selected is too sensitive for manipulation, work on the areas above and below the spot. This procedure can also be performed on the outside of the ankle, midway between the heel and anklebone. Once again, if this point is too delicate, try to use an area nearby.

What to Avoid

It is a good idea for everyone, but if you're concerned about PMS, be sure to avoid caffeine, alcohol and sugar. Since many victims of PMS also suffer from hypoglycemia, sugar intake should be restricted in order to eliminate wide fluctuations in blood sugar levels. When people consume large quantities of sugar, their blood sugar level increases dramatically, and consequently, the body is forced to respond by rapidly diminishing the sugar level. Mood and energy levels plummet as a result.

Note that clinical evidence has correlated the consumption of caffeine with breast tenderness and sleep disorders. Also, the consumption of dairy products should be limited because of their tendency to increase estrogen levels within the body. As discussed, a heightened level of estrogen can lead to a deficiency of progesterone and thus bring on PMS. Foods that are hot, spicy or acidic should be avoided by women who suffer from acute PMS. They should stay away from foods high in sodium and starch, as well.

Treatment Summary

A healthful diet low in animal products and inclusive of snacks, green salad foods and legumes will work to minimize PMS.

Chinese herbs are available that will counter premenstrual symptoms.

Homeopathic remedies, keyed to specific complaints, have proven effective in dealing with PMS.

Research has shown that regular participation in aerobic exercise can prevent mood swings, alleviate cramps, reduce fluid retention and limit sugar cravings.

Reflexology and pressure point therapy are manipulative techniques that can alleviate PMS.

Prostate Conditions

The prostate is a gland found between the bladder and penis. Though small, its functions are vital. Urine leaves the body through a tube in the prostate called the urethra. The prostate also provides seminal fluid, which nourishes sperm. There are two common conditions that affect the prostate, prostatic hypertrophy and prostate cancer.

Prostatic hypertrophy is an enlargement of the prostate. The condition is common in older men. Fifty to 75 percent of men over the age of 50 have prostatic hypertrophy, and 30 percent of these men have an operation for the condition. Prostatic hypertrophy is associated with the excessive intake of fat, especially saturated fat. It is also connected to the production of male hormones. Prostatic hypertrophy may develop into prostate cancer. Symptoms associated with prostatic hypertrophy can include any of the following: urination at night, decreased force of the urinary stream, hesitancy or difficulty in starting urination, dribbling, burning of the urine, discomfort when passing urine and blood in the urine. Sometimes a mass is felt in the area of the prostate. Occasionally, there are problems with sexual potency. When prostatic hypertrophy blocks urinary flow, urine backup can result in kidney damage, bladder infections or kidney stones.

Prostate cancer is almost as prevalent as lung cancer and is quickly becoming the number-one cancer killer of men. The risk is highest for men 65 and older, though 25 percent of all cases occur in men under 65. There are over 180,000 new cases and 35,000 deaths annually from this disease in the U.S. Prostate cancer occurs at higher rates among African Americans and older men, but is not unusual in men in their 30s and 40s. African Americans suffer from prostate cancer 34 percent more than Caucasians; unfortunately, they are two times more likely than their Caucasian counterparts not to survive the disease. Genetics and diet seem to be the main reasons for this alarming statistic.

The disease is unusual in that it is generally very slow growing; many men who have prostate cancer are unaware of it and die of other causes. Prostate cancer is linked to excess testosterone, which is believed to increase with a high-fat diet. An analogous condition in females is breast cancer, where too much fat increases estrogen levels.

If prostate cancer is caught early, when it is confined to the gland, the chances are in favor of its being controlled. Remember, prostate cancer is a slowly developing cancer. It usually takes a period of time to develop. However, if it spreads beyond the prostate, dealing with it will be far more difficult. Like all other diseases, the best strategy is to avoid getting it.

Prostate infection (prostatitis) is an inflammation of the prostate gland. It is usually caused by infectious bacteria that have entered the prostate from other areas of the body. This inflammation can lead to the retention of urine. The retention results in bladder distention, thereby making the bladder more vulnerable to infection. The infection in the bladder can easily spread up through the ureters to the kidneys.

There are basically two kinds of prostate infection: acute and chronic. Acute infections were detailed above. Chronic prostatitis symptoms are generally milder than the acute symptoms.

There are few symptoms associated with prostate cancer. Nodules in the prostate may be felt on digital examination, although these are not necessarily malignancies. Bone pain can indicate an advanced stage of the disease, after there have been metastases to the bones. Other symptoms may include inflammation and difficulty urinating. The presence of the disease is determined by the prostatic specific antigen (PSA) test. A raised PSA level is a marker for cancer, though an elevation in PSA does not always mean that the patient has cancer. Conversely, 30 percent of patients with prostate cancer have normal PSAs.

Interestingly enough, it has been demonstrated that the PSA test is a financial powerhouse. Its sales are estimated at over $350 million annually, representing 40 percent of all yearly cancer serum biomarker revenues.

But there is hope that improved technology is on the way. In a 2004 issue of the *Journal of Urology*, researchers suggest that testing for the protein called EPCA could detect prostate cancer up to five years earlier than the PSA test. The researchers believe that testing for EPCA could assist in diagnosing patients with elevated PSA levels, who are frequently subjected to repeated needle biopsies.

Additional diagnostic methods include transrectal ultrasounds and digital rectal examinations. Note that biopsies potentially spread cancer and are not recommended in the early stages of this disease where the cancer has not spread outside of the prostate.

Treatment

In the case of prostatic hypertrophy, the drug Proscar is the conventional therapy. The FDA warns, however, that the drug may inhibit PSA levels. Since excessive amounts of PSA are a strong indication of prostate cancer, Proscar may obscure this diagnostic sign.

In treating prostate enlargement, it is advisable that one avoid antihistamines and decongestants, for they can exacerbate urinary problems. Taper down on drinks, especially alcoholic and caffeinated, if there is a frequent urge to urinate at night. Don't delay when the urge to urinate strikes. Finally, consider supplementing with saw palmetto or pygeum.

If prostate cancer develops, mainstream medicine typically offers prostatectomy, or removal of the prostate, as well as chemotherapy and radiation. All are ineffective and often dangerous. Surgery, like biopsy, can actually spread cancer cells, and often decreases sexual potency and urinary control. PACT, a prostate support group, advocates hormonal blockers to induce cancer shrinkage, which may hold the disease at bay for several years, followed by a prostatectomy or cryosurgery (freezing of the prostate). The most common hormonal blockers are Lupron and Fludamide. As prostate cancer is generally slow growing, patients, especially those in the early stages, have time to try less harmful methods of treatment.

Nutrition

Low-fat diets are recommended, with special emphasis on complex carbohydrates, chiefly organic fruits and vegetables, raw juices and some whole grains for their alkaline effect. A modest amount of nuts and seeds may be added. (See section on alkaline diet in Cancer section.) Foods specifically related to decreased prostate cancer risk include beans, especially soy beans, lentils, peas tomatoes, raisins, dates and other dried fruits, in some cases, small amounts of organic chicken and fish may be eaten. The following supplements are also recommended:

Zinc...Everyone needs zinc, but it is especially crucial for preventing prostate problems, as zinc inhibits the uptake of testosterone into the prostate. The literature is replete with studies that show zinc's effectiveness in treating prostate diseases. The prostate gland contains a higher concentration of zinc than any other organ in the body, thus zinc is a helpful indicator in the diagnosis of diseases of the prostate. Studies indicate that 40 mg of zinc taken daily not only lessens the risk of prostate cancer but also helps in treatment. Pumpkin seeds are naturally high in zinc. Other good food sources of zinc are sunflower seeds, eggs, poultry, seafood, peas, soybeans and mushrooms. As an extra precaution, a zinc supplement should be taken as well, in conjunction with pyridoxine (vitamin B6), manganese and chromium, to help tissues better absorb the mineral. Vitamin A and phosphorus also increase the body's ability to use zinc efficiently.

Bee Pollen . . . In addition to zinc, try bee pollen. It helps to reduce an enlarged prostate.

Prostate Glandulars . . . Powdered animal prostate is high in zinc and nourishing for the human prostate.

Alanine, Glutamic Acid and Glycine . . . These amino acids, combined in equal measure, have been shown in several studies to relieve many of the symptoms of benign prostatic hypertrophy. In a study reported in the *American Journal of Geriatrics,* half of the 45 men who participated were supplemented with the combination of glutamic acid, glycine and alanine. The other half received a placebo. After only three months, 95 percent of the men who received the amino acid treatment reported an improvement in nighttime urination, 81 percent had a significant decrease in the urgency to urinate, 73 percent had a reduced frequency of urination and 70 percent showed improvement in delayed urination. In addition, this amino acid mix can help shrink the swelling of the prostate gland. In summation, this combination has been shown to reduce nocturia (excess urination at night), urgency, frequency and hesitation.

Vitamin C . . . High doses of vitamin C and the minerals selenium, copper and magnesium provide additional support to a body working to overcome prostate cancer. Intravenous vitamin C drips provide a super-saturated concentration of the vitamin in the body, which cancer patients need. This helps to remove toxic materials, mainly heavy metals, and allows the body to repair itself and return to its normal functioning capacity. Vitamin C is a prime antioxidant that neutralizes toxic free radicals.

Vitamin D . . . Prostate cancer frequently metastasizes to the bone, resulting in extreme pain. Researchers discovered that vitamin D supplements relieve the pain and improve muscle strength. The report from the Veterans Administration Medical Center found that a significant amount of patients suffering from metastatic prostate cancer eventually have a vitamin D deficiency.

Vitamin E (Gamma Tocopherol) . . . A study published in the *Journal of the National Cancer Institute* showed that men with the highest blood levels of gamma tocopherol were five times less likely to get prostate cancer. The study, which took place over seven years, was done at the esteemed Johns Hopkins School of Public Health and involved 10,456 men. In addition, the same study demonstrated that selenium and alpha tocopherol successfully reduced the incidences of prostate cancer. However, they did so only when the gamma tocopherol levels in the blood were high.

A nutrition and preventive medicine specialist at the famed Mayo Clinic stated that approximately 40 percent of men in their 70s have latent prostate cancer. He went on to say that vitamin E (alpha tocopherol) appeared to be effective at stopping small latent tumors from transforming into full-blown cancers. By stopping this transformation, vitamin E could help numerous men avoid cancer.

Proteolytic Enzymes...These help with digestion, and when taken on an empty stomach help dissolve the coating around cancer cells so that normal white blood cells can attack them.

Omega-3 Fatty Acids and Gamma Linolenic Acid...Borage, black currant seed, evening primrose oil and flaxseed oil all have beneficial effects.

Lycopene...More evidence is emerging that lycopene—one of the substances that is found in tomatoes and other fruits and vegetables, and which gives them their red color—can prevent and slow prostate cancer. In one study, researchers from the University of Illinois in Chicago gave tomato sauce to a population of mainly prostate cancer patients from the African American community—which has among the highest incidences of prostate cancer in the world—every day for three weeks. The test patients had a significant decrease in DNA damage to prostate cells and white blood cells.

Lycopene has received much publicity as a food ingredient that reduces the risk of many forms of cancer, including prostate cancer. It also protects against LDL cholesterol oxidation.

The results of a six-year Harvard study involving 50,000 men showed that the men who ate foods high in lycopene were up to 45 percent less likely to develop prostate cancer. Another study showed that patients treated with lycopene had smaller prostates than those who received no lycopene.

Men in the Mediterranean consume more tomato sauce than men in other parts of the world. Consequently, they have shown a lower incidence of prostate cancer. The cooking process involved in making tomato sauce tears down the cells of the tomato to release more lycopene.

Modified Citrus Pectin (MCP)...A 2003 issue of *The Prostate* confirmed earlier research that showed oral consumption of modified citrus pectin (MCP)—citrus pectin that has been hydrolyzed to yield molecules of lower weight, which seems to make them more absorbable—slowed the progression of prostate cancer in humans.

Herbs

Herbs are effective in treating benign prostatic hypertrophy as well as prostate cancer, and they do so without side effects. The following are especially helpful:

Saw Palmetto...Saw palmetto is one of the best herbs for prostate health. It produces the same benefits as Proscar but in a shorter time and without PSA repression. A December 2000 presentation made at an American Society for

Cell Biology meeting showed that saw palmetto inhibited prostate cancer cell growth in the test tube. Recent studies showed that saw palmetto decreased smooth muscle contraction. In so doing, it relaxed the bladder and sphincter muscles, lessening urinary urgency.

American Ginseng and Licorice Root...These herbs are for prostate problems due to low testosterone and androgen levels. They are safe to take on a regular basis, two to three times a day.

Corn Silk...Corn silk relieves inflammation of the prostate. It is also a remedy for inflammatory conditions of the urethra, bladder and kidneys.

Pumpkin Seed Extract...This is an excellent source of zinc and essential fatty acids, both important substances for prostate health. Pumpkin seed extract helps to tone the bladder muscles, relax the sphincter mechanism and decongest the prostate.

Pygeum Africanum...The properties of this African evergreen tree help reduce edema and painful, urgent urination. This is because pygeum is rich in phytosterols, substances that inhibit the biosynthesis of prostaglandins, which is the process responsible for prostate inflammation. Once inhibited, prostaglandins return to normal levels, and tissue swelling decreases. Eliminating the swelling helps to normalize metabolism, blood flow, lymph drainage and nutritional deposition. Some people have ill effects from this herb, but small amounts, used in conjunction with other modalities, usually work quite well.

Though saw palmetto is the better-known herb for reducing the size of an enlarged prostate, pygeum could be a superior treatment for benign prostatic hyperplasia or benign prostatic hypertrophy (BPH), a noncancerous tissue growth of the prostate. In actuality, three herbal medications are well respected for their ability to assist in the urinary flow of older men: saw palmetto, nettle root and pygeum africanum.

Siberian Ginseng, Wintergreen and Hydrangea Root...These may help when there is an overproduction of hormones.

Essiac...This is an herbal preparation that is useful in the treatment of all cancers.

Uva Ursi...This has antiseptic, diuretic and tonic properties that target the bladder, kidneys and urinary tract, benefiting both disorders.

Uncaria Tomensoa...This immune modulator from South America may return PSA levels to normal in the case of prostate cancer and help some people when all else has failed.

Homeopathic Remedies

Homeopathic remedies for particular conditions vary according to symptoms. The following remedies may be appropriate for treating prostatic hypertrophy patients with these indications:

Apis Mellwiga . . . Frequent urination with burning or stinging pain and inflammation.

Chimaphilia . . . Urgency to urinate with burning pain; strain to urinate.

Conium Maculatum . . . Chronic enlargement; difficult urination, urine flow that starts and stops. Helps soften the prostate.

Ferrum Picricum . . . Frequent urination at night; full feeling and retention of urine.

Hepar Sulphuris Calcareum . . . Dribbling urine or poor flow.

Sabal Serrulata . . . Difficult urination with enlarged prostate; constant desire to urinate.

Staphysagria . . . Urge to urinate but inability to urinate fully; feeling of bladder not being empty.

Thuja . . . Enlarged prostate; sudden desire to urinate; stream is split.

Reflexology

In reflexology, the sides of the feet, below the bony part of the ankles, correspond to the reproductive system. The prostate/uterus points are on the idler, insides of the feet, while the testicle ovary reflexes are on the outer sides. These areas are extremely sensitive to touch, especially when there is a problem in the corresponding body parts, so proceed with caution.

Walk the fingers along the areas surrounding the ankles, applying pressure to points at every interval along the way. The finger can also be pressed into the bladder point, on the inside center part of the heels. Working these systems increases circulation and helps to speed up the healing process.

Chelation Therapy

A study performed in Switzerland administered 10 chelation treatments to one group and none to another. Follow-up over the course of 18 years revealed that the subjects receiving chelation had only one-tenth the cancer deaths of the other group.

Lifestyle Considerations

Patients should exercise regularly, and take in much fresh air and light. Stress management programs may also prove invaluable and can include biofeedback, massage and meditation.

What to Avoid

Foods to avoid include alcohol, sugar, starch, caffeine, additives and preservatives, impure water (such as water with chlorine and fluoride), hydrogenated fats (such as margarine) and foods prepared in aluminum cookware. Exposure to tobacco should be avoided as well.

Treatment Summary

A low-fat, organic diet is recommended, with emphasis on alkaline foods. Soybeans, lentils, peas, tomatoes and dried fruits are related to decreased prostate cancer risk.

Zinc is an important nutrient for prostate conditions.

Herbal remedies include saw palmetto, pumpkin seed extract and others.

Homeopathic remedies may be appropriate for prostatic hypertrophy patients with specific symptoms.

Chelation therapy is proven to prevent diseases associated with aging, such as prostate cancer.

Patients should exercise regularly and use techniques that will help manage stress levels.

Respiratory Conditions

Most of us take the ability to breathe for granted. But what should be a natural act for all people can prove difficult for some. Respiratory problems range from mild conditions in which a person occasionally experiences slight difficulty breathing, to more severe levels of illness that can impede a person's ability to deal normally in society or, at the extreme, result in death.

One of the most common respiratory problems is asthma. This is a condition that periodically impairs the ability of a person to breathe. Asthma is characterized by shortness of breath, chest tightness, racing heart, sneezing, coughing, flared nostrils and mucus. The *Morbidity and Mortality Weekly Report* states that in 1996, asthma affected approximately 10.2 million adults (7.2 percent of adults living in the United States have asthma), ranking it among the most common chronic diseases in the U.S.

According to Dr. James Braly, asthma occurs because airways are irritated, supersensitive and inflamed—not just during an asthmatic attack, but all the time. A popular misconception about asthma is that it is primarily an obstructive or constrictive airway disease. This has led to the overprescription of adrenaline-like inhalants to dilate or enlarge these openings. Dr. Braly feels their frequent use may be responsible for the recent 300 percent increase in asthma mortality in the U.S. This distressing statistic, coupled with reports that the incidence of asthma has nearly doubled in the past decade, indicates that we have to take a serious look at our approach to this disease.

Dr. Braly emphasizes that asthma is a condition that can be caused by allergies to foods and pollutants in the environment. The actual asthmatic attack may occur hours or days after exposure, making the allergenic trigger difficult to identify. He advocates, therefore, increased use of the IgG ELISA delayed-onset food allergy assay and/or the IgE ELISA blood test for airborne allergies.

Asthma can also be triggered by emotional stress, and is associated with a sense of fear or losing control. Sometimes children develop asthma after a frightening experience. In addition, the condition has been linked to the pertussis vaccine, as studies indicate that vaccinated children have higher incidences of asthma than do non-vaccinated children.

Bronchitis is another common respiratory problem. This disorder is an obstruction of the bronchi, or breathing tubes, that lead to the lungs. It is a condition wherein the mucous membranes of the lungs swell. Bronchitis can be short-term or long-term, acute or chronic. Factors leading to the condition include childhood infections, smoking, air pollution and long-term infections; the condition produces a dry, nonproductive cough that releases mucus, as well as fever and chest and back pain. A person with bronchitis tends to have difficulty walking briskly or with physical exertion. Other symptoms may include lung infections and blue skin, the latter being a sign that there is less oxygen and more carbon dioxide in the blood.

Chronic obstructive pulmonary disease or COPD, formerly known as emphysema, is a lung disease commonly associated with smoking and inhaling chemical pollutants. The condition manifests as the lungs become restricted or obstructed due to blocked bronchial tubes. The onset of the disease is gradual and the patient gets progressively worse. With time, an individual breathes in less and less air. As the disease advances and oxygen levels in the blood become insufficient, medication and additional oxygen are required. Although the disease targets the lungs, complications in the intestines and liver may contribute to the problem.

Treatment

Some of the natural solutions that help to combat respiratory conditions focus on prevention. Should respiratory illnesses develop, they may require medical attention and drug intervention, although natural solutions can provide supplementary help.

Nutrition

Diet plays a major role in the prevention and treatment of all these respiratory disorders. An appropriate diet is, of course, individualized, based on a person's biochemical makeup, although there are some general dietary rules that may help ease respiratory problems. Essentially, the emphasis should be on complex carbohydrates and fiber, with a variety of organic whole grains, beans, fruit and vegetables included in the diet. Foods rich in omega-3 fatty acids are also encouraged; these include dark-meat fish, such as salmon and tuna.

The rise in the incidence of asthma has recently been tied to the altered consumption of polyunsaturated fatty acids (PUFAs). The Western diet has 10 times more linoleic acid (omega-6 fatty acids) than alpha-linolenic acid (omega-3 fatty acids). This causes an excess production of eicosanoids, which start a chain reaction that ultimately results in the increased production of IgE. According to one study, by limiting eicosanoid production, omega-3 fatty acids assist in the prevention of an asthmatic response. Furthermore, taking gamma linoleic acid (GLA) stimulates production of prostaglandin E1 (PGE1), which dilates the bronchioles and soothes inflammation.

Diets high in chlorophyll are cleansing. This means juicing carrots in combination with a small amount of celery or parsley. Wheatgrass juice is especially rich in chlorophyll. Radishes, horseradish and lemon juice are healing to the lungs and should be eaten often. Foods can be eaten raw or lightly cooked. In addition, onion, garlic, ginger, cardamon, cumin, cloves and cayenne are good herbs and spices to use when cooking.

It is also important to address any food allergies by working with a complementary physician, a doctor trained in nondrug approaches to healing, as well as in traditional medicine. An antiallergy diet can often correct or ameliorate the problem by having the patient eliminate certain foods completely, and eat others on a rotational basis. If the same food is eaten day after day, the body may become sensitized to it, but when the food is spaced four to seven days apart, there is usually no adverse reaction. Three-quarters of asthmatic children and nearly half of all asthmatic adults respond to the removal of allergy-producing foods in the diet. Once allergies are diagnosed and addressed, many individuals can eliminate or greatly reduce their dependency on drugs.

Patients with respiratory illnesses may benefit from taking a teaspoon of cold-pressed virgin olive oil first thing in the morning. This helps to eliminate toxins in the intestines, liver and lungs. Adding flaxseed oil enhances the concentration of fatty acids and can be helpful.

Supplements

A variety of nutritional supplements can be helpful in preventing and alleviating respiratory illnesses:

Nutrients that can help asthma specifically include bee pollen and honey (particularly in attacks brought on by hay fever); bromelein, an enzyme found in pineapples that alleviates inflamed bronchi; and hydrochloric acid, for attacks precipitated by insufficient amounts of stomach acid. Bromelein works even better when combined with quercetin and vitamin C.

Magnesium intake is related to asthma. Lower levels of intake are associated with an increase of allergies and asthma. Magnesium can open the bronchioles, relaxing the muscles inside the air tubes, and stop an acute asthma attack quickly. As a preventive measure, asthmatics can benefit from large amounts of elemental magnesium supplements taken orally. The recommendation for adults is 1000-1500 mg; children and infants can usually tolerate 100-400 mg. However, since magnesium has a laxative effect, it is best taken throughout the day with meals, rather than all at once. And, according to Dr. Alan Gaby, when magnesium is combined with calcium, vitamin C and the B vitamins in an intravenous "cocktail," serious asthmatic symptoms subside within minutes. Magnesium is also excellent for people who are exposed routinely to toxic chemicals and suffer from bronchitis as a result.

Taking higher levels of vitamin E is associated with lower blood IgE concentrations and a lower frequency of allergen sensitization. Tocopherol (vitamin E) and tocopherol acetate inhibit the formation of leukotrienes (substances that regulate allergic and inflammatory reactions) that, when overexpressed, can lead to bronchial constriction and other respiratory reactions.

By preventing the release of histamine, quercetin, a flavonoid, assists in reducing allergic reactions, asthma and hay fever. Quercetin blocks the release of histamine, thereby lessening allergic reactions in a safer way than many of the conventional drugs.

In one European study on people in the age range of 16 to 50, researchers discovered that selenium protected against asthma, and that its use has been declining in Britain. The drop in the blood levels of selenium throughout the United Kingdom and other European Union members may be the reason asthma is on the increase in those countries.

Zinc has also proven to be a helpful mineral in combating asthma.

Chlorophyll is a supplement that purifies the blood overall, enhancing its oxygen-carrying capabilities. It also chelates toxic metals out of the system. Fresh organic (½ dark yellow and ½ green vegetable) juices are a great source.

L-methionine, L-cysteine, N-acetyl-cysteine and glutathione peroxidase help repair damaged tissue in the lungs by counteracting the effects of smoke and other environmental toxins. These substances protect cell membranes from the ravages of free-radical damage, lock up toxic chemicals at the cellular level and speed up the removal of poisons via the liver. In other words, glutathione, NAC, and other antioxidants counter the cellular oxidative damage that takes place at elevated levels in asthmatics.

Other supplements recommended to prevent free radical damage and defend against inhalant lung injury are beta-carotene (50,000 IU or lower if skin turns orange); vitamin C (up to 10,000 mg divided into five doses); vitamin E (300 IU); and coenzyme Q10.

Some nutrients may be helpful when one is being weaned off prescription medications. These include calcium, coenzyme Q10, dimethylglycine GLA, found in evening primrose, black currant seed and borage oils and pantothenic acid.

Herbs

There are numerous herbs that may be beneficial to people with respiratory illnesses. Garlic, for one, helps fight infections. Mullein tea has historically been used in France to treat inflammatory conditions of the lungs. Easter lily is an old bronchial remedy used to expel heavy stagnant mucus from the lungs, and can be purchased as a flower essence. Yerba santa is a Southwestern herb that grows in semi-desert regions. Its shiny leaf is covered with a resin, an indication of a plant that helps the respiratory system. Resins are sticky substances that pick up and expel mucus, so that the air passages can open up. Yerba santa helps clear out the lungs' membranes and linings, and is especially good for people worn out from a deteriorating cough. For this reason, it has been used for the treatment of tuberculosis.

Other good herbs for respiratory clearing are white pine, spruce, marshmallow root, lungwort and comfrey. Licorice root fights coughs and lung congestion, and is a demulcent (it coats and soothes). In fact, it has been known to be as effective as codeine. In addition, licorice is an expectorant that helps coughs by increasing the secretion of the bronchial glands. Fresh thyme, nettles and fenugreek are commonly used throughout Europe for treating various lung conditions. Horseradish, taken with more soothing herbs, helps to get rid of lung debris. It can be prepared by scraping, rinsing, shredding and placing in oil overnight. Ginger is an expectorant herb that clears mucous secretions from the bronchi. One squirt of ginger extract into the mouth will clear the bronchi in a few minutes. For asthma, a hot ginger compress can be applied to the chest to relieve congestion. This method involves soaking a cloth in ginger tea, applying to the chest, and alternating with a cold-water compress several times. Myrrh has also been used successfully for treating lung diseases. However, it should be used in small quantities and only for short periods of time, to prevent toxicity

For asthma patients, the following are also recommended: cayenne pepper, ginkgo biloba, lobelia and slippery elm bark. In addition, wild cherry will work as an expectorant to release mucus, while the relaxation of muscles can be achieved through the use of antispasmodic nervones, such as skullcap and valerian, as well as crampbark.

Echinacea is effective in reducing the duration and the severity of the symptoms of the common cold, coughs, bronchitis and upper respiratory infections.

Alpha-Lipoic Acid

According to a recent report, alpha-lipoic acid (called the "universal" antioxidant) exhibits strong antioxidant action in virtually every tissue in the body. Alpha-lipoic acid also elevates glutathione levels in cells. In its reduced form, glutathione is the most potent intracellular antioxidant. One report suggests that it may be useful in many inflammatory lung processes. The recommended dosage is two 250-mg capsules twice per day.

Green Tea

Green tea has become somewhat of a panacea in the prevention and treatment of an array of diseases. Green tea has repeatedly shown its propensity to inhibit bacteria and viruses, and has proven to be a protective factor on the immune system.

Garlic

From biblical times, garlic has been treasured for its healing properties. Recent studies have shown that garlic—in particular, its active component, allicin—has antifungal, antibacterial and antiviral properties. Additionally, garlic increases the number of natural killer cells and the killer activities of the spleen cells, according to a 2001 report.

Vitamin C

Vitamin C (ascorbic acid) is found in citrus fruits and green vegetables. It has shown effectiveness in stimulating the immune system and in providing relief for cold and flu symptoms. Reports indicate that high doses of vitamin C lessened cold and flu symptoms by 85 percent. In addition, vitamin C levels work to protect bronchial tissues from oxidative damage, which is one of the causes of asthma. One report suggests a daily dose of several grams. Lastly, the blood of asthma patients has lower levels of vitamin C than that of persons who do not have the disease.

Even more promising are the studies that raise the possibility that high doses of vitamin C could combat a virus's effects, and that it is virtually certain to be an effective therapy for HIV.

The suggested dosage of vitamin C is four 1000-mg capsules three times per day.

Detoxification

Healing foods and supplements will not work nearly as well in a toxic system as in a clean one, since weak digestion from the buildup of residues in the bowel can interfere with nutrient absorption and trigger inflammatory responses. For this reason, complementary physicians may recommend enemas, colonics and high-fiber nutrients, such as bran, psyllium and bentonite. A catnip and garlic enema can be taken twice a week with beneficial results. In addition, exercise and deep breathing of fresh air will eliminate mucus from the lungs.

Aromatherapy

The inhalation of volatile herbs with expectorant properties, such as eucalyptus, hyssop and thyme, helps clear the lungs of mucus. In addition, a potpourri of lavender, figwort, mullein, horehound and lungwort can be heated and the steam inhaled. An aromatherapist can guide you in the use of additional essences and techniques.

Homeopathic Remedies

Homeopathic medicines used to restore respiratory health include ipecacuanha, which may be recommended by homeopathic physicians for violent coughing, chest restriction and choking. Natrum sulphuricum may be suggested for rattling in the chest that gets worse in damp weather, and spongia tosta is prescribed for dry hacking coughs, with wheezing and hoarseness that worsen in the cold air. To open bronchial passages, adrealinum is sometimes used. Other homeopathic remedies for respiratory problems include belladonna, which may alleviate breathing difficulty, and soidago virgaurea, which aids in stemming heavy mucus, and curbing coughs.

Stress Management

Research clearly demonstrates that inner-city clinics see increased rates of depression occurring with asthma. A big factor in this correlation is the higher rate of stress experienced by members of this population. Relaxation techniques are helpful in overcoming feelings of fear and loss of control, which can precipitate a breathing crisis. Deep yogic breathing can immediately replace a sense of tightness in the chest with a calming sensation. Relaxation can also be mastered through biofeedback, meditation, self-hypnosis and acupuncture. Specifically, an acupuncture technique called drug accupoint application has proven effective against asthma. In addition, a treatment using topical applications of herbs and heat called moxibustion has also shown positive results in treating asthma sufferers.

Breast-Feeding

A Brazilian study demonstrated the effectiveness of breast-feeding in preventing asthma. Breast-feeding was correlated with a low rate of asthma. The report showed that children who were breast-fed for longer than six months had a lower risk of developing asthma than children who were not. A study from Australia confirmed the results from Brazil. Breast milk contains anti-bodies that are believed to help elevate immune function.

As per one report, newborns have undeveloped immune systems, and the immunological properties in their mother's milk are necessary for the normal development of their immune systems. Gamma linoleic acid (GLA) and pre-formed di-hommo-gamma linoleic acid (DGLA) are present in human breast milk. GLA and DGLA are essential in the production of PGE1 prostaglandins, which are powerful anti-inflammatory compounds.

Magnets

Advocates of magnetic healing report that the negative pole of a magnet can decrease inflammation, and increase oxygen to an area. However, magnets should not be placed directly on the lungs or used on the chest if a pacemaker or defibrillator is present. For best results, wrap three or four stacked plasti-form magnets in an ace bandage and place over the chest area for several min-utes. Magnets should be approximately 4 x 12 inches. This will bathe the whole area in a magnetic field, providing relief. If constriction occurs, remove the magnets and try again later.

Another recommendation is to drink eight to ten glasses of water that is negatively ionized by a magnet. A magnetic bed pad is also helpful, but should not be used for longer than eight to ten hours; otherwise it is weakening.

Chelation Therapy

The EDTA chelation pulls out toxic metals from the body, such as cad-mium, lead and calcium, and therefore promotes healing.

What to Avoid

A prime consideration for those with asthma should be the identification and elimination of allergens in foods and in the environment. Although any food is suspect, the ones most likely to trigger asthma are dairy products, eggs, chocolate, wheat, corn, citrus fruits and fish. Preservatives and additives may also be detrimental. In fact, a commonly used food coloring, yellow dye #5, is believed to trigger asthma in as many as 100,000 Americans. Sulfites, preserva-tives found in many alcoholic beverages and added to salad bar foods in restaurants, are also known to promote asthma attacks. Monosodium gluta-mate (MSG), an ingredient used in Chinese and Indian cooking, can also ex-acerbate symptoms.

In all respiratory conditions, mucous-forming dairy foods, such as milk and cheese, can exacerbate clogging of the lungs and should be avoided. Salt should also be omitted from the diet.

Treatment Summary

A vegetable-foods-based diet is recommended, with any allergy-producing foods identified and eliminated.

Magnesium is one of the nutrients important for those with respiratory problems.

Herbs may be beneficial to people with respiratory illnesses.

Bioflavonoids, such as water-soluble quercetin, isoflavones, pycnogenol and lycopene, may help improve lung function.

Since healing foods and supplements will not work optimally in a toxic system, the following detoxification methods are recommended: colonic therapy, high-fiber nutrients, exercise and deep breathing of fresh air.

Aromatherapy may help promote respiratory healing.

A number of homeopathic remedies are used for patients with respiratory health illnesses.

Stress management is a crucial part of any respiratory health regimen.

Chelation therapy acts as a lung-cleansing agent, and reverses free radical damage.

Exercise can improve lung function and will help with symptoms. However, exercising in cold or polluted air can exacerbate asthma.

Many have also found yoga, massage, biofeedback, acupuncture and moxibustion helpful.

Sickle Cell Anemia

Sickle cell anemia is a genetic disease affecting 1 out of every 400 African Americans. Contrary to popular belief, the disease affects other nationalities, as well. Overall, it affects 8 out of 100,000 people. This painful and disfiguring chronic condition attacks the red blood cells, causing joint pain, fatigue, breathing difficulties, blood clots, fever and long-term anemia.

During a sickle cell crisis, red blood cells lose their shape and elasticity due to oxygen depletion. The characteristic reshaping of the cells into sickle figures causes restricted blood flow, especially to the pelvic region.

There is no cure for sickle cell anemia. The goal of therapy is to manage and control the symptoms connected to the disease. Bed rest to reduce energy expended and oxygen needs during a crisis is highly suggested. Low oxygen levels result in acidosis, which causes the sickling.

Patients are often hospitalized for weeks and are given painkillers and tranquilizers. Repeated crises often lead to physical deformities and severe emotional distress.

Treatment

Drug Therapy

Generally, conventional medicine is used to treat sickle cell anemia. However, alternative therapies may be useful in pain control. Relaxation, application of local warmth and hydration may supplement the conventional therapy. Always recommended is maintaining good health through adequate nutrition and avoiding stress and infection.

In the U.S., the cancer drug hydroxyurea has been prematurely approved for use, based on studies showing it to lessen the incidence of sickle cell crises in patients receiving it. Hydroxyurea reactivates fetal hemoglobin, which is known to decrease the complications caused by sickle cell disease. But what has been ignored is the fact that patients given this drug tend to develop bone marrow depression, and that long-term use has been associated with leukemia. The drug is considered too toxic for children, although it is approved for use by adults.

A recent study in the journal *Blood* indicated that the drug decitabine has been offered as an alternative to hydroxyurea for people with sickle cell disease who cannot endure hydroxyurea. However, it should be noted that not all patients respond well to the medication.

Ozone Therapy

Small amounts of medical ozone added to a patient's blood have been found to prevent flare-ups and to resolve a sickle cell crisis in half the time of existing treatments, with no adverse side effects. This may be due to ozone's ability to make red blood cells more flexible.

Trials in Havana have led to ozone's approval as a treatment modality by the Cuban Ministry of Health. It is currently available throughout the island, where it is used both prophylactically and during crises.

Sinusitis

Sinusitis is an inflammation of the cavities in the skull (which make up about a third of the skull) and are found behind the eyes, forehead, nose and cheekbones. The condition is usually caused by bacteria, viruses or allergic reactions. Allergy-related sinus conditions may begin as allergic rhinitis, an inflammation of the nasal membranes, and then move to the sinuses. People with compromised immune symptoms are more susceptible to sinusitis.

The combination of inflamed sinuses and thick mucus often leads to pressure and pain. Specific symptoms of sinusitis can include headaches—sometimes even migraines—as well as postnasal drip, a cough, facial tenderness and occasionally fever. Infections in the sinuses should be immediately addressed; otherwise, they may spread to other parts of the body.

Treatment

Typical treatment for sinusitis involves the administration of antibiotics, which can have dangerous long-term consequences, and decongestants. Fortunately, safer natural treatments and lifestyle changes are highly effective and without negative side effects.

Diet and Lifestyle

Vegetarian diets that are high in fiber and free of mucus-forming foods can help to prevent and eliminate sinusitis. Freshly squeezed raw juices contain beneficial enzymes for fighting infections. An enzyme that is especially helpful is bromelain, found in pineapple juice.

Remove all dairy products from your diet. A significant majority of patients doing so reported drastic improvement in sinus conditions after only two months.

People who get respiratory infections may also benefit from rest, according to Dr. Thomas Sinclair. They do not need to stop activities completely, but should perform them in moderation for a week following the onset of sinusitis.

In addition to extra rest and a good diet, Dr. Sinclair recommends the following supplements for fighting sinusitis infections: vitamin C, 500 mg every 2 hours; beta-carotene, up to 50,000 IU three times a day; zinc lozenges or zinc picolinate; coenzyme Q10; and quercetin.

Note: Histamine is linked to nasal and sinus congestion. Taking 2000 mg of vitamin C three times per day has been demonstrated to reduce histamine levels in people with either high histamine levels or low blood levels of vitamin C.

Herbs

When a fever is present it is helpful to drink peppermint or elderberry flower tea. For building immunity, echinacea, goldenseal and chaparral can be taken in tincture, capsule or tea form. The best time to take these antibiotic herbs is when symptoms first appear. As many as four to six capsules can be taken at first (less if they cause a digestive upset). Symptoms should decrease within 24 hours. At that point, the amount should be gradually lessened. Cayenne and garlic are also excellent for fighting infection.

Barberry has comparable healing powers to goldenseal, due to the fact that both herbs contain active substances called berberine alkaloids. Berberine alkaloids help to fight infection, stimulate the immune system and reduce fever.

An effective gargle to get rid of a sore throat and the mucus in the sinuses consists of equal parts of powdered clove, cayenne pepper and ginger. One level teaspoon should be added to warm water. To clear clogged nasal passages, horseradish, with a drop of lemon juice, can be placed in the mouth.

Many herbalists use echinacea to combat infections in general and sinusitis specifically. Furthermore, many studies support the use of echinacea for the common cold. Because it shortens the length of a cold, this popular herb may help prevent the development of sinusitis.

Eucalyptus oil has been shown in studies to possess strong antibacterial properties. In studies with animals, it has also demonstrated its ability to perform as an expectorant (it loosens mucus in the respiratory passages) and antiseptic (it thwarts infection).

External Therapies

Moist heat packs applied over the forehead, eyes and nose three times daily provide relief from sinus congestion, many people report. An herbal equivalent of a moist heat pack is dry powdered ginger and pureed lotus root (available in Asian markets), made into a paste. This should be applied to areas above and below the eye; it heats the area, but does not burn it.

Steam inhalation is also effective and is simple to do. Just heat a pot of water on the stove and add a drop of one or more essential oils. Thyme is antibiotic and antifungal, while eucalyptus and peppermint oil are excellent decongestants. Breathing in the vapors is soothing as well as healing.

Severe sinus infections may need nasal irrigation, which involves the use of warm salt water or boiled water with goldenseal. To do this, towels should be placed on the bed. Then, while one is lying on the towels, with the head extending back off the edge of the bed, either of these solutions should be slowly dropped into one nostril and then the other. After treatment, the head should be slowly and carefully raised.

Apply pressure to ease pain and stimulate circulation. For a few minutes, press the top of your nose on either side between two fingers and then release. Perform this a number of times a day.

Examine the likelihood of the cause of your sinusitis being a food or inhalant allergy.

Household dust and mold frequently aggravate sinusitis. Make sure you wash your bed sheets often in hot water. Spend a few extra dollars for pillow covers that protect against the numerous dust mites that thrive inside pillows.

A dehumidifier will help keep the humidity below 50 percent. A humid environment is encouraging to dust mites.

Many have found relief from drinking six to eight glasses of water daily, especially when suffering from a cold or stress. Hot drinks such as herbal tea, broths and soups can be used in place of water.

Reflexology

To combat sinusitis, reflexologist Diane Rooney recommends working on the tops and sides of all of the toes, and the upper part of the left heel that is in line with the fourth toe. Since the toes are far more sensitive than the heel, she notes, work less deeply here. After treatments, more sinus drainage may occur, a sign that the body is healing naturally. Don't take medication to stop drainage at this point, Rooney advises. Just help it along with hot baths and herbs or aromatherapy.

Acupuncture

Acupuncturists usually describe sinusitis as a "dampness" that causes inflammation and congestion in the mucus membranes. By strengthening the spleen meridian and working with the stomach meridian, the dampness is cleared. Acupuncturists often perform needling therapy for this condition.

Exercise

Exercise may provide relief, since it releases adrenaline. Adrenaline constricts blood vessels, thus possibly reducing swelling in the sinuses. A brisk walk while deeply inhaling may be just what the doctor ordered.

What to Avoid

Common foods that tend to produce allergic reactions include those that people generally think of as healthful, such as dairy products and wheat, which are both mucus-forming. Peanuts, corn and sugar are other common culprits. Smoke is another irritant to be avoided, through both direct and passive inhalation. Other irritants to avoid are air pollutants, such as car exhaust and even perfumes.

Treatment Summary

A vegetarian diet, high in fiber and free of mucus-forming foods, is recommended to alleviate or eliminate sinusitis.

Freshly squeezed raw juices are helpful, particularly pineapple juice. Recommended supplements include vitamin C, beta-carotene, zinc, co-enzyme Q1O and quercetin.

Antibiotic herbal teas may be helpful.

Quit smoking, and refrain from smoky environments.

Symptomatic relief from sinusitis can be eased through moist heat packs, steam inhalation and nasal irrigation.

Massaging areas of the foot, using the principles of reflexology, can provide relief of sinusitis.

See also: Allergies, Headaches

Skin Cancer

In the United States, skin cancer is the leading type of malignant disease. Basically, skin cancer is the growth of abnormal cells that are capable of invading and destroying other, linked skin cells. Skin cancer frequently is further divided into either melanoma or non-melanoma. A melanoma usually is a malignant tumor that arises from a skin cell that has the ability to make the pigment melanin (a melanocyte). Non-melanoma skin cancer, in the majority of cases, originates from the external skin surface, from a squamous cell or a basal cell.

Forty to 50 percent of all people develop skin cancer at least once by the time they are 65. Most common is basal cell carcinoma, a benign and slow-growing form of cancer that appears as a roughening on the neck or head, though it can appear on any area exposed to the sun. More than 800,000 people in the U.S. are diagnosed with basal cell carcinoma annually. In actuality, basal cell carcinoma is the most common of *all* the cancers. A third of all new cancers are skin cancers, with the overwhelming majority being basal cell carcinomas. Due to the fact that basal cell carcinoma develops gradually and occasionally resembles psoriasis or eczema, seeing a dermatologist for diagnosis is strongly recommended. If diagnosed in time and treated properly, over 95 percent of all basal cell carcinoma can be cured.

Squamous cell carcinoma is the second most common skin cancer in the U.S. More than 200,000 cases are diagnosed each year. Squamous cell carcinoma is usually a result of too much sun exposure and appears as a red, painless bump, while a melanoma generally appears as a flat, dry, brown or black skin patch with an irregular border, although it can sometimes bear a resemblance to a wart. Like basal cell carcinoma, squamous cell growths often develop on the parts of the body that are exposed to the sun. However, the growths can also appear on skin that has been harmed by burns or other types of injuries. An increased risk of squamous cell carcinoma is associated with people whose immune systems are compromised or who have chronic skin inflammation. While rarely fatal, basal cell carcinoma and squamous cell carcinoma can spread to other parts of the body.

Another, more dangerous skin cancer is malignant melanoma. It grows very quickly and metastasizes to other parts of the body through the lymphatic system. It is the most common fatal skin cancer. It is one of the most frequent skin cancers in young adults. This is due to the fact that it is not caused by prolonged exposure to UV radiation, but by sporadic, intense doses of UV radiation.

As with all chronic diseases, cancers have multiple and long-range causes that can be subsumed under the term lifestyle. These include denatured food, air and water pollution and imbalances brought on by parasites, fungi, bacteria, viruses, toxic chemicals and heavy metals. Skin cancers in particular are directly attributable to sun exposure. Sunny Arizona has the highest incidence of skin cancer anywhere in the world. In addition to more general concerns, such as nutrition, exercise and avoiding exposure to toxins, prevention and treatment of skin cancers involve wearing hats, long-sleeved clothing and sunscreen when out in the sun.

The SPF (sun protection factor) is the system that gives higher numbers to sunscreens that provide higher levels of protection. Yet, the SPF system is based on the ability to prevent erythema, an inflammatory redness of the skin. An SPF of 15 usually indicates a sunblock, since, if correctly used, it will thwart redness. However, ultraviolet damage can still occur.

Note: Before purchasing a sunscreen, check its ingredients, since some of these are carcinogenic.

Treatment

Standard treatment for basal cell carcinoma, the benign form of skin cancer, is removal of the tumor through surgery or freezing. When dealt with early, these tumors rarely pose a problem once removed.

Orthodox approaches for malignant skin cancers are not nearly as successful. These spread quickly and usually reappear, even after removal.

Diet

Attention must be paid to balancing the blood pH, as research indicates that maintenance of proper alkaline balance inhibits the proliferation of cancer cells. The blood's pH should be between 7.2 and 7.4, ideally. To get the desired effect, the diet should consist of 50 percent alkaline foods. Eating raw fruits and vegetables will create this effect. Many nuts, seeds, grains and legumes are also good.

Dr. Gerson's diet therapy has demonstrated success in the treatment of all skin cancers. The program involves extensive cleansing using organic juices, coffee enemas and other means. Research shows that in cases where the cancer had spread to the lymph glands, people who underwent operations to remove as much tumor as possible and then used the Gerson therapy had five-year survival rates of 92 percent (early stage) and 80 percent (late stage). This therapy is practiced today by Dr. Victor Ortuno, who can be reached at 800-759-2966.

Herbs

A classical herbal ointment, commonly referred to as the black salve and made primarily from sanguinaria or bloodroot, is helpful in treating skin cancers, as it causes the lesion to come to a head and fall off. Bloodroot extract must be used under the supervision of a qualified physician; skin must be continually monitored and particular attention paid to preventing and treating secondary infections.

Pau d'arco has long been used by the indigenous peoples of tropical America to heal a variety of serious illnesses, including cancer and syphilis. Scientists have found that this herb contains a substance that works against various kinds of tumors by inducing cancer cell death without harming healthy cells. Another herb used for cancer, chaparral, has potentially toxic properties. It can be beneficial, though, when used under the guidance of a qualified health practitioner.

Supplements

It is important to understand that with skin cancer, alternative medicine's main focus is prevention, as opposed to treatment. Vitamins have demonstrated their ability to prevent sunburn and, perhaps, skin cancer. A number of dermatologists advise their patients to supplement with vitamins E and C, to help prevent sunburn. In one notable study, males and females supplemented with E and C for eight days before they were exposed to UV light. As opposed to those who did not supplement, the people taking the vitamins needed about 20 percent more UV light to cause sunburn. This marks one of the first studies demonstrating that using vitamins E and C increases resistance to sunburn. Vitamins E and C are believed to lessen the risk of skin cancer. Furthermore, lower doses of these vitamins are thought to guard against harm from the sun. Other antioxidants, such as beta-carotene, vitamin A, coenzyme Q10, selenium, zinc and the bioflavonoids quercetin and pycnogenol, could assist in preventing skin cancer. Do not forget to use the antioxidant herbs, such as bilberry, hawthorn, turmeric and ginkgo. Maitake mushrooms are recommended, too.

What to Avoid

Substances to stay away from include pesticides, synthetic hormones and antibiotics, including those used in animal-derived foods. Foods that foster acidity should be minimized, and include meat, dairy products, caffeine, sugar, carbonated beverages, liquor and processed foods.

Treatment Summary

The standard treatment for benign skin cancer is surgery or freezing. Unfortunately, malignant skin cancer is much less responsive to conventional solutions.

A cleansing, highly alkaline diet contributes to success in the treatment of all skin cancers.

Load up on your antioxidants, particularly vitamins E and C.

Several herbs can aid in the treatment of skin cancer, including bloodroot, pau d'arco and chaparral.

Nutrients to use in fighting skin cancer include quercetin, pycnogenol and coenzyme Q1O, among others.

See also: Cancer

Skin Conditions

The skin is a thin layer of tough tissue that comprises the covering of the body. While it protects all of our internal systems, it is also connected to these, so it can react to infections anywhere in the body. Skin is affected by our emotional health. For someone who has gone through an extended period of stress, the aging effects on the skin are apparent. One theory even names cortisol as the culprit behind female adult acne. Further, if a person is not careful, the skin may also be affected when it is exposed to environmental toxins. Regardless of whether skin irritations originate internally or externally, they are not only uncomfortable, but may cause more severe ramifications, such as scarring and bleeding. Thus, it is important to understand how to prevent and treat the most common skin conditions.

Common Conditions

Acne

This common complaint, commonly referred to as pimples, is caused by bacteria and other irritants embedded underneath the skin's oil glands and hair follicles. It is generally a result of improper hygiene and poor diet, i.e., excessive amounts of processed, fatty and fried foods, as well as dairy, meat and sugar. Generally, the liver and kidneys work to cleanse the system of toxins. However, when an excessive amount of germs exist in a person's system, an extra burden is placed on the skin to remove them. If the bacteria are unable to be cleansed from the system, this type of inflammation is the result. Acne tends to develop mainly on the face, chest, back and shoulders. Generally, the condition is associated with adolescence, but in some individuals, it persists into adulthood and can leave permanent scarring.

461

Psoriasis

This is a chronic condition whereby the body produces an excess of skin cells, characterized by thick, dry, red, scaly patches over the skin. It affects fewer than 2 percent of all Americans, occurring in people who are highly toxic—particularly those with poor diet and liver function. It is also believed that many individuals have a genetic predisposition to this problem. It is inclined to appear and reappear, but psoriasis never really goes away. Flare-ups of this condition seem to be brought on by stress. While this problem may present itself anywhere on the body, the most common sites are the arms, scalp, ears, knees and pubic area. It can even cause changes in the fingernails, such as splitting and dimpling. Joint swelling may accompany the disease as well.

Fungal Rashes

These are common rashes caused by infection in various areas of the body. Tinea cruris (more commonly referred to as "jock itch") is a reddened, inflamed and itch rash found on the groin or buttock crease. Tinea versicolor is a result of excessive exposure to the sun and mainly around the chest and back. It appears as a dark, flat, scaly rash that can result in areas of discoloration in dark-skinned individuals. Athlete's foot is a red, itchy rash occurring between the toes and in the web spaces. Ringworm presents itself mainly in children and is identified by a red, circular, ring-like inflammation.

Cysts and Abscesses

When a sebaceous gland becomes clogged, it will start to progressively enlarge to form a bump under the skin, referred to as a sebaceous cyst. It consists of a fluid that, when infected, causes redness and tenderness. Therefore, if a cyst is not treated immediately, it can develop into an abscess, which is a concentrated accumulation of pus. Another cause of abscess can be skin injuries that are left unattended. This problem generally tends to form on the armpits, genital areas, buttocks and lower extremities.

Dermatitis

This covers a broad array of skin irritations. It generally refers to a red, inflammatory rash, which may include scaling and blisters. It can also be accompanied by an itching, burning or painful sensation. One type of dermatitis is contact dermatitis, which is most commonly a result of exposure to poison ivy or poison oak. These are plants that produce irritating oil that, when in contact with the human skin, can cause it to break out in this type of reaction. This same response may also be the result of handling certain common metals, such as nickel, contained in a variety of everyday products.

Another type of skin inflammation in this category is irritant eczema. This is an irritation that is caused by an allergic reaction to impurities or environmental factors (e.g., chemicals in food and soaps, cold weather or heat). Irritant eczema is most common among people who need to wash their hands several times a day and don't allow their hands to dry completely (such as health care and restaurant workers).

Yet another type of dermatitis is seborrheic dermatitis. This is generally due to a genetic predisposition and is typically found in infants and patients with Parkinson's disease. While seborrheic dermatitis produces most of the symptoms common to this category of skin problems, it generally does not produce itching. It tends to occur around the nose, chin, eyebrows, ears and lips.

Treatment

Conventional treatments for these skin conditions typically deal with the problem once it has emerged. The solutions consist mainly of medicated topical creams and ointments to clear the infected area. However, these may produce side effects, given that the medications often contain antibiotics, steroids and hormones. Furthermore, since they do not address the cause of the problem, their effects are usually temporary. Natural solutions, on the other hand, are simple, do not produce side effects and focus on prevention so that individuals may lessen their susceptibility to the problem.

Diet

In order to help the system cleanse toxins from the body to guard against infection related to acne, psoriasis and abscess, a person's diet should be optimized. The best foods for healthy, attractive skin are low in fat and protein and high in complex carbohydrates. Generally, a high-fiber, vegetarian diet is best. Foods should be eaten as close to their natural state as possible, as opposed to being refined or processed. Good foods for the skin are rich in vitamins A and C, beta-carotene and chlorophyll. They include beet greens, carrots, egg yolk, potatoes, yams, peppers, artichokes and dark green vegetables. Pure water is also essential for clear skin. At least five 8-ounce glasses are needed daily. Two to three 8-ounce servings of freshly made juice are important as well. Carrot juice combined with a small amount of green vegetable juice contains an abundant amount of nutrients.

It is important to note, when talking about skin conditions, that allergies to certain foods may aggravate these conditions. Common food allergens are corn, soy, wheat and peanuts. A naturopathic or complementary physician can help you identify these.

Herbs

Herbs can help the skin in numerous ways. Some herbs improve liver and kidney function, thus helping clear the body of toxins that can trigger acne and psoriasis. Other herbs help the skin more directly.

To improve liver function, herbs to consider are agrimony, barberry, dandelion root, echinacea, milk thistle, sassafras, yellow dock, red clover and sarsaparilla. The kidneys benefit from buchu, parsley celery seed, corn silk, cleavers and goldenrod.

To cleanse and nourish the skin directly, one can ingest burdock root, Oregon grape root or yellow dock. One can also nourish the skin externally through steam treatments or baths that help open up pores to push out toxins. Steam treatments can be made by pouring boiled water over a handful of herbs, placing a towel over the head and leaning over the container. Herbs recommended for this type of treatment are strawberry leaves, eucalyptus, thyme and wintergreen. For bathing, herbalist Lynn Newman recommended that hot water be poured over a mixture of chamomile, witch hazel, nettles, echinacea and calendula. After allowing this to steep for an hour, it should be strained and poured into a tub of water.

Herbs that can be applied directly to the skin to help stop itching include aloe vera, lavender, calendula and oats. An herb that can prevent the spread of poison oak or poison ivy and can be applied directly to the skin is jewel weed.

Supplements

Nutrients can be valuable in the prevention and treatment of skin conditions and their symptoms. Consider the following:

Chromium . . . This is perhaps the single most important nutrient for the skin. It balances blood sugar and lowers stress, both of which have an impact on skin problems. Studies have shown that chromium helps fight acne. Refined sugar, white flour and lack of exercise all rob the body of chromium. In addition to supplement form, chromium can be found in brewers yeast, complex carbohydrates and fresh fruit. There is no RDA for chromium, but a daily dose of 200 mcg is suggested to guarantee proper blood sugar regulation.

Zinc . . . When taken in the recommended dosage of 30-150 mg daily, this nutrient can prevent acanthosis, which is a thickening of the skin seen in serious cases of acne, eczema and psoriasis. It is as effective as the antibiotic tetracycline, without the side effects. Zinc's usefulness may be due to the fact that it helps release vitamin A. Good food sources of zinc include eggs and seafood, garlic, onions and sea vegetables.

Vitamin A . . . Taking a minimum of 10,000 IU daily has been shown to cure acne, due to vitamin A's antiviral action. The water-soluble form, palmitate, is proven to cure stubborn plantar warts as well. Since there is no toxicity from water-soluble A, up to 100,000 IU can be safely used.

Vitamin E... In order to heal skin lesions and scar tissue, both internally and on the surface, 200-800 IU daily of vitamin E can be used. This supplement also helps skin stay younger longer.

Vitamin B6... Pyridoxine, or vitamin B6, protects against infection. This nutrient can help prevent or treat acne, especially in premenstrual women.

Lecithin... This supplement provides fatty acids needed for healthy skin, and is effective in treating many dermatological disorders. Lecithin helps the body to better utilize the fat-soluble vitamins A, D and E. Evening primrose oil, borage oil and black currant seed oil are important sources of essential fatty acids, which work well in conjunction with lecithin.

Teas

Most people are familiar with green tea, because of its popularity over the past decade, but remain unfamiliar with its cousin, red tea. Red tea has a number of the most powerful and protective natural antioxidants and enzymes that have been proven to be beneficial for the skin. Leading the way are vitamins C and E, along with beta-carotene. These natural antioxidants help in new skin health following the removal of dead skin cells. Furthermore, red tea has flavonoids, which have been proven effective in treating assorted skin and circulatory problems. Red tea has a huge amount of alpha hydroxy acids, which assist in removing damaged surface skin. Free-radical damage (the principle cause of aging skin) is greatly thwarted when exfoliation is combined with red tea.

Detoxification Methods

Bowel detoxification with enemas or colonics is helpful for improving skin conditions, particularly acne, eczema and psoriasis. When one improves intestinal function and overcomes liver congestion, the skin becomes less burdened and takes on a more healthy appearance. Colonics can help even long-term psoriasis sufferers resolve itching and sores.

Magnetic Therapy

Removing toxic wastes from the body through magnetic therapy is another approach to improving skin problems. Sleeping on a magnetic bed is used as a way to increase oxygen to the entire system and remove acidity. Additionally, magnets help to eliminate inflammation. Magnets can be placed directly on lesions, but to ensure cleanliness, it is suggested that cotton be placed between the magnet and the lesion. If an area is too tender for magnets, spraying magnetically charged water over the area is a good substitute. Be sure to use the negative pole of the magnet only.

Reflexology

Another way of improving eliminative function to help prevent and over-come skin disorders is with reflexology, a type of massage technique that applies pressure to specific points on the feet that correspond to other areas of the body. To aid the liver in removal of toxins, one can massage the under part of the foot from the ball down toward the middle area. To help the kidneys in the process of excreting fluid from the body, pressure should be applied to the area in the middle of the underside of the foot. The nervous system can also be worked to alleviate stress associated with skin conditions. The area to which pressure should be applied is the inner edge of the foot, starting at the heel and moving upward to the top of the toes. Then, one should massage across all toes. This procedure stimulates the spinal cord and brain.

Homeopathic Remedies

When deciding which homeopathic remedy to choose, consider the one that most closely addresses the symptoms. One of the following formulas may prove useful. But if it does not, seek the guidance of a trained homeopathic practitioner.

Calgarea Sulphurica . . . This formula is indicated for boils and acne when there are pimples at the rim of the scalp that bleed when scratched.

Hepar Sulphuris Calcareum . . . This helps moist skin that is very sensitive to dry, cold air and touch. Boils can be treated with this remedy.

Abrotannum . . . This solution is specifically used for boils, particularly those that recur on various parts of the body (sometimes as a reaction to antibiotics in the treatment of acne).

Sulphur . . . This is for dry, itchy skin that feels worse in heat or after bathing.

Belladonna . . . In some cases of contact dermatitis, where a sudden rash is hot, dry, red, burning and occasionally itchy, belladonna, given in pellets that are placed under the tongue, may provide relief.

Apis Mollifica . . . For heat rashes that are bright red and inflamed, this remedy should reverse the condition.

Pulsatilla . . . This can be used in some cases of dermatitis, where an itchy rash may worsen with heat or when exposed to air.

Utica Urens . . . This is another solution for contact dermatitis in which the rash may be itchy and prickly and where red blotches are present. This can either be taken as pellets placed under the tongue or used in a tincture applied directly on the rash.

Dulcamara . . . For cases of dermatitis in which the skin reacts to an upset stomach or after exposure to cold, wet weather, this remedy is helpful. Usually, this kind of skin irritation is present on the hands, arms and face and is characterized by red spots and eruptions.

Calendula . . . This can be applied directly to the skin for general skin irritations, after the infection has cleared.

Rhus Toxicodendron . . . For the prevention of poison ivy, rhus tox should be used in pellets only and taken prior to exposure to the plant. It can also be used in the very early stages of this rash.

Croton Tiglium . . . This should be used in the more advanced stages of poison ivy, where there is extreme itching, where burning occurs after scratching and where there may be blisters that leak.

Anacardium . . . This is another treatment for extreme cases of poison ivy. While the symptoms are the same as for croton tiglium, they also tend to become exacerbated when warm water is applied. This remedy should be taken in pellets placed under the tongue.

What to Avoid

Avoid refined foods, which are devoid of trace minerals needed for healing the skin. Also, beware of fried and fatty foods, chocolate, other sweets, soft thinks, alcohol and milk. These contain substances that the body converts into prostaglandin-E2. This, in turn, suppresses the immune system and causes an inflammatory reaction.

Stress should also be avoided, since many skin problems are aggravated when an individual is tense and upset.

Treatment Summary

A diet that is low in fat, moderate in protein and high in complex carbohydrates is recommended to help cleanse toxins from the body and thus decrease the chance of skin problems.

A variety of herbs, taken internally or used externally, can improve skin health.

Chromium is an important nutrient for the skin. Others that are helpful are zinc, vitamins A, C and B6 and lecithin.

Detoxification methods such as enemas or colonics can be helpful for clearing up skin conditions.

Magnetic therapy and reflexology are additional techniques used to improve the condition of the skin.

Homeopathic remedies are keyed to specific skin conditions and symptoms.

Stroke

Because of the similarity between heart attacks and strokes, the two are sometimes confused. Traditionally, strokes have been given less attention than heart attacks. Both involve a cutoff of blood supply: In a heart attack, the supply to the heart—and consequently to all the other organs—is cut off, while with a stroke, blood supply to the brain is cut off, as a result of a clot or a hemorrhage. Consequently, many feel it more accurate to classify a stroke as a "brain attack." Once this happens, oxygen becomes depleted and brain tissue dies. This can ultimately result in paralysis, blindness, speech difficulties, loss of function in an arm or leg and other serious disabilities. There may also be cognitive impairment—the person cannot think or remember as well as before.

In the U.S., stroke is the third leading cause of death, ranking only behind cancer and heart disease. Approximately a quarter of all stroke victims die as a direct result of the stroke or its ensuing complications. Nearly a half of stroke victims have moderate to extreme bodily impairments and long-range disabilities. Sadly, just about a quarter of those who suffer a stroke recover all or almost all of their former bodily functions and health.

Most strokes occur when a blood clot blocks the flow of oxygenated blood to part of the brain. This kind of stroke, called an ischemic stroke, is caused by a blood clot blocking, or "plugging," a blood vessel. The vast majority (83 percent) of all strokes are ischemic, with over 50 percent of ischemic strokes being thrombotic.

Ischemic clots form either inside the artery of the brain (thrombotic stroke) or in another part of the body, subsequently entering the brain (embolic stroke). Ironically, blood clotting is beneficial in healthy individuals, since blood clots stop a bleeding wound. However, problems arise when the blood clots abnormally. When this happens, clots can block arteries in the brain, effectively halting blood flow, thereby causing a stroke.

Strokes affect people of all ages. In older people they are usually associated with high blood pressure, elevated cholesterol and blocked arteries. Younger people can have strokes as a result of congenital abnormalities. Certain drugs, such as cocaine and amphetamines, can bring them on as well.

Recent estimates of stroke occurrence in the U.S. place the number between 715,000 and 750,000 yearly. These estimates, however, are deceiving, for they do not take into account the incidences of silent strokes and hemorrhages. Reliable studies have estimated that silent stroke takes place 10 to 20 times more than symptomatic stroke!

Risk Factors for Strokes

Heart Disease

Heart disease adds to the risk of a stroke. Those with heart disease have more than twice the risk of suffering a stroke than those without heart disease.

High Blood Pressure

For the past 50 years, no other factor has been more important in predicting stroke than high blood pressure. Many correlate the successful treatment of high blood pressure with the declining death rates from strokes. While high blood *pressure* remains an extremely important harbinger for stroke, recent studies indicate that the importance of blood *analysis* as a means of predicting stroke is increasing. Monitoring the levels of key factors in the blood—homocysteine (a protein in the blood that has been linked to heart disease), fibrinogen, glucose, iron (blood ferritin is an indicator of the full amount of iron stored in the body), LDL-cholesterol, DHEA—to ensure they fall within acceptable parameters is a proactive way of benefiting from the numerous studies showing that most strokes can be prevented. One of the most important levels to monitor is that of C-reactive protein. In fact, C-reactive protein is one of the hottest health topics around. Specifically, many believe that measuring the levels of C-reactive protein in the blood is an accurate way of predicting who will suffer a stroke. According to an article in *Stroke*, elevated C-reactive protein levels cause a two-to-three times greater risk of stroke. By keeping an eye on the levels of all these important factors, one will be able to quickly avail himself or herself of treatments that have demonstrated their effectiveness in lowering these factors.

Gender

Males have approximately a 20-percent greater likelihood of a stroke than females.

Heredity

Those with a family history of stroke have a greater likelihood of stroke than those who do not have such a family history.

High Red Blood Cell Count

Because red blood cells thicken the blood, thereby increasing the chances of clot formation, even a moderate increase in the red blood cell count is a risk factor for stroke.

Race

African American stroke victims have a significantly higher risk of death and disability than do their Caucasian counterparts. This is due, in part, to the fact that African Americans have a greater frequency of high blood pressure.

Cigarette Smoking

If you want to lower your risk of getting a stroke, you should say "Butt out!" to cigarettes. Studies show that cigarette smoking is an important risk factor for stroke. Additionally, female smokers who also use oral contraceptives are at an even higher risk.

Transient Ischemic Attacks (TIAs)

Better known as "mini-strokes." TIAs create stroke-like symptoms, though they produce no long-term damage. They should be heeded, for they are accurate prognosticators of a stroke. Someone with one or more TIAs is roughly *10 times* more likely to be victimized by a stroke than someone similarly situated with no TIAs.

Warning: The importance of TIAs as warning signs cannot be overemphasized. They are extremely important stroke warning signs. Be on the lookout for them!

Other Risk Factors

Other important stroke risk factors include *excessive alcohol consumption* (more than one drink per day for women and more than two drinks per day for men), which can raise blood pressure, increasing the likelihood of stroke. *Cocaine* has been closely linked to strokes. Also, a report based on 15 published studies showed that mild-to-moderate *elevations in homocysteine levels* were associated with an amazing 86-percent increase in the risk of stroke.

Symptoms

A stroke can produce different symptoms depending upon the part of the brain that is affected and the length of time that the brain is without oxygen. Small strokes may escape awareness and produce slight numbness on the face or another part of the body. Severe strokes can cause any number of symptoms, including paralysis, loss of speech, loss of memory, loss of movement, an inability to swallow or death.

According to the Mayo Clinic and the National Stroke Association, the following are stroke symptoms: sudden trouble standing or walking; dizziness; loss of balance or coordination; sudden confusion; trouble speaking or understanding; sudden trouble seeing in one or both eyes; sudden, very severe headaches with no known cause.

Note: Any of these signs may be temporary and last for only a few minutes.

Prevention and Treatment

If an ischemic stroke is happening, it would be helpful to give the patient large doses of antioxidant vitamins, as well as herbs such as ginkgo biloba. A 1500-mg oral dose of magnesium can ease an arterial spasm, which is a frequent problem in thrombotic strokes. By taking high-potency antioxidants a minimum of three times per day, you can considerably enhance the odds of recuperating from an ischemic stroke.

The best way to prevent a stroke is to maximize total systemic health. A complementary physician, one who combines traditional and holistic medicine, can determine whether risk factors for stroke are present and can educate the patient on how to lessen them if they are. Such a doctor helps people to lower cholesterol levels, keep blood pressure down and unblock arteries. Chelation therapy is often recommended for this purpose. A series of treatments can open up the arteries and eliminate the risk of stroke.

The use of computerized tomography (CT), Doppler ultrasonography and magnetic resonance imaging (MRI) have been responsible for drastic improvements in the early detection of strokes. These advances have led directly to declines in stroke mortality.

Hyperbaric Oxygen Therapy

It was once thought that brain cell damage was irreversible. But this is not always so. Hyperbaric (high-pressure) oxygen therapy can produce a successful turnabout in most stroke patients. When this therapy, which delivers pure oxygen to the patient, is used within the first 24 hours of a stroke, aftereffects may never manifest. And even when the treatment is used years later, dramatic improvements can be seen, as many lingering symptoms disappear. In fact, people who have tried every other form of treatment, to no avail, often find success with hyperbaric oxygen therapy.

While this may seem hard to fathom, the reason can be scientifically explained. During a stroke, only a small area of the brain actually dies. This is the part supplied by the blocked artery. Surrounding tissue is injured, but not necrotic. It receives some oxygen from peripheral arteries, but not enough to keep it fully alive and healthy. Hyperbaric oxygen revitalizes this injured tissue, and restores it to fuller function.

Another reason for tissue damage with stroke is brain swelling. During the initial cerobrovascular accident, as a stroke is called, dying tissue swells and squeezes into surrounding areas. Pressure on blood vessels causes loss of oxygen. That, in turn, causes paralysis and other stroke-related injuries. Hyperbaric oxygen reverses the swelling, and in so doing reverses many symptoms, even years later, since brain tissue does not die suddenly. It stays alive many years after the stroke.

Hyperbaric oxygen therapy is more successful when combined with chelation and antioxidant therapies.

Magnesium

The development of a genetically engineered drug called TPA has recently been praised as a significant advance in treating patients who have suffered strokes. But this drug's *expense*, and the possible side effect of brain hemorrhage, have hindered its becoming widely used. Interestingly, the natural substance magnesium sulfate, which costs only about $5, is safer and therefore more beneficial than its unnatural counterpart. Not just a treatment, magnesium sulfite is helpful in avoiding stroke as well. Between 800 and 1500 mg can be taken daily as a preventive measure, and the bulk of that should be taken before bedtime.

Other Supplements

In addition to magnesium, these nutrients can prevent strokes or speed up recovery:

Multivitamin-Mineral Supplement . . . Make sure this contains 3-6 mg of copper, as copper deficiency has been linked to strokes.

B Complex . . . B-complex vitamins nourish the brain and help the mind overcome depression. B vitamins can be obtained from blue-green algae or bee pollen, using 50 mg three times a day. The use of extra vitamins B6, B12 and folic acid is one way of lowering homocysteine levels. Folate, a B-complex vitamin, also reduces the levels of homocysteine, a protein in the blood that has been linked to heart disease. Incredibly, Lorenzo D. Botto, MD, with the National Center on Birth Defects and Developmental Disabilities of the Centers for Disease Control and Prevention, estimated that *17,000* deaths linked to ischemic heart disease and *31,000* stroke-related deaths may have been prevented each year since fortification with the B vitamins was initiated in the U.S. in 1996 to help prevent neural tube birth defects!

Beta-Carotene... The results of a six-year study in Finland prove that beta-carotene lowers the risk of ischemic stroke. The study involved 26,497 male smokers and concluded that beta-carotene remained a significant risk reduction factor against cerebral infarction. The study also confirmed that vegetables and fruits protect against the risk of stroke.

Vitamin E... This powerful antioxidant helps reduce clotting. Start slowly with 200-800 IU a day and increase to 800-1000 IU.

Selenium... Selenium should be taken along with vitamin E to improve its action and to keep tissues elastic. The recommended dosage is 200 mcg.

Pycnogenol...Pycnogenol keeps collagen elastic and softens blood platelets so that they can move more efficiently. The recommended dosage is 400 mg.

Coenzyme Q10... This is one of the most important nutrients for getting oxygen into the tissues, heart and brain. Approximately 200 mg should be taken daily.

Lecithin... Two capsules taken with each meal helps to protect the brain, deter cardiovascular disease and reduce cholesterol.

Vitamin C...Take plenty of this vitamin to strengthen arterial walls, thereby preventing a stroke or heart attack from occurring. Vitamin C should be taken along with bioflavonoids, in a dosage of 3000-20,000 mg. A study published in *Stroke* concluded that high serum vitamin C levels mean a lower risk for stroke. The study, conducted over 20 years, involved 880 men and 1241 women. The participants' serum vitamin C levels were inversely proportional to their incidence of stroke during the follow-up period. This applied to both cerebral infarction (ischemic) and hemorrhagic stroke. The researchers concluded that higher vitamin C levels lowered the risk of both forms of stroke.

Melatonin...Melatonin is one of the most powerful scavengers of free radicals. It easily penetrates the blood-brain barrier. Consider taking 500 mcg-3 mg of melatonin at night as part of an integrated treatment program for thrombotic stroke.

Hydergine

Hydergine is an antioxidant medication known to protect the cells of the brain that the patient may be given under dire circumstances. The recommended dosage is 10 mg sublingually or 10 mg orally. Note: Because the FDA has not yet approved Hydergine for this purpose, the patient needs to specifically ask for it.

Herbs

Ginkgo, at a preventive dose of 125 mg a day or a therapeutic dose of 120-240 mg daily, is recommended for the brain. Based upon the findings of 40 clinical trials, the journal *Neuroreport* stated that "positive results have been reported for ginkgo biloba extracts in the treatment of cerebral insufficiency."

Other herbs that help prevent strokes are the same ones used to help the heart. These include hawthorn, garlic, cayenne and blueberry leaves.

Green Tea Extract

Green tea is a powerful antioxidant and has antithrombotic properties. A dosage of 350 mg per day is recommended. According to a study in the *Proceedings of the National Academy of Sciences*, the tannin called gallotannin, which is derived from green tea, and another tannin, nobotannin B, prevented stroke damage to brain cells in culture.

Whole Grains

According to the *Journal of the American Medical Association*, women who increased their intake of whole grains reduced their risk of ischemic stroke. As noted above, ischemic stroke occurs when a blood clot blocks one of the arteries supplying blood to the brain, resulting in damage to the brain because of a lack of oxygen.

Aromatherapy

Essential oils can play a vital role in the recovery of stroke patients. Oils that stimulate circulation can be highly effective in helping patients overcome the temporary paralysis that often accompanies strokes. In English intensive ward units, essential oils of lavender, lemon and geranium are used for this purpose. For stimulating a return of memory, rosemary, clary sage, peppermint, rose or basil can be given. Under the guidance of an aromatherapist, a few drops of the pure essence can be added to water and taken two or three times a day. Essences can also be placed on a tissue and breathed in, or vaporized in the room.

Emotional Support

People who suffer from depression have an increased risk of stroke, according to a study by the Centers for Disease Control published in the journal

Psychosomatic Medicine. As noted above, several physical risk factors for stroke have been firmly established over the years. However, this seminal study also shows the importance of emotional risk factors, particularly depression.

In the study, researchers analyzed information from 6095 individuals. They found that people with elevated levels of depression symptoms had a significantly increased chance of suffering a stroke. Incredibly, the risk was increased by 73 percent! Moderate levels of depression increased the risk by 25 percent.

The willingness of friends and family to help means a lot to the patient in recovery, and can speed up the healing process. It is important to smile, and it is helpful to think positively, say affirmations, pray, meditate and find other ways to keep upbeat.

Exercise

According to an article in the June 2000 issue of the *Journal of the American Medical Association (JAMA)*, walking reduces the risk of stroke in women. The study, involving 72,000 women, showed that regular exercise, such as moderately brisk walking, can considerably lower the risk of stroke in middle-aged women. Women who walked frequently and at a quick pace lessened their risk of stroke—the kind caused by blocked blood vessels (ischemic)—by over a third. These results were probably obtained because exercise reduces blood pressure and increases HDL (the good cholesterol) levels, thereby decreasing the risk of blood clots.

What to Avoid

When in the presence of a person who has had a stroke, never offer the person anything to drink. If the ability to swallow has been lost, the person could choke.

Treatment Summary

While monitoring high blood pressure is critical, go one step further and monitor the levels of homocysteine, C-reactive protein, fibrinogen, glucose, iron, LDL-cholesterol and DHEA. These are key factors in the blood that predict the likelihood of stroke.

To prevent stroke, a complementary physician can determine risk factors and recommend ways to lessen them.

Exercise.

Stop smoking.

Pay attention to stroke symptoms.

Magnesium supplementation is preventative.

Other anti-stroke nutrients are the B-complex vitamins, vitamins E and C, selenium, pycnogenol, coenzyme Q1O and lecithin. A multivitamin/mineral supplement containing copper is a good idea. The use of extra vitamins B6, B12, trimethylglycine and folic acid is one way of lowering homocysteine levels.

Helpful herbs are ginkgo, hawthorn, garlic, cayenne and blueberry leaves.

Remedies effective in treating stroke patients are hyperbaric oxygen therapy and magnesium sulfate.

Aromatherapy can aid in stroke patients' recovery.

Emotional support of the stroke patient can speed the healing process.

Remember, new studies indicate that by following sound advice, strokes can be prevented.

Tinnitus

Tinnitus is a major medical problem that affects roughly 50 million Americans, 12 million of them severely. There are two main categories of tinnitus: subjective and objective. Subjective tinnitus, the more common form, can be heard only by the person who has it. Objective tinnitus can be heard by the examiner.

Many of us who live in excessively noisy surroundings learn to acclimate to this lifestyle, not aware of the consequences that could eventually develop. One of these is tinnitus, a ringing or tinkling sound in one or both ears.

Causes

Blaring music, gunshots, explosions and other extremely loud sounds can create ear injury and cause tinnitus. Additional factors are exposure to toxic chemicals in foods, medicines and the environment.

Symptoms

Tinnitus is characterized by a noise resembling that of a fuzzy television set, and ranging from barely audible to quite loud. The sound may be continuous or heard at intervals. Symptoms accompanying tinnitus can include headaches, digestive disorders, learning disabilities, irritability, insomnia and fatigue.

Treatment

Nutrition

There is a high correlation between tinnitus and poor nutrition. Diets high in fat, cholesterol and refined sugars are particularly detrimental to ear health. Switching to a diet that is rich in vegetable proteins and complex carbohydrates is important. In addition, freshly made juices are concentrated sources of healing vitamins and minerals and of valuable enzymes, all in an easily assimilated form. (Unlike store-bought juices, just-squeezed juice contains live, healing nutrients and no chemical additives.)

Supplements

The inner ear contains thousands of specialized sensory cells, which need water, oxygen and nutrients in order to effectively deliver complete electrical information to the brain. Some of the more important nutrients for this condition are as follows:

Vitamin A—about 25,000 IU
Vitamin B1 (thiamin)—100-500 mg daily
Vitamin B3 (non-flush niacin)—50 mg twice daily to start, moving up to 500 mg maximum twice daily, along with 25 mg of zinc twice daily and 2 mg of copper daily
Vitamin B12 (cyanocobalamin)—1-5 mcg daily in lozenge form
Vitamin B complex—50 mg twice daily
Vitamin E—400-800 IU
Vitamin D—500-1000 IU
Ionized calcium—500-1000 mg
Magnesium—up to 500 mg
Potassium—500 mg
Zinc sulfate—60 mg

Sometimes an iron deficiency is associated with tinnitus, in which case 75 mg of iron each day for two weeks is recommended. After that period, reduce iron intake to a normal level. Exact dosages of all nutrients should always be given by a physician.

Patients who suffer from ear ringing have improved their condition by supplementing with B vitamins. In particular, vitamins B12, B6 and B5 (pantothenic acid) have proven effective in improving tinnitus. Tinnitus sufferers frequently have a vitamin B12 deficiency. A number of these sufferers have found their condition improved through intramuscular injections of vitamin B12.

In one experiment, patients who had difficulty sleeping because of subjective tinnitus were given 3 mg of melatonin each night for 30 consecutive days. Roughly 50 percent of the patients reported their condition improved.

Ginkgo biloba, or maidenhair, is the oldest living tree on earth. It is proven to increase circulation throughout the body. Many studies have shown the efficacy of ginkgo on tinnitus.

Stress Reduction

Stress and tension have been found to cause or exacerbate tinnitus. Consequently, many tinnitus sufferers who have reduced stress and tension in their lives have found their condition ameliorated.

Biofeedback

Many patients have not attempted to reduce the stress in their lives, but have attempted to deal with their reaction to such stress. They have done so with the relaxation technique of biofeedback, which shows people how to control specific autonomic body functions, such as pulse, muscle tension and brain wave activity.

Magnetic Therapy

The results of a small experiment in Germany offers hope that the use of magnets to stimulate the area of the brain that processes sound could provide relief to tinnitus sufferers by "jamming" this part of the brain. They tested the theory on 14 patients with severe and intractable tinnitus. The majority of the patients indicated the noise in their ears lessened while the magnets were stimulating the left temporoparietal cortex, a part of the brain that contains a number of regions proven to be involved in the processing of sound.

TMJ Treatment

Tinnitus can be a warning sign of a dysfunctional jaw joint (temporomandibular joint, or TMJ). The muscles and nerves of the jaw are closely linked to the muscles and nerves of the ear. Consequently, in certain situations, problems with the jaw lead directly to complications in the muscles and nerves of the ear. When this circumstance arises, dental treatment or bite realignment often provides relief for tinnitus sufferers. See your dentist if you think you have this problem.

Transcutaneous Electric Nerve Stimulation (TENS)

Electrical stimulation treatment for tinnitus has been shown to be effective in approximately 50 percent of patients with tinnitus of various causes. TENS is a safe method for treating tinnitus if administered by a trained professional.

What to Avoid

Avoid excessive exposure to loud noises. Refrain from the damaging chemicals found in alcohol, cigarettes, caffeine and tap water. Home and office environments should be cleaned as much as possible. Exposure to copy machines, household cleansers and common toxins such as formaldehyde can help bring on or exacerbate tinnitus. Medicines known to be toxic to the ear include certain antibiotics, contraceptives and Novacain. Poor diet is a major contributor to tinnitus, especially a high-fat, high-cholesterol and sugary diet. Reduce your intake of salt. Salt can contribute to the increase of fluid in the ear. Refined carbohydrates should be replaced by complex carbohydrates. Acidic foods, such as meats, should be reduced. In their place, more alkaline foods, such as fruits and vegetables, should be eaten.

Treatment Summary

Remember, before treating tinnitus, it is important to discover the cause of it. Sometimes your doctor can alleviate the condition by simply removing earwax or treating an ear infection.

Switching to a diet that is rich in vegetable proteins, complex carbohydrates and fresh juices creates an environment conducive to healing.

Supplements of important nutrients can build ear health.

Avoid loud noises and common pollutants as much as possible.

TMJ Dysfunction

The temporomandibular joint (TMJ) is the joint where the mandible (the lower jaw) joins the temporal bone of the skull, immediately in front of the ears, on both sides of the head. A small disk of cartilage, very similar to knee cartilage, separates the bones. Each time you talk, chew, yawn or swallow, this disk permits the mandible to move easily. Consequently, it is one of the most used joints in the body, and one of the most complex.

In reality, TMJ Disorder is a catchall phrase used to describe the dysfunctioning of the muscles and joints of the jaw. Such dysfunctions can range from a slight clicking or popping sensation that occurs when the mouth is opened and closed to a serious, unrelenting pain that extends into the face, neck and shoulders, affecting posture and mobility.

The dysfunctioning jaw muscles and joints represent an abnormal condition characterized by facial pain and problems associated with the use of the lower jaw. The clicking or popping noises can accompany chewing or other movement of the jaw, and the resulting pain may not be limited to the jaw itself, but may shoot up into the neck, face, ear and shoulder. Headaches and toothaches are sometimes part of the TMJ dysfunction picture—even if all the teeth are healthy. There can also be dizziness, difficulty with opening the mouth and inflammation of the muscles around the mouth, to the extent that they may spasm and prevent closing of the mouth. An estimated 50 million Americans suffer from TMJ problems. TMJ troubles are widespread enough that Americans spend about $1 billion yearly on treatment and drugs to alleviate them.

Causes

Poor bite is one cause of TMJ problems; typically, new dental work, such as braces, can alter the alignment of teeth, which will then result in TMJ dysfunction. Stress is another common cause of TMJ dysfunction, and the stress caused by hormonal changes, as with premenstrual tension, can bring on or exacerbate the condition.

Trauma can cause TMJ problems, as well. An injury to the joint or to the head and neck can trigger a TMJ problem. For instance, a serious blow to the side of the face can cause the bones of the joint to fracture. Such a blow can even displace the disk (place it in an abnormal position), thereby leading to TMJ problems. A person suffering whiplash from a car accident can have his or her tissues and ligaments stretched or torn, leading to TMJ problems.

In addition, TMJ problems can arise from inflammatory or degenerative arthritis, poor dental work or structural defects that push the mandible back towards the ears whenever the patient chews or swallows. Stress-induced grinding or clenching of the teeth is also a frequent cause. Occasionally, muscles around the TMJ that are used for chewing will go into spasm, causing head and neck pain and difficulty opening the mouth in the normal manner.

TMJ dysfunction occurs more frequently in women than in men. In fact, 90 percent of patients seeking treatment for TMJ are women, most between puberty and menopause. A University of Washington in Seattle study showed that women on hormone replacement therapy were 77 percent more likely to seek treatment for jaw pain than those not receiving this treatment. Additionally, women taking oral contraceptives were 19 percent more likely to come in for treatment.

In addition to premenstrual changes, the physiological changes of pregnancy—hormonal shifts, weight gain, the loosening of ligaments and general stress—can foster TMJ dysfunction. And nursing mothers sometimes experience TMJ problems if they throw their bodily alignment out of whack by habitually nursing without proper postural support. The problem stems from the fact that the jaw is not an isolated joint; it's part of the craniosacral system, which extends from the feet upwards and lies along the center of the body. So misalignment occurring in any part of this system, such as in the upper back or neck, can get translated into TMJ pain.

Symptoms

The symptoms of TMJ disorder include the following:

Pain or soreness in the jaw, more noticeable in the morning and afternoon.

Pain in the jaw while chewing, biting or yawning.

Earache not accompanied by an infection, occasionally spreading into the face.

A clicking or grinding noise when opening and closing the mouth.

Difficulty opening and closing the mouth.

Stiffness of the jaw when eating, talking or yawning.
Sensitivity of the teeth without any signs of dental problems.

Treatment

There are a number of approaches to alleviating TMJ dysfunction, with surgery being the treatment of very last resort. (This is because there is no guarantee of success with surgery and it too often leaves patients with worse jaw problems than they had before they underwent the procedures. Also, most TMJ patients do get better with less drastic remedies.)

One of the less drastic approaches to the condition is craniosacral therapy, usually undertaken by an osteopath or chiropractor. What the doctor does is to try to establish the correct balance between the pelvis, spine and cranium; breathing techniques may be incorporated into this approach, in order to effect musculoskeletal changes.

Other effective treatments of jaw dysfunction include acupuncture; progressive relaxation training, which has been shown effective both with and without biofeedback; intraoral appliances, especially in combination with biofeedback; isotonic exercises; the use of moist heat; ice; and self-massage.

Healthy Diet

A healthy, whole-foods diet and nutritional supplements are often suggested. Some supplements that may alleviate TMJ problems are calcium and magnesium (to relax muscles) and the B-complex vitamins.

Herbs

Antispasmodic herbs, such as the herbal mixture called Euphytose, can help relieve jaw pain.

Soft Diet

Soft or blended foods allow the jaw to rest temporarily. Remember to avoid hard, crunchy and chewy foods. Do not stretch your mouth to accommodate corn on the cob or whole fruits.

Jaw Exercises

Slow, gentle jaw exercises may help increase jaw mobility. Your health care provider or a physical therapist can evaluate your condition and suggest appropriate exercises based on your individual needs.

Relaxation Techniques

Relaxation and guided imagery can be helpful in dealing with the pain that accompanies TMJ dysfunction. Deep, slow breathing enhances relaxation and modulates pain sensations.

Patient Education

Remember the proper jaw posture. The suggested sleeping position is *not* on the stomach. Always try to relax the jaw.

Toxic Shock Syndrome

Toxic shock syndrome (TSS) is a rare but dangerous condition that affects individuals with jeopardized immune systems. It occurs unexpectedly; as a result of poisoning by a strain of bacteria called Staphylococcus aureus. This type of staph sometimes creates a poisonous substance called enterotoxin F, which damages cell walls, allowing blood to seep into tissues.

Most cases of TSS occur in menstruating women who are using tampons, although children, men and women who are not menstruating do sometimes get the disease. Teenage girls and women under 30 have a higher risk of TSS than do older women. Though tampons are implicated in many cases of the disease, they do not directly cause it. Rather, they seem to create a breeding ground for the bacteria that do.

In the early 1980s, toxic shock syndrome was linked to the introduction of tampons containing four new ingredients: highly absorbent polyester cellulose, carboxymethyl cellulose, polyacrylate rayon and viscose rayon. Up until that time, tampons had been made mainly of cotton. Today, all but one of these new ingredients, viscose rayon, have been taken off of the market.

Symptoms

TSS is characterized by headaches, a sore throat, high fever, diarrhea, nausea, vomiting and rashes that look like red skin blotches or sunburn. These symptoms may then progress to include low blood pressure, fainting, confusion, acute kidney failure and abnormal liver function. Occasionally, death may result.

Treatment

If you suspect you may have toxic shock syndrome, seek medical care immediately, and if you are using a tampon, remove it. Once a person is diagnosed with TSS, hospitalization may be necessary, depending upon the severity of the case. However, several natural solutions are available once the critical period resolves; they can also be used to achieve quick recovery in less severe cases. There are also ways to avoid recurrence of the condition.

Herbs

Dr. Linda Page, author of *Healthy Healing: An Alternative Healing Reference*, reports that the following herbs have been proven to combat toxicity, reestablish a healthy immune system and restore the patient to health.

Ginseng . . . This will help to equalize and tone all systems within the body as well as strengthen circulation. However, people are strongly advised to refrain from taking this herb when a high fever exists.

Cayenne and Ginger . . . These aid the body in recuperating from shock. They are nervous system energizers that can be consumed or used as compresses placed directly on the skin.

Hawthorn Extract . . . Hawthorn accelerates and regulates circulation while reestablishing an overall sense of well-being.

Dr. Page recommends nutritious foods that are easily digested and rapidly utilized. Foods such as high-potency royal jelly, bee pollen, wheat germ, brewer's yeast and unsulfured molasses rank at the top of her list. The doctor also supplemented her diet with green drinks, including chlorella, barley grass, spirulina and wheatgrass. These drinks are powerhouses of vital minerals.

Diet

TSS necessitates a diet in which healthful foods can be readily digested and immediately used by the progressively weakening system. Considering this, Dr. Page suggests incorporating the following foods into the diet: high-potency royal jelly, bee pollen, wheat germ, brewer's yeast and unsulfured molasses. Additionally, important minerals should be included in the diet. These can be consumed in the form of green drinks, such as chlorella, barley grass, spirulina and wheatgrass juices.

What to Avoid

Women who wear tampons should choose only the absorbency necessary to meet their needs, since tampons with higher levels of absorbency present a higher risk of TSS. Also, women may want to alternate use of tampons with the use of sanitary pads. Tampons should be changed no less frequently than every four to eight hours.

Treatment Summary

Any instance of suspected TSS should receive medical attention, as this can be a life-threatening condition.

Some herbs and foods are recommended to combat toxicity, reestablish a healthy immune system and restore patient to health.

Trauma

As Americans entered the twenty-first century, they did so with a familiar companion: stress. The realities of a new world have made Americans among the most stressed peoples on earth. Some of the stress is self-imposed and some is not, but the bottom line is that most of us suffer from multiple pressures every day. There is the stress from unhappy relationships, poor health, working, traveling, living too closely to too many people, artificial time requirements, accepting too much responsibility, job-related issues and, recently, the threat of terrorist attacks. If left unchecked, these stresses can eventually lead to a whole spectrum of physical illnesses, including heart disease, mental illness, high blood pressure, obesity and insomnia, just to name a few.

Prolonged stress can produce a state of trauma. Physical and emotional trauma can also be induced by an accident, illness or shocking personal event. Even after muscles and tissues that were injured in an accident are completely healed, symptoms of trauma can manifest.

Treatment

Nutrition

During periods of stress and recovery from trauma, it is particularly important to be kind to yourself nutritionally. Diets should be high in fiber, full of wholesome, organic foods. Stress reactions thicken the blood; therefore, foods with a blood-thinning effect, such as ginger, garlic and cantaloupe, should be included in the diet.

When dealing with stress and trauma, supplementation is vital in restoring the plasma levels of the antioxidants necessary for assisting the body's forces responsible for repairing body tissues. Trauma can frequently produce a domino effect that jeopardizes the multiple organ systems of the body. Trauma can also lead to widespread infection. Supplementation with antioxidants such as vitamins C and E; the mineral selenium; and the amino acids L-arginine, N-acetyl-cysteine and L-glutamine, can assist in protecting and restoring tissues and reducing infection.

In one study, 18 patients suffering from trauma were placed in either a control group or given vitamins C and E along with selenium and N-acetyl-cysteine for seven days. As measured against the control group, the group that received the antioxidants had less organ dysfunction and fewer infection-related complications.

In addition, tissue damage has been linked to elevated levels of lipid peroxides, as well as other types of free radicals. Antioxidant supplementation can assist the body in combating such free-radical damage.

Vitamin E has been shown to neutralize the effects of free-radical damage and to strengthen the immune system by protecting the T-cells. Take two 400-mg capsules or a dry powder (d-alpha tocopherol) supplement once a day, 200 mg of gamma tocopherol (in an oil base), and plus at least 50 mg of tocotrienols (derived from palm oil).

In one study, the examiners looked at the formation of reactive oxygen species[1] in humans by measuring antioxidant depletion. Six female and seven male head trauma patients, with one woman and 14 men with intracerebral hemorrhage, were enrolled in the study within 24 hours of receiving their injuries. Blood samples from the patients were taken. These patients, along with 40 control patients, were examined by a CT scan of the brain to determine the severity of their injuries. The lab results established that *all* of the patients with brain injuries had appreciably lower vitamin C levels than those in the control group.

The best antistress nutrients are the B-complex vitamins. One member of the B family, pantothenic acid, is particularly important, as it quickly dissipates during stress reactions. Plenty of vitamin C, renowned as a free-radical scavenger, is important, as well, in its role as an antioxidant that helps protect the body against stress reactions and many associated diseases. Beta-carotene is another antioxidant that will protect the body during periods of stress. Minerals that need replenishing include zinc, potassium, magnesium and chromium.

In instances where it is necessary to protect the brain cells against oxygen deprivation or permanent damage caused by head trauma, 10 mg of sublingual Hydergine (an FDA-approved drug to treat dementia), along with 10 mg

[1.] In aerobic organisms, such as humans, oxygen is converted to water at the end of the respiratory chain in the mitochondria. The mitochondria provide the energy necessary to maintain normal body function and metabolism. But, in the mitochondria respiratory chain, oxygen is reduced partially to form superoxide. Superoxide is a radical, i.e., a chemical containing an unpaired electron. Radicals typically are an extremely reactive species, because electrons like to pair up to form stable two-electron bonds. Due to its radical nature, superoxide is referred to as a "reactive oxygen species" (ROS).

of Hydergine tablets, should be administered immediately. A potent antioxidant, Hydergine facilitates oxygenation of the brain cells.

In treating trauma and surgery patients, L-glutamine, the most abundant amino acid in the bloodstream, has been found to be of great importance. It has also demonstrated its ability to decrease infection in these patients.

Animal studies have shown that the damage that occurs with stroke or head injury is in large part caused by the production of reactive oxygen species and excess free radicals, unstable molecules that react with other molecules and damage tissue.

While it is a good idea to take supplements, it is even more important to consume foods rich in these nutrients. For example, broccoli and kale are good vegetable sources of pantothenic acid, while red pepper, strawberries and collards are high in vitamin C. When eating or juicing vitamin C-rich citrus fruits, be sure to include some of the white inner peel for its bioflavonoid content. Ginger, parsley and carrots are rich in zinc, while collard greens have lots of magnesium. Bananas, Swiss chard and spinach contain potassium. Dark green, orange and red fruits and vegetables are high in beta-carotene. More concentrated sources of these nutrients are obtained from juicing fruits and vegetables.

Cherie Calborn, author of *Juicing for Life*, recommends making a mineral-rich juice with lots of potassium. She suggests combining a handful of spinach and parsley with carrots and celery. To get more magnesium, Calborn recommends combining a clove of garlic with some parsley, carrots and celery.

Biofeedback

In treating victims of trauma, biofeedback can produce impressive results. Often, a trauma patient will experience decreased muscle flexibility and a tendency to brace the muscles on the opposite side of the body from where the injury occurred. Using computerized EMG instruments, a biofeedback specialist attaches sensors or electrodes to the patient's body to get detailed feedback, such as the temperature of the skin or amount of muscle tension. Using this data, the specialist can analyze the muscles for the signs of asymmetrical movement that are typical of trauma patients. Then, with repetitive corrective exercises, the patient can restore the body's ability to function symmetrically.

By availing themselves of biofeedback, people can lessen the severity of migraine headaches. Biofeedback can also help stroke victims regain the use of their muscles.

Purification Lodge for Post-Traumatic Stress Disorder

The purification lodge is a Native American traditional ceremony known popularly as the sweat lodge. Native Americans prefer to use the terminology of purification, though, since men and women who participate do more than merely sweat. Experiencing the devastation of war alienates a person from his spirit. The purification ceremony helps one regain a sense of well being. First Americans have long used this ritual to help warriors and now share the process with others.

That's a reality that George Amiotte, an Ogalala Lakota from the Pine Ridge South Dakota Reservation, knows well. Amiotte served in Vietnam and had a near-death experience there. Upon his return home, he searched for ways to restore his own wounded spirit and was guided by Lakota elders to pursue Western medicine and traditional native healing. As a physician's assistant, Amiotte now specializes in helping veterans overcome post-traumatic stress disorder (what used to be called combat fatigue). Interestingly, Amiotte has been able to achieve success where standard Veterans Administration programs have failed. Puzzled Western doctors have questioned Amiotte on his success. Amiotte points out that healing is more than physical. Healing takes place on the physical, mental and spiritual levels, and a medical practitioner needs to consider all three aspects for optimum success. This is something Western medicine fails to do.

Another Native American doing similar work is John Joseph, a shaman with the Chinook tribe and a nurse practitioner in Washington State. Joseph agrees the men in war have lost their spirituality and that the lodge becomes a safe haven for them, a place to find it again. Everything said in the lodge remains there. Nothing is repeated outside of it. This gives a person a real opportunity to cleanse the heart, and so to place things into the fire. The effects are wonderful and long lasting, Joseph says, explaining that once people start to get their spirituality back, their physical appearance changes. They start to pay more attention to personal hygiene and to their clothing. More importantly, their thought patterns become steadier, without constant intrusions. Their sleep patterns begin to normalize. The purification lodge, in short, works to make people's lives cohesive and to calm their minds.

What to Avoid

It's important to stay away from foods that deplete the system, such as sugar, which robs the body of chromium, as well as caffeine, alcohol and over-the-counter drugs. Many medications promise short-term relief, but weaken the system in the long-term, making stress and trauma worse.

Treatment Summary

During periods of stress and trauma, it is especially important to eat foods rich in the vitamins, minerals and enzymes that will nourish the immune system and build health.

Supplementation with antioxidants, powerful free-radical scavengers, can combat some of the major damage (organ dysfunction and infection) caused by trauma.

Since stress thickens the blood, foods that thin it should be eaten; these include ginger, garlic and cantaloupe.

After trauma, biofeedback can help the body return to normal functioning.

The Native American purification ceremony helps those suffering from posttraumatic stress disorders move toward normalcy.

Urinary Tract Infections

Statistics from the *Journal of the American Medical Association* (*JAMA*) indicate that urinary tract infections (UTIs) account for more than 11 million physician visits annually in the United States. Most of these visits are by females. Next to respiratory infections, UTIs are the most commonly occurring infections among women. Unbelievably, 80 percent of women who get a UTI will experience another such infection during their life. Urinary tract infection, known to many as cystitis or bladder infection, is commonly caused by E. coli (a bacterium usually present in the digestive tract and on the skin around the rectal area) and other forms of bacteria, viruses (herpes simplex type 2), fungi (Candida) and a variety of parasites (worms and protozoa) that develop inside the large intestine and contaminate the nearby urethra and vagina.

Essentially, there are two kinds of UTIs: lower and upper. The lower type usually occurs in the urethra or bladder, and happens more frequently in females than males (the female urethra is much shorter, measuring about half an inch, thereby providing less of a defense against invading bacteria). Although men do get UTIs, the likelihood of infection is greatly reduced because the male urethra is much longer. In addition, prostate gland secretions afford a defense against this kind of infection.

Upwards of one-third of all women will have a UTI in their lifetime. Ideally, urine that is in the bladder should be sterile. However, even in healthy adults, the large bowel is not sterile. Bacteria flowing from normal intestinal flora can enter into the bladder. When bacteria from the large bowel settles in the bladder, cystitis or a bladder infection results.

Note: Though cystitis is rare in young men, they can contract it as a result of urethral obstruction from a previous infection of a sexually transmitted disease.

Infections in the kidneys or ureters indicate an upper UTI. An upper UTI is not as gender discriminating as its lower counterpart: upper UTIs typically occur in both males and females. Though a problem with a lower UTI can cause an upper UTI, it is important to understand that a UTI can arise without lower urinary tract complications. For example, an obstruction in the urinary tract can lead to an upper UTI.

As already mentioned, males are not generally predisposed to lower UTIs. However, they can contract upper UTIs because, as they age, the prostate enlarges, thereby preventing them from fully emptying their bladders. After an extended period of time in the bladder, urine loses its sterile quality. Retaining unsterile urine is a recipe for disaster.

In general, there are several categories of women who are at especially high risk for contracting urinary tract infection, with young, sexually active women topping the list as the most likely candidates. Young women often acquire a UTI after they begin having sexual intercourse, when bacteria that usually inhabit the vaginal region are relocated further inside the body in the urethra. Although sexual intercourse may promote the onset of infection, sexually active women should be aware that their partners are not transferring the bacteria from their own bodies; they are merely pushing bacteria that were already present deeper inside the body.

In addition, because of the proximity of the urethral opening to the anus, which is a petri dish for bacteria, the bacteria from the anus can cross the perineum (the bridge of flesh separating the anus from the vagina) to the urethra. When this occurs, acute cystitis, the most common type of UTI, can result.

Women who have experienced menopause are also at a heightened risk for UTI, as studies show that 8 to 10 percent of all women over the age of 60 will contract bladder infection at some time during their elder years. People with multiple sclerosis and other neurological disorders are at high risk, since they often are unable to fully drain their bladders during the excretion process.

Causes

Although many sexually active women contract bladder infections at some point in their lives, there are large numbers of females who seem to magically escape this irritating problem. This phenomenon can be explained by the development of hormonal imbalances in certain women. Estrogen and progesterone, which reinforce the urethral cells, attract and entrap bacterial bodies that are propelled into the region. Under normal circumstances the invasive microorganisms are expelled during urination, but in women with hormonal imbalances the bacteria cannot effectively be discharged, leading to recurrent bladder infections. This explains why women who have experienced menopause are often susceptible to this condition; the reduced level of estrogen in the body tends to enhance the adhesive qualities of the urethral lining and, consequently; prevent proper bacterial emission.

Urinary tract infection is often an indication of faulty nutritional habits and a debilitated immune system. Usually the presence of bacteria within the body can effectively be combated by the body's immune system, but when the system becomes weakened the widespread reproduction of disease-producing microorganisms is encouraged, resulting in the appearance of acute symptoms. Prolonged exposure to stress or the occurrence of a traumatic situation, such as a divorce or a family death, can further debilitate the immune system, adding to the chances of illness.

The muscles of the pelvic floor are often weakened after childbirth, causing the bladder to protrude closer to the vaginal region and the rear portion of the bladder to sag below its neck. When this occurs the bladder cannot be properly drained, resulting in the accumulation of stagnant urine and the growth of bacterial communities. This condition is responsible for the multitude of UTI patients who visit the doctor shortly after termination of pregnancy. In addition, a prolapsed transverse colon, which can result from childbirth; aging; poor posture; spinal disorders; and excessive abdominal fat are factors that can contribute to the compression of the bladder, with consequent obstruction of the flow of blood to this organ. Consequently, the bladder, which is deprived of an adequate supply of oxygen, becomes prone to disease-causing bacteria.

Our body eliminates waste products in several ways, including the excretion of feces by the bowels, the expulsion of carbon dioxide by the lungs, perspiration of the skin and finally, the discharge of urine by the kidneys and bladder. When a malfunction occurs in any of these processes, an excessive burden is placed upon the other systems. For instance, if a person suffers from constipation, hazardous waste that builds in the body must be eliminated by an alternative method. Medical evidence shows that recurrent urinary tract infections can often be correlated with persistent bowel problems.

Practitioners of Asian medicine explain that urinary tract infection results from the presence of damp and warm conditions within the bladder. They say that a weak flow of energy in the spleen and kidney is frequently accompanied by stagnation and a damp environment, which eventually leads to friction and the production of heat. The weakening of the spleen and the depletion of energy is commonly caused by an excessive diet, drinking during meals and over-consumption of greasy foods. In addition, certain foods, such as dairy and chilled foods or drinks, can exacerbate damp conditions within the organs, while prolonged exposure to stressful situations, including extended periods of studying, promotes spleen damage and continuous energy drainage. According to the Asian view, the presence of overexertion, anxiety, exhaustion, inordinate alcohol intake and too much sexual intercourse can hamper the proper functioning of the kidneys.

Interstitial cystitis is a bladder inflammation that is a result of autoimmune or allergic responses, which can result in inflammations of the pelvis and bladder and heightened blood flow in the region. In addition, candida has been found to promote antibody reactions that irritate the bladder.

Furthermore, we are a nation that wipes but does not wash. The bidet (rhymes with "relay") has long been recognized in many European, Middle Eastern, Latin and Asian homes and hotels as a far healthier and more comfortable choice to standard toilet paper. The bidet propels a gentle stream of cleansing water toward the genital and anal areas. Many health care providers tout the bidet's cleaning powers over that of toilet paper. They claim it helps prevent not only urinary tract infections, but vaginitis and other ailments, while leaving the area cleaner and fresher smelling after sex and during menstruation. Additionally, bidets provide relief for people with hemorrhoids, diarrhea and rashes, conditions that toilet paper can aggravate by hastening the spread of bacteria. Many have found that wiping with a little hydrogen peroxide has left them feeling cleaner and fresher.

Lastly, UTIs are inadvertently contracted by females who, while exercising (and not having properly cleansed their rectal area), have the sweat from the anal region transport bacteria to the vaginal area. Again, this can be avoided by properly cleansing the area prior to exercise.

Symptoms

Urinary tract infections and inflammations are frequently characterized by increased urination, accompanied by a constant feeling of urgency or that the bladder has not been completely drained. In addition, a burning sensation during the excretion process usually develops; along with an intense need to urinate during the later hours of the night. Additional symptoms may include cramps and dark, foul-smelling urine, while more serious cases may involve the presence of blood in the urine.

If you suspect that you suffer from urinary tract infection or inflammation, be sure to seek medical attention so that the problem can be effectively treated before it becomes compounded. The examination for an infection is relatively simple, consisting of having a midstream urine sample analyzed for bacterial infection. The presence of an inflammation is more difficult to assess due to the lack of bacterial evidence in the urinalysis.

Treatment

The traditional medical approach to treating UTI involves the administration of antibiotics. Predictably, UTIs have become more and more resistant to antibiotics, the traditional first line of defense. Prolonged exposure to these drugs can have adverse long-term effects due to their tendency to attack microorganisms that actually aid the body. A major problem is that the undiscriminating nature of antibiotics often results in the destruction of helpful gut bacteria, which in turn allows the propagation of harmful bacterial strains, including E. coli and Candida albicans, in the gastrointestinal region.

Ideally, then, reliance on prescription medication should be avoided in favor of alternative modalities. If the holistic approach repeatedly fails, the condition may necessitate a small dosage of bacteriostatic antibiotics. This form of treatment is less severe than traditional antibiotics because bacteriostatic agents simply restrain bacterial development, rather than kill these organisms. Thus, bacteriostatic antibiotics do not provoke yeast infection and the resultant gastrointestinal disorders. Some members of the medical community prescribe surgery, hormonal therapy and antidepressant drugs to treat more severe cases of chronic urinary tract infection. However, these therapies should only be used under extreme circumstances, when all else has failed.

Nutrition

There are a variety of natural remedies that can alleviate urinary tract disorders without the risk of harmful side effects. To begin with, the consumption of one 8-ounce glass of water per hour can aid in the treatment of an infection by diluting the bacteria in the urine, and is especially helpful in ameliorating severe pain. Unsweetened cranberry juice or cranberry capsules contain natural antibacterial agents and increase the acidity of urine, creating an unpleasant environment for bacterial communities to develop. Recent studies have demonstrated that 15 ounces of cranberry juice can hamper bacterial growth by up to 80 percent because the bacteria are no longer able to adhere to the urethral wall and, consequently, are excreted during urination. According to one study reported in *JAMA*, within two hours of drinking cranberry juice, the bacteria-fighting ability was present in the urine and lasted for up to 10 hours. Other research has demonstrated that the consumption of vitamin C along with the cranberries can further heighten the acidity of urine. Some other beneficial drinks that tend to alter the pH level of urine are lemon juice mixed with water, buttermilk and a mixture of two teaspoons of apple cider vinegar and water. These concoctions should be consumed three to four times a day.

Severe UTI symptoms can also be alleviated by temporary changes in diet. Increased intake of acidic foods, such as certain grains, seeds, nuts, fish, dairy products and bread, and reduced consumption of fruits and vegetables is recommended during acute attacks, but it is important to remember that this dietary modification should be short-term only. Usually, foods that are low in acidity, such as whole grains, vegetables, flax oil, fish oils and beans, are recommended to prevent irritation.

After taking antibiotics for a UTI, plain yogurt should be consumed to help control the development of a yeast infection. In addition, the regular use of a probiotic (such as lactobacillus, acidophilus, or bifidus) supports good and healthy intestinal bacterial flora. Probiotics are good bacteria that naturally colonize in the colon and vagina. Probiotics allow you to maintain balanced bacterial flora in the intestine. Studies show that the presence of probiotics in the gut and vagina are connected with a reduced risk of UTIs. Seemingly, the presence of probiotics hinders the formation of the pathogenic bacteria.

Supplements

Vitamin C, also known as ascorbic acid, can intensify the acidity of urine and in the expulsion of infectious bacteria. For maximum results it should be administered to bowel tolerance, or when the stool becomes soft and almost diarrhea-like. When fighting an infection, the body can require up to 15,000 mg of vitamin C daily and sometimes even more intravenously. Since it is water-soluble, vitamin C should be taken every two to three hours to prevent nutritional loss during excretion. People who do not suffer from an infection but wish to take vitamin C as a preventive agent should take between 2000 and 6000 mg daily. Vitamin C serves as an effective combatant of urinary tract infection because of its antibacterial attributes and its ability to enhance the operation of the immune system by encouraging the production of infection-fighting white blood cells.

During acute attacks, a daily dose of 50 mg of zinc can assist the body in white blood cell production and the elimination of bacterial intruders. In addition to zinc and vitamin C, vitamin A can fortify the mucous membrane lining of the bladder, prevent irritation of the bladder and improve functioning of natural antibodies and white blood cells. Note, though, that pregnant women, or those who may be pregnant, should substitute vitamin A supplements with risk-free beta-carotene, as studies have correlated high maternal dosages of vitamin A with birth defects. Other people can receive sufficient quantities of vitamin A by consuming up to 25,000 IU in halibut or cod liver oil capsules daily. Some additional preventive agents that can be used daily include 100 to 200 mg of vitamin B6 and up to six capsules of evening primrose oil.

Herbs

Antiseptic herbs, including buchu, goldenseal, uva ursi, juniper and garlic, are helpful in curbing the onset of cystitis. Marshmallow root, juniper berry, corn silk, which are classified as demulcents, soothe the mucous membranes of the urethra and bladder, while diuretic herbs, such as parsley and goldenrod, encourage the production of urine and the elimination of bacteria. A mixture of equal quantities of burdock, fennel and slippery elm can be effective when a teaspoon of the mixture is added to a cup of boiling water and allowed to sit for 20 minutes. This herbal solution should be consumed after each meal and before retiring for the evening. Other efficacious natural remedies include flaxseed tea and uva ursi/buchu tea, which should be prepared in a similar fashion to that described above. These solutions should also be consumed three to four times per day. Although they may have an unpleasant taste, herbal teas can often produce dramatic results in the battle with UTI. In addition, the homeopathic remedy cantharis can be used to alleviate irritations of the bladder and urethra. A final suggestion for preventing urinary tract infection: After having sexual intercourse, women may want to gently cleanse the opening of the urethra with a dilute solution of Betadine or a potent solution of goldenseal tea in order to remove harmful bacteria that may have been pushed into the region during intercourse.

Exercise

Participation in aerobic exercise, including jogging, walking, swimming and bicycling, can enhance circulation and aid in the elimination of blood congestion in the pelvic area. Inverted-position exercises, such as yoga headstands and shoulderstands, and rotating the legs in a bicycle-like motion, are also beneficial for improving circulatory functioning. If you suffer from back or neck pain and are unable to perform these exercises, you can use an old door or a couple of wooden boards to support the body by bracing one end on your couch and the other on the floor. The slanted position of the body facilitates the transport of blood away from the pelvic region and toward the head. It is advisable to limit such exercises to three to five minutes at a time because remaining in a slanted position for extended periods can cause dizziness.

Additional Treatment Modalities

Sitz baths and hot compresses enhance blood flow, allowing for the removal of hazardous waste in the pelvic region. In addition, these natural remedies can alleviate some of the pain of urinary tract infection. The preparation of a hot compress consists of dipping a small towel into a tub of hot water, squeezing out the excess, and applying the towel just above the pubic bone. When the cloth eventually cools, prepare another compress and reapply. After applying approximately eight or nine compresses, take a rest for several hours, and then repeat the procedure two or three additional times later in the day.

Norwegian researchers conducted a six-month clinical trial to evaluate the effect of acupuncture on 67 women with recurrent cystitis. The women were divided into three groups. After six months, 85 percent of the women in the acupuncture group were free of cystitis. These results indicate that acupuncture treatment could be a feasible alternative in combating UTIs.

What to Avoid

There are numerous preventive measures that will hinder urinary infections and inflammations. First of all, after urination, women should wipe from front to back (remember the urethra's close proximity to the anus), rather than vice versa. Also, before engaging in sexual intercourse your partner should clean his hands. In addition, try to avoid the transportation of bacteria from the anus to the vagina during intercourse, and remember to change pads or tampons frequently during menstruation. Tight-fitting jeans and nylon pantyhose can facilitate the spread of bacterial infections, so try to wear clothes that will allow ventilation, such as loose-fitting cotton pants or skirts and stockings with garter belts. Chemical irritation to the urethra can be prevented by avoiding perfumed and artificially colored hygiene products. Women susceptible to infections should substitute use of birth control pills and diaphragms with condoms or fitted cervical caps to avoid further infection. Those with urinary tract infection brought on or exacerbated by spinal disorders should seek the guidance of an osteopath or chiropractor.

The consumption of seven to eight glasses of water can dilute the urine and discourage bacterial development. Urination should be encouraged because it rids the system of harmful bacteria. Women who neglect their need to urinate are at an increased risk of infection. It is important to urinate after sex in order to eliminate bacteria forced into the urethra. It is therefore advised to avoid urinating before sex. In addition, drinking a glass of water prior to intercourse will increase bladder content, allowing more bacteria to be eliminated during postcoital urination. If you suffer from persistent infections you may wish to cleanse the vagina with a direct stream of water from a handheld shower unit prior to sex. This technique will eliminate a significant portion of vaginal bacteria, hence reducing the quantity of bacteria available for transportation to the urethra. Consequently, showers are preferable to baths.

Excessive consumption of tea, coffee, alcohol, spicy foods and soda should be avoided. Furthermore, intake of red meat, dairy products, citrus fruits and shellfish should be limited because prolonged exposure to these foods can increase the acidity of the body and promote bacterial infection. As discussed earlier, acidic foods and drinks can sometimes aid in combating UTI, but only when the body is experiencing acute symptoms and needs to be immediately flushed. Long-term acidic dietary modifications can have adverse effects and, so, should be avoided.

Treatment Summary

The conventional medical approach to treating urinary tract infection generally involves antibiotics, which tend to produce adverse side effects. In the case of chronic UTI, hormone therapy and antidepressant drugs may be prescribed. Natural solutions present excellent alternatives in both cases, although, if they do not work, a small dosage of bacteriostatic antibiotics may prove beneficial.

There are a variety of drinks and foods that can alleviate urinary disorders: These include cranberry juice and acidic foods (for acute attacks).

Herbs will prevent UTI as well as alleviate symptoms. Some useful herbs are uva ursi, goldenseal, buchu, juniper and garlic.

Cleanliness is next to godliness. Make sure you and your partner thoroughly cleanse with soap and water before and after sexual activity.

Exercise can enhance the circulation and aid in the elimination of blood congestion in the pelvic area. Inverted-position exercises are helpful.

Among supplements recommended for UTI are vitamins C, A and B6 and zinc.

Sitz baths and hot compresses are recommended.

II.

The Gary Null Protocol and Participant Testimonials

The Gary Null Protocol

This is the protocol I use for all the people who participate in my health support groups. For best results, I advise strict adherence to it. The remainder of Part II presents 182 of the hundreds of testimonials I have received from those who have followed my protocol. To view the complete list of testimonials, please visit my website at www.GaryNull.com.

Note: This information is presented for educational purposes only. It is not intended as a substitute for diagnosis and treatment by a qualified, licensed professional.

1. Drink Green Juices

Drink two 10-oz glasses of organic green juice per day, each consisting of:

- 4 oz of dark and light green vegetables plus 6 oz of water, or
  1 tbsp of chlorophyll-rich green powder plus 10 oz of water
- 1 oz of aloe concentrate
- 1 tsp of red fruit powder

2. Take Supplements

Each night, take:

- Antioxidant complex—read the label
- Garlic complex—read the label
- Comprehensive fiber formula—read the label

In divided doses throughout the day, take:

- Vitamin C—2500-5000 mg total

Always read the label on any product you purchase.

3. Follow a Healthy Diet

Eat primarily during the day. Have a light breakfast, your main meal between 1:00 and 3:00 P.M. and a light dinner (grains, a salad with dressing, a sea vegetable and/or soup).

Follow this elimination diet:

- **Eliminate meat**, including beef, poultry and shellfish. Replace with cold-water fishes (tuna, salmon, trout, mackerel, sardines and cod, all fresh) four times a week. Eat nuts, nut butters, seeds, soybeans and soy products; organic eggs; and quinoa (a high-protein grain). Mix beans and grains (such as brown rice, kamut, buckwheat, millet and amaranth).
- **Eliminate dairy** This includes milk, yogurt, cheese, butter, ice cream and cream sauces. **Replace with** rice milk, soy milk, amazake, silken tofu and oat milk. Do not consume anything with cassein among the ingredients.
- **Eliminate caffeine and alcohol**, including chocolate, coffee, tea, wine and hard liquor. **Replace with** herb teas, grain beverages (such as Postum, Cafix and Raj's Cup), lemon water and green tea.

4. Eliminate Sugar and Artificial Sweeteners

Replace with stevia root, raw honey, molasses, brown rice syrup, beet sugar and natural fruit sweeteners. You may use chromium picolinate (200 mcg) for sugar cravings.

5. Eliminate Carbonated Drinks

This includes soda and seltzer. **Replace with** spring water, distilled water, filtered water and fresh-squeezed organic fruit juice.

6. Eliminate Wheat

Replace with spelt bread, sprouted whole grain bread, rice bread and Essene bread.

7. Eliminate Nonorganic Produce

Replace with organic produce, including potatoes again, organic potatoes are fine, squash, sweet potatoes, yams, grains, beans, fruits and vegetables.

8. Eliminate Fried and Processed Foods

Replace with steamed, sautéed, stir-fried, grilled or broiled foods. Use the following oils for cooking: coconut, macadamia and safflower. Use the following oils for baking: hazelnut and macadamia nut. Use the following oils for salads: walnut, flax seed and extra virgin cold-pressed olive oil. Do not cook with olive oil.

9. Eliminate Chemicals

This includes food additives, preservatives, coloring agents and flavorings.

10. Avoid MSG and Miso

Testimonials

1. Alston D.

Aging
90 years old and self-sufficient

Before

I retired from the Merchant Marines at age 65. I have always been very active and considered myself to be healthy, but considered my future health. I heard Gary Null on the radio and began to read books on health and nutrition.

Now

I follow a vegetarian diet, and I juice. I use a rebounder every morning. I get on the train and travel to Manhattan to buy supplements.

I do not see many people my age these days. Most of them have caretakers and are dependent. I am totally self-sufficient; I care for my home and shop, wash my clothes, and even take my curtains down to wash and replace them alone. I do not need anyone to take care of me. I can accomplish my tasks alone.

I believe my diet and nutritional supplements are responsible for maintaining my health.

2. Carol J.

Arthritis gone

Before

Overweight
Low energy
Beginning to get wrinkled skin
Arthritis
Would get involved in negative situations
Liked to eat until very full

Now

Lost 60 pounds
More stamina
Skin less wrinkled
Arthritis gone
Will not acknowledge negative people or situations
Positive outlook
Does not overreact anymore

3. John E.

Cancer stopped
Basal cell and colon cancer reversed

Hepatitis halted. Normalized blood triglycerides, HDL and LDL. Blood pressure 180/128 to 117/63.

Improvements: Stopped basal cell cancer, lost 15 lbs, reversed colon cancer, halted hepatitis C, normalized blood triglycerides (HDL and LDL), blood pressure significantly dropped.

Mental Changes: Memory has improved greatly.

4. Jean K.

72 years old
Cancer gone
Arthritis diminished

Before

I am a lung cancer survivor. I had radiation, chemotherapy and several body scans, which left me anemic. I also developed osteoarthritis, which incapacitated me. Walking was difficult, and I needed help to board a bus. I used pain medication. My blood pressure was slightly elevated. Although I considered myself to be nutritionally aware, I used dairy. My energy was quite low after cancer treatment. I joined a support group to rebuild my immune system. I wanted to be healthy.

Now

The arthritis has diminished. I no longer require medication. I take walks and practice yoga. I am totally vegan, drink juices and follow Gary's protocol totally. The group homework assignments expanded my self-awareness and created new insights.

I am delighted with the results of each new blood test. I am cancer-free and optimistic. My work, in the wardrobe department of a theatrical company, is enjoyable, and I look forward to a good season with the crew again.

5. Diane P.

Cervical dysplasia improving

I was diagnosed with cervical dysplasia (cin2-moderate). After following Gary's protocol, the cervical dysplasia went to con1, which is classified as mild. On the last culposcopy, the gynecologist saw nothing to biopsy. I am confident that the cervical dysplasia will be reversed.

I now have radiant skin and hair, more energy, a general sense of well-being and no more colds and flu.

6. Frantz V.

Diabetes improving

Before

I had severe diabetes. I was taking insulin and glucophage. I also had high blood pressure and asthma. I then went on the protocol/lifetime diet.

Now

My life has changed tremendously. I have learned to balance my job and my personal life. I have increased my energy levels. I sleep a lot less. My high blood pressure went down. My asthma is gone. I no longer am on any medication for diabetes. And I lost weight: I went from 240 lbs to 205-210 lbs.

7. Christopher B.

Ulcerative colitis healed

Following your protocol, I had my ulcerative colitis healed. Prior to going to your retreat, I was unaware that there were people out there who could actually heal other people. My life has changed immeasurably.

8. Hozana B.

Acid reflux healed

Before

I was slightly overweight and had acute heartburn, acid reflux, and stress and anger toward my teenage son. I am a massage therapist, and I wanted to change my life and learn proper nutrition, so I joined Gary's support group.

Now

I've lost 8 lbs and now have the body I've always wanted. I take organic, vegetarian juices. I no longer have acid reflux. My mind is clearer. I have a successful relationship with my son, and I handle coworkers without anger.

I exercise by powerwalking, and my body is alive and energetic. I've uncluttered my mind and my home. Now, I am more open and accepting, less critical, more optimistic and helpful to people.

9. Jean D.

Digestive problems cleared
Memory has improved

Before

My husband and I began to notice our bodies were not in good condition. He was a meat-and-potatoes man and a very picky eater.

Over the years, he was exposed to lead, paint and cadmium on his job and developed nocturnal seizures, low energy, digestive discomfort and memory loss. I handled stress badly and was often intolerant. I had a bad accident: my breasts were caught between two doors and throbbed for two years.

We followed Gary's protocol in one of his books. We studied urine therapy and acupuncture, and used colonics and sprouts.

Now

Today, my husband has fewer seizures, more energy and enhanced memory, and he enjoys his new diet. He is enthusiastic and looking forward to his seventy-fifth birthday. We are energetic and without intestinal problems. We handle stress well, because we are no longer toxic. My female organs function as well as they did in my younger years. Our naturopath told me I avoided fracturing a hip during a fall because my bones were well mineralized. We are vegan, eat raw vegetables, juice and invent nutritious recipes using a dehydrator. I am involved in community affairs.

Our outlook is cheerful. We love spreading the word.

10. Doug

No more heartburn

I was scheduled for gallbladder surgery to relieve chronic heartburn. My pre-operation EKG was abnormal, and I had a quadruple bypass. I decided to change everything and started adopting Gary Null's protocol.

I lost weight, have no more heartburn and enjoy a good sense of health. I am on a strictly vegan protocol.

11. Kurt H.

Before

I was fairly healthy. I had seasonal allergies and took Celdane and Claritin. I had digestive problems: food would often get trapped in my esophagus. I drank a lot of caffeine. Then I listened to Gary's radio program. I decided to become vegetarian. I took supplements. I increased my exercising. I went into Gary's 1½-year detox program (with the wellness support group).

Now

I sleep less. My digestive problem went away. I do not get colds anymore. I have eliminated caffeine and alcohol.

12. Zara B.

Retinopathy in remission

Before

I was a vegetarian and had juvenile diabetes. I consumed coffee, junk food, sodas and such. I had diabetic retinopathy and fatty deposits in my eye. I consulted a "health coach" for alternatives and to control my diabetes, but saw this as a bandage rather than healing. I wanted a mind-body-spirit approach.

I began Gary's protocol, and this opened me up to spiritual meditation and personal strength.

Now

My retinopathy is in remission. I no longer have fatty deposits after three months on supplements. I use acupuncture and drink green juices that are organic. Medical examinations revealed that my eye vessels are stronger and that a thicker membrane is growing.

13. Bob W.

No more headaches

Before

I had allergies, suffered from upper respiratory infections and headaches, ate junk food and had elevated cholesterol and blood pressure. Then I went on Gary's protocol.

Now

I have increased energy levels, sleep less and have no more headaches. My blood pressure and cholesterol levels have decreased. I exercise (lift weights, do deep breathing), and I feel better all-around.

14. Art G.

67 years old
Blood pressure normalized
No more hemorrhoids

My cholesterol went from 260 to 180. My hemorrhoids have gone. My vision has improved. I have no more constipation. I have lost 18 lbs and run three marathons.

15. Warnetta A.

Thyroid normalized
Carpal tunnel syndrome and cataracts gone

Before

I listened to Gary's show for many years before I actualized the information.

My cholesterol and blood pressure were elevated, but my primary concern was obesity: my weight was 209. I wore a size 22, and I was diagnosed with an underactive thyroid, low energy, osteoporosis, osteoarthritis, cataracts and carpal tunnel syndrome. Gary explained that detoxification must precede dieting in order for the dieting to be effective. That made a lot of sense to me, so I went with the protocol.

Now

I weigh 150 lbs and maintain it. Recent physical examinations ruled out an abnormal thyroid, carpal tunnel syndrome and cataracts. I take lutein and blueberry capsules, and I threaded a fine needle today without difficulty. My cholesterol and blood pressure are slightly elevated but not abnormal. I have no symptoms of osteoarthritis or osteoporosis.

I exercise three times a week with a senior class in a Buddhist temple. I buy organic food, and I stopped eating meat and eat fish instead.

Ingredient labels shocked me. I am more aware of the unnecessary amount of salt in products. I share my new knowledge with people interested in regaining their health.

I was determined to enjoy life in good health, and I do now, with great, positive energy.

16. Janet F.

Was perimenopausal but now gets hot flashes and her period

Before

A college teacher, I was a longtime listener of *Natural Living*. I was never totally committed to change. I had low energy, I saw aging in my future, and I wanted group support. Though I was a vegetarian, I ate dairy, sugar and wheat. I had insomnia and indigestion, and I was constipatcd.

Now

I joined a health support group in August 1999 and gave up dairy, sugar and wheat. At first, I felt weird. I lost 15 lbs slowly. My hair is 3 inches longer, shinier and thicker. I was perimenopausal but began to get hot flashes and my period. My period continues to come and go. I lost my sugar craving. I have charges of energy. I eat my big meal at midday. I use green powders. My skin texture has improved, and I get no more age spots. My eye floaters are gone. I feel the writing and homework are as important as the dietary aspect and are responsible for my life changes. I create an area for introspection, and I love being in a group of positive people.

17. Ernestina P.

Fatty tumors gone

Before

I had fatty tumors under my arm and on my thighs. I was overweight, with low energy and joint pain. I took pain relievers, and I was tense. I held onto past angers.

Now

I am pain-free, and the fatty tumors are gone. I have lost 30 lbs.

18. Thomas G.

70 years old
Parkinson's symptoms improved

Before

I suffered from Parkinson's disease, hypertension, skin problems, herpes simplex outbreaks and arthritis. I became aware of the importance of nutrition and studied various theories, but my physical problems continued.

My Parkinson's symptoms caused me shame in public. I could not write. I typed with two fingers. My hands trembled when I put food in my mouth. I was advised to take medications. My past experiences with drugs were unpleasant. I refused them. I went on Gary's protocol and learned the specifics of diet and organics, the biochemical necessity of green juices and grasses, and the importance of attitude and beliefs.

Now

It was when I combined supplements with my diet that things began to look up. I honor myself, unclutter my life of people and objects, and share this important knowledge with others. I am alert, without past negative influences. Green and red powders keep me going.

These are my happiest and proudest times. I intend to live another 70 years.

19. Robert A.

Before

I had problems with gum swelling and infection (almost always following stress). My dentist told me nothing except that I had a chocolate allergy. I took antibiotics, which caused intestinal problems (candida). Then I had eight fillings removed over the course of 1½ years.

Now

I have no more mouth eruptions. My stress levels are still high (I lost my parents), but mouth remains healthy.

I just recently found a solution to my intestinal problems at the Metropolitan Wellness Center.

20. Dolly F.

Bell's palsy reversed
Low energy corrected

Before

Although we considered ourselves nutritionally aware and healthy for seniors, my husband and I felt something was missing. We knew our lives and health could improve, but we found no satisfaction in traditional guidelines.

We did not want our vitality to diminish as we aged. After listening to Gary Null on the radio, we decided to join one of the first Reversing the Aging Support Groups.

Now

It was easy following the protocol cold turkey. We had vitamin drips. We eliminated all meat, dairy and chicken from our diet. We are now organic and vegetarian, and we use air, water and shower filters. We have magnetic appliances. Our amalgam fillings were removed, and we make our home healthier by removing our shoes at the door. When a neurologist confirmed I had Bell's palsy, I had a consult with Gary.

We meditate, practice yoga and run. Our physician daughter now runs. I am a nurse teacher and busier than ever. We feel great juicing and using green, red and protein powders.

My Bell's palsy symptoms subsided within 10 days on the protocol. Our energy is strong, and our bodies feel vital and healthy from the juices and healthy food. We use alternative physicians for diagnosis and treatment if problems occur. This program was very successful for us.

21. Job T.

71 years old

My mother introduced me to good diet and healthy living. Although I listened to Gary Null for 23 years, I did not actualize the information. I weighed 210 lbs, smoked three packs of cigarettes a day, drank alcohol, felt depressed and had knee pains and upper respiratory infections. One day, I looked at the very aged man in the mirror and was shocked.

Today, I follow the protocol and use Gary's green, red and protein powders. The shakes keep me feeling full and satisfied all day. I drink "clean" water, use supplements and feel terrific. I did not get a cold in five years, and I have no more upper respiratory infections.

I am organic, vegan and do not take vaccines. My neighbors tell me I look 45 years old. They admire my changes. I appreciate my healthy lifestyle. It makes me quite aware of the tremendous amount of obesity today. I am confident, and I am pleased with my life.

22. Alice D.

Before

I had upper respiratory infections. I required long sleep, and I had alopecia. I had acute allergies from a cortisone shot. I had dry eyes.

Now

My upper respiratory infections are gone. I sleep less. My alopecia is gone. My symptoms from the cortisone shot are gone. My allergies have lessened. My eyes are healthier.

23. Diane G.

Sinusitis, hypertension and asthma gone

I was a New York City paramedic diagnosed with occupational asthma. I inhaled a mixture of bleach and ammonia during a medical pickup and developed a condition called osteopenia from prednisone. My vision diminished, my hair began to turn gray, and my skin peeled as if it were ash. I was stressed, had insomnia and sinusitis, and slept three hours a night. I retired from the fire department because of the accident, and I joined a support group.

Today, I am a vegetarian, I am organic, and I juice. I am no longer suffering with sinusitis, hypertension or asthma. My black hair is returning, my skin is lovely, and my vision has improved. I sleep six hours a night, and I am calm and happy. My family joined a food coop. My vitality and energy have zoomed up.

I work out in an adult ballet class, study flamenco and will perform in a recital. I also Rollerblade, do spin cycles and am studying toward a rabbinical career.

24. Marey C.

Before

I was overweight and had weak hair. My skin was wrinkling, and I had herniated disks in my neck that caused severe pain. My muscle tone was low, and I suffered from upper respiratory infections. I was always fatigued and pessimistic.

Now

Following Gary's protocol, I have lost 20 lbs, my hair is healthier, and I have fewer wrinkles. I have less pain from the herniated disks in my neck. My muscle tone has improved, and I no longer have head colds or sinus infections. I feel I am stronger, calmer and more positive.

25. Charles L.

64 years old

Before

I ate the typical American diet: meat, dairy, sugars. I thought my primary health concern was not being able to gain weight.

I began to listen to *Natural Living*. Gary presented valid research. People spoke about their experiences in health support groups. They sounded energetic and happy, as if they created new, free lives. Many of these speakers were my age or older. Their testimonials influenced me to change my life.

Now

I follow a protocol on my own from a book. I use green, red and protein powders. I no longer put poison in my system from meat. Mine is a natural way of eating. I walk 6 to 8 miles a day and use supplements.

Gary Null is my classroom on the air. I gather information daily and put it to use. My health is better today than it was in my younger years.

26. Jerome G.

Before

I was overweight, and my mental outlook was negative. I was introduced to Gary's show in 1980 by my wife. After meeting Gary in Central Park, I became a vegan. I went to Gary's ranch with the goal of improving, learning and reaching my full potential in order to run in the New York City Marathon.

Now

I have lost 20 lbs. My attitude is better, and I am more decisive. I focus on what I can and cannot obtain and on what is in my best interests. I have eliminated toxic people. I forgave my mother and myself by writing forgiveness letters. I can go on. I find reaffirmation in the support group.

Actualizing

I am involved in social and political issues. I took action in the passage of a school referendum, and I am creating social situations in the new development that I moved into.

27. Kate

Period returned

Before

I was a vegetarian for years but ate dairy, sugar and wheat. I was an insomniac, had indigestion, was constipated and had floaters in my eyes. I had age spots on my skin, and my hair and skin were unhealthy.

I was a college teacher and a longtime listener of Gary's show, but I never totally committed. I needed a group support.

With low energy and aging in my future, my career as a professional singer was out the door.

Now

I have lost 15 lbs and no longer have a sugar craving. My hair is longer and thicker, and my age spots are gone. My skin improved, I am more energetic, and my eye floaters have disappeared.

I joined a support group and love being with positive people. I follow the protocol and have eliminated toxic foods. At first I felt weird. I eat a large meal at midday. The green powder gives me a large charge of energy. Although I have been perimenopausal for many years, my hot flashes have resumed and my period has returned. I feel my hormones are active.

I ended a toxic marriage and healed my relationship with my son. I uncluttered, cleaned up my finances and feel responsible for my life.

28. Debbie T.

My breast cysts are decreasing in size. I have lost 10 lbs. My gray hairs are returning to their natural color.

29. Fran M.

Senior
Moles fell off
Age spots gone
65 years old

Before

Moles on skin
Skin beginning to sag
Dark age spots on body
Decreased energy
LDL
Hair color changing
Mental function slowing

Now

Skin tighter
More youthful in looks and attitude
Moles fell off
Age spots gone
New hair growth dark brown

LDL normalized
Energetic
Mental function improved

30. Rick C.

77 years old

Before

I had surgery many years ago for a hiatal hernia. My diet of vegetables and juices controls this condition. My father and two sisters died from aortal abdominal aneurisms. My brother had one repaired successfully. I was diagnosed with this condition. Surgery was indicated. I prepared myself for six months with a specific protocol. This included good vitamin intakes, mental and attitudinal insights, and healthy food.

During that time, I obtained a copy of the surgical procedure from a medical library and realized it was an extensive operation. My internal organs would be removed from the ribs to the pubic bone. My aorta had a balloon type defect and would be opened and patched. My organs would then be replaced. I meditated on every organ in my body several times before surgery. I was relaxed before and after the procedure. I demanded my body to heal itself. My immune system was at its peak.

Now

I survived the surgery well, in excellent condition. I left intensive care in two days and took a bus home a few days later. My physicians were amazed. I explained how I obtained my strong immune system with diet, supplements and respect for my body.

Actualizing

I am now in the process of creating the biggest project of my life: building the world's largest wind farm. Following the Gary Null protocol gave me the strength and energy I must call upon to complete this mission.

I encourage seniors to build your energies, both mental and physical, and create new goals, exercise, build your immune system, study and be a part of your environment.

31. Felicia P.

Before

>   Arthritis
>   Joint pain
>   Overweight
>   Anxious
>   Depressed
>   Stressed because son using drugs
>   Fatigue

Now

>   No longer has arthritis or joint pain
>   Increased energy
>   Sleeps less
>   Looks great
>   Lost 20 lbs
>   No longer anxious and depressed
>   Finding connection to self
>   Uncluttering
>   Detaching from son

32. Glenroy A.

>   68 years old

Before

I was diabetic, developed cellulitis while serving in the military and had severe knee and lower back disk pain. I could not climb stairs, and I used crutches, a cane. For two months, I was paralyzed and in a wheelchair. My blood pressure and cholesterol were elevated. I ate the typical American diet: flesh foods, wheat and dairy. Underneath it all, I wanted to be healthy.

Now

My legs are no longer swollen from cellulitis. My backache has subsided. My circulation is normal. I can easily walk up the three flights of steps to my apartment. I buy organic food and follow the protocol: eat fish and use green and red powders and supplementation.

My life is active. I am retired and work on a veteran's council. It is wonderful to babysit my granddaughter, feeling lighter and energetic. All my past symptoms are gone. The homework we did in the support group caused me to focus on myself. I learned to be tolerant, less pushy and more humble. This teaching enhanced my body and my life.

33. Gloria F.

No more upper respiratory infections
77 years old

Before

She was hypoglycemic, used dairy and wheat, and ate flesh foods. She had poor concentration and mental clarity, low energy and upper respiratory infections.

She joined a 1½-year support group because she was a college senior and needed more energy to complete her degree

Now

She lost 8 pounds, and now wears size 4 or 6. She is energetic, has no more upper respiratory infections, does not need stronger glasses and has less wrinkles. Her skin is bright, her hair is thicker, and she uses juices throughout the day, without a desire for meals.

She learned to honor herself. She developed solutions for daily problems. She keeps a positive outlook. She is an active walker.

She convinced her daughter to use an alternative physician for her granddaughter, who was diagnosed as psychotic. The child returned to school within two weeks.

34. Amy S.

Cysts and acne gone

Before

Double heartbeat
Ganglian cyst on wrist, with surgery advised
Nocturnal teeth grinder
Cystic acne
Unhappy with relationships

Now

Double heartbeat rarely occurs
Ganglian wrist cyst gone
Does not grind teeth at night
Cystic acne gone
Takes stronger role in relationships, no longer following the other person's expectations
Cleaning out life and environment

35. Eileen F.

Before

Overweight
Hair thin
Nails fragile
Knee would swell due to several accidents
Skin eruptions
Did not sleep soundly

After

Lost substantial amount of weight
Hair healthy
Nails growing
Knee condition improving
Skin clear
Sleeps well
Is actualizing a new career

36. Etta B.

Cancer seems to be in full remission

Before

She had a hysterectomy for uterine cancer, but the cancer returned. She went through chemotherapy and radiation. She had arthritis, psoriasis and low energy, and she was overweight and unhappy at work.

Now

Her cancer seems to be in full remission. She lost 26 lbs. Her psoriasis is gone. Her hair and skin are healthy, her arthritis is gone, and her immune system is strong.

It was through class assignments and other workbook activities that she learned she was hard on herself and came to experience the positive relief of forgiveness of self and others.

Etta left her toxic job. She meditates twice daily, exercises, practices yoga and lifts weights.

37. Beatrice C.

Yeast infection gone

Before

I had lupus for eight years and used prednisone and 13 other pills, which caused me to have an upset stomach. I felt horrible. I had a yeast infection, with liver problems and headaches. I also had low energy. I had five surgeries, and I underwent chemotherapy for my kidney condition. My physicians never suggested diet changes.

Now

Following a specific protocol that uses glutamine, flaxseed oil and DHEA, and after three hydrogen peroxide injections, I suspended all but one medication. I have higher energy, decreased joint pain and an improved stomach condition, and my yeast infection has totally cleared up.

I do tai chi and yoga, and my depression has gone. My relationships with my friends and family are stronger.

38. Adele M.

77 years old

Before

Low energy
Allergies
Hair graying
Housewife who wanted to get out

Now

> More energy
> Original hair color returning
> Allergies not as severe
> Has job
> Leads her group, keeps a daily journal and actualizes change
> Developed self-confidence
> Enjoys time alone
> Engages in self-exploration

39. Angelo Q.

> Lost 100 lbs

Before

He was 300 lbs and had high cholesterol and blood pressure. He had high hemoconiosis (abnormal hemoconia count in blood), hepatitis B and discoloration around his eyes. He used an inhaler and had eczema, bleeding knuckles and elbows, and hemorrhoids. He felt sluggish and fatigued, and had pain with simple movements.

He listened to *Natural Living* and joined a support group with his wife in 1999.

Now

All the above-mentioned ailments are gone. He lost 100 lbs. He has constant energy and runs, racewalks, powerwalks, skates, does aerobics and trains in a gym. He lost one shoe width size. His skin and hair improved, and he needs more frequent haircuts. He has had no additional graying of his hair.

He follows the protocol, juicing and using green and red powders. He creates organic vegetarian menus with his wife. He finds he easily completes tasks, and he is on a wild uncluttering spree. He does image consulting today. His children are slowly adapting to his lifestyle.

40. Athena P.

I heard Gary Null's support group members speak on the radio about experiences in the group and on the protocol. I had several conditions to improve and decided to join a group. I suffered with PMS, cystic breasts, depression, eye floaters, fatigue and graying hair, and I usually was involved in bad relationships.

I entered a group with many other people also seeking true health naturally. I detoxified and rebuilt my immune system. The results are no more PMS, cystic breasts, fatigue and depression, all within six weeks on the program. Uncluttering was crucial. It enabled me to rid my life of negative people and to get closer to those I desired to be with. The eye floaters diminished. I detect no new gray hairs. I changed jobs and have a better salary and work in a happier environment.

41. David E.

Before

He listened to *Natural Living* for two years.

He had 13-percent body fat. He felt the effects of middle age: he was cynical, had low energy, was dissatisfied with his physical self, felt he looked old and ate the typical American diet. He was worried about cholesterol but ate meat and restaurant food, and had a poor diet.

He was very stressed and had many problems. The shows on *Natural Living* began to influence him to change his life. He abstained from fast food, drank less alcohol and began to juice organic greens.

Now

He went to Paradise Gardens. He is less self-critical, gave up bad foods and alcohol, and easily accepts himself with a positive attitude. He increased his exercising: he powerwalks, runs 4-5 miles, is training for a marathon with Gary Null, participates in a running and walking club on Sundays and did 14 miles. He read *Who Are You Really* and realizes it was his attitude that once made him feel old.

He was asked for proof of age recently to enter a bar to hear a band he enjoys.

42. Andre D.

Before

High weight
Low muscle mass
High blood pressure
Cholesterol not in normal range
Worked in law firm and was unhappy there
Cynical

Now

> Lost 25 pounds
> Gained 7 pounds of muscle
> Blood pressure normal
> Cholesterol normal
> Left his job
> No longer cynical
> Feels complete and alive
> Uncluttered
> Sees others as equals
> Positive attitude
> Is now a personal trainer

43. Andrea V.

> Lost 75 lbs

Before

She weighed 300 lbs. and wore size 24-26. Although she had no diagnosed illnesses, she was exhausted, had painful varicose veins and back problems, was nauseated after meals, had bad digestion and was lactose intolerant. She ate flesh foods and dairy.

She listened to *Natural Living* and joined a support group.

Now

She lost weight, going down to 225 pounds and size 18. She developed a sense of values in the group and can say no. She feels centered and empowered within her truth. She juices, uses powders and takes supplements. She discovered a new world of health food stores. She chooses products carefully, reads labels and does not use canned products. As a creative cook, she enjoys translating old recipes into vegan meals, using grains. She discusses the availability of this lifestyle with others. Her family acknowledges her progress. Her mother now uses supplements.

44. Alexandra M.

Before

I was dissatisfied with my body. My energy was low, and I was very overweight. My acquaintances and friends were depressing me to the point of irritability. I had a fear of public speaking and did not know where to turn for guidance.

I joined a health support group. Gary Null was informative on the radio, but I could not apply this information in a constructive way.

Now

I lost 16 lbs without dieting. My increased energy made me feel young again. I need less sleep, and I find I am not distracted by other people's petty, unimportant issues. My house was uncluttered; having fewer objects gave me space and a feeling of freedom. My toxic relationships were dismissed; my self-esteem replaced them.

I learned to be the real me, healthy and vital.

45. Alice

Before

I was concerned about my health. My blood pressure and cholesterol were elevated. I had a stressful life and could not control these feelings. I disliked my varicose veins. I suffered with an acid reflux condition that I assumed was caused by my job. My body was falling apart.

Now

I detoxed and carefully followed Gary's protocol. I felt stronger each week and released stress each day. My blood pressure is normal today. My digestion improved, and I have no more acid reflux. I lost 15 lbs. My blood tests are good, and my figure is leaner. I am shapelier. I feel cleaner. I do aerobics at home in the morning, yoga during the evening hours, and bike, walk and run. My uncluttered environment and journal writing give me a new constructive outlook. I use green juices and green and red powders with supplements. My water is pure. I am organic. I am goal-oriented.

46. Clara

I had four children and felt old and unhealthy. I wore size 20. My blood pressure was elevated. I lived a fast and stressful life on an organic farm the city wants to confiscate for open land. I wanted to join a support group for a while, but this time I followed my determination.

The support group was a classroom in biology, nutrition and human potential. I learned quickly. Today, I wear size 13. We are an organic family and use the green and red powders. Sugar and dairy are out. My daughter had one asthma attack that was not repeated after we eliminated sugar and dairy. I am focused and energetic, and I look forward to my exercises, which I do four to six times a week.

47. Connie

I am 65 years old and thought fatigue, arthritis, high blood pressure, high cholesterol, cataracts, osteoporosis and overweight were part of aging. My hair and nails were weaker, and I was sensitive to the opinions of others.

I decided to go with Gary's research and knowledge. I wanted to be well and happy.

I no longer am tired and sluggish. I have no more aches and pains. I lost 20 lbs and look younger. My hair and nails grow in strong, and most of all, I am indifferent to the opinions and criticisms of other people. Look what I did! Bravo for me.

48. Damon

I felt frustrated, and I could not muster up energy. I overslept, my hair was graying, my sinus infections drove me mad, and my cholesterol and blood pressure were elevated. This was not me; I had to find a method of true reversal.

I went on Gary's protocol carefully. It was easy. I enjoyed new foods. I learned to understand my body mechanisms. My elevated blood levels are normal now. My sinus problems are gone. I sleep less and awake with energy. My hair texture has improved, and I have less graying. I am determined to achieve and to have relationships with my family.

49. Fatimah

I was a sugar addict and ate 2 pounds of it per day, creating a sick, uncomfortable body. I overate using junk food. My energy was low, my skin was bad, and my blood pressure and cholesterol were high. This inability to control myself stressed me. As I listened to Gary, I thought about freeing myself from these habits. I joined a support group.

It is wonderful to be free of compulsive eating. I lost 50 lbs. I do not crave sugar. My cholesterol and blood pressure are lower, and I have real, vital energy. Problem solving comes easily, my marriage is happier, and I meditate. The foods I eat are healthy, and so is my outlook.

50. James

I procrastinated myself into a severe cardiac condition. After my angioplasty, I took blood pressure medication and joined Gary's walking club. I was amazed that the walkers and runners, some of whom overcame serious illnesses, were fit and healthy. They made major lifestyle changes. I looked at my life, working 7 A.M. to 9 P.M. without exercise. I was a coffee addict and felt stuck. A change was in order. I joined a group.

If you're going with the protocol, go with it all the way ... and I did. Organic, juicing, powders, vegan and life changes. We were a great team, the support group people and I. We are different people today. That's what knowledge does. I am aware of labeling and chemicals. I no longer crave caffeine for energy. I ran in two marathons, and I confronted my procrastination. I believe in the power of actualization: "speak the words, live by the words."

51. Henry Q.

My life was unmanageable, and my stress was overwhelming. I had many allergies and frequent upper respiratory infections. My blood pressure and cholesterol were elevated. I heard about Gary Null's support groups and detoxification. I needed to change, and I decided to enter a group as soon as one was formed. That was the beginning of the best part of my life.

How could green juices clean toxins from one's body? Well, that's exactly what happened with good results. My energy built, my headaches stopped, and my cholesterol and blood pressure lowered. I have a new body since exercising, using weights and doing gi gong and deep breathing. I feel calm, more patient and less irritable. I love my food and progressive life.

52. Glen

I wanted an improved future without illness. My cholesterol was high, and I had great pain from herniated disks, which also prevented my exercising. I was a compulsive eater and chose an unhealthy diet. I snored, and I simply did not care for myself. When Gary Null talked about a support group on his radio show, I did not hold back and I joined in 2000.

I was a student again. The entire time was amazing to me. I learned why my body had problems and what I can do to reverse them. I understood the impact of meditation and forgiveness. I lost 18 lbs and am pain-free. I exercise three times a week, practice martial arts and do not snore. I recover quickly from illness, and I feel happy and alert.

53. Irene

I was overwhelmed by possessions. My home was very large and cluttered. It became too much for my husband and me. My weight, cholesterol and blood pressure went up. I developed cardiac arrhythmia and lost energy. My nails became weak. We were lost in indecision.

Joining a support group gave us the tools to create a new life and future. Detoxing returned my body to health. I lost 30 lbs, which normalized my cholesterol and blood pressure. I am no longer a cardiac patient. My nails are growing in strong. We are energetic, and most of all, we sold our large home, dividing the unessential items among our family, and now live in a four-room house and love it.

54. Peggy

I was slightly overweight. My symptoms were uncomfortable: skin outbreaks, cysts and eruptions on my arms and premenstral syndrome. These conditions did not fit into my projection of a happy future. That is why I joined a support group and learned a totally new way of life.

Today, my facial skin is clear, the eruptions on my arms are gone and the annoying sinusitis is over. It is a pleasure to be healthy. I intend to remain so.

55. Brian C.

I listened to support group members on the radio and decided I would change my life and my body. I had many symptoms of early aging: graying hair, eye-color change, nails growing slowly, scars not healing, hypertension, pock marks on my face, eczema, tension after years in the corporate world. My personal relationships were not going well.

I followed the detox protocol, attending meetings, to cleanse my body physically and emotionally, and the results are wonderful. My blood pressure is normal, my skin condition is gone, my hair is growing in blonde (my childhood color), and my hairline is reversing. My eyes are returning to their blue color. My nails grow quickly, and the wound scars have disappeared. I left the corporate world, and I find my relationships and attitudes are happier.

56. Janice

I had a 10-year-old son but was diagnosed as infertile. I miscarried and could not become pregnant. My periods were heavy. I had Lyme disease, with headaches and joint pain. I was exhausted from all these conditions plus allergies. We ate the typical American nonorganic diet.

Good changes came with a Gary Null support group in 2000. I see a 95-

percent improvement in all the areas of my health and my life. My periods are normal, my vision is improved, and my allergies are lessened. We eat an organic diet and follow the protocol using Gary's green and red powders. Our family relationships are better, because we are healthy and optimistic.

57. John F.

I developed psoriatic arthritis 30 years ago. I underwent surgery to fuse my right wrist. My knees and neck were deteriorating, so I used heavy medications and over-the-counter analgesics. My blood pressure became elevated, and I was advised to change careers.

My daughter motivated me to join a health support group. Today, I am vegan and eat no sugar or wheat. After I began the protocol and juicing, I became pain-free in four weeks. I take no more medications, and all swelling subsided. My doctor commented that the condition of my knee joints is the best he has observed, and my blood pressure is normal. I am able to take long walks. I have reclaimed my life. Neighbors who have observed my improvement now follow the protocol. One couple, a diabetic and his wife who has multiple sclerosis, report physical improvements. By following the protocol, my cousin lost 10 lbs in two weeks and no longer has heartburn.

58. Karen

I would often have swollen glands, and I had frequent upper respiratory infections. My energy was low, my hair began to gray, and I was overly tired before my period. My life was complicated by people I today call toxic.

I joined a support group and decided to give it all I had. I juiced, became organic and was very careful with my food plan. I did the homework, and carefully listened to the lectures and guest speakers. Today, I am in excellent health, without colds, premenstrual discomfort, or the impact of annoying people. My energy is high, and I forgive past errors.

59. Karina

I was quite ill before I learned how to detoxify. My skin condition was unsightly, my gums bled, and I had neuropathy in my hands and knees, pain from arthritis and kidney disease. Floaters and retinopathy caused sight problems. Tests showed abnormal thyroid levels, and my blood pressure and cholesterol were high.

Today, after completing the support group, following Gary's directions and carefully going with it day by day, I do not have bad skin. My teeth and gums are fine. I no longer have pain from neuropathy or arthritis. Tests determined that my kidney disease is reduced. My eye problems have disappeared. My thyroid tests read normal, as do my blood pressure and cholesterol blood tests. I have a normal life, and I am thankful for the experience, education and caring I received.

60. Kenneth

I carried around too much weight on my body. I was uncomfortable, with pain in my shoulder from an injury. My asthma often held me back. These problems made me angry and pessimistic. I often had temper tantrums—sometimes with violence. My confidence and esteem were low.

The juicing, homework, vegetarian diet, lectures and confidence in me the people in the group showed got me through the first few weeks. I am vegan and enjoy my lifestyle now. I learned a lot about myself by answering the questions. I thought about my relationships. I lost over 35 lbs. My nose no longer runs all day, my asthma seems to be controlled, and I do not try to keep up with others. My life is uncluttered, and so is my head.

61. Keith

I was quite unhappy with my life. I had to lose weight and thought that was the problem. I did not feel I could accomplish much. Where was I going, not doing anything constructive? I was not sure lectures and a change of diet would help. Things were that bad, so what did I have to lose? I joined a support group.

Many group participants entered that door wondering if this would work. We knew the information and teaching would be correct, but could we do it? I did it, and so did everyone else. What a change from day one to graduation. I lost 10 lbs and maintain it. I don't feel alone, and I look forward to planning a better future. I actually feel happy and have learned to listen to my inner voice. The experience has reshaped me. I know I have self-determination, and I am wild about the protocol.

62. Larry

Carrying around a heavy body caused me exhaustion and fatigue. I never exercised, and I ate the typical American diet. I often had heartburn, probably from the sugar in sodas and the bad food.

It took me some time to get used to drinking juices, but the explanations and respect shown to the people in the group made me enthusiastic. I began to feel the energy growing. I went with it totally: I am organic, vegan and exercise. I run and powerwalk. My hair is growing in darker. I lost 20 lbs, and my digestion improved. I still follow the protocol, using the powders and supplements, and I love my new body and lifestyle. Thank you, Luanne and Gary, for helping us understand that our lives are in our hands.

63. Marie

After my husband died, I tried to adjust to a new lifestyle. I smoked and ate flesh foods, dairy and sugar. My energy was low, my hair was thinning, and I had scars from earlier acne. I was exposed to asbestos and other chemicals, and developed emphysema, Epstein-Barr disease and bronchiocytosis. I was a sculptor and inhaled clay dust. Being overweight added to my burden. I felt my energy declining.

Listening to *Natural Living* for 10 years opened the world of alternative medicine. I began to take supplements, changed my diet and had chelation therapy. My response to the food on the protocol was immediate and positive. I am now organic and vegan. Everything tastes so good. I create wonderful desserts: fresh fruit with honey and nuts.

I no longer need a leg brace. My hair is thicker, and my skin is lovely. My pulmonary problems have lessened. I lost 8 lbs and will continue to lose weight. I exercise by swimming and walking. Without this protocol, I would have been on an antibiotic one week a month for the rest of my life.

64. Luis

At the time I joined a support group, I weighed 155 pounds. My blood pressure was high, and so was my cholesterol. I was not sharp anymore. My memory was not as good as it once was. My hair was growing in thinner, and I felt tired. I listened to Gary Null on the radio and read his books, but when a new support group began, I joined immediately.

I was enthusiastic and optimistic immediately. I stayed after class to pass my good feelings on to the group members. I knew I could improve my health and help them improve theirs. Today, I weigh 145 pounds. I am totally organic, juice, use pure water and have great energy. My hair and eyebrows are thicker. My blood pressure and cholesterol tests are normal. My memory improved, my skin looks great, and I can read without glasses. I eat my last meal before 6 P.M. This experience gave me a new lease on life.

65. Marcia

77 years old

I was sad about entering old age. I could not recognize myself, with my overweight problem and white, thin hair that was falling out. The hair under my arms and my pubic hair fell out after menopause. I lacked energy and had no sensual emotions.

The Gary Null protocol has changed all that and changed my emotional attitude. Just seeing my hair growing back thick and in its original color returned my femininity. My body hair has grown back, too. My libido returned as it was in my early 40s. My energy is phenomenal, and I sleep only four to five hours a night. This is a clean, healthy, youth-preserving program, and it gave me back my life and womanhood.

66. Marina

I had several problems and wanted a solution. The medical community did not have that solution. I was overweight, and that sapped my energy. After menopause, my hair and nails became weak, and I felt very depressed. I was given Prozac for multimenopause syndrome. I was still depressed. Wasn't there anyplace to go for help for people like me? Finally, I heard about a health support group, and without knowing exactly what it was, I signed up.

I joined the group, and it was so interesting, and it was an intelligent class that respected the people attending. I learned how diet affects mood and the body. I followed the protocol and lost weight. I kept it off. I have lots of energy, and my hair and nails are coming back to their premenopausal thickness. I stopped Prozac when I began the protocol, and I feel great. I sleep well, and I have no more depression.

67. Mary Ann C.

I began to display the signs of aging. My weight went up with my fatigue, my hair was weaker, and my skin was wrinkling. I was pessimistic about losing my looks. I was in pain because of herniated disks in my neck. I noticed my muscle tone was not as it was just a few years ago. I was determined to turn these conditions around and joined a support group after I heard group members speak about their positive experiences.

The group experience was exciting. The group participants were wonderful, optimistic and helpful to me and each other. We were a family. I lost 20 lbs and have fewer wrinkles today. My hair is healthier. I have less pain in my neck, and with exercise, my muscle tone improved. I do not get colds or flu, and I feel stronger, calmer and more positive. It's a miracle, but not really. It's cleaning out, building up and keeping to the protocol.

68. Moira

I had an eating disorder. My body fat level was low. I was an athlete: a runner and a hockey player. I could not ovulate and was diagnosed as infertile. I tried the orthodox treatment and found it ineffective, with unpleasant side effects. My husband and I joined a health support group in 2000.

After four months on the protocol, I ovulated and conceived. I feel my hormonal system is now stronger. I had a natural birth, but I experienced postpartum depression. My doctor labeled me clinically depressed. I was advised to discontinue nursing and to use medication. I rejected this and continued nursing. My health returned six months postpartum with exercise and meditation. My family and I are vegan. We juice and use only organic food. We stick to the protocol. I research postpartum depression and reach out to women suffering with this condition.

69. Michael

62 years old

I attended a Gary Null retreat. I learned the benefits of vegetarianism, juicing, supplements and meditation. In 1994, I became disabled because of carbon monoxide poisoning. I am still in the process of recovery. I no longer work. I cannot see the computer screen. Surgery for two detached retinas affected my eyesight. My blood pressure was extremely high. My heartbeat accelerated to a dangerous level. I took several pharmaceutical drugs to control these conditions. A few years later, I began having seizures and Alzheimer's-like symptoms. Abnormally severe edema in my legs incapacitated me. I was in a coma for 60 days. Nursing home care was considered. My health took an upward turn on the Gary Null protocol. Juicing, stress management and homework opened me to my potential and purpose in life. I discovered the best of what works, and I realized I was not doing anything worthwhile. Today, I no longer need a compressor for leg edema. My leg size decreased by 30 percent. I sleep less, lost 23 lbs and exercise with hand weights. I recently received a Bowflex to build my upper body. My blood pressure is lower. My brain speed seems to be faster.

70. Nellie

My blood pressure was 140/90, and my cholesterol read 268. I had large fibroids and was warned of possible cancer. Excess stress created chest pain, possibly angina. I felt this was due to business tension, but with it all, my husband and I adopted two children. Tension began to affect my family life.

I enjoyed listening to *Natural Living*. It opened me to the possibility of turning my health and life around. I could not see how I could attend a group—my business and children absorbed each day completely—but I signed up anyway. After the first meeting, I knew I was committed. My family and I are vegetarians. I do not allow my children to eat junk food. We use juices, and I cook healthy meals. I lost 15 lbs. My cholesterol is 198, and my blood pressure is 120/80. My last medical exam was excellent. I had no trace of fibroids. I powerwalk, feel energetic and work out in a gym. People compliment my healthy skin. I handle stress with humor, and I do not react to other people's indifference. I am patient with my children. All in all, my life is healthier.

71. Oliver

I weighed 238 pounds. My cholesterol and blood pressure were elevated. I had pain in my chest, pain in my knees and ankles, and frequent heartburn. I was embarrassed by brown age spots on my skin. My eyesight was off, and an examination revealed astigmatism. An Internet acquaintance suggested I listen to Gary Null on the radio. I did, and I decided to try a new way of dealing with health issues. I joined a health support group.

I was impressed by the enthusiasm of my fellow group members and the scientific research that went into creating Gary's magnificent protocol. My weight went from 238 to 188 lbs within five months. My blood pressure and cholesterol values were lower. I exercise one to two hours daily, meditate and use juices and supplements with great enthusiasm. No longer do I have chest pains or heartburn. I feel energetic, my eyes are less astigmatic, and my hair and nails are healthier. The support group ended, but my life just began.

72. Owen

I was an unhealthy vegetarian. I ate sugar foods and dairy. I assumed my health was good. I never got sick. I listened to *Natural Living* since 1985. One day, I decided to change my health and my life, but I needed parameters. I could not do it alone. I heard testimonials from support group members. They did what I intended to do. They understood the reasoning behind detoxification and rebuilding the body. I wanted to understand it, too. I joined a group.

Today, I am not just vegan and organic, but I am an organic cook aware of my reaction to toxic foods. I designed an efficient meal program, and I juice two to three times a day. My body fat is 3 percent, I sleep six hours, and I awake with good energy. I seem to be thinner. We learned to unclutter our lives by uncluttering our environment, and I did that with great benefit. I exercise five times a week and may begin feng shui. Luanne, Gary and guest speakers gave me an education and stable future. I thank them.

73. Ricardo

I was a good candidate for health reform, so I jumped into a support group the day Gary announced a new one was beginning. I felt just awful. I constantly was sick with colds and flu, my hair was thinning, I lost my energy, and I was getting fat. I overreacted to people who were critical of me, and I never dealt with situations correctly.

I sat in a big room with people who had their own problems and, like me, needed to learn about real life and real health. We all wanted to be happy and feel well. Most of us did not know where or when we spoiled our lives. I changed my eating according to the protocol, became aware of the terrible horror of factory farming and slaughter, and learned real nutrition. The results are more than I imagined. I never get a cold or flu, my hair is thicker, and I have the energy of my youth. I did not diet, just followed the protocol, and I lost weight. I feel clarity, and I handle people effectively. That may be because I found my self-esteem. It was a major improvement for me.

74. Richard

I noticed that I got a lot of upper respiratory infections when I gained weight. Also, my energy dropped, and I needed more sleep. My skin was dry and often was problematic. I was not happy, and I had a negative outlook. I heard about Gary Null and listened to his show. The results of the people who completed the support groups were too good to be true, but I gave it a shot and joined.

I learned many things, but most of all, I learned it is not difficult to become healthy. It is simple and enjoyable. Physical and emotional health developed for the first time in my life. I lost 20 lbs, and I have good energy because of it. I do not need to sleep as long as I used to. I no longer cough up phlegm. My skin is smooth and moist. I threw out unnecessary objects and people. These are positive actions that I handled successfully without stress. I am proud of that.

75. Robert

I felt I lost control of myself. I was getting heavier each year, and my muscle tone was decreasing. I did not have the vital energy I once experienced, and I was worried and fearful about my financial situation. I needed guidance to get me back on track. I was not happy with the claims I saw on television or with the many books I read. I did respect Gary Null and entered his support group.

The detoxing affected not only my body but also my mind. I shed over 35 lbs and built muscle. I sleep less and have more energy. The lectures and homework opened the true me to myself. I found the strength to forgive, which improved my family relationships. I can do whatever it takes without fear today. This experience is the most effective method of understanding human potential and of gaining respect for our planet. I thank everyone.

76. Rosalind

My blood pressure shot up. That was just one of the frightening aspects of aging that hit me. I was tired during the day and wanted my vitality back. The best way was to go into a Gary Null group. He always used the term "reversing the aging." They were golden words to a fatigued woman. I joined the study.

The body is remarkable. Mine immediately responded to the green juices. I eliminated dairy, flesh foods, wheat and everything Gary and Luanne suggested. In a short amount of time, my blood pressure normalized. I felt more energetic, and after a while, I realized I was younger than my contemporaries. I now exercise five times a week. I was held back by an automobile accident and had to eat hospital food for a while. I recovered quickly, thanks to my healthy immune system. I came home and immediately went back on the protocol. There is no other choice, and I love it.

77. Ruben

I did not like the way I felt or looked. I ate the typical American diet, thinking that was the rule. My skin broke out with infectious cysts. I needed long nighttime rests. My weight gain coincided with frequent outbreaks of colds and flu, and my hair developed a dry, unpleasant texture. Was this aging, or did I do something wrong? Could I reverse these problems? I was not sure, but I respected Gary Null and knew that if anyone had the answer, he did. I heard about his group from past participants. They convinced me I could help myself with his coaching. I joined a study group.

I began juicing, and I eliminated toxic food and substances. In a short amount of time, I lost 12 lbs and the skin cysts cleared up. My hair is softer and healthier. I do not have upper respiratory infections, and I seem to have developed a sensitivity to mainstream food. I sleep less and enjoy my waking hours more. The protocol really worked for me.

78. Sondra

The night my son brought me to the emergency room, I was told I would not have awakened the next day. I had three bleeding ulcers, and I felt angry at my illness. The anemia caused me extreme fatigue, and the daily weight loss I experienced was somewhat of a joke to me. I just did not take it seriously. I was told I might lose 30 percent of my stomach if the condition persisted. I was sent home with medications. Being a vegetarian and researching medical conditions, I used only one medication for my thyroid. I was very stressed without an out. My children suggested I listen to *Natural Living*. The first day I tuned in, Gary mentioned aloe and cabbage juice for ulcers. I bought a juicer and aloe, and I drank the combination. All medication was discarded that day. Eventually, I joined a support group.

Aloe, cabbage juice and sometimes sauerkraut soothed my problem, but it was the green juices and elimination of dairy, wheat and other products that really built me up. I am totally organic, vegan and healthy. My endoscopy revealed no ulcers. I think that is remarkable. I lost 15 lbs on the protocol, and my body began to reshape. At this point, never straying from the program, I have reversed the aging and am emotionally stronger. I made peace with myself and the past by journal writing and powerwalking, and I enjoy a happy family life with my children and animals. The many support group participants I meet are wonderful, happy and free people. I am one of them.

79. Summer

I always felt tired. I was sick each day, and I had a chronic walking problem because of hip displacement, which fatigued me. I suffered from various allergies. My cholesterol was high. I was depressed. When a health support group started, I felt this was one chance I would not pass up.

I had to learn to eat and choose foods according to their compatibility with my body and their nutritional value. I learned how to cleanse my system of toxins and of the abuse of a bad diet. I found peace doing the homework, which forced me to confront painful but important issues that held me back in life. I was motivated and even went on a watermelon fast three times without hunger or fatigue. I use the green powders and juice. Exercising several times a week gives me energy and enthusiasm about life. I can do headstands, and my body is flexible. I go dancing. Also, I am 16 lbs lighter and do not have discomfort walking. My allergies improved. My physician is amazed by my younger, youthful body.

80. Veronica

I ate junk food and was a heavy coffee drinker. I was hypoglycemic and fainted frequently. My skin had ugly eruptions. I cried easily and had low energy. I had several allergies. I heard Gary speak about Paradise Gardens and the experiences people had there, improving their insights and health. It sounded beautiful. I signed up for the trip. That was the beginning of a new, wonderful life.

I learned how to powerwalk and exercise, how to juice and prepare healthy foods and fruits, and how to plan meals. I lost 15 lbs. Eventually, all my upper respiratory infections and skin problems disappeared. I still follow the diet, juice during the day, eat fruits in the evening and make one well-planned meal a day. I am now a marathon runner. My energy is without limit. I am healthy.

81. Cheryl

I developed severe allergies and upper respiratory infections. I was consumed with family issues, which made me angry and anxious. Negative people annoyed me. My past caused anger. I could not express my feelings or deal with them.

The support group and protocol allowed me to see myself and my life on many levels. I developed a healthier life, without colds and other respiratory illnesses. I am now vegetarian, juice, meditate and see my loved ones with compassion. I understand my anger and anxieties. They are gone. The past no longer plays over and over again in my mind. I actualized a new, successful career as a freelance editor, which means no toxic office environment. I am active in political causes, especially violence against women, using hotlines and shelters.

82. Sara

I was interested in avoiding the illnesses my mother suffered in her old age. I had PMS symptoms for 14 years. My sagging skin aged prematurely with pimples, cysts and scars. My digestive problems caused bloating. My personal relationships were unpleasant. I read *Get Healthy Now,* which motivated me to explore sensible methods to relieve my symptoms. I joined the next support group that opened up.

I followed the detox protocol, and in time, the results I longed for manifested. I no longer have PMS problems. My skin is tight and less lined. The pimples and discoloration from cysts are fading. I believe the detox cleared these problems, too. My energy increased. The journals and letter writing self-empowered me. I take risks with confidence, not fear. I bicycle, use a rebounder and belly dance. The new man in my life is far superior to those of the past.

83. Dora

I considered my eating plan to be healthy. I thought meat and dairy gave me good protein and calcium. I enjoyed wheat breads. As time went on, I developed cysts in my breasts and was diagnosed as hypoglycemic. I did not feel well, and I wondered if my diet impacted my physical system. Motivated by a fear of future illnesses, I joined a support group.

The teachings and protocol gave me the answers I needed. I quickly lost 8 lbs. The lumps in my breast are gone, and I have no more pain. I am vegan and organic. My dog and I enjoy green and red juices and powders. I do not test as hypoglycemic. I can skip meals. With daily yoga and exercise, I have wonderful energy. My skin is moist; people compliment my glow and happier attitude. My hair and nails are healthy. I sleep well, and I am aware of potential toxic people and situations. My goals are financial independence and business success. My family is beginning to follow the protocol.

84. Medina

I am truly a survivor. I had breast cancer 11 years ago and refused chemotherapy and radiation but used Tamoxifen, which impaired my vision and emotions. I developed polyps, an inflammatory digestive problem and an ulcer. I was taking too much medication, and it was making me sick. I sought a natural approach to healing—immune enhancement. I gained weight without cause, and my abdomen bloated. It was all wrong, so then I tuned into *Natural Living* and joined a health support group.

After three months on the protocol, my immune system shot up. My digestion improved, without bloating, as I eliminated many foods. The weight is slowly coming off. I feel radiant and wake up 5 A.M. each morning with phenomenal energy to do breathing and meditations with a naturopath. I realize that suppressed emotions of the past and holding on to nonexistant obstacles made me ill. All aspects of my life have fused. I am where I should be.

85. Scott D.

I am a construction worker. I felt I was losing stamina and did not know if I could handle my work. I felt my body age. I ate the typical American diet, without labeled illnesses. One day, I listened to *Natural Living* and discussed the show with a friend. I decided to join a group.

Today, I can keep up with younger coworkers, my physical endurance has increased. Injuries and pulled muscles heal quickly. I juice, and I keep to the protocol more and more as time goes by. I exercise and find myself seeking new directions. My forgiveness letters allowed me true introspection, and I focus on myself, avoiding all toxic situations.

86. Jay

I am a holistic dentist and vegetarian for 32 years. I had mood swings and problems concentrating at times, most likely due to sugar and dairy. I was negative on occasion. My hair was graying.

My wife and I joined a health support group. We follow the protocol: powders, juices, a lot of liquids, totally organic. My energy increased dramatically, and my mood swings are gone. I maintain a good, positive mental attitude for long periods of time. My concentration stabilized. I notice less gray hair in new growth. We use affirmations, uncluttering, exercise, powerwalking and Nordic Trac. Four of our six children are vegetarians. Gary Null put it all together by formatting a nutritional plan, condensing it and making it clear. Going to the ranch in Florida caused a major positive change in our lives, and attending the classes, experiencing other energies in a support network, made our successes possible. I recommend the protocol to my patients.

87. Jose

I studied radiography for two years and worked with nuclear isotopes. My radiation badge determined I was exposed. I worried about my health. Information was withheld at work. Prevention training was improper. I ate some vegetables, flesh foods, rice and beans, but deep within, I knew I had to change my life.

I was unable to attend support group meetings, but I followed Gary's information and began the protocol. I used green and red powders, and purchased the weekly specials. I read Gary's books, juice and research supplements and new teas. I became aware of my allergies as I eliminated toxic substances in my diet. My energy is high, my hair is thicker, and my receding hairline is filling in. I teach my family about nutrition and proper diet. Today, I work as a limo driver and tape *Natural Living* to play in my car during the day.

88. Hank

I was introduced to *Natural Living* in 1980 by my wife. I became vegan at Gary's Texas ranch. I wanted to educate myself and reach my full potential in order to run the 1995 New York City Marathon. I was evolving one step at a time and joined a support group in 1999.

I lost 20 lbs. My mental outlook improved, I am decisive, and I focus on realistic goals. I eliminate toxic situations and people. Forgiveness letters cleared the past, and I can enter a free future. Group support was essential. I am now involved in social and political issues, most recently the passage of a school referendum.

89. Sherry

I wanted to get my life on track. I overextended myself to others, without reciprocation. I ate junk food and had a broken vein in my leg. I joined a health support group to learn about health through nutrition.

I learned not only how to eat, and what to eat but why we choose this new diet. I began to understand the relationship between the physical and the metaphysical. My family and I are vegan and organic. The vein in my leg healed. I eliminated toxic friends and family from our lives, which allowed me to focus on myself. I use visualization. The relationship with my husband and children is closer, warmer and more affectionate. We do affirmations and uncluttered our home. With new insights and peace with the past, we are a cohesive family.

90. Terry

I tried to be vegetarian. I did not eat flesh foods, but I did eat fried foods, breads, pizza and muffins. I had asthma and refused to use an inhaler. My hair was thinning. My intake of water was low, and my job stressed me.

I joined a support group in 2000. I lost 7 lbs detoxing, and I became organic. My energy increased. I am calmer and sleep less. My hair grows in thicker, and I seem to be less stressed between jobs. I discovered my spiritual side, and I use quality time well. By uncluttering, I set boundaries. Now, I handle people well, without getting involved in toxic situations. I make thought-out meals for family dinners and do not react to adverse remarks. I find I am attracted to people on a cellular level. Exercising and sports are on my agenda. My asthma attacks come faster and leave easier. I identify their cause. Respiratory infections heal quickly. I returned to school, and I made a list of future accomplishments.

91. Monty

I was an overweight semi-vegetarian. I used dairy and had digestive discomfort. I felt healthy, but I angered easily. I am a trained psychologist and studied Chinese medicine, herbology and German electro-acupuncture. I lived in Italy for many years.

I joined Gary's support group to learn the protocol for myself and my patients. I recognized my defensive anger. Today, living vegan, juicing and enjoying changed eating patterns, I find life to be quite different. I meditate, am self-empowered, set boundaries and will not expose myself to abuse. My career is beginning to be successful. I make contacts easily. Recalling my former behavior and anger, I realize the support group and detox protocol remolded my life.

92. Barbara

I weighed 168 lbs and gained weight without overeating. I used pain medication for a spinal disk injury and was in rehab, badly stressed, with anxiety attacks. I was swollen after eating my usual meat, wheat, sugar, coffee and dairy. My cholesterol was high, and migraine headaches caused me to be bedridden. I was labeled disabled for four years. Candida plagued my body. I threw up after meals. One day, after reading one of Gary's books, I saw him on PBS. I joined a support group in 1994.

I attended classes, open to change, and after two weeks on the protocol, being vegan and organic, and never returning to toxic foods, the change began. I exercise in a rehab center for my back problem. Probiotics and sensible eating eliminated my throwing up. I am a vegetarian cook and intend to study vegetarian meal preparation. My back pain is sporadic and not as acute. I am still in recovery, but I use no medication. I never looked at life as I do now.

93. Stuart

I ate flesh foods, but I did not use dairy. I believed this was a sensible diet. I had colitis and cardiac valve prolapse, which required antibiotics before dental work. Although I did get frequent upper respiratory infections, however, so I considered myself healthy. Something was missing, however, so I decided to join a support group in 1999.

I certainly changed my life patterns. Since I became vegan, my energy improved and my perspectives on life issues are healthier. The homework made me aware of my mortality. I get fewer and milder upper respiratory infections. My colitis is less severe. I work out six days a week, and I use green and red powders. I retired and use my free time to give back to society. I am active in local community affairs.

94. Cathy T.

I was bedridden for two weeks with Epstein-Barr disease and could not walk more than three minutes at a time. I lost some of my memory. I returned to work, but only put in five hours a day and went to bed as soon as I returned home. Stair-climbing was difficult. My physician could do no more for me and suggested I do independent research. A homeopathic examination revealed food sensitivities. The day I watched Gary on PBS changed my life. I donated to the station, and soon I joined a support group.

Today, I carefully follow the protocol. I gave up chocolate without difficulty. At first, the new food choices were difficult to accept, but today I am vegan and feel 1000 percent better. I work seven hours a day and exercise after work. I walk 1½ hours and am training to racewalk in the New York City Marathon. I still need eight hours of sleep, possibly because of Epstein-Barr, but my waking hours are productive. With a clear mind and good memory, energy and concentration, I plan future occupations in art and volunteer work.

95. Joseph I.

63 years old

I read Gary Null's books and listened to *Natural Living* for many years with good results. I have hepatitis, high blood pressure, diabetes and damaged nerves, and I recently had a bout of Bell's palsy. I also have three bulging disks on my spine. With all of these problems, I sought relief and healing.

I decided to follow the protocol. The people that stick to it had good results. Today, I juice, I no longer use eyeglasses during the day, and I am delighted that my blood pressure and diabetes are controlled and that the Bell's Palsy did not return for two years. I discontinued weight lifting when my back was injured 10 years ago. I recently resumed lifting weights. I have a lot of energy, and the skin on my face is strong and my nails are healthy and pink. As a senior on a fixed income, I cannot afford a nutritionist. However, I study nutrition with Gary's shows and books. Thank you.

96. Fred M.

I used drugs and was melancholy, with tendencies to cling to and control people. I reacted to others with anger and felt unpleasant toward them. My decisions were based on that which was best for others. I could not understand why I behaved this way. I wanted a happy life.

I discovered my body was reacting to the drugs and toxic foods I consumed. The protocol provided me with a method of starting all over again, cleaning my body and my mind out. Little by little, I lost my need to control people and to strike out in anger. Uncluttering my environment made me aware of the rational possibilities ahead, beginning with a clean slate. I now think before reacting to people. I feel positive. My relationships improved.

97. Pat

63 years old

I was hospitalized three times for congestive heart disease. I was on oxygen 24 hours a day for emphysema. I weighed 225 pounds. I had arthritis, diabetes, sciatica and glaucoma, and I used steroids.

I came to support group meetings in a wheelchair, with oxygen hookups. Today, I call myself a walking miracle. I follow the protocol, walk daily, no longer use steroids and even traveled to New York City. It took a while to clean my system out, but vegan organic living was the answer. My neighbors are happy to see me as I leave for my daily stroll. Detoxification works.

98. Ralph

I felt well-balanced and healthy even though I functioned in a hyperactive mode. I slept eight hours a night but awoke feeling tired. I was slightly overweight and needed good dietary and behavioral changes. What better way toward health than a Gary Null support group? I jumped right in.

Detoxing brought miracles to my life. I lost weight and am now 6.2-percent body fat. I feel clean, healthy and energetic when I awake and throughout the day. I sold my company and entered a PhD program. I created a method of teaching the trumpet. I believe these changes were manifested by uncluttering my home and life.

99. Alan S.

If anyone was ready to rearrange his life, it was me. I was under heavy stress and felt totally fatigued by midday. I developed allergies. Life was about hurry-hurry-hurry and making money. I did not want to continue at this pace.

I entered a support group and embarked on a life-enhancing program. The protocol addresses the physical, spiritual and emotional self. It is life-enhancing. My body feels lighter and cleaner. I have energy all day. I handle stressful situations without internalizing. I discovered that I do not need as many "things" for happiness. Although I make less money, I gain a great deal more on another level. I am exploring life confident. If failures come, they are not major complications. I read *Who Are You Really* and discovered I am a dynamic assertive and should not work with others. I am now creating a business venture.

100. Nora

I was plagued with a urinary tract infection that would not clear up. I had infections in my mouth and was tired most of the day. My skin began to look older, and my hair, weaker. I held a fast-paced job, which exhausted me, and I held on to anger from the past.

I became part of an active health support group. The group energy and lectures were of great benefit. I keep to the protocol and drink juices, take supplements and eat organic and vegan. All my infections cleared up. I am less tired, my skin improved, and my hair grows in healthier and thicker. Doing less, slowing my pace, simplifies my day. I have a positive outlook and put the past where it belongs—in the past, not in my mind.

101. Joe G.

I was under major stress and developed twitching muscles. I refused medication. Nocturnal cold sweats and anxiety were difficult. My walking was affected by an Achilles tendon injury. I did not understand true nutrition and needed guidance. There was no better source than Gary Null, and I joined in.

The group was a class for me. It was optimism and discovery. As my body cleaned out with the protocol, I improved, as did my behavior. Each meeting taught me the mechanics of our life systems. My muscle twitching stopped. I no longer have cold sweats or feel anxious. The Achilles injury is healing quickly. I enjoy stamina. My family is benefiting from my experience and uses the protocol, too.

102. Kenneth L.

I was reticent about meeting with a group of people to improve my life, but I did, and my progress was enhanced by these people.

The group kept me on the protocol and prevented my usual fear of isolation. I used to feel that no one understands my problem. I lost 10 lbs and feel joy, happiness, really good about myself. I can now easily help other people. Praying and listening to my inner voice brought good results. The protocol cleaned my body and mind.

103. Yvonne

Brain surgery left me with numb fingers and cold extremities. I had flulike symptoms, a constant "frog" in my throat, fatigue in the morning, tinnitus, dizziness, constipation and a general lack of motivation that interfered with my work performance. I was angry and soon went on disability. The first time Gary Null spoke about support groups on his show, I listened but did nothing. At that stage, I could not really help myself. Feeling totally locked in, I pulled up some inner courage and went to the first meeting.

I began the protocol. In a short amount of time, it was evident the protocol was working. I began to feel better, the pains and other symptoms lessened. As I continued and listened to the lectures, which were quite penetrating and motivating, I noticed all the symptoms I once had were gone. I am a functioning, healthy woman.

104. Joanne

I was quite negative. This drained my energy. My skin was not clear, I had backaches, and I could not confront heavy emotional issues. I did not help myself or others. I was not certain if detoxification could help these problems, but I joined a support group.

I really enjoyed and benefited from the group meetings. I became organic and vegan, and I love the lifestyle. I feel healthy, and my skin looks wonderful. The lectures and writing assignments were educational and psychologically healing. Exercise improved my back problems and energized me. I now look at life with a positive eye and can undertake world issues that will help others. I let my negativity go.

105. Maria R.

I was prescribed Prozac for multimenopause syndrome by my gynecologist. I gained weight and lost energy. My hair and nails were weak. I had difficulty sleeping, and I felt depressed. I thought I followed a sensible eating plan. I did not connect food and aging.

I began the detox protocol carefully and followed it diligently. I wanted to reverse my aging and clean my system out. I lost weight and am keeping it off. I have good energy. My hair and nails are growing to premenopausal thickness and strength. I discontinued the Prozac when I began the protocol and am not depressed. I sleep well, look well and get healthier each day.

106. Moishe

I was not energetic at all. My skin was rough, and I had fungus infections on my nails and several allergies. A chronic, dry, burning eye problem persisted. I feared loneliness and did not travel or live alone. I isolated myself. I heard support members speak of their improvements when I visited Gary Null's office, and I decided I would enter a support group.

Initially, after a short time of detoxing, my energy and endurance shot up. As I continued, my skin and nails healed. I do not have allergic reactions today. My eye problems have healed, and my hair grows quickly. The lectures and homework made me look deep within. I live alone today. I do not fear loneliness. I attend activities and feel open to people.

107. Dorothy

During the program, I lost 50 lbs and many inches. My bra and shoe sizes are reduced, and I am five dress sizes smaller. My skin tone and elasticity improved, and my energy level increased. I had several haircuts in the past month.

I handle stress and negativity; this increased my self-esteem. Meditation time is important, as is reading and reflection, not only at the end of the day but whenever I require it. I set future goals, focusing on solutions and personal needs. I use affirmations in the present tense during the day, accepting myself without denial. I am confident of positive solutions, without negative factors. My strengths are far greater than I once thought. I am a work in progress, and forgive, learn my lessons and leave the garbage.

108. Cynthia

I was a dancer and became an interior designer. I was organic and vegan. I used sugar occasionally and had hypoglycemia. Although I felt disgusted with the waste, toxicity of materials and disregard in the design field, I was a workaholic and developed septicemia from overwork, travel and a bad diet. When I left that field, I set out to find myself, and I entered a Gary Null Woman's Issue workshop and studied energy types.

Today, I am an accupressure therapist and garden designer. I follow the protocol with more detail, and my hypoglycemia improved. I am energetic, and I have no more bitterness. I am proud and happy in my new professions, and I am in touch with myself. Not honoring oneself allows others to intimidate you.

109. Kim

I was a smoker. I worked hard, and I internalized negative issues and work problems. I developed cancer.

I followed Gary Null's protocol and used Dr. Revici's methods. I do not smoke today, nor do I internalize negative thoughts. I meditate, exercise, use a rebounder and feel happier and more peaceful. I work less and take quality time for myself.

110. Gloria

78 years old

I came into a support group with several physical ailments. I was somewhat overweight. My hair was graying. I had macular degeneration, hypoglycemia, periodontal disease, varicose veins in my legs and a spinal curvature that, I was told, could become degenerative. I joined a support group.

I shed 10 lbs and am filled with renewed self-confidence. My sparse hair is fuller and growing back in a dark color. There is an improvement in the macular degeneration problem I feared would be permanent. I do not have hypo-glycemia or periodontal disease. The leg varicosity decreased, and my spinal curvature feels less acute. My amalgam fillings were removed. I returned to school for a degree, and best of all, my family is proud of these reversals. They prepare my special protocol foods when I visit, and they respect my choices.

111. Wilma and Myron

75 years old each

We were not happy with the symptoms of getting old. We both had memory difficulties. I did not like to be a homebody, and I wanted this part of our lives to be active. There is so much to experience and learn.

We joined a support group and feel we have reversed aging. We follow the protocol and noticed we have increased brain power. It is sad watching our friends fail physically. They are closed to detoxification and diet changes. We are the only couple in our group not taking medications. I study piano and am writing a book. This is a wonderful time of life.

112. Margaret W.

I was plagued with a long-term yeast infection. My personal relationship did not satisfy me, but I held onto it. Life was not empowering. I felt I was not going anywhere.

I joined a support group and was amazed to see other people like me searching for a happier and healthier life. None of us understood where we went wrong. I juiced and detoxed with optimism. My yeast infection and the accompanying lethargy is over. I feel happy and energetic. I ended my toxic re-lationship without guilt. I am mentally and spiritually awakened. I fell in love with running and powerwalking, and I am training other people to use them. This is a wonderful time.

113. John C.

My body changed with each birthday. My skin tone was sallow, almost yel-low. I had a general, daylong fatigue and would get hay fever, which drained my energy. My body could not defend itself, and I was ready to commit to change. I signed up for a support group.

The protocol and meetings expanded my reasoning, thinking and sensitivi-ties. I am energetic; I have no more fatigue. My skin is healthy. My hay fever bouts lessened and are manageable. Uncluttering changed me emotionally. I dream less, feel well-grounded and have released past angers with forgiveness letters, meditation and prayer.

114. Janice Q

I had major skin eruptions and cysts on my arms. I would get unpleasant PMS symptoms each month. Sinusitis was persistent. I wanted to lose weight and sought a sensible approach to end these symptoms without medications. I felt optimistic about Gary Null's approach. He certainly expanded my knowledge through his radio show. I jumped at the chance to enroll in a support group.

I found the detoxification aspect pleasant to follow. The spiritual lessons changed my attitude. My skin is clear and eruption-free, and the arm cysts are gone. I have no more sinusitis and my PMS symptoms are less severe. I lost 10 lbs, and I am focused and more positive. I meditate with tai chi.

115. Linda O.

I did not have a disease or major symptoms. I wanted to improve my life and use my physical self in a healthy way. I wanted to grow stronger with age. The protocol made me stronger physically. I feel my health in my energy. I run additional miles without fatigue. My hair and nails are stronger. Keeping a journal made me introspective. I observe life positively. I feel courageous and attempt new projects.

116. Bob

I was curious about this thing called a detox protocol. I did not feel unhealthy, but I decided to attend a group and see if it impacts in any way. I wanted to lose some weight but did not like dieting. My blood pressure was a bit high, and I did get headaches.

I came to each meeting, and listened and learned. I lost weight without dieting. My waistline is smaller. My blood pressure is normal. I need less sleep, and my headaches are gone. The protocol and science behind it are valid. It was a wonderful experience.

117. Linda L.

I was able to eliminate several problems with Gary Null's protocol in a healthy, normal way. My acne and cysts cleared up. I used to produce a lot of phlegm, and I do not now. My hands and feet are not cold. The spider veins in my legs are less apparent. The dark circles and broken blood vessels around my eyes are reduced. The intestinal bloating of the past is gone. How's that for success?

118. Ann L.

My concern for several medical conditions brought me into a detoxification group. We met weekly. The group dynamic was powerful. I wanted to participate in rebuilding and regaining health. I had mitral valve prolapse, and I had several upper respiratory infections and gum problems each year.

Cleaning my body and rebuilding my immune system turned my health around. I follow the protocol carefully. It is all in my hands. I do not have mitral valve prolapse or colds and flu. I have no more gum problems. My energy returned. I participate in new activities, such as studing botany and leading bird-watching groups. I can control old, negative habits, and carefully choose people who will enhance my life.

119. Ted J.

I made many positive changes as a result of attending Gary Null's support group. I always used nutritional supplements. Today, I understand the relationship between the emotional, spiritual and physical. I used to have upper respiratory infections and needed naps during the day. I endured stress in my professional life, and I wasted time on petty things.

I increased my knowledge of the interdependence of food, biochemistry, and emotional and environmental factors in the support group. Upper respiratory infections ceased when I gave up dairy. My energy is maintained all day without naps or long sleeps. I changed my professional life. I own my own business—professional training. It is very satisfying. I often demonstrate techniques in the new support groups. I no longer waste time.

120. Omar

My wife and I joined a support group together. We did not want to lose our stamina as we aged, and we respected Gary Null's knowledge. We intend to raise our family in a healthy environment. I was overweight, which fatigued me. Gastric problems kept me awake at night. My work was stressful, with long hours. I felt annoyed with the friends and family members who interfered in our lives.

We embarked on the detox with enthusiasm. Our children enjoyed exploring new foods. I lost 37 lbs, which gave me the energy to enter races. Today, I work fewer days at the hospital and I feel happier. My gastritis is gone. Life is simpler without negative, toxic people in my environment.

121. Mary E.

I decided to get my life together, lose weight and enjoy life. I just did not know how to do it. One day, Gary announced the opening of a health support group. Several people spoke about their positive changes in the group and their ongoing accomplishments. I registered, and my life is not the same. I had fibroids, painful periods and bloating. I wore a size 20 dress and could not stick to a "diet." I was not happy spending long hours on a job I did not like.

Detoxification and eliminating dairy and other allergens seemed more difficult than it actually was. I found many choices to replace the old foods. My new diet is varied and delicious. No longer do I get painful periods and bloating. I do not have fibroids, and I wear a size 10 dress. I still lose weight just eating naturally. I will not interact with negative people, and I have a job I enjoy.

122. Joe M.

I sought healing for my allergies and loss of hair. I did not turn to medications. I felt there had to be another way to stop these conditions. I came into a support group for these problems but learned much more.

My experiences in a health support group opened me to my potential and unexplored strengths and joy. I follow the protocol and use juices. I can feel my body react to the detox. My allergies are greatly relieved. I feel energetic, and I require less sleep. My hair loss stopped. Today, I eat more than ever, and I experience real taste and health. I read my body.

123. Paul P.

I wanted to feel healthy. Medications did not do the trick, they could not make me healthy, only relieve discomfort for a short period of time. I had high blood pressure and frequent muscle pulls. If a health support group worked for so many other people, I decided to give it a try.

The dietary changes created physical improvements in three days. I follow the protocol and writing exercises. I listen to the lectures, and then one day I am told my blood pressure medication is cut in half. I no longer have muscle pulls. The spiritual aspect of our teachings had an impact, and I decided to slow my pace and unclutter my home. It made me feel free. I now consider myself as important as my clients, and I am beginning to understand myself.

124. Maria T.

I was depressed and overweight, uncomfortable with the extra pounds. I held anger in and did not discuss, understand or share my feelings with anyone. I was afraid to take risks, such as asking for a raise. Being timid and angry was not a good place to be. I knew and trusted Gary Null, so I joined a group to see if I could be happy and make changes.

I am on the protocol and love it. My depression lifted as my health increased. I exercise without fear of injury. I lost 20 lbs, and my energy is high. I cope, do not hold anger in and speak my mind. I spoke up at work and got a raise.

125. Larry P.

I use the cancer protocol for a testicular tumor. I follow it carefully, and I find I have more energy and feel alive and relaxed. In addition, the skin around my eyes was dry but is now supple, with fewer wrinkles. I am more spiritual and express myself. I focus on weight by simply eating naturally. I do not interact with negative people. I enjoy my job.

126. Jerome D.

I lost some weight and feel healthier. My skin is softer and more youthful-looking. My energy level is way up. My mentality is improving every day. I am now able to cope with events in my life.

127. Joyce C.

My energy level has gone up. I can get through the day without feeling drowsy. The eczema and constipation improved. My tinnitus symptoms greatly diminished. I lost weight after two months on the program, and my percent of body fat went down almost 10 percent. I did not gain any weight back. My memory has significantly improved. I can now connect the names and faces of my friends. I am calmer and more relaxed.

128. Mark M.

The pain I once had in my left testicle has decreased significantly. My energy level has increased. I am energetic all day, into the night. I no longer have to wake up in the middle of the night to urinate. My gray hair is beginning to turn black in areas. I have a great deal of inner peace throughout the day. My memory is sharper. I can remember things that need to be done for myself and others. My focus and concentration are sharper.

129. Alim A.

Three of the tumors I once had are no more; another one has decreased in size. My skin is softer and smoother. My stomach is smaller. I feel more energetic. I exercise regularly.

130. Jan S.

Since I started the program, my bowel movements have improved and become more regular. I am more focused, and my anxiety and depression have lessened. My eyesight has improved. I have more energy and sleep better. I lost some weight and feel much better.

131. Carol G.

I sleep better and am better able to cope with my nightmares. My depression decreased, and my energy levels have improved. My appetite has improved, and I have lost some weight. My memory and concentration are slowly improving.

132. Rochelle K.

My PMS symptoms drastically declined. I no longer feel sad, and I have little fatigue and almost no bloating, cravings or feelings of nausea. Overall, I feel good energy and sleep fewer hours at night. I lost about 10 lbs after cutting out junk food and improving my diet.

133. Gary L.

My blood pressure improved significantly. My triglycerides dropped to the normal range. I raised my good cholesterol and lowered the bad cholesterol. My homocysteine levels are better than before. I am less depressed and have a more positive outlook on life, with more energy. I also lost 15 lbs so far.

134. Edwin M.

My hepatitis C viral load reduced from 7 million to 4 million since following Gary Null's protocol. I think clearer; my brain fog and mental and physical fatigue are reduced. The aches and pains in my knees and ankles are gone. My weight reduced by 40 lbs. I find my mental and physical clarity enhanced, and I have more energy and strength. I seem to need at least two hours less sleep.

135. Michael C.

The results of my following Gary's protocol are phenomenal. I lost 23 lbs and trimmed over 5 inches from my waist. I eliminated two blood pressure medications. I sleep at least an hour less, and I experience a strong feeling of well-being. My rate of hair loss decreased. I have strength and energy. My joint aches and back pains disappeared. I breathe easier, and my sinuses have cleared up.

136. Theresa

I proudly list the following improvements in my health since I began Gary Null's protocol. My poor digestion has improved. I do not feel bloated or suffer from flatulence. I lost 13 lbs. My energy levels have gone way up. I do not require as much sleep as I used to, and I am much happier.

137. David P.

My skin color returned to normal. My nails are now growing properly. I have less mucus, and I require $\frac{1}{3}$ less diabetes medication. The sinus problems that caused such discomfort are gone. My hair and eyebrows grew back in their original color. My voice is strong and firm today.

138. Lillian R.

I have had remarkable results since going on Gary Null's detoxification protocol. My energy level is greatly increased. My blood pressure dropped to a stable, measurable reading. I am no longer constipated. I am totally motivated to heal myself, body and mind, and to bring joy into my life.

139. Ruth K.

To date, I can happily report wonderful changes on Gary's protocol. I lost 18 lbs, and my blood pressure returned to normal. My energy level increased, and I am not sluggish after meals. Feeling and thinking in a positive mode has increased my self-esteem; I feel good about myself. I did not regain weight, because I am determined to continue the program.

140. Dimitrios

I was too heavy and wanted to lose weight in a healthy way. I worried about things more than they required, and I would get involved in bad relationships, without the proper tools to handle them. I joined a support group and immediately began the protocol.

I lost 15 lbs, and I retained this loss when the group ended. I work out three times a week and have built new muscle. I developed confidence and self-esteem. Doctors do not intimidate me anymore. I no longer listen to commercial radio. I hardly watch television, but fill my time with soccer, dance lessons and learning new languages. I listen to books on tape while I am at work. Running a 5-mile race, something I never even considered doing years ago, made me feel the health I built. I love running and walking. Nonessential, unpleasant people and situations are outside of me. I weeded out all toxic relationships.

Today, I can truthfully say, I hardly ever get sick, and when I do, it does not last as long. I have detoxed, and it feels wonderful.

141. Andrea

Participating in Gary Null's antiaging program improved my health physically and emotionally. After I gave up dairy, sugar and fried foods, my allergies improved. I have fewer colds and better elimination. My energy increased, and I lost some weight.

The behavior modification aspect of the program taught me to be more assertive and confident. I am closer to achieving my goals.

142. Carol

I went to Paradise Gardens during the time I had been a support group member for six months. My weight was stable. It was my first step toward fulfillment. Watching the videotapes and attending Gary's talks led me to the pain I kept in my subconscious. This process made the difference between living an existence and living life to its fullest, at a high energy level. I enjoyed each challenge and learned the joy of walking. At first, I felt I could not do it. Then I stopped thinking and turned the walks into meditations. This unique approach helped me to continue my health journey.

I expect I never did anything more important in my life.

143. Beatrice

My arthritis often prevented me from walking. My hair was thinning, and I had a fungal infection on my right heel. I barely had enough energy to get through my daily tasks. I noticed ridges on my fingernails.

When I compare myself now to what I was 1½ years ago, I see a woman without fear and doubt, with hope and optimism, constructing a new life. I have more inspiring dreams than I did in the past, even though my path, at the moment, is not truly constructive. My hair is growing in healthier, the nail ridges have lessened, and I do not have arthritic pain. The heel fungus disappeared. My energy level is high. The homework questions gave me the opportunity to deal with issues directly. Just thinking of an answer redirected my life. My future is a good place. No one can push my buttons anymore.

144. Susan M.

Although I was health-conscious, I knew there was room for improvement. I overslept but was low on vitality. I am a busy businesswoman.

In the eight months since I began the antiaging program, I sleep 1½ to two hours less each night and awake with great energy. I lost 20 lbs. My skin is smooth, my nails are strong, and my hair is shiny. I built muscle tone by powerwalking, yoga, cycling and Nautilus. I feel more appreciative, with a better perspective. I manage two hectic businesses and four employees calmly, and I enjoy it. I research and pursue new ventures, including a book that may help people. I make time-out and laughter a priority. I am a spur-of-the-moment person, ready for action. Focusing on nontoxic people, I detach with love from the others. Family and friends are curious about my younger look and lifestyle, and I share the protocol with them.

145. Mildred L.

I entered a support group to rid my body of an acute bladder infection that had taken over my life. I sought a natural approach. I did not have good energy and required long hours of sleep each night. I was overly sensitive and easily hurt. I did not stand up for myself. My family was critical of me. This continued during my marriage.

I do not have a bladder infection today and can go to museums, on automobile trips, anywhere I wish without running to a bathroom. I learned to appreciate myself and burst into song without realizing it. Finally, I told my family and my husband, "Enough." I will not tolerate their nonsense. Not only did I reverse the emotional and physical conditions in my life, but my husband takes care not to hurt my feelings. I speak my mind and challenge people. Uncluttering opened valuable space in my home and life.

146. Lou L.

I had a negative outlook, dealing with chronic fatigue, driving 10 hours a day and spending time with my children, who whined and nagged. At times, I lost my temper from exhaustion. My hair was turning gray and white, my vision was getting worse, and I experienced frequent body pains. Committing to a time allotment twice weekly to commute to the city and attend a support group challenged me at first. I had to adjust to my lifestyle changes and my family's reaction to it.

Today, my outlook is more positive. I adjusted to the exercise regimen. I do not make decisions with anger, and I control my temper. I admit to making mistakes without embarrassment. I am patient with my children, and I find myself courteous on the road. I know my positive attitude will lead to total well-being. My eczema improved, and my energy level seems to be longer-lasting. I desire less sweet and salty foods, and I notice fewer graying hairs on my head. My vision improved. Spiritually, I respect and help others, even at my personal inconvenience. Living guilt-free, without condemnation toward others, has opened my mind to new experiences. Eliminating wheat and sugar was difficult at first. My wife has become a creative vegan cook.

147. Mutaba H.

The biggest change I have experienced since beginning this program has come through focus and eliminating toxic people from my life. I can say no without guilt. My body requires less sleep. My elimination is regular. I have also learned so much more about healing the human body through detoxification. I am truly grateful for this lesson in healing.

148. Patrick H.

I have experienced many positive changes following the protocol and anti-aging program. My mental clarity and sense of calm and relaxation increased. My outlook is wider. I am less cranky and not fatigued. My recall and memory are sharp. I cope successfully with stress. My skin is clear. I have less nasal mucus and an improved resting heart rate. I rejuvenate with less sleep. My tonsil size decreased. No longer do I have dark circles under my eyes, and the pain from peripheral neuropathy in both my legs has diminished, as has my arthritic pain. I have not been ill since I began the program. Thank you for the knowledge you bestowed upon me. I am grateful and will continue to actualize it.

149. Elaine

The changes I made since the onset of the protocol exceed any I made in several years. For a month or two, I had a difficult time sticking to the program. In that short time, I gained a few pounds and experienced exhaustion. My headaches returned. Now that I am fully committed to the protocol, I lose 1 lb a week and inches from my hips and waist. My blood pressure dropped to 102/60. My self-confidence, energy and sense of security increased. My hair is shiny. I am not dehydrated, nor do I get headaches. I feel competent, confident, positive and clear-headed, with an ability to focus on life goals.

150. Philip G.

My health began to improve six years ago when I was introduced to Gary Null's nutritional protocol. I had symptoms of Lyme's disease. Being physically ill and exhausted, I had a rotten attitude. I did want to improve my life. I gradually experimented with Gary's concepts and became healthier. I took responsibility for myself and did not depend on others for care. I will not hand myself over to professionals anymore—auto mechanics or medical. I research and listen to their advice before taking action. I feel better since beginning this journey, and I continue to improve.

151. Sigrid

I came into the antiaging program with several problems. My knuckles cracked from arthritis. My gums were damaged. I felt my eyesight weaken. I was overweight, and I never considered my spiritual needs. It was because of the above, as well as diminished energy, that I joined the antiaging group.

During the course of the program, I felt as I did many years ago: young, happy and thinner after a 30-lb weight loss. My relationship with my father improved, and I eliminated very toxic people from my life. I can tolerate long intervals between meals. My spiritual needs have awakened. I read the Bible again, and I pay attention to the present, to the tasks at hand. I look forward to happiness, without need for approval or reward. I truly believe everything falls into place if the spiritual is acknowledged. My life is easier.

152. Trelline G.

Stress, weight, hypertension, anemia and a heavy menstrual period brought me into a study group.

The regenerative powers of my system tapped into the protocol. I experienced a return to overall health. My hair, skin and nails are strong and healthy. The anemia was life-threatening. Today, I no longer have this condition, and my periods are normal. I have not met my ideal weight or controlled my hypertension yet, but I will continue the program diligently with success. This is a life-sustaining protocol, and I am on the road to wellness.

153. O. L.

I was underweight, and I had behavior problems. I had a lot of unresolved past issues that caused anger and brooding. I often engaged in negative thinking. It was time to change.

Since following the protocol, my emotional and physical health improved. My skin is smooth, and I have more energy. I gained 10 lbs and lift weights. Recovery from heavy exercise is faster today. I wake up mornings with clarity. The homework questions helped me eliminate unpleasant memories and resentments. I let go of people who do not accept me, and I find myself seeking and obtaining new relationships, having fun, laughing. The guidance of Gary, Luanne and my fellow group members is appreciated. I am very thankful.

154. Marcia D.

I required eight hours of sleep each night and still awoke with low energy. I used to overeat and craved sweets. I often had pains in my body. I did not handle stress well and often worked longer hours, which caused exhaustion. It was difficult saying no to people.

The protocol changed these obstacles. My life is far happier and healthier. I require six hours of sleep and feel well-rested in the morning. My mind is clear and focused. The exercises defined my leaner body. I am in tune with this healthier eating plan and feel the difference if I go off even slightly. Sugar is not my sweetener. I worked through that addiction using the allowed sweeteners on the protocol. Not overeating and keeping myself clean builds energy. My body pains are gone. My most apparent progress is that I believe in myself, consider my well-being and say no. I can focus and remain unstressed and calm. I did that with work, and today I enjoy leisure time.

155. Eugene

Three months before joining the study, I was diagnosed with a small melanoma in my right eye. I am legally blind in my left eye. The cancer options were horrendous: removing the eye, treating it with radiation or leaving it alone, with the chance the cancer would metastasize to my liver. I often had migraine headaches, chronic lower back pain, prostate problems, pain from a rotator cuff injury in my right shoulder and arthritis in a toe. I was overweight. It was time to change strategies and rid myself of these conditions.

Gary's words were powerful. I had to become my own authority. Since beginning the protocol, the cancer has not grown in eight months. My migraine headaches virtually disappeared about two months after changing my diet. I lost 35 lbs, and my back has improved. Saw palmetto and other herbs did not relieve my prostate problem in the past, but they are quite effective now. My body is receptive to healing. The other minor conditions have improved. Although my energy level varies, I feel more energetic and younger in a body that knows how to heal itself.

156. Nevea

I eliminated food allergies when I eliminated wheat, dairy and processed foods. I learned about, and now feel the benefits of, eating a healthy diet. I no longer have sinus infections or colds, my skin looks great, and my menstrual periods are normal. One major change is listening to my body. If I feel a major change, it is because I consumed something I am allergic to. The program and protocol put me on the right track.

157. Tom G.

I joined the group to get healthy, regain energy and develop self-motivation. I have gained far more.

My energy returned as I exercised, followed the protocol and made the appropriate dietary adjustments. My skin is younger looking, and I see the world differently. An old injury that turned into varicose veins is healing. The veins are smaller. I require fewer hours of sleep. Uncluttering really put everything in order. I cleaned my basement for the first time in 15 years and just threw everything out. My wife and I argue less; I bought her a copy of *Who Are You Really*, which helped. I intend to stay on the protocol and go to the next level. My family and I thank you. Our lives are happier.

158. Natalie K.

I suffered with bothersome tension-type headaches, which sometimes became debilitating migraines. I also had recurrent cold sores; one episode involved one of my eyes, resulting in a cornea-scraping procedure.

Since joining the group, I am eating a primarily vegetarian diet, including fish. I eliminated caffeine and sugar. I can state that I no longer have tension headaches, and the severity of my cold sores has diminished. I will continue working on eliminating them. I feel very fortunate. I am an optimistic person, and I feel loved and respected in all of my relationships. I am an intelligent, supportive woman with a natural desire to learn new things. I have learned many new concepts in the group and by reading *Who Are You Really*. I see changes in my physical health and awareness of my surroundings. Understanding my life energies further empowered me, with insight and understanding.

159. Stacey T.

I came into a support group six months ago, and, in that time, my health and behavior have progressed considerably.

I can walk a 15-minute mile today and lost more than 60 lbs. I sleep less, with more morning energy. I have eliminated toxic people in my life. My skin cleared up, and I have bladder control. By practicing yoga and meditation, I spend free time quietly at home. This sense of joy and happiness is passed to my patients as a better doctor, healer and wiser human being.

160. Eleanor H.

Before coming into a support group, I had physical disorders. My adrenal and thyroid functions were low, leaving me exhausted, stressed, cold and tired.

Hypoglycemia caused a constant hunger until the evening. I did not have energy for exercise. I would wake up in the middle of the night and would not be able to fall back to sleep.

The protocol reversed these problems. I enjoy strong energy and a sense of integration with tai chi and gi gong exercises. I have not had a sinus infection in ages. My hypoglycemia is practically gone. I wake up early, without stress, feeling happy and alert. I no longer use prescription medications; my body will heal itself. I focus on the future, integrating my work with my friends. A healthy body and life are part of my mission to aid people on a personal and environmental level. I look forward to the rest of my life with joy and love.

161. Samuel N.

Since I joined the program, I have experienced wonderful changes. I understand the members of my group and I are all from the same source. We receive the same benefits, breathe the same air, receive the same sunshine and rain, and desire the same inner peace.

By attending this group, I developed a spiritual awareness I never felt before. I am able to control my emotions, because I am aware that I can return to the spiritual source for guidance. I discovered my mental attitude relaxes my physical body. When interacting with other people, I am less anxious and impatient. I developed an understanding of people. I am most grateful for these improvements in my life within this short amount of time.

162. Rich V.

I came into a support group with long-term negative habits. I eliminated alcohol and cigarettes from my life years ago, but I did eat flesh foods. I indulged in negative emotions, and I dwelled on the worst of a given situation while ignoring any positives. My home was full of objects that I considered to be junk. My self-esteem and energy were low, and there were signs of aging on my skin.

I have made progress through vegan living, support group lectures and detoxification. I detoxed my body and mind; this improved my skin tone. I will not be in the company of negative, complaining people. I post affirmations on my mirror and in my car. They are very beneficial. The supplements have given me new health and vitality. I lost weight and now run 8 miles, not the 5 miles I used to. My sense of smell is improving. New hair grows in with fewer grays. I no longer feel a slump in energy at 3 P.M. each day. My self-esteem is blossoming, and I sing and perform again. My home is uncluttered, and my future priorities are on my agenda.

163. Marc C.

I joined a support group to lose weight and change my life for the better. Years ago, I was able to cause positive changes. I seemed to have lost this ability. The homework and group interaction returned this aspect to me. I am an avid skier and ski instructor. Being on the protocol gave me the most rewarding ski season of my life. My students brought an overwhelming amount of positive feedback. I taught the best lessons and received the best tips to date. I received an award for excellence in ski instruction. This year, I was relatively injury-free. During the last four seasons, I experienced injuries that lessened my abilities on the slopes for weeks at a time. I failed a high-level certification exam 14 years ago, but I will retake it this year. The exam will be a learning experience, and my athletic performance is at a high level. My surroundings will be detoxed soon. The group has given me the power to make wonderful changes.

164. Liz M.

I lost 20 lbs during the first six months in the support group. I work out four to five days a week, with incredible energy and no exhaustion. I sleep fewer hours but have restful sleep. I think clearly, making personal and business decisions quickly. I am not depressed. Affirmations developed a general feeling of grounding and balance. I own an organic, vegan home-delivery business, which has tripled in size. This is an extension of me, organized without procrastination. I am careful with my free time, and I recently moved out of a long-term relationship into a studio apartment that belongs to me, serene, peaceful and beautiful. I choose only positive relationships. Each day develops enjoyment within. The support group was the catalyst that changed my life to a positive, peaceful state of being.

165. Tom

I came into a support group to reach my potential and establish goals. I entered the group after a divorce. My job and apartment loss soon followed because I allowed other people to make decisions for me. I gave them power.

I entered a study group with an objective of developing the spiritual, physical and emotional potentials I could not muster alone. An uncompromising commitment to the program would, hopefully, give me the power to make my own choices. I want control, and I have it now by controlling what I will or will not put into my body. I feel my energy without using sugar. Now that I am single and possess the solitude necessary for reflection and spiritual growth, I follow a path toward discovery and wholeness. Positive changes in one aspect of life lead to positive changes in other areas. Good changes can build on each other.

166. Liza S.

I am a teacher, and I would get angry with my students and other people at times. I had pain from fibromyalgia and arthritis. I joined a support group to improve my health and found other changes.

I lost 25 lbs and have more strength and less pain. People tell me my skin looks good and want to know what I am doing. I use the green powders and follow the protocol. I feel focused and mentally clear, and find my teaching has improved. I can tolerate students without anger, but keep toxic relatives at a distance. My new viewpoints and positive energy seem to be rubbing off on them. During the past six months, several unfortunate circumstances hit my family. I know that without the changes I have made, I could not have coped as well as I did. I continue to work on detoxifying my body, remain aware of anger and have become more playful.

167. Cris M.

I have followed Gary's protocol for the last two years. I entered the anti-aging program with fatigue, which impacted my exercise program. Eventually, my strength and endurance increased. My complexion is clearer. My hair loss has reversed. I have a great sense of well-being and personal satisfaction. My outlook has improved in work and in my personal life. Areas of importance have shifted, and I feel focused, alert and aware.

168. Rose V.

I would like to thank you, Gary, for your constructive criticism of my power-walking, as well as for encouraging me to compete eventually in this sport. As for my foot problems, I will follow your advice, because I trust you. I know I will be cured. I would like to let you know, based on my perception, that you are a perfect example of "mens sana in corpore sana." You have given me inspiration to strive for the same, although I wonder how far I will get or when I will feel complete.

169. Brian B.

I could not prioritize my life. I worked 12 hours a day and did not honor my belief system. I used vitamins, exercise and reaching out to others as my spiritual focus.

I will continue to use my supplements and follow the program. I do honor my health and have found comfort in a spiritual power. I will face my problems without fear, because I am more of a complete person. Gary and the group gave me inspiration, insight and their generosity. I will pass this on to the people in my life. Thank you.

170. Laura

My stay at Gary's Florida ranch helped me find a new direction in life. I arrived with my past and present, and came home an enlightened woman. I made permanent changes in my life and feel terrific. My changes are numerous. I feel I can do anything I wish.

171. Nancy A.

My illness was undiagnosed for a year and a half. It was debilitating. During my stay at Paradise Gardens, I looked at deeper issues. I was able to understand the issues preventing me from achieving health. Gary made me aware of my right to live joyfully and strong. His fierce and unflagging dedication was inspirational, and I am grateful. I look forward to a healthy, strong life.

172. Mike C.

I am detoxing for the past year. My life keeps getting better and better. In some ways, I feel like a child again. Gary's uncompromising passion for his beliefs and work, and his dedication to the mastery of each day set a powerful role model in my life. I plan to help others grow and improve their lives.

173. Gina S.

I am at peace and harmony today. My spirit awakened for the first time since childhood. I have come full circle. Body, mind and spirit are one. My family has made many life-affirming changes. My father-in-law is beginning to heal. Our children are healthy again. The effects are endless and go much deeper than mere words can express.

174. Dorothea M.

67 years old

A new beginning at 67 years of age. I am so grateful to you for showing me how to improve life for myself and others. You opened my life to the joy of exploration for myself and others. I now realize there is a world of joy to learn about as I follow my bliss. Thank you for leading me to a healthy body, mind and spirit.

175. Florence H.

I wanted to live a healthy life but could not keep on track. I lacked motivation and discipline. I developed both of these skills when I entered a support group. I learned to exercise three times a week, and I began to enjoy and make this my personal routine. I lost weight and feel energetic. I follow the protocol with enjoyment. I foresee a healthier and more vital future.

176. David Y.

The antiaging program gave me a pathway toward life expansion. I am happy to be away from the typical American diet. The support group taught me strategies for coping when I am perceived to be different. My body is cleaner. I understand that there are other paths on the road of life.

177. Yanick

I had a history of fibrocystic breasts for 20 years. I was underweight and had hair loss. I took Synthroid and was told I was facing possible thyroid cancer.

After six months on the program, my fibrocystic breasts decreased by 50 percent. I gained 2 pounds and exercise five to six days a week. I built muscle. My hair loss lessened, and I no longer use Synthroid.

178. Patricia B.

I came into the study detoxing from a 28-year abusive marriage. After a stressful legal battle, my husband was removed from the home and the court awarded me custody of our child. I was diagnosed with myelogenous leukemia during my separation. I was in remission with chemotherapy and attended a Gary Null lecture on "Who Are You Really." It was there, as an answer to my question, that Gary suggested I detox, and I joined a support group as soon as one opened. My defenses were gone. My nails, hair, skin, muscles and strength were weak, and I did not exercise. I worked 30 hours a week and raised three teenagers, in addition to attending interior design classes at the Fashion Institute of Technology and doing drapery design work on the side. I drank coffee, ate flesh foods and walked only when home pressures built up.

The decision to live healthier, happier and holier, and to renew my faith in

God came to me. We moved, and I began juicing and rebuilding my immune system.

Today, I powerwalk and run 3 miles five times a week. I do 200 crunches or sit-ups daily. People tell me I look well. The study has been an important part of my recovery. I could not believe I would find the energy to make myself well, but I did.

179. Helen

60 years old

I've been listening to Gary for 25 years. I use Gary's website and read his books. I follow the protocol. I decided I could use a boost of health and joined the retreat group. The impact was tremendous. I was able to understand myself, the relationships in my life and my fears better. I began powerwalking, doing yoga exercises and establishing new social contacts. The eye-health lecture was informative. This was a new space for me. The chiropractic treatments were healing. I never felt uncomfortable about my body size.

I made new friends, all of them enlightened.

180. Inez

She joined the retreat week as a work-study participant. After a consult with Luanne, she had a desire to learn more as she created an organic home. Hypertension and a low thyroid caused her to be cautious about exercise, but she wanted to learn more about physical fitness.

She learned how to juice in the kitchen, be totally organic and prepare vegan meals. Luanne taught her to focus on home hygiene. Andre's exercise class was exceptional, and the eye-health lecture improved her eyesight. She found peace and calm that week.

With new skills (how to listen to her inner self and create calm), she meditates and creates introspection. Inappropriate issues do not cause her upset when looking beyond and planning a future. Today, she is thinner, healthier, vegan, organic and working to eliminate occasional "cheating."

181. Andre B.

He was in a support group years ago but did not follow the protocol. He decided to go to the retreat because he was mentally fatigued and could not give up marijuana.

He learned to exercise in a workshop and began drinking juices to rebuild his body. He needed this push to establish self-confidence and gain the will-power to stop using marijuana. The people, environment and lectures made a positive impact.

He has not smoked marijuana since he left the retreat. He is following the protocol, and he is juicing. In order to stick to the program, he eliminated toxic and negative people from his life. His positive attitude and determination to renew his life intelligently, without emotions, reveals the building of self-respect.

182. Julie C.

She attended one retreat in the past. She was ready for a new beginning. Her dog was 10 years in remission from cancer, thanks to an alternative veterinarian. There was much to learn about health and nutrition.

Gary's lectures expanded her mind. She learned that life does not have to be routine and boring. The issues were exactly what she needed to explore: energy dynamics and alternative dimensions. She wanted to apply these issues practically and went on a media fast for one week, listening to music but not television. She had choices and was not alone. During this time, she was diagnosed with hepatitis C.

Today, she works as a buyer and is an environmental activist. She and her husband decluttered their home, rescued five cats and adopted two dogs. She admits to following the protocol 98 percent, tempted by the free-range chicken she prepares for her animals. The family, human and nonhuman, uses green and red powders, juices and many supplements. She sees an alternative physician for her hepatitis, and the mercury level in her blood is half the level of two years ago. Her last eye examination revealed 20/20 vision for the first time.

III

Treatments and Patient Experiences

There is more than one way to heal from a disease. This section describes a variety of nontoxic noninvasive therapies that permit the body to heal itself.

Usually, in a book like this one, the scientist's or doctor's view is presented and the patient's outlook ignored. But here, patient stories are included to elucidate the benefits of the treatment modalities. We feel this perspective is valid and can offer valuable information and insight.

Acupuncture

Acupuncture has been used successfully for thousands of years to heal the body of specific diseases, relieve pain, and enhance well-being. During treatment, hair-like needles are placed into the skin on specific points along a series of lines known as meridians. Exact placements are determined by pulse diagnosis. Needles open up congestion and allow energy to flow freely into these areas so that healing can occur. While not a cure-all, acupuncture is remarkably effective when used in conjunction with other therapies, such as diet, herbs, and homeopathy.

Patient Stories:

Cathy on seasonal allergies

I was first diagnosed with allergies about seven years ago. It got to the point where I was suffering for over half a year; I had allergies from March to the first frost. . . . It got to the point where I had to sleep with an air purifier on at night and take medication first thing in the morning. Despite all this, I was absolutely exhausted. I was sleeping a lot and had trouble getting through the day. Last year, I was so physically drained that I lost about two weeks of work.

Last summer I became fed up and decided I could not take it anymore, especially after the allergist said that this would get worse as I got older. The diagnosis was not encouraging. I basically felt that I had two options. One was to get allergy shots. The other was acupuncture. I decided to try the acupuncture.

As a journalist, I have written some articles on asthma and acupuncture. The research I did impressed me. I spoke to several acupuncturists in Boulder last summer and learned that I should try the acupuncture before the allergy season started, so I waited until February. It's been remarkable.

When I went in to see the acupuncturist, at first we talked about my main concern, which was allergies. He explained a little bit about the philosophy behind acupuncture and about energy patterns in the body. Regarding allergies, he basically said that most people do not have a reaction to pollen in the air but for some reason my body was reacting to it. There was something out of alignment with the way the energy flows were working in my body. He told me that the first treatment would get my body into alignment and that the second one would get rid of negative energy.

I was comfortable with his explanation and said I wanted to get started. On the first treatment, he placed one needle on the inside of my elbow. I didn't really feel anything. When he hit the meridian point there was a flare of intensity but it was very brief, maybe 10 seconds. I was surprised and asked, "Is that it?" He said a lot more happened than I realized.

Leaving the office, I felt giddy. I couldn't decide if it was my excitement at having done something for myself or if something was happening in my system. By the time I got home, I was completely exhausted and decided to take a nap.

The next week I went back and he did the treatment to release negative energy. This involved a number of points on my back and was quite intense since the needles remained there for a longer time. I asked him to cut the treatment short since it was painful. He said that it was not pain but an intense sensation. I thought that was funny and said, "You can call it what you want but it hurts." He cut the treatment short and I had to have it repeated at another time.

Since that time, I have had a series of treatments, about 12 in all, and it has never been as intense as the second one. At most, I would feel a flare sensation where the needle would go in and come out. I would never come away from it feeling sick.

After the first three or four treatments I became really tired afterwards but that shifted. Now, I usually come away feeling very energized.

The reduction of my allergies is amazing. Every day I look forward to getting out of bed. I still have a little bit of an allergic reaction where my eyes sometimes are bloodshot in the morning. And sometimes I get a little bit of a headache. But it in no way compares to what I had to put up with over the last five years.

For the first time in five years I have actually enjoyed spring. I didn't realize that I hadn't been enjoying it until this spring when I was looking at the grass growing and the trees blooming and saying, "Isn't this beautiful" instead of wishing for snow.

Joe on allergies

My allergies that I had gotten in my mid-20's were getting worse and worse. I was gradually losing weight. I was physically cold a lot of the time, even in the summer heat. Different types of foods were increasingly bothering me. I had strange body odors that came and went that were obnoxious to me and other people. I had unreasonable levels of fear that just didn't seem appropriate to the circumstances. My thinking was foggy and I needed to concentrate to get things done on the job.

I went to a number of doctors and chiropractors and found little bits of help here and there. Finally, I found a physician who said that I had indications of problems but that she did not know what to do for them. She suggested that I try some other types of healing paradigms as some of her other clients found help from alternative forms of therapy. I finally decided to try acupuncture in the fall of 1993 and have been receiving treatments now for the past two years.

This is the best I have felt in 15 years or more. I am seldom cold. I think better. I have what I believe to be excellent energy levels. I no longer have unreasonable fears. I see great changes.

I am absolutely convinced that my condition was not psychosomatic and that the therapy is not a placebo. I kept journals and logs where I measured and tracked my condition. I can go back and pull stuff out and tell you what I did and ate on certain days, what my responses were, and how bad I felt from my allergies. I have an engineering and computer background and am very analytical. Since then, I have given up tracking because my condition has improved so much. There is no question that I am better.

Joanne on allergies, skin problems, and candida

I had a terrible case of allergies where I would break out in rashes and hives all over my body. This went on for a number of years, and I tried all kinds of treatments. Acupuncture and Chinese herbs were the only treatments that helped me. I was going to my acupuncturist for less than a year when the skin rash disappeared. It has never returned.

I'm still getting treatments but I don't need to get them every week anymore. Now, I just go to stay healthy, energized, and in balance.

The cost is very little. The other treatments I tried were much more expensive. . . . There is no question in my mind as to whether acupuncture works. After using the treatment, my allergies and candida have completely disappeared.

Michelle on Cushing's disease

Once my pituitary tumor was diagnosed, the doctor recommended surgery. I had the surgery but was also taking herbs. I attribute the lack of any dire side effects to the herbs I was taking. I never got the diabetes that the doctor predicted I would get, and I didn't have to live on hormones.

However, I still had a lot of residual hormonal discomfort. I was tired most of the time, and I had sleep disturbances that kept me awake during the night and made me want to sleep during the day. That was difficult because my daughter was two years old. I was still very overweight and with the adenoma I gained 30 pounds in three weeks. I still had a lot of hair that you get from this illness.

After a while, I found a doctor who did acupuncture. The acupuncture seemed to assist me further in balancing. He recommended herbs, homeopathic remedies at times, as well as the acupuncture. Together, these treatments have been very helpful in alleviating my symptoms. I lost some weight and, as a result, my whole body looks and feels better. Also, I have more energy. Whenever I get a flu or cold, I bounce back very quickly and am never out for more than a day.

The acupuncture also assists me emotionally. When there are deaths in the family and other upsets, acupuncture helps to calm me down. I also go to my doctor's wife for private mediation and yoga classes. One thing we have to remember is that a person is not just a body but a mind and spirit as well. When you address all three spheres, the healing, joy, and potential for growth are enhanced.

Acupuncture has helped my whole family. My husband was diagnosed as having a hernia and was supposed to have surgery immediately. Instead, he went to the acupuncturist and worked with herbs. As a result, he has not needed surgery. Acupuncture and herbs have also helped my daughter when she tested positive for TB. The doctors wanted to place her on an antibiotic regime. We were very anxious about this. We brought her to the acupuncturist instead and to a doctor who uses homeopathic remedies. She is tested every six months to make sure that her TB does not become active.

I feel that acupuncture has benefited me on two levels. It has had a preventive effect because I never manifested the side effects that I was expected to get from Cushing's disease—the heart, liver, and kidney problems. I also think it has helped with some chronic issues. For instance, when I had a gallbladder attack, I didn't need to take any medicine. The acupuncture relieved the discomfort. So, it has alleviated chronic conditions and acute conditions at the same time.

Maxine on skin problems

It started with an itch on my foot. There was nothing there to see, and yet, it was persistent. I was in a Feldenkrais training at the time so I was aware of the depths of changes I was going through. One of my classmates recommended acupuncture. Originally, I began with herbs because I was a little nervous about the needles. At some point, my doctor said that it could go a lot faster if we had acupuncture as well. I lost my fear after the first session. The symptoms disappeared within a month.

I continued with the sessions in order to deal with chronic, long-term issues, particularly issues around a certain pattern of pain. It had never occurred to me to approach this through acupuncture but once I started to know more about acupuncture as a way of looking at the human being as a system, it made perfect sense that this could be useful. So, it evolved from being about relatively superficial symptoms to becoming about how I could be more of who I really am. It helped me to work through all of the different compensations that I had adopted over the years.

In the past, any small change or trauma caused me a lot of anxiety. One of the things that I have been learning through all of this is how to ride with the waves more comfortably. I may have a reaction of anxiety or a reaction of joy and come back to a kind of more comfortable neutral.

I firmly believe that disease is an outcome of many small decisions that we make, many refusals to take chances, and many refusals to look at certain issues. So, for me, the idea of a medical system that deals with the whole person—the spirit, the body, and the intellect—and deals with it in a way that can help you through the process, makes perfect sense. I always felt that, in Western medicine, they were all so quick to give you an antibiotic or to make a particular symptom go away without looking at . . . what the role of the symptom is in the whole picture.

I feel that acupuncture is, first of all, truly a preventive medicine. Second, it makes the quality of life much better. I am much more out there in the world and out there in a way that is comfortable for me.

Ruth on yeast

I went to a Western doctor because I was quite tired. I was given an extensive blood test and the results indicated that I was positive for yeast. After that, I went to see an acupuncturist. At the end of three months, I went back to the doctor to be retested and was negative for yeast. Actually, my doctor was surprised to learn that she completely cured the problem with a combination of acupuncture and cooking herbs.

I have been going for acupuncture treatments for about a year and a half. Although the yeast cleared up in a three-month period, I find that ongoing treatments continue to help me with my whole life. I feel much stronger and calmer and better able to deal with issues. It has returned me to me. I also find that acupuncture works as an immune system booster. I have two small children and tend to get every virus that comes down the pike. Now, when I do get something, it moves through my system faster. My body is definitely more on the offensive.

Lorraine on hepatitis A

I got very frightened one day after going to the bathroom and discovering that my urine was completely orange. I called the doctor, who said that I had hepatitis. I went to see him and he confirmed this with some blood tests. There was nothing I could do, I was told, but to wait it out. Months later, the worst was over, but my liver enzymes were not dropping back to normal. I was having terrible mood swings and could not pull myself out of them.

I decided to give an acupuncturist/Chinese herbalist a call. After the first session, my mood swings stopped and my mood stabilized. That was such a relief. She told me that certain things would happen along certain timetables, and they did. She said my liver enzymes would go down in a couple of months and that is exactly what happened.

I am positive that this is from the treatment. After the acupuncture, I would feel a release under my right rib cage, which is where the liver is. I also took a lot of herbs in the evening before bedtime to cleanse the liver. Then I would switch to herbs for building it up.

Acupuncture, combined with herbs and diet, cured me of hepatitis. Now I am absolutely in the normal range.

Donna on pain

Two years ago, out of the blue, I had excruciating, relentless pain in my left shoulder. I can't describe how bad it was. I couldn't do anything. I couldn't sleep or eat or function in any way. I was aware of nothing but the pain.

This went on for several days before I sought medical help. I didn't want to go to a doctor, but I did. I was x-rayed and the doctor told me that I had calcium deposits on my shoulder, which were pressing on a nerve. He said that there was really nothing that could be done other than surgery. The surgery might impair the use of my arm slightly. I consulted a few other doctors to see if there was anything else that could be done. The general consensus was that there was no other way.

Fortunately, someone gave me the name of an acupuncturist. I called and he said he thought he could help. When I went to see him, I was literally bent over from all the pain. The treatment consisted of placing a few needles in my shoulder, hand, feet and other areas. I left there with an 80 percent reduction of pain.

It wasn't just an anesthesia to get rid of pain; the treatment got to the cause of the pain. Once a week, I would return for treatment. I went back four or five times. In between treatments I noticed myself getting slowly but steadily better. It's more than two years now and I've been fine ever since.

Alexander Technique

The 19th-century actor Frederick Alexander created the Alexander technique while attempting to overcome a physical problem that no doctor could cure. The problem was that Alexander would lose his voice whenever he needed to perform a long recitation. After several physicians said that nothing was physically wrong, Alexander decided that the problem must reside in his presentation. So, he began to observe himself in a three-way mirror as he rehearsed, and noticed that his nose and chin lifted in such a way as to place pressure on the back of his neck, which cut the wind off from his vocal cords. He also noticed that by lifting his chest and pushing his lumbar spine forward, he was narrowing his back and imposing on his diaphragm. Alexander's self-observations continued for 11 years, during which time he discovered a more natural way for the body to be in space.

Alexander developed a system wherein the whole person, not just the body, is involved in movement. His technique particularly looks at the relation of the head to the spine. When the head is out of balance with the spine, negative consequences can result. Too much pressure is placed on the internal organs and there is interference with breathing, as the diaphragm is not free enough to move.

The Alexander technique helps people rediscover their natural ease and balance. Through simple verbal and hands-on guidance, students get in touch with patterns that they naturally had as children, but lost. Students are made aware of their styles of movement; then, they are taught to release incorrect patterns, and to organize new ones that are in line with their center of gravity.

Alexander's work is profound in that it is a psychological, physical, and neurological reeducation. Some people feel it has a spiritual quality as well in that it takes an enormous amount of trust to give up old ways of sitting, standing, and moving and to form new ways of being.

Patient Story

Mimi on back injury

I have been studying the Alexander technique for about 20 years. When I started, I had just had a child, and I would get tired a lot, with no particular symptoms. But within a short time, I injured my back, and it helped me enormously in that area.

When I started, I was in my early 30s. I needed help for working long hours standing up. Now, 20 years later, this is the same technique that has made it possible for me to work well all the time and feel strong. It's a balance, an ease. The better you learn the technique—and anyone can learn it—you learn to do what you do in everyday life with less tension and better balance.

Applied Kinesiology

In the 1960s, chiropractic physician Dr. George Goodheart founded the practice of applied kinesiology after observing that muscles correspond to specific organs and weak muscles indicate organ weaknesses. Applied kinesiology is a system of diagnosis that uses manual muscle testing to identify various organ dysfunctions in the body. The technique does not necessarily replace conventional forms of testing, as it can be used in conjunction with standard procedures, such as X-rays and blood tests. It is particularly valuable when a patient has symptoms of a problem that are not explained by medical tests. Applied kinesiology can be used to treat problems in a very early stage or to treat problems that conventional methods often fail to find, like chronic fatigue or environmental illness.

Besides manual muscle testing for organ weakness, the health care provider may place certain foods, vitamins, minerals, herbs, or homeopathic formulas under a person's tongue and test for muscle strength. An immediate improvement indicates that the remedy will help correct the person's condition. Conversely, sustained weakness indicates that the remedy will not work. Applied kinesiology can also be used to test the effects of other noninvasive modalities, including acupuncture, biofeedback, and chiropractic adjustments.

Patient Stories

Ellie on environmental illness

I thought I might have had chronic fatigue or Lyme disease. I was always tired and depressed, and unable to keep up with my life. I had joint pains, digestive problems, depression—severe unwellness, as I put it. I started going to a lot of different doctors trying to determine the problem because I knew there was something wrong. I went to many traditional doctors who told me that my tests were good and that everything looked okay. They pretty much were saying that the problem was all in my head. But I was really in bad shape. And I was very frustrated and becoming desperate.

I had heard about Dr. Silverman through a local health food store. I spoke to some of his clients who told me that they had chronic fatigue or Epstein-Barr and that Dr. Silverman had helped them. I made an appointment to see him because I was getting sicker and sicker.

Dr. Silverman has a holistic and environmental approach. First, he would have me come in twice a week for three or four months and he would muscle test me for all my foods. Each time I would bring in 10 to 12 foods and he would muscle test me to see whether or not the foods strengthened or weakened me. If the foods weakened me, I would eliminate them from my diet. In addition, he would have me bring in all of the products I used—face creams, deodorants, etc.—and he would test these as well. Right away, he tested the drinking water and determined that I must stay away from tap water, and drink only good filtered water. That made a very big difference because I actually had an accumulation of toxic metals in my system from the water. Another thing I learned was that my digestion was very bad, which prevented me from assimilating food properly.

Homeopathic remedies worked very well for me. They helped to leach out the metals in my system and improve my ability to assimilate foods. Within a few weeks, I started feeling an improvement. That really lifted my spirits because I was feeling like nobody out there would be able to help me. With Dr. Silverman, I started to feel more and more encouraged and life just got better and better.

One of the most important things Dr. Silverman does, in my opinion, is go to your home and work environment, and muscle test you in that space. You could have a rug next to your bed, or you could be sleeping on a pillow or a quilt that outgasses chemicals and adversely affects your health. Don't forget, you're sleeping 12 hours a night in your bedroom, and if your surroundings are hurting you, it can have a severe impact on your system. Dr. Silverman helped me out with that.

I started making more and more improvements to the point now where I feel that my health is good. If I feel I am slipping a little, for whatever reason, I go in for a tune-up. If I am beginning to use some new products, I go to Dr. Silverman and he tests me. He says this is good and this isn't. I just feel that I am on a much, much better track. My outlook is much more positive now. I am encouraged about facing the world in a dynamic manner. And it's just great. I have more energy, no more joint pains, better digestion, just general, all-over improvement.

Elaine on chronic pain and Lyme disease

I have been bothered with chronic pain for many years. It started when I was 17 and I'm 47 now, so that's 30 years. I've spent many years going to a lot of different doctors. They did the traditional things—x-rays and lab work—and everything always came back negative. I went for years without knowing what was wrong. About five years ago, I went to a rheumatologist. After ruling everything else out, he came up with a diagnosis of fibromyalgia. That's where a whole list of medications came in. I was taking loads of medicine which weren't doing much good. They helped a little, but not very much. Somewhere around four years ago, I started to develop a lot of new symptoms other than just generalized body pain. New things like headaches and a sleep disorder started to come into play one at a time. My doctor suspected there might be Lyme, so he tested and it came back negative. From there, we just kept on treating the symptoms of fibromyalgia.

About January of this year, my pharmacist started to become very concerned about all the medications I was taking. They really weren't having a very big effect. He had seen an ad for Dr. Silverman's lecture, and it mentioned fibromyalgia, so he asked me if I would like to go to the lecture. You get to a point in time where you think, I'll do anything. So we went to the lecture and listened, and most of the things he talked about were kind of foreign, like kinesiology, and homeopathic remedies. But he does a demonstration at the lecture. And that kind of convinced me that there were possibilities there.

I made an appointment for that night, and I started to see Dr. Silverman twice a week. A couple of weeks after I started to see him, he kept reminding me that one negative Lyme test really doesn't mean that you don't have Lyme. And I really had the classic symptoms of Lyme disease. So we decided to test again, and this time it came back positive.

So right now, I'm being treated for Lyme disease, and I'm continuing to see Dr. Silverman two times a week. He realigns my spine. Each time I go, I take 10 items with me to find out if they are making me weak or strong or whatever. And as you go along, you take out the things that make you weak. He gives you things that makes you strong. I'm taking nutrients for bone and tissue repair, arthritis and muscle pain, and liver detox. I'm also taking a multivitamin and mineral supplement. And I do aerobic exercise every day, which really seems to help the pain a great deal. I'm about a month into treatment for Lyme, which is Doxycycline. And I'm continuing to feel better. Compared to how I felt when I first went to Dr. Silverman, there is less pain and few symptoms. I would say that probably the best thing is that I have a very dramatic increase in my energy level. I used to wake up in the morning and just drag through the day. Now I'm at a point to where I'm getting up and living each day. I expect that it's bound to get better if I continue.

Aromatherapy

Aromatherapy is the application of essential oils for healing purposes. Essential oils are volatile materials, which means they evaporate. An example is a peppermint leaf, fresh out of the garden. Squeeze it, and you smell an aroma. That smell is the essential oil. These oils differ from cooking oils, which do not vaporize.

Over the centuries, aromatherapy has been a part of various civilizations. Ancient Egyptians, who are considered the fathers of medicine, prized essential oils and incorporated them into religious rituals central to their culture. The oils were also valued for their everyday uses, and utilized in the treatment of emotional and physical ailments, such as diabetes, cancer, ulcers, and depression. Early Greeks and Romans respected the therapy as well. In the first century, the Greek physician Dioscorides praised the essence of onion for its diuretic and tonic properties, and its effectiveness against infection. Fortunately, thousands of plant oil recipes were recorded and are being rediscovered today. In France, where the therapy is used widely, many physicians never resort to antibiotic prescriptions, using aromatic substances instead.

Research confirms that essential oils have many advantages over antibiotics. First, the patient does not acquire a resistance to an oil; essences remain efficient for long periods of time. Second, there are no negative side effects. Third, aromatics successfully treat a number of diseases that pharmaceuticals have little success with.

Aromatics are widely available and fun to experiment with. However, a few guidelines should be followed:

Only use oils that are pure and natural.

Use oils sparingly. They are highly concentrated, powerful substances.

Learn to use oils properly. Some should be ingested, some should be applied topically, and some should be dispersed into a room with a diffuser. Although oils are generally safe, some oils are contraindicated for certain conditions. It is wise to begin aromatherapy under the guidance of an aromatherapist or other health practitioner well-versed in this field.

586

Ayurvedic Medicine

This medical system has been used for thousands of years in India, and has recently gained popularity in the United States through lecturer and best-selling author Deepak Chopra. Ayurveda means the science of life, and this practice uses various modalities, such as herbs, diet, exercise, aromatherapy, and massage, to overcome sickness and enhance well-being. Disease is treated as an imbalance of the elements (earth, air, fire, and water), and specific recommendations are made according to an individual's constitution. Individuals are classified into one of three types: pitta, vata, and kapha. Pitta types tend to be excessively hot, vata types tend to be restless, and kapha types tend to be lethargic. Getting well is a matter of correcting imbalances in these types. More than a medicine, Ayurveda is a knowledge about how to live correctly for optimal health and longevity.

Patient Stories

Lavonn on idiopathic pulmonary fibrosis and fibromyalgia

I had been seeing doctors for about seven years and they had yet to diagnose me according to their tests. Everything is by tests. If they can find a test to diagnose you, then that's what you have. Diagnosis was a long process. There was a six-week wait here, and a six-week wait there. I was going down and had to sell my business. I couldn't work anymore, and I felt that the doctors were looking at me as if I was nuts. In fact, one prescribed Prozac. Needless to say, I was depressed, because at one time I had worked 70 hours a week with my business and now I could hardly take a shower and get dressed in less than a couple of hours.

I was in the bookstore one day looking at the health books when I came upon *Perfect Health* by Dr. Chopra. I read through it and thought that it sounded very interesting. I tried one of the recommendations, boiling ginger root, and found that it helped clear out mucus. I wondered what more Ayurveda could do for me. Three to four months later, I went to their clinic in Lancaster, PA. It's a very interesting program that involves cleansing toxins that build up in the body and cause illness after many years. The system is guided by the seasons and the time of day. It works through natural processes rather than a lot of pills.

My father was ill at the same time. By the time he passed away he was on $500 of medication a month. I felt that I did not want to go down that road. I really feel your physician needs to be behind you 100 percent. And I found that this was very true with Ayurvedic medicine.

When I arrived home from Lancaster, I started seeing some differences within two months. Four months later, I went down to Fairfield, Iowa, and went to the clinic there for another week. They recommend you do it twice a year, but the first year I needed to go three times.

The whole idea of Ayurvedic revolves around the digestive system. If the digestive system is not working, the body gets ill. This is very important. What nourishment you put in your body is vital. Schedule is very important, and the main meal should be eaten between eleven and two.

The first thing I learned about was meditation, and that has been very helpful. The mind is a positive force you need in your life because what you think about comes about. This is where the medical doctors have been so wonderful.

They prescribe many combinations of Indian herbs. I eat fresh basil leaves three times a day and that is helping to balance the body. Licorice powder and ginger root boiled together takes care of a lot of the mucus too. Before doing this, I was using aloe vera, which I also recommend highly.

Ayurveda works on balancing the elements or doshas in the body. Once they get balanced, you get well. They don't really like to talk about the fibrosis or fibromyalgia because these are just symptoms in the body.

The doctors are very supportive and call to check on me. I never had that with my regular M.D. It's a wonderful program. I could not say anything more positive.

Bema on maximizing energy

I was a competitive athlete in college and I wanted to continue playing basketball and soccer, and weight lifting. Of course, working full-time in New York, it takes a lot of energy to continue sports. I have been a vegetarian since 1970 and have studied meditation since that time as well. This goes right along with my interest in natural foods and meditation. It has given me a lot more energy to pursue sports. I'm not sick, but I use it for my training.

The therapy consists mainly of herbs and natural foods. You go to an

Ayurvedic store and you get the proper herbs from the people there. They try to balance you depending on your constitution. That's what I did. I went for an interview where they questioned me about the different foods I eat, my energy, and other things. Then they would prescribe depending upon my nature. The herbs they gave me really increased my energy level, which I put into sports as well as my workday.

Matt on psoriasis

I had a severe case that began in 1987 and peaked in 1990. Ninety-nine percent of my body was covered. There were not too many places that were not. What wasn't red and inflamed was white and flaky and falling off. I couldn't even sleep at night. I went to Western doctors, and they told me it was incurable.

Then I went to an Ayurvedic doctor. I was introduced to him through a friend who was a registered nurse. According to Ayurveda, just about anything is curable. It's just an imbalance somewhere in the system. So I opted for the system of medicine that said it was curable. And it worked!

Ayurveda just nicely said, it's toxins coming out of the body. They can't find any other way out. Ayurveda is very big on proper digestion and proper elimination. They recommended a specific diet for me, a specific exercise program, and a cleansing program.

I grew up on a very tough meat diet—meat and potatoes, meat and fries, you name it. I don't think I touched a vegetable until my mid-20's. Then I started transcendental meditation. It took me 10 years but I slowly became vegetarian. Today, I don't eat any meat at all. Apparently, for my particular constitution, it was a blessing. I couldn't digest the things that were in that meat, and that was coming out through the skin. I weaned off meat to fish and turkey for a couple of years, and then less and less of that.

Also, according to Ayurveda, there are three particular doshas, or predominant qualities in the body. And that is pitta, vata, and kapha. I was diagnosed with a particular tendency toward one of those called pitta, which is hot and moist. So, I should stay away from those foods. No salsa, no onions, no garlic—nothing that would inflame the internal because that was being reflected through the external, through the skin. . . . And if you buy into the concept that what comes in has to eventually come out, I was then, through Ayurveda, put on this road of taking in less and less that was bad for me. I was going through purification techniques as well.

I literally woke up one day and 80 percent of it was gone. As quickly as it came, it left. It was amazing. Nobody has to sell me in Ayurveda. I'm a firm believer in it.

Hubbard on chronic sickness

I tried a number of other approaches. I did acupuncture and I also tried Western medicine. They couldn't find anything wrong with me and it was very frustrating. I had horrible hay fever. Nothing was life-threatening, but I had one cold after the next. Six months out of the year I was sick. I didn't know what it was, only that I felt lousy and that I couldn't do anything for it.

A friend of mine went to the Raj in Fairfield, Iowa, and had had miraculous results. His cholesterol dropped 50 points in seven days. He told me to go and I was so desperate that I did.

It's truly amazing. As I said, I tried all these other ways of going and nothing has helped like this. I have not been sick once in two years. It is such a restful experience.

I have changed my diet a little bit, but not as much as some other people. So, I really think it depends on the person. But what I can say is that this technique works. I learned about cycles of rest and activity. I used to live in New York City, where I was a night bird who would stay up all night long. I would paint and work all the time. Now I go to bed before ten. For my physiology, it's really important that I get sleep. I also meditate, which I never did before. And I eat my biggest meal of the day at noon, because it's when the digestion is the strongest.

I would say that everyone should start with where they are at. You make the adjustments slowly. The whole philosophy is to be gentle and to do it in your own time. It's not at all a rigid thing.

What they do is they unblock. They feel the reason you get sick is that things get blocked up. They give you massages. You lie on these tables. The temperature in the room is body temperature. If you are a woman you will have two women working on you. You are massaged with warm sesame oil. And it's all done in silence. I think a combination of going there, changing your diet a little bit, taking some supplements, and just living a natural life, exercising, and getting enough sleep, can make a difference. It's not all that difficult or demanding. It's really quite a natural process.

Sharon on Epstein-Barr virus and menstrual pain

I was getting sick every two weeks when I found out that I had the Epstein-Barr virus. I also had severe menstrual problems. Conventional medicine did not help. I even went for a laparoscopy just to determine what was causing all of this. Nothing was found. I also had irritable bowel syndrome.

All this led me to seek out alternative ways of healing. I discovered Ayurveda at a health fair and started taking one of the formulas, which helped me a great deal. That led me to find Dr. Chopra's book. As I read it, the whole concept made a lot of sense to me. So I decided to go to the school and become a practitioner. I have seen tremendous success, not only with myself, but with a lot of my clients and family members and friends.

I used to eat raw broccoli and cauliflower, but I learned through Ayurveda that this was the worst thing for me because I'm a vata type, an air type, and this increases air. I realized that if I only knew how to cook these vegetables, using various digestive spices and herbs, it would be a lot easier on my digestive system. Cardamom, ginger, coriander, fennel: These are all things that I have learned to cook with that basically help my digestive system to work a lot better.

Epstein-Barr is basically related to a very stressful life. That's where meditation helped me a lot. It brings the body into focus and helps calm the mind down. It keeps you in touch with the higher self. If you just take the time to meditate, two times a day, 15 to 20 minutes, it is very beneficial, as is yoga, massage, and aromatherapy.

David on maintaining nervous system balance

There are a lot of different things you can do in your daily routine to help keep your nervous system in balance. They include keeping regular hours in terms of when you eat, when you get to sleep, and when you get up in the morning. When I get up in the morning, I have a routine that I follow. In terms of the Ayurvedic practices, one thing I do every morning is an oil massage. Usually it lasts for about five to ten minutes. This is a routine that I learned the first time that I went to the Ayurvedic clinic. I also take an herb called amrit kalash, which is a free radical scavenger.

I probably would be a lot more stressed if I didn't meditate. That I do every single day, twice a day. It is part of my Ayurvedic routine in terms of preventive medicine. I am not someone who has any particular illnesses. I have some minor things that bother me occasionally, but overall, I would consider myself a very healthy person, and I would like to stay that way. The way I look at it is that there are a lot of things that one can do to preserve one's health, and Ayurveda is one of those things. It's an ongoing process.

Biofeedback

Biofeedback teaches relaxation skills to patients with a variety of problems in which stress plays a role. The modality uses instruments to measure certain functions of the body, such as blood pressure, muscle tension, and brain wave activity. The patient is taught how to recognize different physiological states, and how to alleviate signs of stress through relaxation techniques. If a person has tension headaches, for example, he may learn how to relax the muscles of the forehead, neck, and shoulders. At the same time, the person hears a tone or sees waves on a screen that indicate the physiological changes taking place. In time, the person learns how to differentiate between tension and relaxation and how to create the latter state. Biofeedback is used to help alleviate pain and to correct a variety of conditions, including high blood pressure, insomnia, and migraines.

Patient Stories

Julie on patients with hypertension and low back pain

I'm working with somebody right now to lower his hypertension. Learning diaphragmatic breathing, and learning to warm your hands—which is getting some control of your cardiovascular system—can help in lowering blood pressure. It's important to apply those skills in situations where you tend to get tense.

I've also done a lot of work with patients with low back pain. The pain can come from an accident, like an injury on the job, or it can appear just all of a sudden. The back pain appears one day, or little by little it creeps up. Very frequently, much more frequently than people realize, there's a muscle tension component to back pain. A lot of physicians just look for disk problems or pressure on a nerve. But much more often we find that back pain is related to muscle tension. So again, using biofeedback to learn specifically to relax the muscles of the back in the area of discomfort can help people to control their pain.

Another very interesting aspect of the physiology that we can look at now with computerized biofeedback is to look at whether people recruit the muscles of their back say, when they're moving or when they're standing still, whether they recruit the muscles in a symmetrical or an asymmetrical pattern. If you think about it, if you're just standing straight and then you bend over straight forward and then bring your head back to center it ought to be the case that the muscles on the right side of your back and the muscles on the left side of your back do an equal amount of work if you're standing centered.

In a lot of cases with muscle pain in which the amount of muscle tension that appears on one side will be 20, 40, 50, 100 percent greater. Sometimes what we do that helps is to teach people to deliberately tense the side that's too relaxed, and then, when they learn to do that, the muscles on the other side don't have to bear such a heavy burden. That can result in a reduction in pain.

Affrine on severe migraines

I've had migraines for about three years now. So far, I would say that biofeedback training has been the one thing that has helped me. . . .

We did a lot of the hand warming and the surface electromyography and relaxation techniques. What I've learned is basically that your whole body is disposed to respond a certain way after many years. Biofeedback helps you to take control of how you are going to respond to certain triggers. Sometimes, with me, just being on the subway will trigger a headache. I've learned that the trigger is not necessarily the cause. Just getting a hold of these triggers has actually helped me tremendously.

At the very beginning when I started this I was not successful at all. It took a lot of practice; it's a lot of work and a lot of time. But nothing else has helped me.

I do it every day and I have different techniques. I have a comfort cycle tape which features a type of relaxation. I also have hypnotherapy and imagery. That's another tape that I listen to. I'm in the pain program at Lenox Hill Hospital and so I do those three things every single day. I think it's worth the effort because I used to get headaches all the time. Sometimes I'd get three a day, and sometimes I wouldn't get one for three days. I haven't had one in two weeks, so I think the success is really high for me.

Biological Dentistry

Your mouth is the gateway to your entire system. It is involved in every part of your total well-being. Biological dentistry takes this into account and is guided by the philosophy "do no harm." This is accomplished by paying attention to what type of work is performed on teeth and gums, and what substances are placed in the mouth. Dental work is meant to last a lifetime. It is therefore important that it has no ill effects.

One of the biggest concerns are metals used in fillings. Most people receive amalgams, which contain a high percentage of mercury. Nickel, beryllium, and other metals may be placed in the mouth as well. These can be harmful for a number of reasons. People may have sensitivities and develop allergic responses. Also, metals can give off ions and cause damage throughout the body; they can depress the immune system, overstimulate the cardiovascular system and affect the nervous system, causing a variety of disorders. There can also be energy disturbances from different metals, where a battery effect is created. Electrical currents are formed that are much stronger than the body needs for nerve transmission. Consequently, the metals become interference fields along the acupuncture meridians in the mouth, which flow to every organ, muscle, gland, and tissue in the body. Biological dentists test the effects of metals, and recommend replacement with biocompatible materials. In the past decade, thousands of people have chosen this route and have reported substantial health improvements.

Attention is also paid to infections, known as cavitations. Bacterial pockets can form under the teeth, and fester silently for years. The person may be totally unaware of the problem; yet gradual damage goes on.

Just as the teeth affect all areas of the body, so does the health of the entire system affect the teeth. Health-centered dentists may therefore advise patients on the importance of a healthy diet and supplementation. In addition, patients are taught how to participate in their own dental health so that their need for dentistry diminishes.

Patient Stories

Kasha on mercury poisoning

I'm 40 years old now, and I was in good health until five years ago, after the birth of my second child. I was always getting headaches and feeling tired. I was fatigued no matter how much I rested. I started to get other symptoms too. There was numbness and pain in my legs, pain in my joints, irritability, depression, memory loss, insomnia. And my immune system was low. I also got a lot of colds and flus.

I saw an M.D. in 1991, who diagnosed me as having arthritis, which didn't seem right. In 1992, I found a naturopathic doctor, who thought I might have chronic fatigue syndrome. I tested positive for Epstein-Barr virus, low adrenal function, and abnormal intestinal flora. The doctor started me on a lot of vitamins and supplements for my immune system and intestinal tract. I took colonics too. My condition stabilized, but I did not improve a great deal. I still felt ill a great deal of the time. I was also seeing a chiropractor for sciatic pain.

Another year passed. In late 1993, I saw a Dr. Chan in Manhattan. He looked into my eyes and said that he could see a heavy metal toxic ring around the iris. He tested me using bio-energetic analysis, which is an FDA-registered device that measures electrical factors in the body with the help of computer mathematical analysis. It assesses the most stressed part of the body. That testing also showed metal toxicity. So, it was Dr. Chan who discovered the underlying source of my problem as mercury toxicity from my amalgam fillings.

I was really in shock. I couldn't believe that that was causing my problem. I hadn't heard much about it, so I had to do a lot of research. In early 1994, I found out about the work of Dr. Huggins in Colorado, and I read his book, *It's All in Your Head.* Then I came across some other bulletins from the Foundation for Toxic-Free Dentistry. I found out that the so-called silver fillings in my mouth were really 50 percent mercury, and that mercury is more toxic than lead, cadmium, or arsenic. Contrary to what the American Dental Association puts out, there's a lot of research stating that mercury is not stable in the mouth. It will migrate to other parts of the body.

In February 1994, I found a holistic dentist in Orange, Connecticut. He and his staff were terrific in helping me to understand this. He tested me using an acupoint testing device, which showed elevated metals in my body. He also ordered a standard urine mercury test, which is used in cases of industrial mercury exposure. Even this test showed elevated mercury levels. Then and there I decided what had to be done. All these fillings had to come out. I had 11 teeth with major fillings. All my molars were metal.

Before he did the work, I was placed on a diet which excluded all seafood. I ate foods that were high in sulfur, such as eggs and garlic. Sulfur binds with the mercury and aids in its elimination. I used supplements such as digestive enzymes, coenzyme Q10, super blue-green algae, a lot of things to help detoxify.

In April 1994, I had all the fillings taken out in two three-hour sessions. I was given an IV drip with vitamin C during the process.

It was not particularly uncomfortable, and I managed to get through it. I felt I was doing the right thing getting all this stuff out of my mouth. That kept me going.

Once all the metal was taken out of my mouth, the sciatic nerve discomfort that I had felt for three years almost disappeared right in the chair. From what I understand, the metal fillings can create minor electrical currents in the body, which interfere with the nervous system. By the second session, after all the fillings were taken out, I felt the tension in my leg immediately go away.

About three days after that, I started detoxifying, and needed almost total rest. I had lots of headaches for almost two weeks, and a strange metallic taste in my mouth. I drank lots of fluids to get this stuff out. My urine was dark and it had a strange odor. This was all a part of the cleansing process that was going on. I had faith that this was all working to my benefit. And it did.

About two weeks later, I woke up one day feeling great. I couldn't believe it. I didn't have a headache. I felt clear and energetic. And my body didn't hurt. It was just wonderful. Over the year, I had several more periods of cleansing, mostly lasting three to five days, with similar symptoms. There were headaches and the strange, metallic taste in my mouth. After every round of cleansing, I felt even better. I felt a new sense of wellness.

Now, it's almost 14 months since the removal of the mercury, and I really feel great. I feel like 18 instead of 40. I'm not sick and my health and energy are reliable. I can really get a lot done. As supplements, I still take coenzyme Q10, 60 mg a day, and super blue-green algae, 3 g a day. I am grateful to have found out what was making me ill, after nearly five years of looking.

Eric on mercury fillings

My initial awareness of another possibility in dentistry goes all the way back to Carlton Fredericks, who used to say in his program that based upon the admonition to dentists by the American Dental Association on how they were to handle mercury, the only apparent safe place for the mercury was in your mouth. He made me aware that there were other possibilities. But moving from that to actually finding a holistic dentist at that time was something else. I investigated, and quite frankly, found some that talk the talk but don't walk the walk. In other words, they appeared holistic until I got in there. It was a gradual learning process that involved the gathering of more and more information.

I found myself that I prefer a one-on-one situation with a dentist. I went to a group office and it seemed to me that the partners were placing their economic returns before the interests of the patient.

I finally found a woman dentist, named Elmira Godall. There was an instant rapport. She presented options. She made her recommendations very clear, but she empowered me to take responsibility for the choices I made. She, herself, went to the trouble to learn Huggins's protocol. She went to Colorado to learn about mercury removal, and essentially followed his protocol.

When she removed mercury amalgam from my teeth, she simultaneously administered a vitamin C drip. She put a composite filling in a tooth that had an awful lot of mercury amalgam in it. My previous dentist insisted that the only option was a crown. The composite is holding up very well indeed.

She happened to be so sensitive in her skills with the drill that I have never had to have Novocain. With my previous dentist, I found that after leaving the office, I always ended up with a bunch of canker sores in my mouth. I haven't had a single canker sore since [switching to this] dentist.

In general, I found that being able to deal on a one-to-one basis with a person who respects you and who considers your ability to take responsibility for your own care to be an important factor. She is not lording it over you, but you are making a joint decision. That seems to be the critical factor here. I will conclude by saying that I am exceedingly pleased with the results I have attained.

Patricia on periodontal disease

I went to a dental hygienist on a referral from my dentist. She told me that I had periodontal disease and suggested a vitamin protocol, an herbal rinse, and a particular toothpaste with no sugar. She showed me how to floss all my teeth, including the ones that have crowns.

At that time, my gums bled whenever I brushed my teeth. I had bad breath. I had pockets with trapped food. I had never been informed about ways to clean my teeth.

Now when I brush my teeth, they seldom bleed. I no longer have bad breath. I have an awareness about dental hygiene that I never had before. I think that she's a very good hygienist and I have seen major improvements in my own dental hygiene.

Patty on candidiasis

I've had years and years of the traditional approach and I've had lots of mercury put in my mouth. As a kid, I lived on sugar, which gave me major cavities. At 16 I had my first root canal, and two years ago, I had another one. I have been suffering for about 10 years with chronic candidiasis and chemical sensitivity from a lowered immune system.

I have been seeing Dr. Levin for about two years now, and he recommended that I have the root canal taken out, as well as the mercury. I just had the root canal removed about eight months ago and I'm in the process of removing the mercury. I need to get eight or nine more fillings taken out. I know that it's good to get vitamin C drips along with the treatment, but since I can't afford that right now I take lots of C orally, and sometimes charcoal tablets, to help absorb the mercury that otherwise might go into my system.

My dentist uses a dental dam. She is extremely conscientious. She herself has suffered from candida and knows a lot about holistic healing.

When the root canal was removed, they found an infection in that part of the gum. I'm glad that I had it taken out, because I think in the long run it is a healthy thing to do. I've read a lot of literature on the disadvantages of root canals and I will never have another one. . . . I believe that they have definitely contributed to my lowered immune system.

Marjorie on sinus problems, arthritis, rashes, and high cholesterol

I had been having rashes and allergies for over 30 years. I had hay fever, I was lethargic, I had chronic arthritis, and my cholesterol was high.

A nutritionist, who was also an M.D., started me on the macrobiotic diet about five and a half years ago. That helped me a lot, but I still couldn't tolerate certain foods. I had lost weight and couldn't gain any back.

I went to Sherry Rogers, up in Syracuse. She was the first to introduce me to the idea of getting the mercury amalgams out of my mouth. My initial reaction was how could something so prevalent, that everybody has some of, possibly be a problem? So I let it go for a couple of years.

And then a year ago, another doctor also recommended it. He sent me to Dr. Bryner. I did have the amalgams removed and the composites put in. At the same time he tested me for mercury toxicity and my measured level then was 9, which borders on a toxic level, consistent with industrial exposure, because the expected range is less than 2.

At the same time he did an electric test to see what organs were harboring the mercury, and recommended the DMPS treatment. And that's used for the treatment of heavy metal toxicity. It binds, I guess, to the heavy metals, and washes them out of your system.

So I've had three of these DMPS treatments following getting the mercury out and I've never felt better in my life. I'm more alert. I've gained back a few pounds. Initially I went from 135 down to 99, and I'm back up to about 106. I can now tolerate more food.

Nancy on pleurisy and pneumonia

I was unaware of the fact that my jawbone was being eaten away. I had a little tingling in the spot where I had a root canal previously done, four, five years earlier. I'd think, "Gee, that's funny," and then I wouldn't think any more about it. I think maybe one of the dangers of root canals is that without a nerve there, you cannot sense the pain, and pain is nature's signal that something is wrong. So it's kind of a scary thing when you can't tell that there's something wrong.

I went for a regular dental check-up and had x-rays. Dr. Bryner said, "We've got a major problem here." This root canal was apparently infected and was eating away at the jawbone. And I was what I considered to be healthy at that time. So I went home and scheduled an appointment to have this root canal taken out—I mean remove the tooth.

Before I could get back for my next appointment, I came down with pleurisy, and that developed into pneumonia. So I had to delay my appointment a couple of weeks. Eventually I did go in. I had two root canal teeth right next to each other, on two lower molars. The one farthest back was the one that was infected. I decided to have him take both of them out. Why wait until the next one has a problem?

In the meantime I had read a book on root canals which really opened my eyes to the problems. Apparently, there are bacteria there all the time. When a root canal is performed, they can't ever get it totally sterile, so they do their best. Then they close that area off. We assume that these bacteria die when they are cut off from oxygen. But what in fact seems to happen is that they mutate and become anaerobic, which is really scary because then they can live anywhere in your body and you don't know it. They can gravitate anywhere, maybe to a weaker organ.

Anyway, when I went back for my appointment I had both of those root canals taken out. Dr. Bryner had told me some time before that every tooth is related to an internal organ. I originally went to Dr. Bryner because I had had twenty years of chronic headaches and I had heard that amalgam removal could possibly help that. When he took out my two root canal teeth I said, "I'm just curious. What are these teeth related to?" These were two lower molars that happened to be on my right side. He looked it up on the chart and said, "The lower molars are related to the sinuses and the lungs." I was amazed. I had had sinus headaches all those years, and sure enough, with this infection and these anaerobic bacteria gone, I had no more problems in my lungs.

Dr. Bryner was good enough to give me a homeopathic remedy to follow up with that. I went back to my walk-in clinic where I had had the original x-ray and my lungs were clear! I hate to think what would have happened had I been going to an ordinary dentist. They probably would have tried to save the tooth, which is what dentists always try to do. I think I would have made a trade-off to keep the tooth and lose my health. I'm grateful that I found Dr. Bryner because although I may have lost a tooth, I have my health.

Sherry Dodson-Puziss (dentist) on mercury poisoning

My story is a story of being poisoned through my work, but I hope it talks to people who are also poisoned through their fillings and their lifestyles because it's really a story of poisoning.

I worked in an old, old dental clinic. The room had lots of mercury spills—five times higher than what the U.S. laws allow for mercury vapor. The mercury was not vacuumed out of carpets; it just stayed. It's odorless and tasteless and you absorb it through the lungs and your skin. That's where I got my exposure for about six years.

I probably went to 10 or 15 doctors who felt I was just stressed from having a baby and working. They never got the diagnosis right, and they wanted to give me phenobarbital and things like that.

Instead, I went to the medical books, read up on the symptoms, and found out that I had the classical symptoms of mercury poisoning. We had someone come in and test the air, which was highly toxic. We got rid of the carpeting.

I worked for a large, traditional clinic where it was not politically proper to do further reading on mercury toxicity. There was a political move to keep this rather quiet, and so I let it go and continued to practice my dentistry, thinking that the problems were taken care of. I wanted to keep my job because I had a family, and I was supporting a husband through school back then. So I didn't do too much reading on mercury toxicity at that time.

Over the course of 18 years, I got sicker and sicker. What happens is your liver gets killed. So do your organs of digestion. It's like a slow starvation. I became more and more ill without knowing why, and didn't realize it was still the mercury until I finally totally broke and fell apart in 1991.

I was in bed for two and a half years with immune system problems. During that time, I began reading. I got access to the Library of Congress, where I was able to read abstracts on mercury research dating back up to 30 years. I learned that both my children were born poisoned with mercury. A lot of these poisons pass the placental barrier and also come through the nursing milk. Children are far more susceptible to the effects of the toxins than adults.

Basically, I realized that you have to remove environmental toxins. You have to look around and that's what I did. I stopped spraying my lawn with insecticides. I stopped bringing poisons into the home, like laundry fabric softeners. I got my drinking and showering water filtered. Water filters on the shower absorb tons of chlorine, a toxin that adds to the mercury. You've got basic mercury poisoning and then everything else added to it makes it worse.

After this is where you need professional help from complementary physicians, naturopaths, chiropractors, clinical ecologists, somebody who understands toxins. You have to get your liver restored. The liver is the organ that cleanses the body and so it gets all the poisons, and it backs up. You get too much poison. So the liver's got to be cleansed and healed and get healthy. Then after that you have to go after the stored body toxins, because these things stay in your fat cells and in all your body cells, your brain cells, your bone cells, everything.

I went through chelation therapy. . . . You may need as many as 15 IV or IM treatments, after you've had your fillings removed. And you have vitamin and mineral supplements in between because mercury depletes these from the body. At the same time, the supplements pull mercury out of the body. Chlorella is a green algae supplement that removes mercury from the body. We know the foods cilantro and asparagus do as well.

. . . We know that sweating works too. If you take a dry sauna, sweat profusely, and shower afterwards, assays on the sweat find metals coming out. Baking soda and epsom salt baths can also help. You can take two cups of baking soda and two cups of epsom salts in a hot, hot bath and soak. That helps pull out the metals.

So I did that. Had I not done the alternative complementary route I feel I wouldn't be alive today. Experts in this field say that. I think it's extremely important to self-advocate. The prognosis for mercury poisoning is generally good, I think, although you may be left with some central nervous system damage, including numb fingers and toes. I don't know if the ability to memorize fully comes back or not, because I'm still in the process of healing and getting better.

I implore people to self-advocate because nobody's going to do it for them. In my case, I saw 25 doctors, and nobody picked this up.

Nancy on headaches

I had had incapacitating headaches, the kind where you just have to go lay down. I guess you could call them migraines. I had visual disturbances and I would get nauseous. After my amalgam removal, I had fewer headaches and they were less intense. But I still would get some.

Following the root canal removals, I have far fewer headaches, and the ones I have are very mild. I guess you call them tension headaches. They're sort of the run-of-the-mill things that everybody gets. I don't have to stop what I'm doing with a headache now.

Let me just give one little detail on the headaches. I tend to get them at the approach of a storm. I think I'm sensitive to barometric changes. I had my root canals removed in December of 1993. That was a terrible winter with storm after storm here in the northeast. Where I live, in Connecticut, we had 17 major snowstorms. Yet I did not get a single headache the entire winter. Now, that is phenomenal, because for 20 years I had been getting headaches whenever a major low pressure system came through my area. That's probably the most significant improvement for me.

Flip on periodontal care

I'm in my 40's, and I've been going to my childhood dentist for years. He is a very nice fellow but he paid very little attention to my gums over the years. I don't hold that against him because back in those days nobody was really talking about that. Anyway, he discovered some pockets and asked me to have them checked out by a periodontist. I went to a periodontist who dipped little needles down into the pockets that I had between my teeth. He asked me to come back a couple of days later for the diagnosis.

When I returned, he said that I needed about $5000 worth of gum surgery. At the time, I was not inclined to do that, and I didn't really want to spend money I didn't have. Then he added that I needed a root canal for a problem tooth before he could do surgery. Not knowing anything about the ill effects of root canals I went ahead and got it.

I went to a new dentist, who gave me a perfectly fine root canal. While I was sitting in the chair, I said, "I've had surgery recommended, and I wonder if you know of any alternative hygienist that I could talk to." That's when he told me about someone in the next-door office. I made an appointment with her, which is what changed my—I can't say life, but I can say that it certainly changed my mouth.

She gave me a deep cleaning and talked to me, saying that this was not about my mouth, but about my stomach, my intestines, and my entire system. She recommended that I transform my diet and my nutrition, which would both cleanse my system and boost my immunity. That, in turn, might help to reverse the bone loss that I was having and actually improve my periodontal condition.

I started in on this, although I was kind of skeptical at the time. It involved something I had never heard of before called coenzyme Q10, and an entire regimen. To cleanse my system, I stopped drinking coffee and cut dairy out of my diet. I'm kind of addicted to pasta so I never did get the wheat out of my diet entirely, but I drink a lot less coffee and I am almost completely off cheese.

In addition to the coenzyme Q10, I started to take a group of minerals and vitamins that included lots of vitamin C with bioflavonoids, zinc, B complex, and vitamin E. I began drinking water with half a lime or lemon every night to help my liver. I still do this, and it is quite pleasant.

After she cleaned, she sent me home with an herbal rinse made from echinacea, goldenseal and cayenne and a couple of other things. At first it was kind of a bitter brew but I got used to it, and after about a week I began to think that this was the most delicious thing I had ever taken.

Over the course of a few years, with a lot of flossing, my bone loss never got any worse and my mouth has completely changed. I feel comfortable with it, and my gums don't bleed anymore.

Now this has become a daily routine for me. When I'm under a lot of stress I might boost up my vitamin C intake and possibly take another Q10 or something like that because I find that when I'm under a lot of stress it affects my gums. And I really notice a difference. Anyway, that's my experience. My mouth feels very healthy right now.

Karen on husband's heart condition and her clinical depression and menopausal problems

It started about seven years ago. We were given an Ayurvedic preparation that came into the country, probably not in a kosher way, you might say. Anyhow it was given for indigestion and we didn't know that it contained mercury at the time. He took it for indigestion and he experienced low atrial fibrillation. And he was quite symptomatic. His pulse was about 40; he was ashen; he was nauseated. Blood pressure was about 50 over God knows what. He was hospitalized.

The medical profession didn't understand why he was low atrial fib. He was about 32. It was Christmastime, actually Christmas Day. And so they allowed me to bring him home from the hospital since I was a cardiac nurse, and we just monitored him. We were kind of wondering, what did we do different? You know, why is this happening?

And so one of the things we decided was to stop taking some of these Ayurvedic preparations that we had gotten. We called a friend, and she did identify, in some formula that she had, that the preparation that we had had mercury in it. It was commonly used in India with no problems, but it did cause my husband a problem. We stopped and four days later he converted on his own, and he was in normal sinus rhythm. We had done a little chiropractic work in the meantime to help his body cleanse, but that's all we did. That's all we knew.

About two years later he went into atrial fib again. And this time . . . we didn't know what was going on. It was again even more serious than it was the last time. He had to be cardioverted and he was on all kinds of cardiac drugs. He had terrible reactions to them and I really thought he was going to die once. It was just awful. And then he was on a drug—a heavy-duty cardiac drug—for about four years. But it was really giving him a very difficult time with his intestines. So we felt we've got to go off this. The cardiologist agreed. He didn't like it, but he agreed, and he tapered Gary off his drug.

Gary was good for about a year and a half. Then he went into slow atrial fib again. Again, extremely symptomatic. Absolutely no energy. He would be exhausted just picking up the telephone and saying hello and, you know, we're only talking 40 years old now, so we were really concerned.

We went to an alternative M.D. She dealt in other things, other than just your standard medical fare. She did a couple of tests and discovered that indeed, there were a lot of mercury problems in Gary's system. She suggested that Dr. Bryner could help him. We went to Dr. Bryner. He did some testing on Gary, and felt that he was a good candidate to have his mercury out. We did it, and his digestion got stronger. Before, he wasn't absorbing magnesium or calcium, which is essential for good cardiac function, and they thought the mercury was interfering with that because of his intestines. . . . To make a long story short, it's been a year for Gary, a little over a year. He's on no cardiac drugs. He did not have to be cardioverted.

Nine months into that process, because I saw how wonderful he was doing, I did the same. I had some menopausal problems, some clinical depression, which was just awful. I had the mercury taken out of my mouth and right in the chair, like somebody turned a light switch on, while he worked on my teeth my depression left. I mean I wasn't even thinking that was going to happen. He told me that my intestines were going to get better but he said nothing about depression whatsoever. And I just got so happy and I've been happy ever since. So my husband's got a good heart and I have a happy mind.

Sharon on dental problems

I've gone to several dentists in the last eight years who let me know that I had a potential problem, that the pockets in my teeth were increasing. I really didn't understand what that meant until my present doctor told me that if that continued the bone underneath would melt away and disappear. I let these dentists know that I wanted to participate in my own healing. They always gave me certain exercises to do, but unfortunately it didn't get better.

This past January, my former dentist, a very nice person, said that there was nothing else to do but surgery. I let him know that that would be the last thing I would do, and asked him if he could tell me about something else. He couldn't, but he gave me the names of other dentists. I was in a quandary because I had the feeling that the people he told me about wouldn't know how to do anything except surgery.

But I asked around and learned of a dentist in Brooklyn. I started treatment with her . . . on a holistic regime. Basically the first thing that had to be done was amalgam removal. That was difficult because it was expensive, especially since vitamin C drips were given at the same time. But I decided to do it anyway. I think there were about seven to eight treatments. In addition to that I started to use magnets in the evening. I had magnets on either side of my cheeks.

I saw her a few days ago, and what's been happening is very, very interesting. It seems that clinically I regained—this is what she said—extra attachments in the pockets. My pockets are shallower. This is really interesting because I've asked all over and everybody has told me that that's absolutely impossible. It just can't happen. But it's happening to me.

Claire on periodontal disease

I've had periodontal disease for quite some time, and I was told by a dentist, at least 10 or 12 years ago, that I needed to have periodontal surgery, which I wasn't very happy about.

By accident I discovered the International Dental Health Foundation. Since I was having so much trouble with my teeth, I decided that I might as well go. So I beat my path to the foundation, which is located in Reston, Virginia, and there I saw Dr. Keyes and Dr. Watts.

First they took a culture of my gum which they studied under a microscope and at the same time projected onto a large screen. This enabled me to see what was going on in my mouth. There were a lot of bacteria at that time.

Dr. Keyes taught me how to use a peroxide and baking soda paste. He instructed me on making the paste to the consistency of honey and using it twice a day with a small toothbrush.

In addition, Dr. Keyes sold me a Swiss irrigator, called the Porpoise, and told me to use it twice a day with a salt solution or diluted peroxide. That seems to work very, very well. Here in New York the dentists have told me not to use the irrigator because it pushes the food particles under the gum, but Dr. Keyes laughed at this and said it is not so. The irrigator helps to control the bacterial population in the mouth.

I have been using the irrigator for the past 11 years, and have been able to maintain my natural dentition. I've been having problems on and off, but I'm able to control them. These Swiss-made irrigators are not available in the United States, but they are available all over the world. The Colgate company is producing their own brand of irrigators in Hong Kong, but they are facsimiles of the Swiss machine. They work for a while, but they tend to break down a lot. The public is not aware of the Swiss type.

Recently I went to see a Dr. Resnik in Edison, New Jersey, who is on the board of directors of the Dental Health Foundation. Through him I obtained a Swiss machine which is the latest of the irrigators, called a Hydrofloss. This Hydrofloss comes with three different picks: the regular pick, the perio pick, which has a smaller opening and is able to deliver the solution deep under the gum, and a third irrigating device, called a cannula. I call it a needle. This really delivers the antimicrobial solution deep under the gum. And what I'm using is chlorhexadine. This is very effective in controlling the bacteria and in just helping me to maintain my natural teeth.

And it's really unfortunate, but our society seems to ignore dental health issues and it's quite a [problem] because a person cannot chew their food properly without teeth. Poor chewing causes malabsorption and this causes all kinds of diseases. I consider myself extremely lucky that I was able to maintain my natural teeth. . . . If you need information about the Dental Health Foundation, their telephone numbers are 703-471-8349 and 800-368-3396.

Bob on periodontal disease

I neglected my mouth for years, sort of thinking of it as something that would just disappear, a separate entity. In the meantime, my gums had been receding and bleeding. I was horrified at the expense of gum surgery.

After a number of years of feeling more and more tired and sluggish from the overall neglect, I decided to start looking at the factors contributing to my poor state of health. I was persuaded by a homeopath that I see to go to a dental hygienist. I went to a great one, who was horrified by what she saw in my mouth. After a few minutes, I became ashamed of my condition, and that shame would have kept me from doing anything, but her attitude was extremely positive. She assured me that my condition could be reversed and that gum surgery was absolutely not necessary provided that I followed her protocol. This sounded much better than gum surgery. . . .

I basically followed a whole regimen, relearning basic habits that I had never really integrated as a kid. I started flossing morning and night. She literally showed me how to brush my teeth correctly. Since old habits don't change overnight, there was some backsliding, but seeing her a few times would reinforce some of the basics. It all sounds very primitive and it was. She also told me to brush my tongue because it is a great repository and breeding ground for germs and gum disease.

She gave me an herbal rinse to use after flossing. Then I got on a protocol of multivitamins, calcium, coenzyme Q10, beta-carotene and so on to boost the immune system.

In a nutshell, it took me two weeks to stop the bleeding in the gums that had been going on for years. That, in itself, was a great incentive to keep going with this. I have noticed some regrowth of the gums, which feels miraculous to me. But it's no miracle. What's happening just makes sense. By following this regimen, my mouth is refreshed and it makes a difference head-wise.

Annette on silver and mercury amalgam extraction

Well, first of all my mouth feels entirely different. It's so much cleaner, which is not the most important thing, but I'm aware of it every day. The really big thing is that in these three years I haven't been sick. I haven't had a cold. I haven't had a sore throat. I haven't had the flu. I haven't missed any work because of sickness. It's been absolutely amazing, and there's been no other change in my life. I eat the same way, I live in the same place, I have the same job.

Prior to the mercury coming out, I had nothing out of the ordinary. But every year I had at least one or two colds or the flu. That wasn't the reason that I went to Dr. Bryner, but that was certainly an unexpected benefit.

Marcia on fatigue, allergies and headaches

I had my mercury fillings removed about four years ago. My symptoms were tiredness, allergies, headaches, and a metallic taste in my mouth. After removal of the fillings, it took approximately six months to a year until all of these symptoms went away. The metallic taste naturally disappeared right away. Then I found that the headaches and allergies took a longer time. So did the fatigue. But they all did disappear.

I believe this is all due to the mercury being removed from my mouth. I went to a holistic doctor who specialized in this. He tested me and they found that I had a high mercury level. Mercury was being released when I chewed at a much higher rate than was acceptable. So, I would attribute my results to that, since basically I hadn't done anything differently. I was taking vitamins and I had a good diet before that. But I still had those symptoms and they did seem to gradually go away.

Chelation Therapy

Chelation therapy is one of the most exciting healing therapies available. If it was used more widely, it could be saving hundreds of thousands of lives each year, and improving the lives of millions more by treating conditions such as strokes, cardiovascular disease, diabetes, peripheral vascular disease, memory loss, and damage due to long-term smoking, drinking, and exposure to toxic metals.

Chelation therapy is an intravenous treatment for the removal of toxins and metabolic wastes from the bloodstream. The process involves the slow drip of a drug called ethylene diamine tetraacetic acid (EDTA) and various nutrients into a vein in the arm over the course of approximately three hours. The word chelation stems from the Greek term "chela," meaning claw, and implies that heavy metals and excess calcium bind to carrier molecules after they are picked up in a pincer-like fashion. Substances exit the body through the kidneys, preventing the formation of stones and hardened tissue. Generally, a series of 30 treatments is initially given, and a smaller number are given each year thereafter as maintenance. This, of course, can vary depending on the patient's state of health.

It was in 1948 that the benefits of chelation therapy first became apparent, when a group of Detroit physicians who were employing the modality as an antidote for lead poisoning noticed positive side effects in their patients. These included better vision, better hearing, loss of or decreased angina, less pain, an ability to walk farther, and a reduction of intermittent claudication. They related these improvements to a reduction in arteriosclerosis.

In 1950, Norman Clark, M.D. confirmed these observations in clinical research when he found the therapy effective in removing calcium deposits from the human body. He reported in the medical literature that EDTA might dissolve plaque and improve blood circulation. As a result, pioneering doctors began using chelation therapy for the treatment of arteriosclerosis, with great success. The holistic medical community now considers chelation therapy a safe alternative to coronary bypass surgery and angioplasty, and one that is actually more effective than those invasive procedures.

Chelation therapy also acts to reverse the aging process in three senses. First, chelation keeps free radicals in check, resulting in slowed cellular destruction. Second, oxygenation to the heart and blood vessels is strengthened, so that organ systems are revitalized. And third, osteoporosis is prevented or diminished as excess calcium is transferred from the arteries and joints to the bones. Many health practitioners recommend that chelation therapy be used by everyone over the age of 30 to slow down the aging process and to prevent the onset of disease. The treatment is not a "magic bullet," but rather works best as part of a comprehensive program that includes proper diet, supplements, and exercise.

Patient Stories

Lee on heart disease

I had two bypass operations, one during Christmas 1975 and a second in July 1981. In September of that year Social Security forced me to go back to work at the Post Office once a week. Even though I was working with great constant chest pain, they removed me from Social Security because I looked so healthy. They had a local clerk say that, as far as they were concerned, there was nothing wrong with me even though I had blocked arteries and constant pain shooting throughout my chest.

A year and a half later I ended up in the local VA hospital. While there, they told me I had four arteries blocked 100 percent. I was only able to get from my bed to my bathroom. That was it. I was given a handful of pills and told to go home. Three weeks later I had a real bad spell where I had to sit up in the chair the whole night because I couldn't catch my breath. My arms, legs, my whole body, swelled up like a basketball and I turned just as blue as the car that I drive. I had to concentrate to get every breath. I felt like I had one foot in the pine box and the other one on a banana peel. I promised myself that if I woke up in the morning I would go to see Dr. Sessions, whom I had known for about 10 years.

I did start to see Dr. Sessions who gave me chelation treatments. I can't tell if it was psychological or physical, but the very first bottle I was given removed the shooting-star chest pain that I had for over five months.

I have learned from Dr. Sessions that previous to treatment I had an unbelievable amount of iron, zinc, cadmium, and lead in my system. Now I have changed my diet. Previously I was a heavy beef eater, but I no longer eat red meat.

Claude on intermittent claudication

I had a blockage in the bend of my leg. My leg circulation was so bad that I could hardly walk. After running an arteriogram on me the doctor said I should take an aspirin a day. Then I went to Dr. Sessions, and I have had no trouble since. I have had 95 chelation sessions, and I can now walk. My legs don't hurt me like they did and I can do almost anything I want to. I believe that Dr. Sessions's chelation therapy kept me from having my leg amputated. I was also right on the verge of a stroke when I went to him and he straightened that out. I am over 81 years old.

Randolph on advanced arteriosclerosis

I am 66 years old. Back in 1989 I had artery blockage for which I had an operation. After the operation I still had blockage in my main artery because it was that bad. A friend of mine told me about chelation. I have had 40 treatments; a treadmill test given by my cardiologist shows no sign of blockage anymore.

Chelation therapy has made a substantial difference in the quality of my life. Before I took chelation I couldn't walk a block. Now I have no problem walking. I can walk two miles three times a week. Also, my eyesight has gotten better. In fact, I hardly have to wear glasses at all, even to read, whereas before I had to have them with me all the time. I would start chelation all over again if I needed to.

Mr. H. on diabetes, heart disease, glaucoma, and kidney stones

Approximately 12 years ago I suffered from diabetes, hypertension, high blood pressure (250/110), glaucoma, and kidney stones. There were weeks of time where I did not get out of bed. Evidently my condition was terrible. My kidney stones were so large that I was told they could not be removed except surgically. Dr. Sessions suggested that he might have a treatment for me and I started taking it right away. After the 20th treatment I began to feel better and I have continued to take chelation ever since once a month. In all, I have had 300 treatments.

I am 83 years old and currently I have no kidney stones. This morning my blood pressure was 130/60 and I feel great. . . .

In addition to chelation treatments I have changed my diet. I take vitamins and do not eat animal fats. I exercise as well.

If it had not been for chelation treatments I do not believe I would be alive today. I intend to take one treatment each month for as long as I live.

I have seen many, many people come through Dr. Sessions' office, and almost everyone, including those who were facing amputation, have suffered no ill effects.

I think this is a treatment most of us need since all of us have been contaminated in some manner with lead and other chemicals that chelation removes.

Dr. B. on arteriosclerosis

I was going through a period in life where a lot of my friends, who are in the over-50 age group, were experiencing heart attacks, angina, and associated symptoms. That prompted me to think about my own condition, so as a precautionary move I took a thallium stress test.

To my surprise, they found a blocked major coronary artery. The hospital recommended at that time that I do an angioplasty where they open up the artery. I felt that that was an invasive procedure which should be used as a last resort.

I discussed this with Dr. Corsello, who suggested I try chelation for a year or so. She said I could always have the angioplasty done later because it was not yet at a serious stage. I agreed. In fact, I had wanted to take chelation therapy for another reason. As a dentist I had been exposed to a lot of heavy metals over the years.

I went through a year's chelation therapy. During that year I had a tremendous increase in my energy level. I had younger-looking skin and I felt younger and everyone said I looked great. A year later I went back for another thallium stress test and to the doctor's surprise the blockage was no longer there. I have had two successive thallium stress tests since then with the same results. I have maintained a schedule of having chelation therapy once or twice a month since that time and my heavy metal level has decreased almost 80 percent. I feel great.

Some of my patients have used chelation and the results are equally positive. It alleviates tiredness and it restores the immune system. I have even seen people suffering from Lyme disease have equally good results. And I have seen other people who were intoxicated with heavy metals who have all had favorable experiences. We had one person with Epstein-Barr who was walking around with a cane for years because nobody was able to ascertain what he had or give him a definitive treatment. He calls me up every month to thank me.

Don on lead poisoning and carpal tunnel syndrome

When I first came to Dr. Corsello I had lead toxicity that measured in the upper 300 category. She brought it down during a period of less than a year to about 77 or so, at which point I decided to stop chelation for a while. One of the curious byproducts of the treatment was that it has a remarkable effect on alleviating the bilateral carpal tunnel syndrome that I was suffering from for almost 10 years. After chelation, it disappeared.

Chris on angina and bursitis

I am 75 years old. In 1975, I had a massive heart attack that left me practically a cripple and forced me into early retirement. I could hardly walk even one city block; the pain would get so bad that I would have to stop and wait approximately 15 minutes before going another block. I went to see one of the famous cardiologists in New York and the diagnosis was that if I lasted five years I would lose both legs. I didn't like those odds at all.

In the meantime I heard of something called the Dr. Rinse formula and I started with that. It seemed to help a bit but I still had no pulse in either ankle.

Then I finally heard about a Dr. Levin at the World Health Center and I went to him. I went through his course of chelation and I suddenly realized that I was able to walk as many blocks as I wanted. My angina disappeared. My bursitis, which had made it very painful for me to get into or out of a shirt, just vanished. At the end of the treatments with Dr. Levin I was able to walk several miles with no leg pain and I have a pulse in both ankles. It has worked wonders for me. I am positive I would not be alive today if it were not for chelation.

George on arteriosclerosis

Before therapy I had a heart attack. They found that two of my blood vessels leaving the heart were restricted, one 95 percent and one 45 percent. After leaving critical care, I was not able to walk without experiencing pain. They had me on a couple of drug programs to control my blood pressure and heart action and they told me I should take nitroglycerin for the pain. I couldn't walk more than a half mile without pain after my heart attack.

After I had 9 or 10 treatments of chelation therapy I was able to walk without pain. I could walk 3 miles in 45 minutes. My cardiologist is monitoring me and my injection fraction (which is the cardiac output), has gone from 49 to 54 percent. This astonished the cardiologist, who still to this day will not acknowledge the fact that my progress is due to the chelation therapy.

Originally, I was a fire-fighter and I built houses in my spare time. Since the chelation therapy I have been able to maintain activities similar to that. In fact I recently helped a friend put up a building. I have done carpentry work in my own home and I have completely finished my basement.

Paul on high blood pressure

My blood pressure was elevated all the time so my doctor suggested I take a stress test; it showed that I indeed had some problems. I ended up having a catheterization and they found some blockages in my heart.

Having had 28 years of experience in the pharmaceutical field, and having heard of chelating agents, I started inquiring about them. Dr. Scarchilli was recommended to me by my family physician. He took tests prior to my treatment and there were several things that were wrong other than blockages in the heart. He put me on a program of chelation therapy and diet and exercise. I rode an exercise bike all winter long, 45 minutes each night, while doing some weight-lifting exercise and maintaining a very rigid diet.

I have made progress. I notice my memory has improved. I do power walking now at the doctor's suggestion and I can walk one and four tenths of a mile in 18 minutes. I take my pulse immediately afterwards and it is 88. That is excellent and indicates that my blood flow and overall physical condition is good. I have stopped using my heart medications almost altogether. I carry them with me just in case I need them, but I'm going to stop carrying them pretty soon because I feel a whole lot better.

Ziegfried on blocked arteries

I had a massive heart attack that left me in the hospital for months. One artery was 100 percent blocked and the other two were 60 percent and 40 percent blocked. Of course, the doctors recommended a bypass operation, which I was not very keen on doing. I thought I would try other possibilities, with chelation being at the top of the list.

Since that time I started taking chelation therapy and am now on my 23rd treatment. As a result I feel a lot better and I have increased my walking ability. When I first started I couldn't even walk 100 yards without getting chest pains. Now I can walk three to four miles every morning.

I changed to a completely vegetarian diet and cut out all my fat intake. It took a little getting used to but after three to four weeks I was able to adjust. I have lost 42 pounds in the last three months just from changing my diet.

Leo on blocked arteries

Approximately two years ago, I was suffering from dizzy spells, which at times were just unbearable. I went to see a few physicians who couldn't find out the cause of my trouble. Finally, one suggested that I go to a vascular surgeon and I did. He gave me a thorough examination with all his technology and equipment and then told me that my condition was very discouraging, as one carotid artery was 100 percent blocked and the other was blocked 75 percent. He said my condition was inoperable and that I would have to wait for the inevitable to happen. That was in February 1990.

I then heard of chelation therapy through a friend of the family who gave me the name of Dr. Dan Roehm in Florida. I have since received between 75 and 80 treatments, and as of March 1991 the results have been remarkable. My right carotid artery has gone from 100 percent to 83 percent blocked and the left one has gone from 75 percent to between 44 and 48 percent blocked.

All in all, I have found that this has done me a world of good, as I am able to get around and do my work. I can highly recommend the treatment to anyone in the same position as myself. I am 85 years old and feel that chelation therapy has added quality to my life. In fact, I feel I would be dead today without it because they couldn't operate on me and I was going downhill at the time.

Steve on heart attacks

I had a couple of heart attacks about six or seven years ago and I pulled through those in fair condition. Then I had a bad one where I had an infarct and I checked into a hospital with that. After that I couldn't walk too far or do too much work because I would get angina and a heavy chest.

I accidentally heard about Dr. Schachter on the radio. I went to see him and after several chelation treatments, I began to feel a lot better. It took a little time, but after a couple of years, I could reduce the treatments from two a week to one a week, to once a month.

Now I am feeling fine and can do a lot of work around the yard. I do gardening, I walk better, and I don't have the angina the way I used to have it. I used to walk half a block and take nitroglycerin. Now, I'm doing pretty well on the supplements that they instructed me to take plus the treatment. I recommend chelation highly to anyone with a problem of the vascular system.

Charles on angina and arthritis

In 1984, I was diagnosed as requiring a quadruple bypass. My left ventricle was 85 percent blocked and the rest of my body wasn't too good either.

I was barely able to walk when I started out. Now I am 71 and can walk two miles without any great sweat. Also, I can exercise for 45 minutes or more every day, and I do. I also found that what little arthritis I had left me and I am free from pain. I hardly ever have any angina now.

I have had over 80 treatments by now and I still continue maintenance treatments once a month. I would say that chelation, coupled with exercise and supplements and keeping control of your diet, is pretty much the path to success.

Mrs. K on strokes

Two years ago, at the age of 70, my husband had many strokes which affected his mental capacity. He couldn't remember things and was having difficulty in general.

We took him to our local doctor, who gave him an MRI test and sent him to a neurologist. The outcome was that they decided he had atherosclerosis. When I asked what could be done for that, he said there was really nothing except medication for high blood pressure. We had him on five pills a day until one day I decided that perhaps, since both my husband's parents had lived well into their 90's and had been well and sharp, I should try to do some research to see what I could do with diet and other means.

A year ago last May I found a book on chelation in the library and read about what it could do for the brain. I called medical establishments in Nassau County but they gave me no information on it at all. They thought I was talking a foreign language. Then I found out about Dr. Yurkovsky through a friend and we went to see him.

My husband has had about 40 half treatments and I have seen major improvements in his condition. On a scale of one to ten we have gone from about three to eight, and that makes life much more comfortable.

Florence on blocked carotid artery

My problem was a clogged carotid and I think that chelation therapy saved me from having a stroke. I went for chelation after the Mayo Clinic wanted to put me on Valium for the change of life. I asked the doctor there what tests they took to show I had a Valium deficiency and we were downhill all the way from that point.

My husband had severe rheumatoid arthritis and after five treatments he improved tremendously. We had no idea this would do anything for arthritis. He also started to go for treatments after the Mayo Clinic told him to take 15 aspirins a day and that he would be in a wheelchair in six months to a year. Since the treatments, he has worked 11 years without missing a day. . . .

I can't praise this enough and I just can't believe that the doctors and insurance companies are not allowing this to be spread and accepted.

Mitch on heart disease

I started chelation therapy in March 1987 after having had three open heart surgeries from 1975 to 1987. In all, I have had a total of 11 bypass operations. In March 1987, I went to my cardiologist and he told me to have a heart transplant. I would not hear of it and he just said that I should go home and get my affairs in order.

I heard about chelation therapy from Dr. McDonagh's book *Chelation Can Cure* and got an appointment the day after talking to my cardiologist. By the way, I am 54 years old and was 50 at the time. I had my first heart attack at 36. By the time I got to Dr. McDonagh's office I was taking 29 heart pills a day and my total bill for medication was $394 a month.

In January 1988, Dr. McDonagh began taking me gradually off all my heart pills. Since that time, I have had 100 chelation sessions; I no longer take even one heart pill, and I have never been in the hospital. I work between 12 and 15 hours a day and I travel over 80,000 miles a year making my own deliveries. I do carry nitros but I do not use them. I go back to Dr. McDonagh three times a year for maintenance and I take three bottles every time I go back. I never get a cold or flu or anything like that.

Ed on arteriosclerosis

I started with Dr. McDonagh in 1978. Previously, I had a history of severe leg itching where I would scratch my leg so much that it would sometimes bleed. And I would get out of breath from walking 15 minutes or longer.

I finally decided to do something to help my body so I made an appointment with a well-known physician in Kansas City and had a physical. He diagnosed me as having hardening of the arteries and said that I was 50 to 60 percent blocked. After some tests, he recommended that I have bypass surgery.

I gave it some thought and decided it would be better to get a second opinion so I went to another well-known cardiologist who likewise diagnosed my condition as being 50 to 60 percent blocked in the left femoral artery. He suggested immediate bypass surgery as well. A third opinion was the same.

I decided instead to try chelation therapy. That was in December of 1978 and since that time I have had about 60 chelation treatments. As a result I have never in my life felt better.

Chiropractic

Chiropractic is one of the most important and universally available therapies. It is based on the principle that there is an innate wisdom in the body, which promotes health and healing. Chiropractic's founder and developer, B. J. Palmar, describes it this way: "The master maker of the human body did not create you and then run off and leave you masterless. He stayed on the job as the fellow within, as nerve transmission, controlling every function of life."

The goal of the chiropractor is to unblock energy so that inner intelligence can work better. This is done by determining the state of the musculoskeletal and nervous systems. Then, physical imbalances are corrected by manipulating the spinal column to correct partial dislocations known as subluxations. These adjustments allow the brain's messages to flow freely down the entire spinal cord. This, in turn, can promote self-healing of numerous afflictions.

There are approximately 20 different chiropractic techniques. Chiropractors try to fit the technique to the patient's needs. Some chiropractors integrate nutrition and lifestyle counseling into their therapy. Accounting for individual needs and combining various approaches makes chiropractic an excellent form of preventive care.

Though this modality is widely accepted today, this was not always the case. For decades, chiropractic care was maligned by the orthodox medical community. In its darkest hour, the American Medical Association made a concerted effort to completely eliminate the profession, and employed over 70 people full-time for this sole purpose. Fortunately, they were found guilty of violating the Sherman Antitrust Act, and chiropractic survived.

Today the specialty not only survives, it thrives. Chiropractic is widely accepted as a legitimate science and is the largest alternative healing profession in America. Chiropractors are highly trained professionals. Several years of premedical training followed by specialized education results in a D.C. (Doctor of Chiropractic) degree.

Patient Stories

Ben on psoriasis

I had a severe case of psoriasis. In addition, I had headaches and stomach pains of unknown etiology. Allopathic doctors tried all kinds of medications but were not able to help me. It was so bad that I almost committed suicide.

I went to see a chiropractor who helped educate me about nutrition, exercise, and stress management. I was worried and upset about my problem and what I learned helped me to calm down. Little by little I have been able to overcome my problems. Recently, at the age of 47, I was able to run the New York City marathon.

Now my psoriasis is under control. It's not gone yet but it is much better than it was. My stomach pains and headaches have disappeared. I feel like a new person and feel like I belong here once again.

I believe my success is due to the fact that chiropractic medicine specifically and holistic medicine in general helps. Chiropractic care works with you and doesn't cause problems.

Elaine on ear infections

When my son, Alexander, complains of pain in his ear, our chiropractor, Gary, adjusts him. Sometimes the earache leaves immediately; other times, it takes a couple of adjustments but he always helps to break down the congestion that causes the inflammation.

I'm certain this is not a placebo effect because you cannot trick children. I've witnessed Alexander getting onto the table with a lot of pain and getting off with none.

Fernando on overcoming physical handicaps

Ever since I was a teenager, I have suffered with lower back pain and a knee problem. For 20 years, I was convinced that I had a physical handicap and that I would have to live with my condition for the rest of my life. Thinking this way rationalized my avoidance of physical activities.

Three years ago, I met a podiatrist who began to educate me about my physical weaknesses. I started to learn about my body structure and how I did not have to suffer or avoid physical activities. I also learned that I had a misaligned right hip and that I would have to seek chiropractic care.

At first, I was skeptical. I'm the type of person who needs proof that something will work. Actually, I was looking for someone to tell me that I needed an operation or medicine. Luckily, I met people who recommended holistic care.

Out of curiosity, I went to a chiropractor. At first, I didn't feel any benefit.

After a few months of treatment, I started to lose interest because I didn't think that this was going to work.

Then one day, I went to see him with a really bad stiff neck. This was a turning point for me because he was able to help me. In a matter of hours, I was feeling great. In the past, I had suffered from stiff necks that ruined my days and weekends.

This was proof for me that chiropractic care works. Because of that, I decided to continue treatments, hoping that one day I would feel the same effects on my lower back. I decided to give it about two years or so.

At the same time, I was seeking help from the podiatrist and changing my diet. My chiropractor helped me to improve my nutrition. I was actually knocking down a lot of old walls that kept me from being physically active for so long. I started running for exercise.

One day, I realized that I was running better and longer. I was becoming a marathon runner and decided to run the 1994 marathon. Being able to prepare for and race in the marathon is what ultimately convinced me that chiropractic care works. Before treatments, I never thought I would be able to run 20 miles in my training. I kept my appointments when it got close to the race and stayed with the treatments.

Finally, the day arrived when I was lined up with some of the best runners in the world because I pushed my way to the front of the line. Here I was waiting for a 26-mile race to begin. What's interesting is my chiropractor is also a marathon runner so he understands what I was going through. The support he gave me was great. He even gave me a final adjustment before the gun went off. This was a blessing for me which left me fully prepared to race and helped me finish the race. At the 25th mile, my knee gave me a little problem, which just showed me that I needed to do more work.

I definitely attribute [my success to] a program that includes chiropractic care. This treatment helped me to break through the old walls that I had built around my life and allowed me to let out the spirit of a runner.

Bill on headaches and a liver disorder

Over the years, I was in a lot of car accidents. The worst one was in 1978. As a result, I lived with severe headaches for a number of years, up to four times a day. Sometimes I would scream at the top of my lungs. The pain was so severe that at times I became suicidal.

At first I went to orthopedists and neurologists who gave me a bunch of pills that just worked for short amounts of time. Then, luckily, through a friend, I found chiropractic and I have been getting better. I haven't had a bad headache in seven months. All liver problems have subsided. The tests have shown the improvement. I feel chiropractic care has saved my life.

Besides chiropractic care I actively take care of my health in other ways. I exercise and have become a vegetarian. I also seek out homeopathic care when I need it.

Alma on skin problems

I never believed in holistic medicine until a friend of mine referred me to a holistic doctor back in 1989. One of the most serious problems I had throughout my life was a dermatological problem where my scalp would break out in sores and scabs. I spent thousands of dollars seeking help. As a child, my mother did the same. All the treatments ever did was make my head greasy. They never healed the problem. After just three sessions with my chiropractor, the sores went away. I never had to use anything on my scalp. I have stopped seeing a dermatologist for my scalp because there is no need to see him. Three adjustments took care of the problem, which turned out to be allergy-related.

Then, in June 1991, I was caught in an armed robbery on the job. The robbers really did a number on me. My chiropractor is now treating me for herniated disks in my neck and lower back. I also have other medical problems. He treats me for high blood pressure and for allergies. Treatments relieve me of stress. I see him on the average of three to four times per week. He is wonderful and has convinced me that holistic medicine really works.

Donna on complications during pregnancy

Initially, when I found out that I was pregnant, I had gotten very bad sciatica. My leg was drawn up; I couldn't put it down. I went to my chiropractor for a couple of visits. I still was uncomfortable but I was able to walk around and get around.

He also helped me during my pregnancy with carpal tunnel syndrome. Initially, I was told by my medical doctor to get surgery on my neck to see if it was coming from the neck. Then they would check the elbow.

Overall, it helped improve my well-being during my pregnancy. It helped everything move and go much better. I had a 100 percent wonderful pregnancy. Now, I'm on my second pregnancy and at this point I am really doing fantastic—a little uncomfortable here and there but I keep getting adjusted and I'm doing great.

Sherry on neck and back pain

I suffered for many years and was on all kinds of medication. When it got to the point that medication didn't help anymore, and they wanted to put me in traction, a friend suggested that I see a chiropractor. Not knowing too much about them, I wasn't that willing to go but I spoke to the doctor on the phone. He said he couldn't guarantee that I would run out of his office but he could guarantee that I would walk.

I went and it certainly helped. I'm off medication. I have arthritis in the neck and it's quite painful. When it gets bad, I start my treatments again and it helps so much. I couldn't bear being without a chiropractor.

Before getting treatment, I never believed that chiropractors could be this helpful. You could have never convinced me because it's not something that's talked about. A doctor tells you to take pills to feel better. Of course, you do these things because a doctor tells you to. But when I went to the chiropractor I soon learned that I did not need these pills. All the pills did was upset my stomach. As soon as the medication wore off the pain was back again. With chiropractic treatment, you do get helped and the pain stays away.

Eileen on Bell's palsy

Last year I began to have seizure-like symptoms. I had an MRI done because I had what appeared to be Bell's palsy on the right side of my face and I tended to walk to my left side. The hospital found nothing wrong and said it was Bell's palsy. That was the end of it.

The episodes continued. I finally sought the care of a holistic doctor who gave me some supplementation. The episodes didn't completely go away so he referred me to a homeopathic doctor who referred me to a chiropractor. I was a little skeptical in the beginning about going, but willing to try anything. The doctor did some adjustments on me and amazingly I didn't have any more episodes. When I stopped going, the episodes began again. I went back to him and after my adjustment the episodes dissipated. Thus far, they have not returned. I am very grateful that I don't have them because they're a little on the scary side. I think holistically between the chiropractic work and a combination of a lot of other modalities, I have been helped a lot.

Pat on knee pain and sciatica

About a year ago, I was actively exercising and taking dance classes about three or four times a week. Unfortunately, I injured myself in class. The injury resulted in pain and numbness in my leg. I had difficulty walking, going up and down stairs and driving. Also, I felt that the strength in my legs was gone. If I tried to run, it felt as if my legs would give out underneath me.

At this point, I went to see several doctors. I was in an HMO at the time. The doctors tested me but couldn't find anything wrong. A neurologist ordered a couple of very painful tests. Basically, I was given electric shock for about 45 minutes on and off. Also, a needle was inserted into my leg and I was told to flex my muscle. The test came back normal and they could draw no conclusions from them. Basically, all they did was put me on Motrin for some time. I found it not to be helpful and discontinued that.

In the meantime, from about June to September, I found that the traumatic part of my injury got better. I could function okay but I wasn't back to my normal self. From about October to April, my leg was achy on and off. I also had numbness on and off. I was not exercising.

Finally, in the spring, someone suggested that I see a chiropractor. I went to a chiropractor who suspected that I had sciatica. The improvement I saw over those six weeks was significant whereas the six months prior to that did not show any major change. He said I should visit twice a week for four to six weeks. During that time, I noticed subtle but significant differences in my leg. I also started exercising very, very gradually. At this point, I am doing a lot more exercise.

There were a couple of other positive side effects which I did not expect. I noticed immediately after the first visit that I had a lot more mobility in my neck from side to side. After adjustments, I could also feel energy flow throughout my whole body. Overall, I have had a very positive experience with chiropractic.

Suzanne on knee, hip, and neck pain, and hormonal imbalance

I'm a runner. Last March, I had to stop running due to pain in my right knee and right hip. My neck had been giving me problems for some time as well. The movement in my neck was more and more constricted. It felt like it was constantly misaligned. I heard about Dr. Gary Deutchman through the running club. I saw him giving other runners ankle and knee adjustments. I was very impressed so I started to see him last March. He suggested a program for me to correct the curvature in my neck and inquired about my overall health.

I take very good care of myself regarding diet and exercise and the taking of supplements. I also have an excellent physician who has helped me a lot. Still, I had a low thyroid condition for about two years that I had been unable to correct and very, very painful menstrual periods practically my whole life.

Dr. Deutchman suggested I take an herb called wild yam to help balance my diet's hormone systems. He also gave me special adjustments for the menstrual pain.

Last month, for the first time in my life, I had no menstrual pain. I saw my regular physician last week and he told me that my thyroid condition was normal for the first time. This is a remarkable, major change for me. I have more energy and I've lost some weight. My complexion is better and people are commenting on the way I look. Gradually, I've been able to run again, little by little, with no pain. Now, I'm in training for the New York City marathon. This weekend I did my first race since my injury in March and set a personal record. I'm very pleased about all these changes. I feel the adjustments have helped my body to correct and heal itself.

Ann on torn cartilage

About three years ago, I tore the cartilage in my knee. Several surgeons suggested that I have surgery. I heard about Dr. Robbins and consulted with him. He said that surgery should be the last alternative and that we should try other things first.

First, I tried placing an orthotic device in my sneakers. That worked fine. The only problem was that I became a little overconfident and twisted a knee in my aerobics class.

When I went back to Dr. Robbins, he suggested that I go for chiropractic treatments with Dr. Proffman because my knee was locking three or four times a day.

I liked that Dr. Proffman explained the chiropractic treatment. He analyzed my posture and my walking, and told me that I was out of alignment, and trying to compensate for the pain. He adjusted my back and that seemed to help. That first weekend was very active. It wasn't until Sunday evening that I realized, not once did my knee lock. From then on, I was sold on the chiropractic treatment.

I have been going to Dr. Proffman twice a week, and I have had no problems with my knee. I feel it saved me from surgery. I feel much more energetic now that I am in alignment.

Dorothy on pain and general health and wellness

I began chiropractic care late last year with a desire to improve my overall health, but also for specific discomfort in my neck, lower back, and hip.

I feel that chiropractic treatment has significantly lessened the frequency of the pain I was experiencing. It specifically improved the strength of my arms and legs by relieving the interference on my nerves. I feel that it has improved my energy level as well. I racewalk for exercise and find that the chiropractic adjustments help my ankles and hips when they feel strained or out of position.

Chiropractic care has also helped me to increase my awareness of my body. I find that I am more diligent about attending to stress or injury. I pay more attention to my posture and to my position while sleeping.

I find the entire approach to healing helpful. The lifestyle recommendations, the atmosphere of the office, everything about it has made me very happy.

Some time ago, I had a few chiropractic adjustments with a different health practitioner and it was not the same experience at all. The other individual's approach was to use only chiropractic. He treated me for one subluxation in my lower back area, and that was the extent of the treatment. There were no discussions of lifestyle, nutrition, or stress. It was just more of a mechanical adjustment rather than a holistic approach.

Elise on headaches

I have been seeing a chiropractor for about two years now. I started going because I was experiencing daily tension headaches. The conventional route didn't appeal to me because I had the feeling that my headaches would be treated with medication.

The results were not immediate. I would like to emphasize that because many times people think a treatment is going to work like magic. After a while, there was a significant decrease in the number of headaches that I was experiencing. Before I began the adjustments, I had a headache every day. After two months, I could go for seven or eight days without a headache. This was a new and wonderful experience for me.

At the same time, I started examining my diet. I worked with my doctor to see if some of the headaches were caused by food allergies. The change in my diet, which was a gradual elimination of meat, dairy, sugar, and salt, contributed to a further decrease in headaches.

My son, who is three, started this journey with me, two years ago. He gets adjusted right along with me. As a result he is very, very healthy. I believe that the combination of our weekly adjustments and good diet has contributed to my headaches going away and to the good health of my son.

Maji on degenerative arthritis and sciatica

I became a disabled Vietnam Veteran after receiving an overdose of Thorazine for a nervous breakdown after the war. I was very toxic and later developed painful arthritis. I started to use medication to relieve the pain, thinking that this was the only alternative. I believed that arthritis was a totally irreversible, terminal condition. Every medication I was given for pain gradually wore off and left me with more pain.

I thought I was headed for the wheelchair because I had sciatica as well. I even bought a ground floor apartment so that I could have wheelchair access. I was using a cane for four years and reached a point where I could not go up stairs at all. I had to quit a job in real estate which required stair climbing. Two months ago, I started going to a chiropractor on the recommendation of a friend. I was skeptical but desperate. When I first met the doctor, he told me that the adjustments would release subluxations. As a result, nerve energy would flow more freely and my health would improve. At the time, I had several subluxations. All my joints were affected. It was up and down my spine, especially in my neck and low back.

After my first adjustment, I went to a restaurant to have lunch. When it was quiet, I was aware of a tremendous feeling of activity in my neck. It was as if a little river was flowing through it. I realized that it must be the nerve energy my doctor had talked about. When I saw him again, I asked about it and he confirmed my thoughts. He said my neck was really subluxated and that the treatment released nerve energy.

Now the healing process has taken hold and my body is running more efficiently. In two months, I've lost 10 pounds due to improved metabolism. I am also walking better. In fact, I'm fast-walking and climbing stairs a little bit. My knees feel stronger and no longer shaky. I can sleep well, whereas before I had insomnia. My headaches are gone.

I still experience some pain and realize that it is going to take a while to reverse a lot of my problems. The Thorazine overdose caused tardive dyskinesia and made one leg shorter than the other. Fortunately, this is beginning to release. My sciatica pain has been cut down to a third of what it was.

I am trying to get the Veterans Administration Hospital to introduce chiropractic into their program as part of their physical therapy. I have met a lot of vets in my physical therapy program at the VA who could really use it. When I was in physical therapy, the difference from before my chiropractic and physical therapy and after was really noticeable. My therapist at the VA even noted that I was a lot stronger.

Before chiropractic care, I was using the yellow theraband, a stretch band that exercises the muscles. The yellow is the weakest and the blue is next to the heaviest. I went from the yellow to blue in two days after my first adjustment.

I'm very grateful for chiropractic and would advise anyone to try it to see if the treatment works for them.

Sonia on multiple sclerosis

It started about six years ago. I had extreme fatigue, nervousness, and panic attacks that escalated to the point where I couldn't leave my home. I saw many doctors who said that I was undergoing a lot of stress. They prescribed Valium.

My symptoms progressed; after a year, the doctors suggested that I see a psychiatrist. In my heart, I knew that there was something physically wrong with me. One day, I awoke with paralysis of my right eye. It was at that point that I knew that there was something wrong.

I saw a neurologist, and he suggested that I have an MRI. This revealed that I had the beginning stages of multiple sclerosis. My doctor told me that there was no cure for multiple sclerosis. There was nothing that he could do. My husband and I left the office feeling very upset. In our hearts, we knew that there had to be something that we could do. My husband was listening to the radio, and came across a program one afternoon. He became encouraged by what he heard when he realized that there was some things that we could do. He heard of a Dr. Schwank, who did a lot of research in multiple sclerosis. We decided to go to the library and take out every book that we could find on multiple sclerosis. We started to apply some of the protocols that were in the books, and we realized that these alternative treatments were really helping.

We saw a homeopathic doctor who was also a chiropractor. Those were two methods that we were going to concentrate on. We found a chiropractor who spent a lot of time with me. He suggested that I eat organic foods, that I go on a detox program, that I have regular and strengthening exercises, and also a stress management class. . . .

After trying his protocol, I saw a remarkable difference in my health. I became stronger; I had no more fatigue; I was able to leave my home and go back to work. I had no more limitations. The doctors told me that I would get progressively worse and probably wind up in a wheelchair. But as a result of his treatments, I'm able to continue in my profession as a physical education teacher working with special education children. I have no limitations and was even able to have a child a year and a half ago, which the doctors told me I would never have. I feel completely excellent as far as my health goes.

Mary on osteoarthritis

I have had a bad back since I was 29 years old. Over the years I saw many orthopedic doctors who only prescribed drug therapy to deaden the pain.

One day, I decided to see a chiropractic doctor. In addition to the adjustments, he gave me vitamin supplements, and showed me how to change my diet and exercise habits. Now I take lots of vitamins. I eat lots of green vegetables, lots of fruits, and no red meat. I drink lots of water, up to eight glasses a day. My exercise includes walking and playing tennis.

This has helped immensely. Now my pain is gone. I am able to sit, whereas before I was never able to sit without very bad pain. Now I can sit and watch TV, and I can sit to knit and sew. For those who do not believe that they can reverse arthritis naturally, I am here to say that after 40 years, you can. I am living proof. Now I can play tennis without the pain.

Robert on osteoarthritis

I was experiencing stiffness in my shoulder, lower back, and hip area. After I had x-rays taken by a chiropractor, I learned that I had arthritis. I received chiropractic treatments and started eating more fruits, vegetables, vitamins, and juices. I take magnesium, potassium, vitamin E, garlic, a lot of herbs, echinacea, shark cartilage, bovine cartilage, and chondroital sulfate. I have stopped eating a lot of red meat and a lot of dairy. And I exercise more.

All this has given me a tremendous surge of energy. I don't have stiffness anymore. In damp weather I used to have quite a few cramps as well as cracking and popping of the bones. But I don't experience that anymore.

Chiropractic care, a vegetarian diet, and the other changes have made quite a big difference. I'm glad I started listening to people who said that chiropractic worked. That's something that I will continue to do for the remainder of my days on earth.

Barbara on osteoarthritis

I'm no stranger to chiropractic. I've been using it for 20 or 22 years, but I always used it for a crisis because I had an extremely bad back. Later I learned that I had arthritis. I finally decided to use chiropractic regularly as a preventive measure. I just decided, "Let me go see if this is going to make a difference." And it's made a tremendous difference in just weeks.

Before, I couldn't walk two blocks without pain. I would have to stop and sit down. I would stay home because walking was too uncomfortable. And I was really upset because I went from being 5'10" to 5'4½". I was startled by how much I lost in height. I knew some of it came from aging but that some of it had to do with accommodating for my pain.

Chiropractic has given me back some of my posture. Now I'm 5'7½". I don't expect to regain my full height from when I had no arthritis and was far younger, but I'm hopeful that I will feel far better. The pain is diminished. It's wonderful to be able to lean over quickly. The difference is quite stunning. People I know have commented on the change these past weeks. One neighbor chased me down the street, saying, "I almost didn't know that was you. I didn't realize you were so tall." That's no kidding.

Colon Therapy

Colon cleansing is an ancient and time-honored health practice, initially used by the Egyptians and the Essenes thousands of years ago, and later recommended by Hippocrates, the father of modern medicine. It works on the principle that disease starts in the colon, since most foods, drugs, and other chemicals that do not leave the body are stored there. At first, there are few or no symptoms, but after years of putrefaction, subclinical signs graduate to disease status. This is because several pounds of fecal material laden with millions of bacteria can attach itself to the colon walls. This toxic waste can generate all kinds of havoc with the system. By cleansing the large intestine, colon therapy restores the organ to its natural size, shape, and correct function, thus preventing disease.

During treatment, water is gently infused into the large bowel so that it is thoroughly washed. This allows old encrustations and fecal material to loosen, dislodge, and be swept away. As body pollution is eliminated, many conditions are alleviated, including severe skin disorders, breathing difficulties, constipation, depression, chronic fatigue, nervousness, flatulence, bloating, and arthritis. As people become physically unstuck, they become emotionally lighter, freer, and better able to express their feelings. Colonics provide great relief, especially when accompanied by dietary changes.

A qualified colon therapist uses pure water that is administered at body temperature and a sterilizing device known as an autoclave. The person knows reflexology, as massaging points on the body that relate to the colon enhance the therapy. The practitioner should also test the ileocecal valve, the small valve between the small and large intestines, using kinesiology. If this is jammed open or closed, the therapist can correct it, which will make the session more comfortable.

Patient Stories

Edwina on aging

This is something that I believe in very strongly and have had really good results with. It's wonderful for the skin as well as the colon and all the organs. It also is good for cellulite because oftentimes cellulite is just an accumulation of toxins. So you see, this really works in a multitude of ways.

I found someone who is really quite good through an advertisement. The name of his company is Nature's Path. He's extremely clean and very, very thorough, and not rushing people is really important. It's important to have a full treatment, which could be up to 45 minutes for the average client.

All it really is is water going into the colon and water going out. And of course, when water goes out, waste also goes with it. It's important to do, even if you are going to the bathroom; you can be going two to three times a day, but your body still might not be cleansing properly. . . . Even if a person has a really good balanced diet, there are certain stresses involved that can take away from a full cleansing process.

Not only did it help my body, I felt that my mind also was clearer and more focused. I felt happier and lighter, not just physically, but also mentally. It's wonderful. I would call it the fountain of youth and the greatest thing known to man.

Jill on allergies

I was feeling quite miserable. Then I was lucky enough to find the treatment I'm presently in. In just two days, I'm already feeling a thousand percent better in that my stomach is not distended, gas is eliminated, and my runny nose is gone. I'm no longer walking around with tissues in hand. This treatment is pretty new to me and I was a little apprehensive, but I'm a believer right now.

Once I'm finished with this treatment, my allergies should be gone if I change my eating habits. I am really trying to learn how to eat healthier to avoid this problem again. I may always have this problem, but at least I will be able to avoid the severity of symptoms that I have been feeling up until now.

Dorothy on diverticulitis

Prior to colonics, I tried laxatives and other drugs. Nothing seemed to work. There was no real bowel movement. It was all building up inside of me and I was constantly bloated. It was very discomforting.

Then I got my first colonic. I was a little leery but I was anxious to get it because I figured it would work. And it worked. After all this time.

I only had two treatments and I only took about a quart of water each time.

I couldn't hold more. But I had a bowel movement each day for the last month and four days, a total of 60 inches throughout the day, heavy. Unbelievable.

In addition to the colonic, I was taking bentonite and psyllium. I was told to avoid half and half and carbonated drinks and processed foods. By eliminating all of that, I've really improved and feel like a million dollars now. I am 76 years old and feel like 36.

Linda on eczema

I had a really severe case on my hands and feet. I went from doctor to doctor, trying to clear it up, but was really never successful at it. This winter, when I was in Florida, I showed it to my brother who had been doing colonics for the last ten years. He said, "Your body is toxic. You've got to get to a colonic therapist and have this procedure done." I wasn't really thrilled about doing it, but he's a wise person and I listened to him. I also had no energy and was not able to lose weight. I kept gaining weight even though I was exercising my brains out.

Well, I went through a colonic series. I had 15 done. I have lost 20 pounds and my eczema is almost totally cleared up. I have energy again. I think this is one of the best things that I have ever done for my health.

Jerry on congenital conditions

I was born with twisted intestines. In my early days, I was deathly ill. Even getting up in the morning was painful, and my mother had to put drops in my eyes to get them to open due to the toxins forming all night long. I could not physically open them until the drops were put in.

Ultimately I became a naturopathic physician. And I can let people know that good health is achievable but that it just doesn't happen overnight. Part of my early studies included being sent by Dr. Bernard Jensen to a clinic outside of Guadalajara, Mexico, up in the mountains. There I learned not only proper eating methods, but the cleansing principles of using colonics and enemas and so forth. I learned what to mix in there to help break up the impacted matter, as well as have proper elimination.

Interestingly, they had their own version of a colonic board. Everything was made out of marble because marble in Mexico is very inexpensive. They had a large table that a patient would lay upon to have a tube inserted. The tube came down from a marble 5-gallon holding tank with the turnstile for the water down at the base. Patients could virtually turn on the water themselves, fill the bucket, and go through the process. Everything was easy to clean therefore. It was a remarkable idea.

I got used to the use of this kind of method instead of the normal small enema, which is a bit uncomfortable, and eventually was able to correct my condition, in spite of the many impactions and surgeries that I had at a much earlier age. To this day, if I am fairly careful, I have no major problems with my digestive system anymore. I'm much older now but it has held up very well for all these years.

I would like to tell people that anything less than two or three bowel movements a day is not normal. Even once a day is holding too much waste material and can become very dangerous. To those of you who are getting on in years, I would like to say from my own experience, that the use of an enema or colonic once a week, whether needed or not, can be a very good insurance policy.

I have a colonic board at home with a 5-gallon bucket. I add in a chlorophyll and comfrey mixture, as well as some red clover and a tablespoon of an electrolyte solution to help maintain the electrolyte balance of the soft tissue, as well as restore the peristaltic action of the bowel muscle. I try doing this every Sunday afternoon or Saturday evening, and I find this clears out dangerous waste matter from the week before.

I think it is absolutely critical to do upon return from a trip. Taking an enema or colonic immediately will remove all that excess waste matter. I have known of a number of cases of people who return from trips to Europe, who come back with very poor bowel habits. Within a month many of them develop a heart attack and pass on. I find that totally unnecessary. You can take an enema with you, perhaps some herbal laxatives, and get one, upon returning. If you don't want to set up an enema at home, by all means, make an appointment with a colonic expert, and get your digestive system cleaned out. This is critical in today's world with all the additional chemicals, pesticides, and toxic material that can accumulate in your system.

An interesting article from the old *Saturday Evening Post* of April 1982, was titled "Constipation and Breast Cancer." The authors pointed out that women who only have several bowel movements a week have at least a four times higher risk of breast cancer than women who have at least one bowel movement a day.

Regarding the bowel problem itself, one of the important things I learned down at the clinic outside of Guadalajara are that modern toilets are a nemesis in that the bowel was meant to be in a squeezable position so to speak, as we squatted to the ground for hundreds of thousands of years if not millions of years as an upright human. That allows for a total elimination. I remember that as a child being sickly and sent to the farm and not wanting to use the outhouse that much. I used to go in the field very often, and when I went in the field, I did feel better and was healthier. So we recommended in the clinic, in Guadalajara, the use of a footstool to raise the level of the feet for more of a critical v-shape for the bowel track.

The only other nation I know of [besides the U.S.] that is so far behind with digestion and bowel constipation is England, which has a highly refined diet. It is also known that during World War II, when England could not get processed foods shipped to it, they increased the amount of fiber in the diet by grinding grains less, and there was very little sugar or other refined products available. The incidence of heart disease and cancer dropped rapidly. It's ironic, but right after World War II, disease figures went up tremendously.

The use of the enema, in the evening particularly, before going to bed on a full stomach, I think is very important for those who have not moved their bowels that day. Statistics show that most heart attacks occur late at night or early in the morning. And a number of naturopathic physicians, myself included, feel that the end digestion food turns into a toxic gaseous substance, which produces quite a strain on the heart, to make a long story short. Statistics show that a large incidence of massive heart attacks occur late at night or early in the morning, which are usually fatal.

In order to get that peristaltic action back in the bowel muscle, we were taught to give patients flaxseed and/or flaxseed oil every day, as well as psyllium seed. Flaxseed serves two purposes. One is as a fiber and a second is as a lubricant. For bowel health, it is probably one of the least expensive and best ways of keeping things moving along.

Ann on breast cancer

I was diagnosed with breast cancer, two years ago. I knew that my problem was that I didn't go to the bathroom often enough. Throughout my whole life, I only went twice a week. I was told by many, many doctors that that was normal for me because I had a nervous stomach. And unfortunately, I accepted that.

When I look back now, I realize that I had food allergies all my life. That stopped me from ever being normal in the bathroom.

This year, I decided to really attack it. Things were getting better and better over the last few years and I wanted to do colonics. I found someone here in New York and had a series of 15 colonics.

It really made a difference for me. Now I go to the bathroom six to eight times a day. I have a complete emptying feeling. . . . And I feel great.

Charlotte on heart attack

I had a heart attack and I was six blocks from the hospital so I survived it. Two weeks later I was home, again six blocks from the hospital, when I developed a hole in my heart, they tell me, and I got there just in time to have emergency open heart surgery, which they didn't think I'd survive.

It's been about three years of recovery, which I never would have made without . . . colonics. Since that time, I've probably had over 100 colonics and herbal cleansing. And I'm an entirely different person. In fact, the doctors want to know what my secret is. They just can't believe that I've survived these particular situations.

Last year, I was back in the hospital with right-sided heart failure because after having a piece taken out of my heart on the left side, the right side was trying to compensate. The fluid backed up like any plumbing problem. Eventually, it was pumped out of me. . . . This could not be done naturally. I lost 65 pounds of fluid in 16 days. It was the colonics in the end that saved me.

The material that came out of the colon has been photographed. It was remarkably awful. It was black, tar, putrid-looking material. At one point, I had terrible pain in my left side, near the place where I had the surgery. And I always used to say to doctors before and after the surgery, if you could fix this terrible pain, I'd be very thankful. During a colonic, the hygienist was massaging that area and the final debris came out of it. Then that pain was gone forever. So there you are.

Charlotte's son, Matthew, on mother's heart attack

It was just interesting in that if you picture the letter "U" and you picture the top of each side as being good health and the bottom as death, I basically saw mom deteriorate before me, going down the left side of the letter "U" and then having her heart attack in which they had to shock her and bring her back to life, and then build her up on the medications. She started going up the other side. But then she started getting the allergic reactions to the medications, and slowly sank back down to the bottom of the "U" again, or near death, it seemed.

That's when she started to get colonics. It was at that time that she got all that residue out of her system and started to assimilate good health. Then, instead of going back down to the bottom again, she was able to eclipse it and come across the top and work her way back up to the other side of the "U" and back to good health. It has been an amazing experience for me.

I have decided to get a head start, so I started colonics and began to change my eating habits.

Barbara on constipation

I was constipated my whole life and the doctors never thought that was a problem. I guess I was about 19 when I started working. I became lazy and stopped working out as much. I had a desk job and my health became affected. My fatigue started getting very, very intense. I became lethargic and started getting really run down. Then I got into that health craze as far as working out more and doing as much as I could, but I just wasn't getting any better. At that point I was running 18 miles a week. My weight kept going up and up and up. I got up to about 194. Nobody could figure it out. I went to doctor after doctor. I had a lot of female problems. I had no periods and was just a mess. No one ever said anything about the constipation.

I went on a Fit for Life health diet. It was a very healthy diet and was great for helping me to lose weight. But I never felt better. I never got my energy back. Then I was rushed to the hospital and my colon was totally impacted. Their solution didn't sound good.

My husband heard about colonics in the past so we went for a series. I was in my early 20's when I went in, and I felt that if I lived to be 35 it would be a miracle. The colon therapist would tell me to stick to the program and that I would be able to go on my own every day. I told her that I could never do that. The doctor said a lot of people are just naturally constipated. The hygienist said, "No, they just don't know how to tell you to get it to work right." I just stayed with it.

After a long period of time, I got my colon to start working on a daily basis. My female problems totally went away and all my energy returned. I started having regular periods. I can't imagine it's like that for everybody but it totally fixed that problem without me even realizing it was going to do it. It just was outstanding. To this day, I go in for maintenance just because I believe it gave me my life back.

Susan on chronic fatigue syndrome

I had pneumonia and afterwards I was so weak that I couldn't stand up. I had chronic fatigue for three months before I could even crawl. I went to a holistic doctor, who gave me supplements, IV vitamins, and nutritional advice. I was gradually getting back my strength and was able to go to work for an hour a day. By the time I went to Anita, I was working about three hours a day for five days a week. That was the maximum time I could actually work. I was sleeping 12 to 13 hours a night. I couldn't walk up a flight of stairs and I couldn't walk more than half a block without having to stop to catch my breath.

I asked my doctor if I should take enemas because I was constipated. I was going to the bathroom about once a week. He said he didn't believe in enemas and that I should take different powders instead. Meanwhile, I had been on a natural foods diet for 12 years and I didn't eat processed foods for years. But it didn't have any effect on the constipation. In my mind, I was thinking that I should get enemas even though the doctor said not to.

I heard about the Healing Center on Gary Null's shows. I thought I would go there and try it. I went over there for colon therapy, and after the first visit, I felt very, very good. Anita was wonderful and she made me feel relaxed. As soon as I walked out of the office, I felt great. I was able to work the rest of the day without fatigue. That night, I slept seven hours. After that, every single day,

I slept seven or eight hours, which was a tremendous difference from what I was going through before.

I have been to her nine times. Every visit made me feel even better. The chronic fatigue is gone. My energy is still not optimal, but I don't feel that terrible drained feeling that was dragging me down. The constipation is gradually starting to go away. I had acne my whole life, and that disappeared. My eyesight cleared up. I didn't think there was anything wrong with my eyes. According to my exams, it's 20/20. But after the first visit, I noticed that the colors looked bright and clear. I used to have menstrual cramps, and after my visits, I no longer feel any cramps. I have lost about 8 pounds. My appetite has changed. I used to crave sweets and caffeine, even though I tried desperately to stay away from it. But I would give in to sweets just to keep going. Now I have no desire for sweets at all.

Gary on lack of energy, constipation, and baldness

I didn't really have any pre-existing conditions that I was aware of at the time. I just went to the therapy to detoxify my body from things I had eaten over the years that I felt needed to be cleaned out of my system. I have been to Anita four times.

I have seen a lot of results already. I have more energy and less sluggishness. I don't need as much sleep. I used to need seven or eight hours, and now I need four or five hours and then generally, I'm fine. Then I used to have a noontime nod off, and I don't need that anymore. That was one of the conditions I wasn't aware of that the colonics corrected.

The other thing is I have more frequent bowel movements. I used to have one movement every two or three days. So, I was relatively constipated and didn't know it until after the treatments. It's also much quicker. It used to be a big ceremony type thing, 30 or 40 minutes at a time. I would have to take the magazine or newspaper. It almost became a reading library to try to get through. Now that situation is kind of cleared up.

The other thing I found interesting is that I feel my hair is starting to come back. I'm in my 30s right now. I have a small bump right above my left temple. That's been almost like a benchmark as to where my hair has been going. When I was in high school, that bump was completely covered with hair. When I went into college, it was right at the edge. And when I got out of college it started pushing further beyond. The past couple of weeks, I've noticed that the hairline has been starting to push forward. That bump is now starting to be covered with small fine hairs. I believe that is because the intestinal walls are free of debris so that the vitamins, minerals, chlorophyll, everything I've been taking in now has a greater effect to start maintaining my body where it should be. I think the hair growth is a part of it. I find it a little amazing.

Enzyme Therapy

Enzyme therapy may be the best-kept secret in medicine today. An enormous body of research credits enzymes in the prevention and treatment of a variety of conditions, including circulatory problems, cancer, premature aging, skin problems, damage from injury, digestive disorders, back pain, immune deficiencies, arthritis, bursitis, multiple sclerosis, and viruses, including herpes and HIV. Their wide range of effectiveness is due to the fact that enzymes are essential to all life processes. They work as catalysts. Without enzymes, there would be no cellular activity.

Critics of the therapy say that enzymes lose their potency after they are digested. But this is contradicted by studies showing that when enzymes are orally ingested, blood levels of enzymes increase remarkably. As we age, we need more enzymes. In fact, research shows enzymes to be a key factor in staying young.

We get enzymes from live foods, such as raw fruits and vegetables. Some people have difficulty breaking down food enzymes and need to take them in tablet form. The best mineral supplements are plant enzymes in crystalloid form with electrolytes. These penetrate cell walls, strengthen the body, and help the complete digestion process.

Patient Stories

Marianne on yeast infection

In 1990, I had exploratory surgery for endometriosis. Because I had previously been diagnosed with mitral-valve prolapse, it was suggested I take antibiotics for this surgery. Ten days following the surgery, I had a wicked yeast infection, which my doctor gave me vaginal medicine to help cure. Three months later, it recurred. Every month thereafter, just prior to my period, I would get an infection. I was experiencing such pain and discomfort, I didn't know who to turn to. My gynecologist, of course, found no yeast in my culture, and told me there was nothing he could do.

One day, while at the drug store, I came across a book called, *The Yeast Syndrome.* One of the coauthors happened to practice close to where I lived. I called his office to find out he was a podiatrist. However, he was able to recommend another doctor who might be able to help me. . . . This doctor had an allergist in his office test me for all kinds of allergies. It turned out I was not seriously "allergic" to anything. At this point, my doctor said he really had done everything possible and didn't feel a need for me to continue as his patient. His allergist did, however, tell me about a person who might give me additional help. This person was Robin Keuneke.

Robin did an initial phone consultation with me and felt she could help me with proper diet and nutrition. I met Robin to further discuss my situation. Below are Robin's recommendations to me and what eventually helped me clear up the infection and get back on track:

1. The first thing she said was to immediately stop taking any further medication. She felt this was only driving the infection deeper into my gut (medication kills enzymes).
2. She put me on a strict diet, requiring me to eliminate soda, coffee, commercial teas, dairy, eggs, sugar, any meats with hormones.
3. She had me add tofu, more fish (lots of salmon), grains, more vegetables.
4. I bought everything organic and drank only filtered water (pesticides and chemicals kill enzymes).
5. I learned how to use miso correctly (don't boil—boiling destroys enzymes). Initially, I used only dark miso and was able to later add the lighter miso.
6. I used more fresh garlic, ginger, herbs, and spices in recipes.
7. I added more seaweed, kabocha and delicata squash, and very lightly cooked dark leafy greens with umeboshi vinegar and lemon.
8. I had pressed or fresh salad daily.
9. I drank kukicha tea with umeboshi concentrate.
10. Since frying kills enzymes, I eliminated this type of cooking. Robin taught me how to "water saute" my vegetables, which requires much less oil. I use olive and sesame oils sparingly.
11. I later added chicken and lamb which contained no hormones or antibiotics, and was minimally processed, and organic eggs sprinkled with flax oil.

Initially Robin added a very few important supplements to my diet: liquid chlorophyll, a strong probiotic, vitamin C, a dry vitamin E, chromium picolinate, sea vegetation tablets, and garlic. My present supplements are aci-dophilus, chlorella (which contains chlorophyll), a multiple vitamin, vitamin C, a dry vitamin E, chromium picolinate, evening primrose, calcium/magne-sium, and garlic. I also use flaxseeds and flax oil daily.

It probably took about one year to get 100 percent, with Robin's guidance. Remember, I had this ongoing infection (not just before my period) for a few years. Robin was honest with me in saying it could take this long for me to be able to add new things to my diet, like shoyu, tamari, rice vinegar, etc. I am presently able to eat a much wider variety of foods, and even enjoy a glass of wine on occasion. I continue to buy as much organic foods as possible, drink kukicha with ume concentrate, and have my dark greens with ume vinegar. This helps to keep a healthy amount of good bacteria in my intestines. I still avoid dairy and fried foods. Robin has suggested I buy a juicer to take my im-proved health one step further. I hope to do so in the near future.

Herbal Therapy

Herbs have been used as medicine long before recorded history. Generations of trial and error taught prehistoric people which plants to use when treating injuries and diseases, and this life-saving knowledge was passed down through the ages. In China and India, the study and use of herbal medicine has evolved over 5000 years. In ancient Greece, the father of modern medicine, Hippocrates, used hundreds of herbs in his practice, many of which are still popular today. In short, the healing properties of plants are time-tested, which is why herbal therapy is respected in cultures around the world.

As the limitations of modern medicine become increasingly apparent, the medical profession is once again looking to the plant world for help. Scientists around the world, in a desperate search for answers to AIDS, cancer, and other conditions not cured by standard medicine, have begun to study the properties of herbs, and are amazed at their immune-enhancing effects. Astragalus, licorice, and panax ginseng have powerful anticancer properties, for example, while echinacea and goldenseal taken at the first sign of a cold or flu will often stop the disease in its tracks.

How do herbs help us? Some are like super foods whose nutrients are building blocks for the entire body. Others have drug-like actions, and exert specific strengthening or stimulating effects on certain physiological functions. Still others help to detoxify the system. Some herbs perform more than one function; for example, they may cleanse to a degree, but predominantly build up the system.

While herbalists know that specific herbs are helpful in correcting certain disease states, other factors are taken into account as well. The herbalist considers the whole person, and this is especially true in Chinese medicine, where an herbalist will look to see which symptoms are the most outstanding. If a patient is diabetic, for example, a person can exhibit great thirst, hunger, or urination. The herbalist also considers the state of the overall system: the digestion, sleep patterns, energy. In this way a basic formula for a condition is modified to meet the individual needs of the patient.

Herbalist Christopher Trahan sums up the value of plant remedies: "Herbal medicine works very well because they are biological entities which have evolved simultaneously with human beings. When we use herbs, we are using foods that are molecularly and energetically a part of us."

Homeopathy

Homeopathy is a system of healing based on the law of similars. In the late 18th century, homeopathy's founder, Dr. Samuel Hahnemann, discovered that like cures like: Administering a substance that causes a disease in a healthy individual can cure an illness in a person who is sick. So, for example, if someone with rashes is given a substance that creates rashes, it helps to neutralize and thus end the problem.

Homeopathy uses natural substances that are prepared by a process called dilution and succussion. This means that remedies are diluted over and over until they are no longer detectible. When the final product is viewed through a microscope, there appears to be nothing there. Frequently, homeopathic remedies are highly toxic substances in their natural form, and might include snake venom, arsenic, or harmful bacteria. But after being diluted, they are completely nontoxic. In fact, there appears to be nothing left but water.

If nothing is there, how does homeopathy work? Although no physical substance remains, the vibration of the material endures, and stimulates energy systems of the body to address both subtle and obvious causes of disease. Emotional states such as fear, anger, anxiety, and depression, which may underlie physical diseases, are dealt with, as well as physical symptoms. By rebalancing the whole person, emotionally and physically, homeopathy can make a big difference.

Homeopathic medicine differs from the allopathic tradition in that symptoms are viewed as an expression of the body attempting to heal itself, not something to be masked. The body is always faced with numerous stresses, and people are always reacting emotionally, physically, and mentally to regain balance. Covering up symptoms only pushes them to a deeper level, causing more serious consequences in the long-term.

Homeopathic remedies are either taken orally on placed onto the skin. Health food stores sell remedies labeled 12X or 30X, 12c or 30c, to indicate the number of dilutions that the formula has gone through. The X signifies that the formula has been diluted to a proportion of 1:10, while the c potency means it's been diluted to a 1:100 level.

Patient Stories

Lillian on liver cancer

Three years ago, I was diagnosed with a cancer below my rectum for which I received chemotherapy and radiation. That got rid of it for a while but in time it reappeared in my liver. I received 50 chemotherapy treatments but had I known what I understand today, I would never have had any.

I was very sick and waiting to die. I could not hold food or water down and lost a lot of weight. My bowels were totally paralyzed and I could not go to the bathroom at all. The nurses told me I only had a short time to live, and I wanted to die. The pain was so bad that I had to live on morphine and a narcotic pain patch.

Thank God my daughter introduced me to a homeopathic doctor who gave me a new lease on life. My doctor has done an awful lot for me. My therapy consisted of a lot of natural herbs and vitamins. I juiced and ate a diet high in healthy vegetables. Red meats were eliminated. He gave me medicine to alleviate edema and to lessen acidity. In addition, I received colonic therapy to detoxify my bowel.

When I got home, I had renewed strength. I could walk around and even drive, whereas before I needed a wheelchair. In six months, I have been able to gain some weight back and have no more bowel trouble. I had a myelogram last month. The doctors were shocked that I was able to come this far. They can't believe it. My blood pressure is down, and I have no trouble with my blood. I am a totally different person. I am amazed and my whole family is amazed as well. I feel that if I didn't go there, I would be gone. If I had to do it over, I would not have chemotherapy or radiation at all. I would go the homeopathic route.

Patty on accidents

I was introduced to homeopathy by my husband, 17 years ago. I married a man from a little town in Pennsylvania where 80 percent of the people use homeopathy because in the 30's, 40's and 50's, the hometown doctor was a medical homeopath. When I got married, his father handed me belladonna and arnica and said, good luck.

I didn't pay much attention to it until six or seven years ago when my husband put his hand underneath a lawn mower and almost severed a decent-sized piece of his finger. We went to the hospital where they did a lot of surgery and reattached it. He was told that he would never have any sensation there again because the nerves had been severed. They recommended plastic surgery.

I called a very wise old woman from my husband's home town and asked her what she would do. She said hypericum was the remedy that helps regenerate nerve endings. If anything could help, that would be it. We started giving him hypericum. Now, five years later, you would never know that anything had ever happened to his finger.

In my own case, the value of homeopathy was clearly demonstrated one Thanksgiving Day while I was baking the turkey. My daughter was about three months old and it was a lot of effort to make the dinner. I wanted to do everything perfectly and was very anxious. I put the pot holder on my right hand and took the turkey out of the oven with my left hand. I pretty much melted four fingers. They were pink and shiny and the fingerprints were pretty much gone. They were blistering in a matter of seconds. I remembered that the remedy for burns is camphorus. I only had a 30x, which is not incredibly strong, but camphorus is effective at any potency. In homeopathy, the indications on the bottle sometimes say to take it and wait four hours. In an emergency situation like the one I was in, it's important to take it as often as you need it. I was taking a little pellet of camphorus every minute. Then, it got to the point where I could take it every three minutes, every five minutes, every ten minutes. It got better and better all day. By nighttime, I was able to wash dishes and take a hot shower. Usually the pain is so phenomenally excruciating that you can't be near hot water. The next day, there was only a little bit of melted blistery stuff on one finger. The other fingers had totally healed. That amazed me. Not just that the pain was relieved, because that in itself blew my mind. But the fact that my fingers healed, and that quickly—that was amazing.

One of my favorite remedies is arsenicum for food poisoning. This is homeopathically prepared arsenic. When I've had food poisoning in the past, I probably would have voluntarily taken the substance arsenic just to get rid of the pain. I was lying in bed on a heating pad doubled over with horrible, horrible stomach cramps from food poisoning I had gotten that day. I also knew that in the refrigerator was something that I wanted to eat very much from the day before. It wasn't the thing that had caused the food poisoning but I knew that there were oysters and black bean sauce in the refrigerator and that if I didn't get them, someone else might.

As I was lying in bed, I looked up at the bureau and saw my remedy kit, which, at that point, I hadn't used a lot. I thought, wait a minute, arsenicum is a remedy for food poisoning. I took a dose. Again that was 30x. I got back on a heating pad and about 15 minutes later I took another dose. Within an hour I was eating the oysters and black bean sauce. I have never ever had a recovery from food poisoning that quickly in my life.

Alan on infections

About five years ago, I had a serious infection in my tooth. The doctor said I would have to take antibiotics or else I would end up in the hospital. The problem was, the last time I took antibiotics, I almost died from it and ended up setting off all types of alarms in the hospital. I was caught between a rock and a hard place.

A friend suggested that I see a homeopathic doctor. I didn't know what that was but I didn't have a choice so I went. The doctor gave me little brown pills to put under my tongue. The remedy was called hepar sulfuris calcareum. It is very good for infections around the teeth and gums. In a couple of hours the pain was gone. In two days, it completely disappeared.

I was amazed that you could treat an infection without antibiotics and started reading about homeopathy to learn more about it. Since then, I have many different remedies for lots of different things.

My wife had a headache that was so intense that she asked me if I would take her to an emergency room. At the same time, she was very, very angry. She was angry and complaining about unendurable pain at the same time. I remembered that those were the characteristics associated with a remedy called chamomilla. I approached her very gingerly because she was in a very angry and nasty mood and I put a few grains of chamomilla on her tongue. I walked out of the room and came back a few minutes later. She was sitting up and she said, "Do we have any ice cream?" We were walking the dog about 20 minutes later. She was okay. It's amazing how fast it works, especially in an acute situation, when you hit on a remedy.

I have learned that homeopathy is prescribed on an individual basis. While hepar sulfuris calcareum was the appropriate remedy for my infections, some-one else might benefit from mercurius. This is another remedy useful for infections, especially in the mouth or gums, but for other places also. What characterizes the need for this is a very bad odor coming from the mouth and a tremendous amount of saliva, yet at the same time, a great thirst. There is also a creeping chilliness.

Another remedy called puirogenium is very good for septic infections, the kind of thing people are rushed to the hospital for. I've known people who have used that remedy and then were fine in a couple of days.

Thomas on multiple sclerosis

I was diagnosed as having multiple sclerosis at a major university teaching hospital. The M.D.'s did not give me a very optimistic prognosis. It's the old thing that if you don't like the message, shoot the messenger or change mes-sengers. I sought out somebody who would tell me what I wanted to hear.

All this transpired about four or five months ago. I am 56 years old. What brought me to the M.D.s in the first place is that I had developed some M.S. symptoms. My balance was very poor and I had great difficulty in speaking. I would say that my balance was about 75 percent of what it should be and my speech was about 50 percent of what it should be.

After going to Dr. Ken Pitoway, a homeopathic doctor, I've seen considerable improvement. My balance has gone up to about 95 percent and my speech is back up to about 80 or 85 percent. That's my own subjective evaluation.

I feel homeopathy has made a big difference. I feel better and people tell me how good I look. I'm sure it's how good I look in comparison to how I looked before. My color used to be very pale. I was almost like death warmed over.

When I was with the M.D.'s, in essence, there was no hope. They implied that I should start shopping for a motorized wheelchair. Since changing to homeopathy, I'm jogging 25 miles a week. That's better than a wheelchair!

Before homeopathy, I was not jogging. I was a couch potato and I was letting myself deteriorate. Even though homeopathy didn't suggest that I jog, my general well-being improved to the point where I felt I could jog and wanted to. I believe that had I not started this program I would probably be in a wheelchair today.

It can be argued that whenever you have an MS flare-up, you're always going to improve from the worst point. But I feel that I've improved more than I would have because my general health is better. I'm still under treatment, and I look forward to a complete recovery.

Sandi on carpal tunnel syndrome and other problems

I suffered with carpal tunnel syndrome for three years. This caused me great difficulty at work. I owned a restaurant and had trouble holding onto things. At first, I was on some very bad drugs to control the inflammation and pain but the drugs began to bother my stomach. My orthopedic surgeon was going to perform carpal tunnel surgery.

At that time, a friend of mine encouraged me to call a homeopathic physician. I had never been introduced to homeopathy before and was hesitant about going. She kept telling me I could always have my surgery if the homeopathy didn't work. So, I went.

I was put on a homeopathic remedy called rhus tox. Within a couple of weeks, my hands were completely well. It has been five years since I took that homeopathic remedy. I never again suffered from carpal tunnel. I was saved from surgery on both hands and I saved my health because my stomach was beginning to bother me a great deal. I was also starting to have cardiovascular problems and those have also been relieved. So, I have had great success with homeopathy.

Since then, my family has used homeopathy over and over again and has had nothing but success. I have a grandson who was born with difficult breathing problems. Soon afterwards, he developed a hernia of the testicles. The pediatrician wanted to perform surgery immediately but my daughter wanted him to see a homeopathic physician first. Within two weeks of starting the homeopathic remedy, there was no sign of the hernia left. He too was saved from having surgery.

After a cesarean birth, my daughter's blood count went down to 7. The doctors wanted to give her a transfusion but we talked him into waiting at least 24 hours so that she could be administered a homeopathic remedy. She was given ferrum phosphoricum, which is a remedy that helps increase oxygen in the body and raise the blood count. Within that 24 hours, her blood count raised significantly and she did not need a transfusion.

Another daughter had toxemia related to pregnancy. We administered a homeopathic remedy called apis which took all of the poisoning and swelling out of her body within a very short time.

I can't talk enough about our successes and how it has kept us away from surgeries time and again. It just does wonderful things. Our bodies are much more capable of healing than we give them credit for. I'm all for allopathic medicine when other things won't work, or for diagnosis, but it is not needed as much as people think.

Helen on muscle and joint pain, emotional trauma, and sequential homeopathy

I had terrible muscle and joint pain that kept me incapacitated. I tried acupuncture, Chinese herbs, diet, intravenous vitamin therapy, just about everything, and they all helped. They got me about 50 percent better. But then nothing else worked. I got to a point where I was at a standstill; it stayed that way for a few years. I was relatively happy because I was much better.

Then a friend of mine died of AIDS. Two weeks later, my cat died. That sent me right back down the drain and I could no longer get back up. That went on for about two years. I tried a lot of things but nothing worked.

Then I decided to try homeopathy. The person I found does sequential therapy, which treats emotional wounds and removes repercussions from all life traumas. It starts in the present and works back to when your mother was pregnant. I've been doing this for ten months now. It's a slow process and will take about two years to complete. As a result of this therapy, I feel drastically better. I can drive again and do just about everything. At this point, I still have my problems and I still have pain, but, emotionally, I am 100 percent better.

Now, I'm treating my animals sequentially from all the little traumas that they have had from being strays. I treat them the same way a human would be treated. If they've been outside, you have to assume that they've been abused in some way. I give them opium for fear, natmur for grief and staphysagria for anger. It's definitely working. One cat wouldn't get out from under the bed for two months. We treated her and within a week she started coming out. Another cat of mine was biting and doing all kinds of strange things. We treated her this way and she's also much better. It doesn't happen overnight but it works and it's wonderful.

I also treat them with homeopathy for acute problems and it works wonderfully. Also, it is far more economical than going to a veterinarian. Vets have gotten so outrageously expensive and this is a very inexpensive way to treat them.

I just think it's a very dynamic and very wonderful way to heal. If you're going to get to the basis of where most illness come from you need to address emotions. Traumas certainly affect us for the rest of our lives and need to be removed. Sequential homeopathy can do that.

Dory on asthma

Pre-homeopathy, my oldest daughter was four and my youngest daughter was a newborn, less than a year old. Both of them had severe asthma. We tried the usual medical treatment with the bronchodilators and frequent runs of steroids. On the average, we visited the hospital's emergency room once a month for shots of epinephrine. They were also on nebulizer treatments three times a day.

A friend recommended that I take my children to a homeopath. I basically had nothing to lose because they weren't getting any better on any of the medications. On the contrary, they were getting worse and deteriorating rapidly. Our trips to the hospital were much more frequent. It was very frightening because my children would turn blue three o'clock in the morning.

We went to a homeopath, an M.D. Within six months, my oldest daughter was weaned off all medications. She has had no asthma attacks since that time. Previously, allergy tests showed that she had severe allergies to cats. We could not even go near a house with a cat. We now own a cat and she has had no allergy outbreaks and no asthma.

My youngest daughter's course of treatment took about a year. Same story. No asthma. We've had the lung function test repeated. It's perfectly normal and shows the lungs to be functioning 100 percent.

I absolutely know that homeopathy saved my children's lives and it gave them quality of life to boot.

Kim on ear infections

My son was taking antibiotics for chronic ear infections. It ended up being a dependency relationship. He would get better initially, but then it was really just a back-to-back-to-back series of 10-day courses of antibiotics. Sometimes, he would be on his tenth and final day of antibiotic therapy, and that afternoon, his ear infection would be back again. That would happen after taking my son to the doctor to make sure that his ear was okay. It really was just a Band-Aid effect, and not a long-term healing situation.

With homeopathy, once the remedies kick in, he's fine. His ear infections have dropped to maybe one or two a year instead of six or seven. He had one ear infection in February and another one last month. We treated them with pulsatilla over-the-counter eardrops from the health food store and he's fine.

Virginia on multiple sclerosis

First I tried the allopathic medical route but they could do nothing for me. They chose to really downplay what I was already doing, trying to eat right and exercise. I knew there had to be something else out there.

I turned to homeopathy and got tremendous results through a doctor in the Detroit area. He gave me natural homeopathy remedies and taught me how to eat right. I also was taught how to go inside myself to learn how to become well and to want to be well. Through this combination, I have been able to reverse some of my MS symptoms and feel basically well.

Hypnotherapy

Hypnotherapy can alleviate a wide variety of problems by quieting down disturbing and nonproductive thought processes in our conscious mind, and tapping into our subconscious where suggestions and insights allow us to change our perceptions. Among its many uses, hypnotherapy can help increase energy, manage chronic pain, and overcome addictions, such as overeating and smoking. It can also help one build confidence, and get over anxieties and phobias. Women can use hypnotherapy to subdue PMS, cramps, and other pain. Athletes can use it to enhance performance.

Hypnosis is not a total loss of consciousness, as most people believe. A client is aware and relaxed, almost as if his body is asleep but his mind awake and alert. A typical session begins with an interview, in which the patient communicates his or her problem to the therapist. Then the patient is guided to a peaceful state of mind, referred to as a trance. In this state, imagery is much more powerful than usual. The therapist makes suggestions and the person uses his imagination to shift his view of the world. Some changes are substantial. An example would be a person who does not stop smoking because of a deeply ingrained belief that she is unable to do so. By changing that core belief, smoking can be stopped.

Hypnotherapy holds great promise for life-threatening diagnoses. In these situations, a person has often been led to believe that he has no future. By coming into contact with all his beliefs about death and illness, doctors and hospitals, and then creating imaginary situations in which health has returned and he is surviving long into the future, a patient can shift from a point of no return to a turning point, a new beginning.

When hypnotherapy does not work, the failure may at times be attributed to resistance. As illogical as it seems, the problem may be doing something for the person on a subconscious level. It is creating a benefit, perhaps keeping the person from working, or putting the person in a situation where he or she gets more attention than usual.

Generally, the time invested in therapy is brief, and effects are immediate.

Three to six sessions are usually all that are needed, and sometimes only one is sufficient.

While hypnotherapy is a wonderful modality, there are a few words of caution to heed: A client takes in the energy as well as the suggestions of another. It is therefore imperative to work with someone whose intentions are pure, based on references and intuition.

Patient Stories

Cynthia on psychological blocks

For most of my childhood and part of my adult life, I was in traditional psychotherapy, trying to handle issues around my father's death, which happened when I was a child. I always felt that this was a major albatross stopping me from having the life I really wanted.

I met a hypnotherapist who felt that he might help me. We worked on my particular issues, and the results were truly amazing. I had a good job as a corporate recruiter, but I wanted a better one. I would stop myself from going after my goals because I was frightened that no one would hire me. I thought I wasn't smart enough and that I didn't deserve it. Negative ideas kept blocking me. Soon after the session, a company sought me out and I accepted a great job. Now I have an incredible position, something I only dreamed of before.

Other good changes came of this as well. I always wanted to have great relationships with people, but couldn't because I was afraid that they would leave. Now people gravitate toward me without my seeking them out. I have good, strong friendships, and a great relationship with my mother. These were tremendous issues for me.

Susan on multiple sclerosis

I went to sleep perfectly normal one night, and woke up the next day physically unable to move. I lost my vision, was unable to dial a phone, and was in severe back pain. I didn't know what was happening until going for an MRI, which confirmed that it was multiple sclerosis.

I have always believed that the mind has tremendous power. I knew that I had my work cut out for me, but that I would overcome this condition. Unfortunately, I shared this belief with my first doctor, who told me that I was in denial, and who added that I would be in a wheelchair. That made my situation more of a challenge because I certainly wasn't going to buy into a defeatist belief system.

I found a neurologist who understood holistic health and who believed in me. At first I had to take a drug to get my eyesight back. Otherwise there could have been permanent damage. After that I decided not to take anything. I did lots of affirmations at night, where I would say, "I'm getting better and stronger." I visualized myself healthy again, seeing myself exercising and in better shape than I ever was. I kept writing down my thoughts, telling myself that I was bigger than the disease. I was not in denial; I knew what I had, but I wasn't going to let the disease own me. I was very strong about that.

Now it's five years since my diagnosis. And I'm fine. I've had my bouts and moments, but I have always been able to get back on course because I realize that the mind has tremendous power. Whether it's remission or hypnosis or positive thinking or the combination of all three, I don't know. But it's working.

Today, I practice hypnosis and help other people with MS to realize that they don't have to give their power away to doctors. They can heal themselves by having a positive mind-set, a good diet, exercise, and surrounding themselves with positive people. I try to show people that the mind has tremendous power, and that a crisis can turn into an opportunity. I show people how to erase negative thoughts and make new tapes in their minds. I'm not claiming that I have a cure, but I can help people to get to the root of the problem, negative thinking, so that they can stop feeling sorry for themselves and rise above it.

Anthony on obesity

I went to the Hypnosis Institute and worked with Barry Seidman. And I have lost a substantial amount of weight, 46 pounds in six months. Although I'm a strong individual, I still did not believe I could lose weight because I was quite obese. His suggestions taught me how to think, and how to become more confident.

Alicia on resentment

I had been in therapy for many years and had made many improvements in my life, but I still was stuck in a cycle of resenting my mother and other people I knew. I sought hypnosis to try and alleviate the problem, and found that it vanished after one 2½-hour session with George Bien, a really marvelous hypnotherapist.

As far as the session goes, I am not really sure how it helped. I believe that hypnosis starts a process of organic change within body and mind. Over the course of a few weeks, I was simply able to drop it. I found that indeed I loved her again.

I feel that part of it is simply that you go into an altered state of consciousness. The conscious mind quiets down, and the subconscious mind opens up. One thing that happened to me in the course of the session is that we did a visualization in which I spoke to my mother and asked her why she did not love me. It became very clear to me that she would have loved me if she could. At that moment, the realization was so intense that when I came out of trance I suddenly knew and understood her limits as well as my own. I was able to simply accept the situation and move on from there.

I was fortunate to be in the hands of a gifted therapist. That's very important. George is gifted and astute and able to perceive an individual's problem. It's not simply going in and doing some unilateral technical magic play. The therapist has to understand your situation and be able to use techniques of regression so that you, personally, can be helped.

I think that out of the experience of working with George and simply having this moment, this intense physical and emotional moment of realization and recognition, I was able to simply pass through the problem because it affected me on an emotional, physical, and spiritual level. Before, when I was in therapy, I was cognitively aware, and I could do a little word dance. I would say to myself, "I know I should feel better about this," but it never worked. Hypnosis, on the other hand, was a transformative experience.

Maryanna on confidence

About two years ago, I took the Barry Seidman certification course in hypnotherapy, and it really changed my life. I really thought that hypnosis was about mind control and I wouldn't let myself try it. But Barry changed my whole perspective. He was so personable and warm that he was able to convince me that it was the other way around.

I am finally getting someplace now with my acting career. Not only that, I am working with him at the Hypnosis Institute as a hypnotherapist. So you can see how it completely changed my life.

I use it before auditions. As a matter of fact, it helped me land a principal role in a movie before becoming a member of the Screen Actors Guild. Everybody was telling me that I needed to be an extra in a film before I could get into SAG. I said, "No, I don't have to do that. I can get a principal part." Just like that. I was able to get to my higher intelligence through hypnosis, and get the audition without an agent. I got a small part in *Little Odessa,* and now I'm in SAG. I'm also working with Barry. Everything is so wonderful.

Michael on tumors

This is a case of a physical challenge that was tremendously aided and abetted by George Bien's gifted hypnotic skills. Several years ago, I was in Florida, when a healing crisis ensued. Literally overnight, a gigantic tumor appeared on my spine and another near my rectum. I woke up the next morning terrified and extremely upset. These were not small bumps. They were as big as half a tennis ball. I went to the emergency room, where I was told that this was extremely dangerous. I needed surgery and a barrage of x-rays. But I didn't go that route because of a prior incident.

Twenty years earlier, I was told that I had a brain tumor and that something was wrong with my spine, by three different specialists at three separate hospitals. My leg completely withered up as well. I didn't have any money and I was scared stiff. So I went to Weiser's bookstore and found a book called *Your Mind Can Heal You,* which came from the Christian metaphysical tradition. That led me to the mountains, where I remained alone for five months. I lived through a Canadian winter eating raw grains, and repeating positive affirmations.

Fortunately, that ameliorated the condition without any allopathic remedies, though I really didn't understand why until much later. I didn't understand that the subconscious, like a genius or brilliant inductive child, receives suggestions. I was doing meditation to empty my mind and giving myself strong self-suggestions that my body and leg were healed and whole. The subconscious, according to some schools of hypnotic thought, receives these suggestions uncritically. Because I was isolated, I was not getting the propaganda from society or from the medical profession telling me how dangerous everything was. I was less frightened and my leg came back to full strength.

I returned to my doctor who examined me and looked at the results of my test before telling me that I was 90-95 percent healed. He asked me how it happened and I told him in very sincere, but apparently naive terms. His face was a mixture of contempt and disturbed uneasiness, as he asked me to leave his office. He wanted me out. The power of my experience, combined with the neurologist's reaction, opened my eyes to the nature of Western medicine.

This time, I was told that I needed surgery at once, and that this was tremendously dangerous. Although I was in great pain, and really quite frightened, I went to Chinatown to see a really good traditional Chinese doctor. He also said that I had a tumor and told me that I should begin taking herbs. I did but there wasn't much of a change. Meanwhile, I got sicker and sicker to the point of being bedridden with tremendous sweats.

I had trained with George prior to this and had always loved hypnosis. I had done self-hypnosis before, but in this case, I was not capable of dealing with this problem alone. I went to see George, who I would call unique. He is a genuine healer. He saw me the next day. And for a fee, which I can only call beyond reasonable, I had a three-hour session.

The experience was profound. I can only liken it to an exorcism. The man literally had my jaw open at one point. There was dry heaving stuff that had been so ancient, so toxic in me. I can't even give you a map of what took place during that session, but the next day, this thing broke and drained. This took place literally within 24 hours. The whole psychological situation that I had endured for over 40 years, immediately went into a healing modality, and it has remained that way. There has been no recurrence.

People need to know that their body would not do anything to hurt them. They need to know that their own mind is not their enemy. In fact, quite the opposite. With some loving, conducive suggestions, proper, clean, healthy diet, and a few other things, healings happen very quickly.

Vicki on weight loss and chronic back pain

I went to Barry Seidman for weight loss back in January, and since then I have lost a total of 46 pounds. Now the weight is just falling off, and I have much more confidence and self-esteem. I can't buy clothes small enough fast enough. It's just been a wonderful experience. I got so interested in this that I took a certification course in it.

I was a compulsive eater, big-time. After my three back surgeries, food was my salvation. It was my way of making myself feel better about myself, and it was my way of rewarding myself.

I went through the hypnosis, which gave me more self-confidence and esteem . . . but also helped me to know that these fattening foods were bad for me. The suggestions were that I would eat healthy foods and I would eat what was good for me and only enough for my normal body weight. He just suggested that I eat healthy foods and drink plenty of water. I can't get enough water now. I don't drink soft drinks anymore, just water.

Barry also taught me self-hypnosis, so that I can manage this on a daily basis or as needed. Now it's not a daily basis, but as needed. I just don't want the fattening fried foods, and, as you know, down here in the south we eat fried foods continuously. I no longer eat anything that's fried. It's mainly salads and vegetables. In fact, I don't even eat meat anymore.

I have so much energy because I exercise now, whereas before I wasn't able to physically exercise. This hypnosis has helped me tremendously, and I would advise anybody to go for it.

My son brought a pizza home and I had been a pizza fanatic. I looked at it, and I knew it tasted good, but I just didn't want it. It's as simple as that . . . I talked to Barry last week and I've lost another pound since then.

I was bedridden for three years with chronic back pain. Barry did a private session with me to change the energy through forgiveness. That was a big part of it, a very big part. To forgive you just have to mentally visualize the face and the name of every person who has hurt you in your entire life. You just mentally have to say, "I forgive you," and move on. You just move on until your list is complete. The last person you need to forgive is yourself. That's very important. When you do that, it feels like a weight is lifted off of your shoulders. You actually change the energy in your body from negative to positive, and you can actually feel something going on inside of your body. Then you feel even lighter. When I left there I was on cloud nine.

Before I would try to go to the track to walk, and it would take me forever. I mean the little old ladies were passing me two and three times on my one time around. I would have to get back in the car and go home because I couldn't take it. Now I'm doing two miles and it's wonderful. I love it. I don't hurt anymore. My pain was from a botched surgery and I had nerve damage in my right hip and leg, but I don't hurt anymore. And if there should happen to be a little twinge or something all I do is go into self-hypnosis now. We put a switch up there and I just turn the switch off so it doesn't hurt. A lot of people might think that sounds crazy, but it works. My husband cannot believe the change. He says I'm a totally different person.

Peter on combined therapies

Hypnotherapy has clearly illuminated some of the things from my past that have made an impact on my present life. That was through the combined modalities of regression, Gestalt therapy and psychodrama while in the state of hypnosis. Through that, I have some very clear explanations of some of my present behaviors and how I arrived at that position.

I had been in traditional therapy for about two years and that was helpful, but in hypnotherapy, using Gestalt and psychodrama, I reached better insights because traditional therapy is all talk, while these other processes are more emotional. I could really feel what had occurred and how it was affecting my present situation. I saved a lot of time because I was in traditional therapy for about two years, but in hypnotherapy this was all accomplished in a matter of four or five sessions. I have a lot of faith in hypnotherapy, when it is done with a very skilled practitioner who also employs psychodrama and regression.

Dorothy on sugar addictions

I was a sugar addict, eating a quart of ice cream a day, and putting four to six teaspoons of sugar in each cup of tea. My cholesterol and my sugar were high. And even though I was concerned about my health I just couldn't stop.

A friend finally convinced me to try hypnosis. She gave me the name of Barry Seidman. She felt he could help me, and he did.

I've stopped eating sugar. My blood values are now normal and my cravings are gone. I haven't used sugar in a year. I eat ice cream very occasionally at parties only. I was so impressed with my success that I studied hypnosis at the Hypnosis Institute. It's done wonders for me.

One thing that you learn is self-hypnosis and that is the most wonderful tool. Anyone can learn it, anyone can perfect it. I am now healthy. I am a vegetarian. I use self-hypnosis every day to relax. I feel good about myself. My confidence in myself has increased. I'm positive about my future. I now have a five year plan whereas before I didn't know what I would do five years from now. I am going to have my own practice in a year.

I always wanted to fly. It has been a fantasy of mine for a long time. Now, I know I'm going to achieve it within five years. I am going to learn to pilot a helicopter.

Anyone out there who feels that they are held back should try hypnosis. It does wonders. I'm so much happier with myself since I stopped eating sugar.

Dorothy on self-hypnosis

[In self-hypnosis], the first thing that I do is breathing. I breathe to relax. Then I look at an object, usually above eye level, with focused attention, and just concentrate on that until I feel very relaxed. My eyes become heavy. I say one, two, three, relax, and access my subconscious mind. That's when I give myself positive suggestions: "I am confident, I feel good about myself, the world loves me, I love the world, I can be a hypnotherapist, I will get that doctorate in hypnotherapy, I see myself learning to pilot a helicopter."

I was not always a very confident person. I was very insecure. Self-hypnosis has really been wonderful. I repeat these positive affirmations to myself, which only takes about three minutes. Then I just say, "One, two, three, awaken, emerge."

I do this often during the day—when I'm washing my hands, doing the dishes, walking. I'm now walking anywhere from two to four miles a day, except when it rains.

Joe on overcoming obstacles to success

About a year and a half ago or so, my wife became interested in self-hypnosis. I saw some changes going on in the way she approached her life. She's Japanese and it's taken her quite a while to get used to living in a different country.

Very soon after that, I found Barry Seidman, who was giving a course in certification in hypnotherapy. I really didn't know much about it, but it seemed like an opportunity to get started and to do something that I had always wanted to do, which is work in the field of health. So I took Barry's course and did a little work with some people. I realized at one point that I probably needed to undergo some sessions of my own to understand a little more about it and get the feeling of the person who is having the sessions.

So I had some sessions with Barry and many things in my life began to change. Success seemed to come even more quickly. My wife and I had been involved in various ventures. We publish a magazine in Japanese, and the opportunities that have been coming in since then are just incredible.

I have an offer to publish another magazine on natural health in the near future, and we're working with a health product and beginning to export it throughout the world. This is something that I think came through those sessions because for a long time I believe I've been hesitant to use my abilities fully to reach for a certain level of success, for whatever reason. I feel that I have a greater access now to my subconscious mind. The work with Barry, I'm sure, is a large, large part of that.

This is the feeling that I have. It connects you not only with yourself but with other people on a special level. You become more open to things. I feel like now I have an edge. There's a certain level of confidence and a certain demeanor that I think I've acquired that goes beyond what I had expected of myself before, and I really attribute it to the work I've done. The work actually gets done on yourself by yourself, although there's an impetus that comes from someone else. I think that the beauty of it is that you're working with someone to unleash the powers within you, and eventually you're in control of those powers.

Massage Therapy

Swedish massage, a method of manipulating muscle tissue using specific strokes, movements, and pressure, has several therapeutic benefits: relief of pain, relaxation of muscle tension, improved blood and lymph circulation, better absorption and elimination, greater mobility of muscles and joints, and assistance in the repair of injured and damaged tissue.

Massage can help a wide spectrum of individuals. Athletes can relieve over-exhausted muscles after a race, while the bedridden can alleviate muscle fatigue brought on by lack of exercise. Injured individuals heal faster, while average persons function better all around from a reduction in stress. Massage can help relieve sciatica and common backaches, speed up the healing of fractures and sprains, and even alleviate some of the symptoms of diabetes, multiple sclerosis, cardiomyopathy, hypertension, and fibromyalgia.

Many therapists combine massage with aromatherapy. Inhaling sage or lavender can calm a person, for example, while peppermint can get more energy flowing. Oils open up various meridians, or energy pathways, so that greater healing takes place.

Patient Stories

Sonia on car accident

I had a car accident about four years ago which left me with severe whiplash in my neck, and back problems. I started going for massage with a woman named Susan and it was a wonderful experience. At first, I went once a week for three years. Then I started going every other week, and now I go every third week. I have to say that I ended up feeling better than before the accident.

I'm a painter. I spend lots of hours standing at an easel and painting. The tendons going through my neck would affect my shoulder, and that would affect my painting ability. Because everything got loosened and freed up, I was able to be more comfortable when I was painting. That was definitely an advantage.

I even felt that the massage helped me to feel better than going to a chiropractor. I think that's because the total experience was so comfortable, rewarding, and pleasurable, and that she did such good, deep tissue work.

Linda on dance injuries

I used to train and dance professionally. Later on, after having a child, I continued just to stay in shape. I had a couple of injuries and went to Sarah Vogler, who is a neuromuscular therapist. The first one was a knee injury. I saw her for about four months and she helped with the patterning of my knee. I don't know what she did technically, but she relieved my symptoms a lot. However, I later had to have surgery on that knee.

The other thing that happened is that I had a strain of the psoas muscle. This was a dramatic injury that happened during a class. I couldn't walk out, and left on crutches. I thought of Sarah again, who agreed to barter with me since I had no insurance. I went to Sarah on the crutches and after one session didn't need them. I saw her three more times and was well.

Diane on spasmodic torticollis

This is a condition that affects the neck muscles, causing them to spasm and twist. If it is not treated, it can progress and get worse. The neck muscles tighten into a knot, and it is very painful. After a while it shortens and twists. I tried several ways of treating it. My most successful way was through massage.

When I go for my massage, my therapist works into the muscles to elongate and relax them. There are several different techniques that she uses. Her fingers can tell an awful lot. She does Swedish message, which is very relaxing, but a lot of times to work into the knots in my muscles, she does more of a deep tissue therapy with her thumbs and knuckles. It's a matter of upkeep because it does help.

As you know, when you get nervous or upset, the first thing to react are your muscles. With people who do not have problems with their muscles, over time or overnight they relax again. The problem is that my neck muscles don't relax on their own. So massage therapy is definitely a blessing. I have been going about once every two weeks for about three years and it really has helped a lot.

Jerry on car accident

I was involved in a motor vehicle accident. . . . I had severe injuries to the neck, shoulder, and arm on the right side of my body. I was being treated by several physicians, who recommended that I see a massage therapist also.

When I saw my massage therapist, she first took a complete medical history in order to individualize the type of treatment that was required for my type of injuries. The emphasis, in my case, was the neck, shoulder, arm, and leg. When you go into the room, it's dimly lit with soothing music to relax you.

There was limited range of motion in my arm and neck. She massaged certain muscle groups and the injured areas by finding the pressure points affected. She worked out the knots, tightness, stiffness, and soft tissue injuries, and relieved a lot of the pain that I was in.

As a result, I was able to increase some of the range of motion, relieve a lot of pain, and improve the flexibility and mobility of the affected areas. She took away a lot of the stress, which was causing me to be irritable and moody. I was completely relaxed after the treatment. I highly recommend massage therapy.

Wendy on tightness

I practice yoga, which gets me more in tune with my body. I basically know where I need to have releases done. I love body work. It's just wonderful.

Sarah Vogler is my body worker. She does some craniosacral work with me, which is a subtle approach. It's mostly a very gentle touch that works with the neck, the bones, and the head. I go in feeling not too bad, thinking, "I don't really need this today." Then I come out feeling much better.

Janine on stress management

Unfortunately, I lost my parents and my brother within a two-year period. I witnessed illness, and obviously the stress that goes along with that is very high. I felt that I needed to start doing things for myself so I began massage therapy. The therapist started treating me with a technique called AMMA therapy. I don't know much about the scientific end of it, only that she applies pressure to certain points while I am on the table. She will hold a certain spot on my head or my foot or other areas. I don't know exactly what she's doing. All I know is that after I finish I feel a new energy and I feel that physically something does occur. It is helping me a lot.

Laurie on cystic fibrosis

Cystic fibrosis is a lung disease like asthma but a little bit worse. Basically, it causes me coughing and digestive problems. I have found massage to be terrific. It definitely helps because I can feel the difference before I get a massage and afterwards. I feel that my lungs are a lot clearer. I start coughing and I know that it helps to bring everything up.

Pam on insomnia

I was experiencing a lot of fatigue and stress from work obligations. There were also problems with muscle spasms and sciatic nerve. It was all getting compounded because I would drag myself through the day and then fall asleep for two hours. Then I would wake up with a lot of pain in my hips. A bad problem was getting worse.

I thought massage would be a good way to start getting myself back in shape. I went for Swedish massage, which helped me alleviate the aches and pains. Right away I started feeling relaxed and better able to work and sleep. Muscles stopped aching. And the results would last a whole week. Another side benefit was that I realized that I needed to focus on what I needed to change in my environment to be less fatigued. So, there were many benefits that came out of the massage treatments.

Lynn on chronic muscle tightness

I first started having massages when I was traveling as a flight attendant. When you are working those long, hard, stressful hours in toxic conditions, it's a great release to wake up in a foreign city and head to the gym. So, I'd have a workout, a sauna, and a massage.

Because I'm kind of a hyperactive person, it was good to have deep tissue massage. I found shiatsu to be the most effective although I have had Swedish and aromatherapy with crystals, and that was very interesting as well. I understood that it helped to detox because they're stimulating the lymph glands. In particular, my neck and shoulders were always full of these toxic knots. So, usually Japanese ladies would walk up and down my back for twenty minutes or half an hour and then work on my neck for 15 minutes alone. That, in itself, was amazing. Later on, I discovered a masseur who also did acupuncture. He specialized in athletic injuries, so I would have a massage and acupuncture which was amazing. I would be up for 12 hours by the time I got to Japan. After a massage I would wake up revitalized and go out dancing for the evening. So I think it had some very positive effects.

I noticed that when I did that crystal aromatherapy, I would feel euphoric afterwards. I literally felt an electric shock-like feeling go through my head when she would release something by using what she called a sulfur crystal. So there are some amazing things that a masseuse can do to energize the body by releasing blockages and breaking up toxic knots.

The therapist would massage me with oils of various scents that are geared to trigger particular emotional responses, depending on what she felt I needed. She would place the crystal on various parts of my body or adjacent to it. I remember one time, in particular, she said she couldn't determine exactly which crystal I needed until she got to the sulfur. That's when I felt this electricity go through my head. It was just a "ping" moment. That's when I realized this wasn't hocus pocus. Then afterwards, I always felt euphoric for at least an hour. I think it must be similar to the neurological responses that get set off when people listen to chant music.

Seth on sports injuries

Race-walking taxes the hamstrings quite a bit. I decided to combine massage and physical therapy, which worked out very well. Usually, I would get the physical therapy first and follow it with the massage.

I found that my shoulders would loosen up. As a matter of fact, it felt as though they had broadened. And it helped my hamstrings tremendously. I think massage is an excellent way of getting out the knots and the aches and pains. Typical shoulder and leg problems are helped.

I saw my massage therapist a few weeks ago, and I got a terrific massage in a nice quiet, peaceful room, with some meditative music in the background. You really need the quiet. I think the benefit was really tremendous. I certainly do want to come back and get massaged more.

Tom on stress

I had a lot of job-related stress and tightness. Massage helps me to release a lot of the emotional stuff that I tend to hold on to. Since I have been going for massages, I have been able to relax. I do not feel as tight, and I do not feel a lot of pain in my body. Liz is great. She is strong but gentle. She goes in deep, yet she doesn't leave you screaming. Also, one of the things we work with is breath and I try to carry that with me through the week. I tend to hold a lot of stuff in and close up tight, particularly in my shoulders and lower back. By staying with my breath and breathing longer and deeper, I can release a lot of stress.

Gil on hamstring tear

I went to an orthopedist and paid $175 to hear that there was nothing he could do about this for a year and a half, so good-bye and good luck. Since I was nearly at the point of walking with a cane, that was unacceptable. So I decided to try massage to get at least minor relief. Within two weeks of having massage three times a week, there was improvement. Within five weeks, I was pretty much pain-free. And by the end of two months, it was normal.

Nutritional Therapy

Comedian and social activist Dick Gregory says people commonly confront him about his vegetarianism, insisting that meat is necessary. There is a lot of protein in a steak, he agrees, but cow's don't eat steak. Many plant-based foods provide the right vitamins, minerals, and enzymes to help our bodies manufacture everything it needs.

While a strictly vegetarian regimen may not be the answer for everyone, the idea is that many people are uneducated in their nutritional understanding, and do not realize how the foods they eat relate to every variety of chronic, degenerative illness. They may become depressed from a common food to which they are allergic, or hyperactive from sugar, and never make the connection because they have eaten this way all their lives. Most people can therefore benefit from nutritional counseling, which incorporates supplementation and dietary changes for optimal health.

Patient Stories

Mary on hepatitis B

I used to eat any and everything. I became so sick that I didn't think I was going to make it. I didn't know what was going on but then I found out what I had. I must have had it for years. I had a test for something else. Through that, I found out about the hepatitis.

Then I saw a nutritionist and I learned what I was supposed to do. I needed to eat well and to rest. I think rest is most important. So I became more careful. I started taking a whole spectrum of nutrients for strength. I drink soups and eat green vegetables and sometimes fish. I stay away from the red meat as much as I can. I do take a little beef once in a while.

I had a couple of ozone treatments. That helped too. My blood tests looked much better than they did before. With the ozone therapy, I felt much better right away. So, I assume it's a combination of the ozone and the nutrition. All this has helped me. I'm hoping that I'll stay this way for a long time.

Rabbi Jeff on obesity

I have lost a total of 140 pounds, and I have never felt better in my entire life. Before I was lethargic. I was always tired and needed to sleep 12 hours a night. I had trouble walking a flight of stairs. I had trouble walking around the block. I had difficulty breathing. I had difficulty living. Now I walk five miles a day. I exercise vigorously and regularly. I eat voluminously, but I eat totally differently. I have become a total vegetarian. I have even given up eating fish. My sources of protein come from beans, legumes, and rice. I feel invested with a tremendous sense of energy, a very vital dynamic, and have literally never felt better in my entire life.

Years ago, I would go on a diet for three weeks, and the only thing that I lost was 21 days. This time, I did not go on a diet. I completely changed the way in which I think about food, prepare food, consume food, and apparently, the way I now absorb food and deal with it in terms of my nutritional well-being.

I had reason to see a proctologist for a leftover problem, and he was amazed at the cleanliness of the colon. It was just absolutely marvelous. I feel an invigorated sense of vitality. I saw Dolores, my nutritionist, about eight months ago, and she instructed me in terms of various vitamin, mineral, and herbal supplements. I read voraciously and have found the information inspiring and informative. I have become a kind of local focal point for people in my religious community. People who might not otherwise have access to this information have now begun to call me with some degree of regularity. And I refer them to nutritionists.

The most important element of this entire protocol is the fact that I feel wonderful. Having given up meat, chicken, and dairy products, and a whole variety of other foods, I don't wake up with headaches anymore. I used to think that it was appropriate to wake up in the morning with a headache. I now wake up with a clear head. I have a wonderful sense of vitality, a sense of purpose and direction that is literally inspirational. If someone would have told me two years ago that I wouldn't be a carnivore, I would have laughed hysterically. I was the most carnivorous human being on this earth! If it had four legs and rabbinic supervision, I ate it with great glee and in great quantity at all the wrong hours of the day. Today, I feel refreshed and revitalized, in all aspects of my life. I feel a tremendous sense of joy and vitality.

My total cholesterol used to be 297. Without any medication whatsoever, it is now 171. All the other blood work is much improved: kidney function, liver function, blood pressure, everything, is right down the middle now, whereas before I was a major bomb ready to burst.

It has gotten so good. In fact, I recently had a circumcision to perform on a

Sabbath when I'm not allowed to drive. I walked 6½ miles there, did the circumcision, standing at all times, and walked 6½ miles back. I felt great, and realized, "My God, I've just walked half a marathon."

I was all excited and called Dolores. She suggested that I enter the New York City marathon, and I'm pursuing this. For me, to have watched the marathon 140 pounds ago would have been a tiring experience. Now I am at the point where I am entering the marathon. This is a 180-degree change in my life. I owe it to the brilliant science of good, old-fashioned, basic, fundamental nutrition.

Gay on hyperthyroidism

When I first came to the Healing Center, I saw Dolores Perry. She was very helpful in determining whether I had hyperthyroidism or hypothyroidism, and as it turned out I did have the symptoms for hyperthyroidism. I have the bulging eyes, the irritability, the increased perspiration, and things like that. Hyperthyroidism is a disorder where the thyroid gland produces too much of a hormone, which results in overactive metabolic states. Body processes, including digestion, speed up with this disorder. My husband would make fun of me sometimes because I would always be hungry and eating. I guess that was from the hyperthyroidism. Needing to eat so much was unnerving.

Dolores Perry helped me to design a proper diet. I learned how to eat the right foods and to stay away from foods that caused my thyroid to produce too much of its hormone. This helped me with my weight. I was telling Dolores that I was have a problem filling out my jeans. Now I no longer have to wear my leggings underneath my jeans to fill them out.

All the medical establishment wants to do is pump chemicals into your system. And chemicals are not natural. They treat you like a guinea pig, saying, "If that doesn't work, come back and we'll prescribe something else." That's ridiculous. The best thing for the body are natural foods in their natural state. I would definitely recommend that anyone, even people who think they are healthy, go on a natural diet.

Jean on post-polio syndrome, hypoglycemia, and fatigue

I contracted polio when I was very, very young. Then, in the late 80s, I had some weird, weird symptoms, and I was tired all the time. The medical doctors used that six letter word, stress, and put me on a lot of tranquilizers. I knew that wasn't working. Then I began to have a lot of other symptoms, which as far as I was concerned, were not related to my post-polio syndrome. A friend of mine said that I might have hypoglycemia. I went to a health store and got some paperbacks, specifically, Carlton Fredericks, and realized, "Yes, that's what I have."

I was hospitalized briefly for a rapid heartbeat. They started to pump me with heart medications. But I told the doctor I wanted a glucose tolerance test. That proved that I was hypoglycemic. . . . I found an endocrinologist [but] he made me worse because my body needed a very restricted diet.

When I finally found Marilyn, who I call my guru, I found that I had to be careful of complex carbohydrates. My intake had to be very, very low to avoid symptoms. An added bonus was the supplements that she ordered for me. They helped my muscle tone and bone density in my right legs and hips. That was something I didn't expect.

Right now, I'm not going to say that I'm 100 percent better. I do get fatigued and I do have to pace myself. But this is nothing like what I had prior to 1989. I make sure I eat a correct diet. I eat all natural foods and buy a lot of my stuff in the health food store and make sure that I take my supplements.

The doctor is very pleased, even with the pulse in my right leg. I had been wearing an elasticized knee brace, which had absolutely no movement in it. After the supplements, I started going for days without the brace. I realized, "Oh, my God. I don't need it." I have discarded it and only take it with me when I go away or go out, in case I should fall. But it's also affected my hip and arm. I find that I can grasp better with my right arm now. These changes came on gradually. I never realized that those supplements were going to help with that also.

Valerie on dizzy spells and fatigue

I had a lot of dizzy spells and fatigue, which made it difficult to get out of bed. My normal, daily activities were very limited. I also had a lot of infections: upper respiratory infections, sinus infections, yeast infections, and so forth. In general, my health was very poor.

I went through quite a few doctors, but nobody was able to help me. I was tested to see if I had an autoimmune illness. They thought it might be a variety of things, but nothing ever showed up. Nobody could really help me. Meanwhile, I couldn't even get out of bed. Everybody realized I was sick, but they didn't know what to do for me.

For a year, I was on antibiotics, almost constantly. I was also on other medications, like meclizine for the dizziness, and decongestants for the sinus infections. I think I had about 16 different medications that year. And they were pretty potent. At this point, I am not taking any of them.

It all began to change for me after I saw Gary Null at a seminar held through the Learning Annex in Manhattan. He was discussing diet and supplements. It was the only thing left that I could really do at that point. So I went to see a nutritionist.

I saw a nutritionist who told me specifically what to eat, and what not to eat.

It was a very limited diet, but there was enough of a choice for me to still eat normally. At the same time, I cut out things that had been bothering me, but that I didn't know were bothering me. For example, wheat flour and dairy products where things I had been eating all the time that I didn't realize were having an effect on me until I cut them out. Then I had a total reversal of most of my symptoms.

The first was difficult. I guess I was addicted to a lot of foods. I felt very depressed and weak, but once I got past that point, I gained strength. I did a lot of journaling and that helped me to see the progress that I was making. In the beginning the notes read, "Today I was able to get out of bed, and do some light housework." At this point, I am able to do light jogging. I'm more active for an extended period of time.

When I began seeing a nutritionist . . . I saw the results right away. The first week, I noticed that a lot of the mental fogginess I was having was gone. I was alert. My eyes were very clear. These were things I didn't realize until I changed the diet. Then, all of a sudden, I improved.

I think the main problem was that I was eating a lot of wheat and dairy. Now I'm on a vegetarian diet, except for fish. I have a whole list of what I am able to eat and I try to eat everything as natural as possible. I follow the advice in Gary's books. I study them to make the diet more interesting.

I take a variety of supplements too. The main thing helping me is the Green Stuff. I used to have a lot of hair loss. It was becoming very noticeable. I'm only 28, so that was really upsetting me. My skin and hair were dull too. Since I have been taking the Green Stuff, that's totally changed for the first time in a very long time. I also take choline, inositol, antioxidants, and aloe vera juice.

It feels good to know that it's in my control, whereas before I felt like everything was taking me over. So this has helped me mentally as well.

Nina on digestive disorders

From the time I was in my late teens to my early 20s, I had severe digestive difficulties. I would get debilitating abdominal pain from severe gas in response to eating foods. I would get together with friends to eat Chinese food and go out to a movie. Afterwards, I would have to be literally helped into a taxi to get home.

Eventually, I started getting very fatigued, because if you're not digesting food well, eventually, that's what will happen. I experienced depression from having low energy.

I thought my diet was quite good. In my early 20s, I stopped eating dairy, and I started eating a vegetarian diet. But I still had a lot of problems with food allergies.

I started seeing a nutritional doctor in the late 80s. That helped a bit. Then

I worked with a chiropractic nutritionist. She suggested digestive enzymes and that helped even more. But I still had chronic constipation. So about a year and a half ago, I started working with Dolores Perry. She suggested a real high level of supplements and herbs.

It's one thing to have food allergies, but do you have food allergies because your digestive system doesn't work or does your digestive system not work and then you get food allergies? You've got to both work with food allergies and energize your system. So that's what the supplements have done for me.

Now my digestive system works pretty well. And if it doesn't, I can bring it back into balance with supplements and herbs.

It took just a few months to see an improvement. Now, I'm a very happy, outgoing person. For a number of years I was an unhappy and depressed person. A lot of that was due to the fact that I wasn't physically feeling well. It's made a big difference.

I value working with Dolores because I really work with her. I bring in research articles, we discuss them, and she makes suggestions. I'm really working with her and treating myself. I'm in charge, and I really appreciate that.

Greg on brain tumor

I was on chemotherapy for about four and a half months, when I asked to be taken off it. This was about three and a half years ago. I had had a craniotomy, and they resected the tumor from the brain. Then I went through a regimen of radiation. I was led to believe that that was that. Suddenly an oncologist came in and said that I was to go through chemotherapy. I was having some bad reactions to either the chemotherapy or one of the antiepileptic drugs they were giving me. I had scar tissue remaining in my head and it was causing me some minor seizure activity.

I started the chemotherapy in Chicago, but moved out to San Francisco. I was at the University of California, San Francisco, where I was reading a lot of articles from the American Brain Tumor Association about the permeability of the blood brain barrier. I went to the radiologist for an MRI, which at that time was every three months. I asked if they could do an enhancement to show the permeability of my blood brain barrier. They assured me they could, but upon giving me back my films they could not.

I went to my neurologist and asked him to please show me how permeable the blood brain barrier was. He really couldn't show me either. I asked, "What evidence do I have that the chemotherapy is actually going after these cancer cells and eliminating them?" I would go there every month, and all my blood counts would be very high. Then a month later, after the chemotherapy, everything would crash; my platelet counts would crash, and my white blood cell count would crash. That's my immune system. It didn't make a lot of sense to me that no cancer cells were being chased around in there but good cells were dying. I wanted to build up my immune system, rather than tear it down.

I said, "If I were to stop today (which was actually two and a half cycles short of what was recommended), and I were to have a recurrence, would it be because I stopped taking chemotherapy?" The neurologist said, "Absolutely not. In fact, we really don't even know how much chemotherapy you should be getting. All we do know is that after six cycles we could start doing some damage to your other organs." After that, I said, "We're through today."

The other alarming thing about it is that I had asked the oncologist what I should be doing nutritionally, regarding supplements. The first oncologist said something strange, and I quote her: "I really don't think you should be taking supplements while you are on chemotherapy. The object is to make you sick." I thought the object was to make me well. I asked her to explain it further and she said that with the supplements I could be weakening the effectiveness of the chemotherapy by strengthening my cancer cells. I didn't follow. I had some problems with her and stopped going there.

I went to another oncologist who had no problem with me taking supplements. But in the end, when I was out in California I just decided to stop.

From the very beginning, when I was diagnosed in Barcelona, I began studying what the disease was and the little that was known about it. I started studying about nutrition because nobody could ever answer a question about what I should be eating and avoiding. My cousin had the same exact brain tumor at the same exact time that I did. She was in the same chemotherapy protocol that I was, and we were both given lists of foods to avoid. But our lists were very different. I asked the neurologist and oncologist about it. They didn't have an answer. I said, "I have a feeling that some people on chemotherapy call after a bad reaction. You ask them what food they've eaten and it ends up on that list." They said, "Yeah, I think that's what happens." At that point, I started not trusting conventional medicine.

I started to look at how my nutrition can help bolster my immune system and also how I could eat foods that would not detract from it or harm it. At first, I was doing it on my own. It was a long process of reading a lot of materials. I started reading about a lot of supplements and learned what vitamins and minerals are contained in which foods. I learned how much I would have to eat in order to get an amount that would be effective.

I actually did go to one doctor whose book I had read. I told him that I had gone on a strict organic foods diet and that I had quit all forms of caffeine and processed foods. He told me that the whole idea about organically grown food or food without pesticides or growth hormones or whatever is all a bunch of nonsense. He said his daughter and son grow their own food because they believe the same thing, but the stuff can't harm you. This man wrote a book about nutrition for chemotherapy patients. I became skeptical and didn't know if anyone knew anything about nutrition.

Fortunately, I ended up doing some volunteer work at a natural foods store, which happened to be the first collective or food co-op in San Francisco, years and years ago. I was educated well there by people who had been working there for 15 or 20 years. And also by a lot of people who shopped at the store, some of whom were writers. That's where I got my first quasi-professional advice.

Finally, last year I was able to secure some health insurance in New York. That's when I was told about Gary Null from a taxi driver. I went to see Gary. He found my case to be very interesting because I had just run the New York City Marathon. Part of my regimen for getting well was nutrition. I have a pretty strict diet. I seldom eat out; I prepare most of my food and buy only organically grown food. I pay attention to what kind of oils I use. He explained to me how some supplements can help me out. My metabolism really sped up as a result of training for a marathon. I was having a hard time keeping weight on. He introduced me to some products that would help balance my weight. I was complaining about a lack of energy. He said I was putting a lot of stress on my body and that a B complex would really help. The local health food stores have people who can also answer questions. They're pretty well informed.

I think the greatest testimony to nutrition being very helpful is that last week I had my five-year MRI, and it's fine.

Charles on chalazions and allergies

The specific problem I had was something called chalazions, which was something I would get on my eyelid. I had a history of getting these cysts for 14 years. I would try things like hot compresses. But they would often develop into infections. The doctors would give me antibiotics. When that didn't work, they had to be surgically removed, so I had about four or five surgeries. They were treating them, but they just weren't going away.

Imagine having to go to work like this. My eye would be partially closed. And I would be uncomfortable, even in pain sometimes.

It started getting worse. Not only would I get chalazions, but I would also have infections on the eyeball itself, for which they would give me topical antibiotic drops. Sometimes it would clear it up and sometimes it wouldn't. I wasn't getting any answers. All they told me was that it was related to stress and that I needed to calm down.

I picked up Gary's book, *No More Allergies,* and realized that this condition, along with many others that you wouldn't normally associate with an allergy, could be related to an allergen. After that, I went to see Dolores Perry, who told me to stay away from certain facial washes and scrubs that I was using.

She told me to use a specific type of soap and natural cream. More importantly, she told me to avoid wheat and a few other foods. She also told me to use aloe vera in the eye, which helped me tremendously. When I went to see her I was in the acute phase of another attack, and the aloe vera did a much better job of clearing it up than any antibiotic would have done.

Now, there is nothing wrong with either eye whatsoever. Before seeing Dolores, I had never gone for more than 30 days without redness in my right eye. But I have gone now for seven months with no problem. I think it was the wheat because once I stopped, my eye immediately cleared up.

At first, I found the change somewhat difficult because everything I was used to eating had wheat in it. But I learned how to go on a rotation diet and substitute other grains. One day I will eat spelt, the next day barley, and the next quinoa. For breakfast, I might have amaranth with bananas and peaches and coconut milk. There are just so many grains out there and so many wonderful dishes to prepare.

Since following this diet, I have noticed other changes in my health. By eating more complex carbohydrates versus refined carbohydrates, I find that I have a tremendous amount of energy.

Bob on hypoglycemia and lipoma

I became interested in nutrition about 20 years ago. After being an art dealer for 16 years, I had a mentor who got me involved in the health food industry. That led up to my present position of owning a vegetarian restaurant in New York City.

I had many personal miracles that helped my own health in the early days. I got into the field because I was suffering from the classic low blood sugar. I was having the usual mood swings. At the time I was smoking cigarettes and drinking black coffee. Slowly, I weaned myself away from all that and found out that a wonderful, steady energy came up which has stayed with me since.

About 10 months ago I had another personal miracle. We were constructing a restaurant, and working 16 to 18 hours a day. Suddenly, I felt some fatty tissue under my armpit. I had it diagnosed and it turned out to be a lipoma. End of story. It's gone. Completely vanished. As I speak to you, I am touching the area, and it's flat now. That I attribute to my own whole grain diet, which I have been eating for a year now. I've been eating tons of greens and no dairy.

I'm feeling fine now. I'm in my 50's but still dancing around like a 30-year-old.

Joy on increased energy

I just began eating vegetarian food and have noticed that my weight has begun to come down. I was quite lethargic before, but have much more energy now.

I am a nutritionist. I was counseling people and working many, many hours. I was exhausted. Then I started eating at a natural foods restaurant and noticed how good I was feeling. I would finish a meal and say, "Wow, I feel so good. I don't understand why." Then I figured out that it was the food that had been making me lethargic and the food that was making me more energetic than ever. It's amazing. I had an education in the field, and even graduated magna cum laude, but I had to experience the effects in my own body to really understand the power of the food.

Renata on polio and migraines

I had polio, many, many years ago, when I was 40. When it began, I was having terrible, terrible pains. My husband thought I had the flu and didn't call a doctor. When I got my head back, I called the doctor, who asked me to come in as soon as I could walk. But for about six weeks, I was completely bedridden. I couldn't walk at all.

In the meantime, I had dreadful pain and didn't know what to do about it. Everything ached. My older daughter worked in a health food store and told me to take calcium. I did and the pain immediately went away.

It took about three months before I could walk. And it took me the whole day to get dressed. To this day, it amazes me that anyone thought I had the flu. I was completely paralyzed. I couldn't even lift my head.

Somewhere in that period, I started reading Adele Davis and started taking the sorcerer's potion. It was her own mixture of lecithin, vitamin E, garlic, and a whole lot of other stuff. Then in 1975 I started going out to concerts again. To make a long story short, I met my soul mate at one. Then I wanted to live again and really started getting into life again.

Years later, after my mother died I had become depressed again. . . . My daughter always listens to Gary. She said to me, "You know, Mom. You really should go and see a nutritionist." So . . . I found a nutritionist and found me a new friend.

I have changed my diet. Of course the wheat is out. And coming from Germany, that wasn't easy. Germany has got the most wonderful breads, absolutely sublime. And to come here and eat spelt bread didn't exactly thrill me. But I don't get headaches anymore. I have had migraine headaches frequently. Barely a day would pass where I didn't have a headache. The headaches are now 99.99 percent gone. (If the weather changes I still get them.) She put me on a diet, starting off with watermelon. I have lost 20 pounds on it. It was wonderful because you can eat as much watermelon as you like. I'm on all sorts of supplements and they're doing something.

My joy for life is back.

John on malaria and rheumatoid arthritis

In the late 1970s, I was working as a war reporter, traveling with soldiers in a war zone for about 10 months, when I got very ill. My weight dropped from about 180 to 120 pounds from not having much food. I had been faithfully taking the prophylactic medicine that is supposed to prevent malaria the whole time. But we were in an area that was highly infested, and I came down with malaria.

At the time, I was out in the middle of nowhere. It was several months before I got to an area where they could do a blood test. At that point, you can't tell what type of malaria you've got. You have to diagnose it in the first couple of days.

About the third day, they gave me injections of the normal treatment. About two months later, I got back to Sudan where I was able to see a doctor and get blood tests. I was still very ill. My weight had dropped to 100 pounds. Every week, I would have three or four days of vomiting, high fevers, delirium, extreme muscle weakness, anemia, visual distortion. The medicine I was taking just wasn't working.

The doctors said it was no problem. They had injections for resistant strains, which was what I probably had. I took that treatment in Sudan and it didn't clear it up. I got to Egypt on the way home and got very ill the next week. I went to another doctor and he said the same thing. He said the medicine they gave me in Sudan was the normal backup, and usually does the trick, but when it doesn't, he has something else. Well, this went on and on. I went to Egypt, Lebanon, Rome, Paris, London, New York, back to a special hospital in London for tropical diseases. I went through seven different backup treatments. Each one promised to cure the malaria and didn't.

They finally said that there was nothing more they could do for me. My condition was so bad that they thought I would probably get black water fever and die. Or I would have a miracle where my body would just figure out how to solve it on its own. They said there was nothing more they could do.

I came back to New York, and lived for about 18 months like that. Every week, I would be extremely ill for about three or four days. Often, I would be in delirium.

One day, I met a painter who was working in my building. He saw me in the elevator and we talked for a few minutes. When he realized what my condition was, he said, "Come to my girlfriend's house, Friday night, eight o'clock, and I'll show you what to do." I was kind of startled. He said, "Just trust me."

I went. Turns out these people were into raw foods. It's the first time in my life that I had ever seen a juicer. They gave me a little book by Dick Gregory, and they explained fasting and cleansing. That night, they sent me home with a jar of juice, and instructions on what to do in the morning. They basically put me on raw juices for the next two weeks, a half a day on citrus juice, a half a day of vegetable juice.

For the first time in about 18 months, the malaria didn't come back. It didn't come back the first week, and it didn't come the second week. It hasn't returned since in 17 years. That's important because they tell you that malaria is something that always recurs. Once you get it, you never really get rid of it. It's never come back.

After those first two weeks of doing juices and taking enemas to help with side effects, I noticed that all types of other symptoms in my body were better. My hair looked better, my skin looked better. A lot of residual problems that I had from arthritis disappeared as well.

I had developed arthritis when I was 13 or 14, which left me with quite a few deformities. I had bumps on my hands and elbows. There was extensive calcification between all the vertebra. So, I had quite a limited range of motion. I noticed that all the stiffness felt much better. I mentioned it to them and asked if the treatment for the malaria could be helping the residual arthritic damage. They said that it definitely could, and advised me to stay on the program.

For the next two years, I ate a largely raw foods, vegetarian diet. And I did lots of fasting and cleansing. I did two fasts of 120 days, and four fasts of 90 days. About half of each year, I would be in a juice-fasting state. I would go through gallons in a day.

After two years, all the arthritic damage completely disappeared. A couple of times since then I have been x-rayed for injuries. Doctors always say that they don't believe that I had arthritis when I was younger. They say they know the disease and that I should be totally crippled by this point. They also point to the X-rays, saying that there should be evidence of it. But the arthritic damage is totally gone from the body.

As years have gone by, everybody comments that I look much younger than my age. Here I am at 47 now, and people are always guessing that I'm 10 years younger than that. Often people say, it must be my genes, but I have 10 younger brothers and sisters, most of whom eat a conventional meat and white flour diet. About half of them look older than I do. It's very clear to me that the main change is diet, eating really good, healthy food, and fasting and cleansing.

I also noticed that as I did this, especially the long fasts, my frame of mind really changed. I had been a depressive personality and had done therapy for that. I noticed that the longer I could stay on fresh, live, whole food, the better I felt. So, it really affected me from deep in the bones, to a consciousness, to my skin.

Dorothy on periodontal disease and other conditions

About two and a half years ago, I converted to a natural foods diet, and began to take vitamin supplements. I was always fatigued at that time and I was overweight. I had my allergies identified by blood tests, and I stopped eating those foods. At the same time, I began walking regularly for exercise.

Over a period of a few months, I lost about 25 pounds. I slept better, and I woke refreshed. I had much more energy. My digestion and elimination improved. Also, my cholesterol level dropped about 45 points, and my thinking became much clearer. I used to have vertical splits in some of my fingernails and I had cracks at the corners of my mouth, both of which indicated vitamin deficiency, and they're all gone now. The condition of my nails, my skin, and my hair improved, and I regained a pinker color in my cheeks and lips.

. . . Some years ago, I had several surgeries on my gums due to periodontal disease. I wasn't familiar at that time with nutritional approaches nor holistic dentistry. I also had several back teeth extracted at the same time because of the gum disease.

Since improving my diet, taking supplements, getting vitamin drips, my gums became much healthier. In fact, recently my dentist showed me x-rays that I had regrown bone partially in one part of my jaw and completely in another area. These had been two areas with very significant bone loss.

I suspect that had I been knowledgeable about nutrition and holistic dentistry at that time, I could have avoided the surgeries and not lost those teeth.

Overall, I am very pleased because I feel and look much better. I attribute these changes to eating natural foods, getting rid of alcohol and caffeine, and taking vitamin supplements. The vitamins and minerals particularly helpful for the gum disease were coenzyme Q10, vitamin C, vitamin E, calcium, and magnesium. I know that without nutritional changes, these improvements wouldn't have taken place.

Chris on athletics

I went to a nutritionist just to supplement my diet. I was a rower and I do a lot of in-line skating. I train fairly hard. I just wanted to make sure that I was getting everything that I needed in my daily intake of food. I went to a nutritionist, who gave me a great balance of supplements to my diet.

I sense that I am gradually discovering what my body needs and why I need to take these supplements in order to perform and just feel better during the day.

Ron on headaches and runny nose

My whole life I spent with tissues in my hand. Now there are no tissues, no runny nose, no headaches.

I learned more about nutrition and what my body needed in order to improve my whole life. I stopped eating dairy and animal products. After that, I had no more headaches, no more colds. I never get sick.

That made me feel so good that I'm out there helping others now. I opened up a group of organic health food stores and restaurants so that everyone else can eat as well as I do.

Oxygen Therapies

Oxygen therapies are extremely effective in treating a variety of conditions because oxygen creates optimal function in every cell in the body, whether it be muscle, bone, skin, or brain. Inside the cells, mitochondria become activated, and energy increases. Outside the tissues, oxygen mobilizes immune cells to engulf and kill foreign substances. In fact, harmful germs are less abundant in the presence of large amounts of oxygen.

Oxygen therapies are administered in several different ways. One is hyperbaric oxygen therapy. Hyperbaric, or high-pressure, oxygen first became popular in the United States in the 1920s and 1930s, when clinics with metal oxygen chambers were built, and people from around the world sought treatment. Despite its success, oxygen therapy was all but forgotten during World War II, when metals were used by the military to build submarines, rather than oxygen chambers.

Today most doctors are not schooled in the amazing benefits of high-pressure oxygen. But it has many vital uses. Hyperbaric oxygen can be given to treat diving accidents, carbon monoxide poisoning, gangrene, wounds that do not heal, and flesh-eating bacteria. The effects of serious injuries and strokes can be greatly minimized by this modality especially when it's used within the first 24 hours of the accident or stroke. It is excellent for overcoming viral problems, including chronic fatigue, HIV, and hepatitis B and C.

Intravenous peroxide therapy is another way the healing power of oxygen can be used. Many people know the benefits of applying peroxide externally. Some use it to brush their teeth and gums, for destroying harmful plaque. Others use it to dissolve wax in their ears. But it has other therapeutic uses as well. Complementary physicians administer small amounts of pharmaceutical-grade peroxide intravenously to supply extra oxygen to tissues and to kill germs throughout the body.

Ozone therapy is another way oxygen is used. Many regard ozone (O3) as the safest, most effective, and most promising treatment for a wide spectrum of diseases. The therapy has benefited numerous patients over the years and is widely used in Europe, as well as Cuba. Ten million patients have been treated with ozone in Germany alone since the early 60s. Unfortunately, it is currently illegal in most American states.

Medical ozone differs from the atmospheric type in that it is pure and concentrated. This is an important distinction because atmospheric ozone, produced from ultraviolet radiation, is combined with different nitrous oxide and sulfur dioxide products and is harmful. It is not used in medical practice.

There is a strong argument for its legalization. Consider that in Germany it is routinely used for treating hospital patients after every major operation. When small amounts of ozone are introduced into the bloodstream, it kills harmful microorganisms. This helps prevent secondary infections, which are a leading cause of death in the United States. It is estimated that between 10 and 50 thousand Americans die each year due to complications from postsurgical infections.

Not only does ozone kill microbes; it improves blood circulation. Hence, think of all the people with coronary heart disease, pulmonary disease, strokes, clogged arteries, diabetic neuropathy, intermittent claudication and gangrene who can be helped with this mode of treatment. Better circulation means more life-giving oxygen going to the body's tissues. Doctors report particular success with the different types of hepatitis, as well as with candida, allergies, and bladder infections. Other disorders treated with ozone therapy include herpes, arthritis, respiratory conditions, multiple sclerosis, sexually transmitted diseases, and parasitic conditions. Ozone is especially impressive in its effect on frequently debilitating conditions, such as AIDS, HIV, sickle cell anemia, and cancer.

Doctors administer ozone in several ways. A small amount of a patient's blood may be removed from a vein and a small amount of ozone added to the blood, which is then reinfused into the patient. This process, known as autohemotherapy (AHT), is used throughout Europe, where it is reported to have therapeutic value in circulatory disorders, viral diseases, and cancer. Tiny amounts of ozone can also be given to patients in the form of an enema in a process known as rectal insufflation. The mixture is absorbed into the blood through the intestines. Sometimes a plastic bag is placed over the area to be treated, and an ozone/oxygen mixture is pumped into the bag and absorbed into the body. This method is often used to treat skin diseases, diabetic foot problems, and gangrene. Ozone can also be used topically to treat burns. It accelerates wound healing, induces enzyme production, and activates immune system response. Additionally, there is a procedure known as polyatomic aphoresis, which uses O4 instead of O3. Proponents of this method report that it is highly effective, even in end-stage disease.

Healthy people can become more healthy using ozone to rejuvenate cells. Because ozone increases the effectiveness of the antioxidant enzyme system, which scavenges excess free radicals in the body, ozone therapy helps people stay younger longer.

Clinicians usually recommend ozone as part of a larger holistic protocol in the treatment of seriously ill patients. Dr. John Pittman, of North Carolina, explains: "I rarely give ozone treatments unless they are combined with some other supportive therapy. Admittedly, the shortcoming of doing this is that you don't always know which component is most beneficial. But I certainly know from experience which things generally help the most. Combining ozone with proper dietary therapies and addressing other cofactors, particularly in the GI tract, results in tremendous changes in a person's constitution. Their blood work can turn around, and it definitely can improve the quality and length of life."

Patient Stories

Richard on prostate cancer

Before discovering that I had prostate cancer, I had severe pains, especially during sexual relations. I was passing blood and had an awful time urinating. I went to see a specialist. After taking tests, he told me I had a solid cancer and that he needed to operate.

Fortunately, I learned through someone else about a doctor in Mexico. When I got to the clinic, my prostate count was 78. I began ozone treatments and after three weeks, my count was down to 37. I continued treatments at home and after six months, my count was down to zero.

I continue using ozone to this very day. I take it in different ways. I have an ozone machine, and I use it when taking a bath and I ozonate my drinking water as well. I use it a lot because I feel if I don't the cancer will come back.

Since my treatments, I feel better than I have felt in years. Now I can pass water without a problem. I can work and feel very well. I am more than pleased.

If it hadn't been for the ozone treatments, I wouldn't be here today because that cancer would have had me. Surgery would have done no good.

Brian on viral infections

I first found out about ozone from Ed McCabe who directed me to a conference in South Carolina which, in turn, directed me to a conference in Germany. There, I learned first-hand, from the people who had been using this method the longest, how it should be done. I learned about major auto-hemotherapy.

The reason that I did this is because I am a nurse. I got a needle stick from a patient who was infected with HIV, Epstein-Barr, CMV, hepatitis B and C, and several other things, and became very sick within months. I had night sweats, severe diarrhea, and I lost a lot of weight. I couldn't live that way and wanted to be healthy, so I started ozone treatments.

I had 16 treatments over a period of six weeks. By the end of that time, my health was back to normal. I was gaining weight, feeling better, and my symptoms were disappearing. My T-cell counts did some amazing things. At my lowest point, it had dropped down to 371. Two weeks after the ozone treatments, I was tested again and they went up to 671. They more than doubled.

I'm excellent today. I have no symptomatology at all, no night sweats, and no more weight problem. I am very physically active and able to enjoy life. I actually feel better than at the time I got the needle stick. My health is excellent.

I couldn't have done it without the ozone. That's what made the difference. I tried vitamin C therapy for a while and that helped, but I still had the chronic diarrhea four or five times a day, and I still had the weight loss from not being able to keep food down. Then I started the ozone therapy and that brought me back to normal health.

Angelo on colorectal cancer with metastases to the liver

I was feeling tired every day and coming home to take a nap in the afternoon. That wasn't me. I had been a real active person all my life. My wife suggested that I take a blood test to see if anything was wrong. I did and my doctor found that my blood was low. He suggested that I wait another week before taking another test, which I did. My blood was still low so he suggested a colonoscopy. I went and had it done. The colonoscopy found a tumor in my colon. I had it operated on and taken out. The surgeon told me that he successfully removed it and that there was no more cancer there.

About three months later, I had a CT scan done that found spots on my liver. The cancer had metastasized to my liver. I received chemotherapy treatments for approximately six months. After the first set of treatments, another test was taken which found that the chemotherapy hadn't done any good. I continued with the chemotherapy for another three months. When that didn't help, the doctor said that there was nothing more he could do for me. I asked if I should continue with the chemo or just sit and die. He shrugged his shoulders as if to say there was nothing more he could do for me. I asked the doctor how much time he thought I had and he said three to four months.

My son, who was there with me, had heard about a holistic program at Santa Monica Hospital utilizing ozone and vitamin therapy. He said I should take the treatments there, and I did. I received treatments for 21 days. They asked me to wait for eight weeks before having a CT scan. When I finally took the CT scan, the radiologist called my doctor and told him that he had never read a CT scan like mine before. It showed that the cancer cells in my liver had become capsulized. That prevented them from spreading.

The cancer cells have remained encapsulated and I've been in remission for a year and a half. There is no question about it. The ozone treatment saved my life. In fact, I have so much faith in it now that I plan on going there every year and a half just to make sure that it stays that way.

Philip on chronic active hepatitis B

It was a long process getting diagnosed. I had flulike symptoms, diarrhea and fever, and was not feeling well at all. They initially diagnosed it as arthritis. Finally, a rheumatologist thought to do liver work. He did a liver biopsy, and it came back chronic active hepatitis B.

They suggested interferon. . . . That only had a 40 percent efficacy. I had heard a program on vitamin C drips and began with that. I decided to go further. I started ozone treatments. Once I started that, my liver SGPT came down dramatically. I am waiting today to get results and hoping to hear that it has cleared up entirely.

Jane on breast cancer

I was diagnosed in 1989 with breast cancer, for which I had a modified radical mastectomy. I had numerous surgeries before that time as well. I wasn't really having any life at that point in time. I was a sick person waiting to die. They had cut out some of the cancer but I wasn't well. A friend of mine finally advised me not to have any more of those treatments because they were killing me.

I had the book *Third Opinion*, which had something in it about Dr. Donsbach. I called Santa Monica Hospital and went down there. I was astounded by the humaneness at Santa Monica Hospital. In other hospitals, I had some negative experiences where I felt totally robbed of all dignity and where I was treated like a specimen.

Santa Monica had a program that I could tolerate. I had decided that I was not going to have any more cutting, any more radiation, or any more chemo. There would be no more invasive procedures.

The first week I felt really, really sick because I was detoxifying from all the chemicals in my system. I had been on 10 different medications for multiple problems. Besides cancer, I had ulcers, asthma, everything you could possibly imagine. The cancer had set off a systems reaction and I was having problems in every part of my body.

After about the tenth day, I started to feel like getting out of bed. I began to participate in the therapies and started beach walks. I continued to get better and better.

I have been there six or seven times because I had some tumors in the other breast as well. I received ozone, hyperthermia, and thymus injections.

I don't have any tumors now. Most of all I have a life. I work full-time and I play an active role in the lives of my granddaughter and daughters. I am able to go to church. I participate in library programs. I walk on the beach every day. I follow my program.

I learned some things in the hospital that I need to be real careful with. Santa Monica Hospital will be the first place I go to if I begin developing symptoms. I don't think I will, though. I think I'm cured.

Charles on prostate cancer

I had a needle biopsy roughly a year ago which indicated prostate cancer. I never believed in the orthodox approach and sought another method of treatment. Finally, I decided that I would go to Mexico and get treatment which was not available in the United States. After doing a certain amount of research and checking with other people, I decided the Donsbach clinic in Rosarita Beach was the best place to go. I had been familiar with Dr. Donsbach for a number of years and felt that he offered the best options.

I feel that the treatment has been very satisfactory. At present, my prostate has substantially improved. I'm not free of cancer yet nor was there any promise that I would be that quickly. I am on continuing outpatient care. But I feel it has most definitely made a difference. The PSA, for example, has dropped very substantially, which is probably the best measure of prostate cancer. I certainly feel a great deal better than when I first went to Rosarita Beach.

Madge on arthritis

In 1993, I had been in the hospital five times. I had severe pain in my legs and excruciating pain in my back. In addition, I had fever, sweats, and tachycardia. I would go to the hospital and they would send me home not knowing what was wrong. They said that the next time I came back they would do exploratory surgery just to find out what was wrong.

In the meantime, I found out about Dr. Donsbach and went to Santa Monica Hospital for a month. When I left I had to be helped onto the plane. I came back a month later turning cartwheels. A miracle happened to me and I wanted everyone to know.

So now, I'm fine. I seldom take anything for pain. I dance three times a week and play tennis. I was ice skating and broke my shoulder, which gave me a little setback, but I'm getting better now. I believe the ozone insufflations saved my life and that Santa Monica Hospital is a fantastic place.

Debbie on Hodgkin's Disease

I got sick in December 1985. At that time, I had a lump in my neck, which the doctors removed. They diagnosed me as having Hodgkin's disease and gave me radiation treatments. They radiated me from the chin area to the breast area for six weeks and from the breast area to the pelvic area for another six weeks. After that, they told me I needed to come back every three months for a chest x-ray.

About eight months later, they found a tumor on my lung and said that I needed chemotherapy. I got chemo for a year and a half. A year and two or three months later, the tumor started to grow while taking the chemotherapy. They had to change my chemo twice.

They didn't know what to do anymore so they sent me to the Mayo Clinic in Minnesota. There, they said that the only thing I could do was get a bone marrow transplant. That was in February 1988. For three months, I was given massive doses of chemotherapy to prepare for the transplant. That's when terrible things began to happen. I had seizures for three months straight and had to remain in the hospital all that time. I couldn't walk anymore and was like a zombie. They damaged my right hand with chemotherapy and I could no longer use it.

My husband and I finally met with the doctor. When he walked into the room, he wouldn't look at us. We knew that something was definitely wrong. He finally said, I'm sorry, but due to the shape your body is in, you'll never live through this bone marrow transplant. I started to cry. I said, "You guys said this is the only thing left to save my life. What am I supposed to do? I'm only 30 years old and I thought I had a little more time left." I had two small kids at home.

My husband heard about a hospital in Mexico but I couldn't believe that they could do something in Mexico that they couldn't do here. Being brought up in the Midwest, you think that if your doctor can't help you, you can go to the Mayo Clinic. If the Mayo Clinic can't do it for you, that's it.

On our way home from the Mayo Clinic I listened to the tape that my husband had on oxygen therapy. It just sounded too simple. I thought I was doomed.

My husband continued to stay excited about all of this material that he found. He even went to the library to do more research on oxygen therapies. He kept bringing these things home for me to read and I kept telling him that he was crazy.

Finally, one day, I was sitting at home having a pity party for myself. My mother called and advised me to go. She said that I had tried every avenue possible and that she didn't believe they were going to hurt me.

I finally agreed to go to Mexico. We went there in September 1988 and stayed for three weeks. During that time, I had hydrogen peroxide, DMSO, multiple vitamins, ozone, a lot of different therapies. I was always afraid that doing this would make me sick, like the chemo and radiation, so I would finish my treatment and go back to my room. I would lay down expecting to get sick but I never did.

Instead, I got back on my feet. After my therapies, I would walk on the beach with my husband. I felt that I was on a vacation instead of in a hospital. I also was put on a machine that helped with my hand and arm that was numb from the chemo. The feeling, which had been gone for over a year, started to come back. My hair started to grow. I was up and around and not laying around in bed feeling like I was sick and dying. That was back in 1988.

When I came home, I continued to stay on a home program. I would go back to my doctor every six weeks, then every three months, then every six months. Now I go once a year. A year after I was at the hospital, I had scans and blood work. I had been on medical disability while I was getting ready for the bone marrow transplant and had been out of work for a year and a half. After the scans, my doctor said that he couldn't keep me on disability any longer. He couldn't see any tumor growth. He said I was doing fine and that I could go back to work.

It's been six and a half years now and I'm doing great. I feel wonderful and my blood chemistries are completely normal. If not for the treatments, I might have had a year left. I believe that I was dying from the treatment, not the cancer. The seizures were secondary to the massive doses of chemotherapy.

Harold (medical doctor) on circulatory problems and ulcers

I had very bad circulation in my legs, especially varicosities. My legs were very swollen, especially on the left side. I also noticed that they were increasingly discolored and becoming bluish. At times, I had cramping in my calves and legs and I would feel coldness there. It was very, very painful. I also had an ulcer. Nothing was helping and everyone was saying I couldn't do anything about it. One time, my leg was all blown up. I went to a surgeon because I wanted him to drain it but he would not touch it.

I started to take large amounts of vitamins A, C, and E, but that didn't help me. I thought there must be some other answer. I heard about ozone and I started to go to a physician for it. First, my ulcer healed. Then, the pain in my legs gradually began to go away. I started to feel warmth in my feet and the discoloration started to leave.

Now, I am able to walk better. I used to limp and I don't limp anymore. I don't have the pains like someone is crushing my ankle with a noose. I have very good circulation there and I feel like I almost can run. I was even playing a little bit of basketball with my son the other day. I am beginning to get the feeling and strength back in my legs. My energy has also increased tremendously and my clarity of thinking is much better than before.

I have also seen other patients who were very ill. Some of them had hepatitis. The physician, knowing that I am a physician, showed me their lab values and I was astonished to see how much they changed. I could also see improvement in their appearance. When they first came in, they looked half dead. After a few weeks, they left with improved color and energy. There were also tremendous decreases in the enzymes of these patients.

I myself am doing very, very well with this. I want to continue this and I am looking into doing it myself, as I feel that people should have this treatment readily available. I am always, of course, afraid of someone coming down on me, like the FDA, but I feel that if I can do it for myself, why shouldn't I be allowed to do it for others?

Preston on hepatitis

In February of this year, I was very sick. I was about 60 percent bedridden and barely able to function. The liver specialist I was seeing essentially told me that he was at the end of his rope. He said there was no hope for me and that he could perhaps help to keep me alive until some miracle cure appeared. That was February 28.

On March 9, I began ozone therapy twice a week. Within six weeks, my enzyme levels had dropped dramatically. Other blood scores also improved. More important, my quality of life improved immeasurably. I was able to actually get on an airplane and take a three-day business trip to California in the early part of May.

When I went to see my liver specialist again, he did not accept the improvement. He looked at the blood scores and said that it didn't show anything. The analogy he used was "the bees are in the hives," meaning that the virus was still there but not visible. I got the impression that he would be happiest if I died. If I want my insurance company to pay for my blood test, I have to have them ordered by one of their approved physicians. I continue to have only as much contact with that doctor as I need to for insurance purposes.

Gay on colon cancer

I was diagnosed with colon cancer in 1989. After they gave me 18 months to live, I opted to find other alternatives and did so. I never received standard treatments even though they wanted to do surgery and chemotherapy.

Right now, I'm sitting on an IV of hydrogen peroxide with DMSO and all kinds of supplements and vitamins. That, along with a good diet and the help of a good friend, has gotten me this far. According to their predictions, I should have been dead in 1991 by the latest. In 1991, I made my second visit to the Hospital Santa Monica in Rosarita Beach.

Now I am in remission. When I am checked by the M.D.'s they are amazed.

I have no more cancer in my colon. I have literally passed tumors through the rectum. The latest test showed that I have no tumors.

Ricardo on chronic active hepatitis

In 1990, I was diagnosed with hepatitis C and cirrhosis of the liver. I went to a specialist at one of the biggest hospitals in the city. He put me on alpha interferon for six months and told me that if that didn't help, nothing would.

After that, I started researching milk thistle and other remedies for the cirrhosis but I didn't really know what to do for the hepatitis. I drank a lot of fluids to try to flush it but I was basically ignorant.

In March of this year, I had an attack and was hospitalized for five weeks. They told me that I needed a liver transplant and that the cirrhosis was running rampant throughout my body.

I heard about ozone therapy and was wondering how to get it. A neighbor called and I found out that it has been available in this country.

I've been taking it since May and what it has done for me is unbelievable. When I came home from the hospital, I was lethargic and did nothing but sleep. I started treatment on May 4 and took blood tests that same day. My bilirubin count was 12.4. That Tuesday, on May 9, I went to my gastroenterologist and took another blood test. In those five days, my bilirubin fell from 12.4 to 9.42. I'll take another blood test in June again.

I feel like I'm coming back and I believe the ozone has made a difference. I've been able to stop taking all the medications I was on which were causing my liver to become inflamed. I was on five different medications and they weren't doing anything for me.

Now, I'm out and about. I'm even wrestling. I don't even take a nap during the day. My appetite has returned, which is conducive to getting better. I really believe in this thing and I'm going to stick with it because I don't want to go under that knife.

John on foot infection

I started getting direct injections of ozone in February. Just two injections of 5 cc of ozone eliminated the infection I had been fighting for months.

Before that, I had orthodox physicians who wanted me to go on massive doses of antibiotics, who were worried about my foot having to come off because I am diabetic. I took antibiotics for a little while and they were doing nothing. I did some hydrogen peroxide, which was helping to get it under control.

But ozone is what really did it. It totally eliminated the problem. The infection is no longer in my foot. I don't feel pain from it anymore. I can now start working on rehabilitating my leg.

Qi Gong

Qi gong translates from the Chinese as energy cultivating. It is a system of refining, purifying, circulating, and storing energy. Over time, the practice yields many benefits. Health challenges are overcome as positive energy is mentally and physically directed to all systems via meditation, posture, breathing, and relaxation. As blockages are released and abundant energy flows freely, body systems rebalance, stamina improves, and the manifestation of illness disappears.

Qi gong is an integral part of Eastern cultures where several styles are practiced; many forms have been developed by different lineages and handed down from teacher to student since before recorded history. In China, the value of qi gong is acknowledged by the medical establishment. But the practice is largely unknown to Westerners, as information about it has been largely unavailable and highly esoteric. Recently, with the availability of more and more understandable information in books and classes, many Americans are turning to qi gong, and finding that it improves the overall quality of their lives.

Patient Stories

Octavio on nervous disorder

This year, I was very, very bad, and in the hospital because I had nervousness, depression, and paralysis on part of my face, which the doctors called Bell's palsy. My condition was very severe.

After that, I started to do qi gong, and began to feel better and better. In five days the Bell's palsy disappeared. Now I practice almost every day. It's really fantastic. I recommend qi gong to everybody, especially for stress.

Bob on eye disease

A year and a half ago, I developed a rare eye disease called ischemic optic neuropathy. This is a swelling of the optic nerves that progressed quite rapidly.

Each day for two weeks, I would wake up and see less than I had the day before, with the potential of blindness. I had nearly exhausted all the medical assistance that I could get. I had seen some neural ophthalmologists, and I had been to Will's Eye Hospital twice in Philadelphia. I was given little hope. They knew very little about the disease, but they knew the outcome.

I spoke to a friend in Hawaii and he suggested I see a qi gong master. . . . I needed someone to go with me that day because I couldn't see well enough to bring myself down there and back.

What he did was quite remarkable. The first thing he did was diagnose me by looking at me. Through an interpreter, he described that I had a swollen optic nerve and said that he would work on it. What he did with a series of movements around me is he extracted the bad energy (qi) from that area and implanted good qi. He literally reached out with his hand as if he was grasping something very close to my eye and he would pull it away. He would do this any number of times. Then he would hold his hand up to the sky and reach down. It looked like he was pushing energy into my eye. He also gave me some herbs.

I had had a previous doctor's appointment the very next morning with one of the neuro-optomologists I was seeing. She said, "Bob, you have turned the corner on this. The nerve has stopped swelling. It will not get worse even though there is not much chance of it getting better." I continued seeing Master Lee for several months, sometimes two or three times a week. I also contacted a client of mine who taught me qi gong. It's a movement like yoga only there is no stretch involved. I went to see him and I did it on my own. And I learned how to harness that energy and bring it into my eyes and body.

I love happy endings and this is one. Today I am able to drive, read, and work on my computer with no difficulty at all. I do wear glasses, but you would never suspect for a moment that I had had this problem. It took just three to six months to see significant improvement and as I continue to bring qi into my eyes, they continue to heal.

Miriam on joint problems, fatigue, and partial hearing loss

I've had a lot of problems with my joints—chronic aches and pains in my wrist, knees, and elbows. I have been doing the movement form of qi gong since September and find that it increases my circulation, which helps the joint pain clear up faster. It generates a lot more energy because I've also had a lot of problems with constant fatigue. It basically irons out all the kinks in my body so that the energy flows a lot easier. It also gives me a sense of emotional well-being from stress. I tend to be able to deal with my emotional problems in a much more balanced, easy way.

I have been dabbling with energetic healing work and I have taken a couple of introductory courses on that. I never really felt anything, even though you are supposed to feel energy emanating from your hands. I imagined that I felt it but never really felt it in a strong way. Over a period of time from doing qi gong, I have developed a strong sense of energy emanating from my hands, which was really interesting.

One more thing that came as a result was the correction of a blockage in my right ear. I had a partial hearing loss and there was a lot of sloshing around of liquids and stuff. From doing the work and using the energy that I was able to generate from my hands and placing that over my right ear, I was able to start to heal myself in my right ear. Now the blockage has pretty much cleared and the hearing has returned.

In addition to qi gong there are other things I do as well. I see a chiropractor and I take super blue-green algae and I do Feldenkrais movement techniques. All this has contributed to a more energetic and healthy me.

Dan on stomach cramps and anger

I started learning qi gong about two years ago. I learned to feel the energy movement in my body and to accept that everything is energy-based.

This weekend I had some stomach cramps. I went through an affirmation and breathing and was able to shift energy in myself. I found it very effective. The first thing I do is to realize that it's energy-based. I raise my awareness and accept whatever is going on instead of judging it. I tell myself, "Whatever emotion this is I accept it." Then I state my intent, which is to heal and shift this energy. Sometimes I tap into an anger there and am able to move it. Along with mental focus is breathing, which is the physical aspect.

Whenever I get angry, qi gong helps me to shift away from that state. I have learned not to get involved with it because I see that it is energy in motion. First I had to feel it and actually experience it in my body to get it mentally. Practicing the qi gong, I kept saying, "This is energy. This is energy." Then when I felt the shift in my body, my forehead got hot or all of a sudden I had tingling in my hands, and I wasn't really doing anything to facilitate that. But all of a sudden I was sweating and really not moving. When I really started experiencing qi gong physically, that's when it started clicking in.

Another example is where a store clerk gave me the wrong change the other day. It was just a few cents difference. Normally I am a calm person but all of a sudden I became upset and ended up walking out. Standing outside the store, I did my breathing. The first thing I did was to say, "Okay, I'm emotionally upset right now. And for me to confront or throw anger at the person wouldn't be useful to me or to them." I realized I was upset so my awareness went up. Then I moved to acceptance by saying, "I'm allowed to be really angry. Anger is not bad. It's just an emotion." I did my breathing and I continued mentally saying, "It's okay. I'm allowed to do this." And then I released this energy. I stood and I may have put my hands on my stomach or on my heart chakra, just to say, "It's okay, it's safe," and to bring in the energy and state the intent to release this anger coming up without judgment. Or if I am in judgment, saying, "It's bad to be angry," I accept my anger and accept whatever is coming up as I state my intent to release it. I say that I don't choose to hold onto it anymore, without a lot of stuff behind it, like making myself wrong. That, along with the nice, slow breathing made me feel just fine. I looked around and I said, "It's a nice, sunny day." As soon as I noticed that, I knew that I had shifted the energy.

There is no one right method. A lot of what you do is intuitive. Sometimes I will go to a qi gong class and start the exercises and then be physically exhausted. I will sit in the back and do a meditation and work with the energy as it is coming up with me. Sometimes I will need to do the movements. It's different every time. There is no pat answer. It's learning to tune into me. It's learning also the acceptance and stating my intent. That's what qi gong is.

Diane on thyroid cancer

I had radical neck surgery for a thyroid cancer six years ago. Of course, that entailed the loss of half of my left, upper shoulder muscle and the musculature on that side of my neck.

Now I have no cancer left in my body. I have maintained myself very well. But one of the residual things I was left with was some nerve loss, which made me feel very off balance. Of course, I had a shoulder slump on the left side of my body because of the loss of muscle. I was very upset about it and went to physical therapy. I knew there was a good deal that was not going to return to me.

I had taken hatha yoga many years ago and I thought that I would go back to that, but discovered that because of the loss of musculature that I couldn't do any of the inverted poses. Just by chance, I walked into a qi gong class. I started to go and realized after about a month and a half that my balance was returning. The discomfort that I was feeling on my left shoulder was subsiding. Any time I have a problem with it, if I just go through some very basic qi gong exercises, I have relief for a good period of time.

What I think happens to me is I tense up and get myself blocked. This side is much more vulnerable because of the real physical blocks from the surgery. What the qi gong has allowed me to do is find new nerve endings, a new way to connect with the loss and to compensate. It's a very accepting process.

Barbara on insomnia

I had sleeping problems for years. I had a pretty significant sleep disorder and I was diagnosed as having a chronic sleep disorder, etiology unknown. I went to neurologists, psychologists, psychiatrists, internal medicine doctors, even a specialist in the field of psychopharmacology (it cost $500 an hour). But I was desperate. At one point I was awake for six weeks. I tried many different Western medications, but they only exacerbated the problem. I never got any relief. I went to sleep disorder clinics and was wired up with all kinds of machines. But no one was ever able to help me.

I tried several acupuncture doctors and finally hit upon one in Rhode Island who also used diet and Chinese medicine and herbs along with acupuncture. He was the one who told me about qi gong. I went to a conference at his insistence. He said that this would be the thing that would really cure me. So I went to the qi gong conference in Boston and met a qi gong master. I practiced the qi gong there.

It really helped when I went to the prescription seminar that he held during his conference. He was able to give me a prescription for Chinese herbs which I had filled in Chinatown. It's probably about 27 Chinese herbs and it comes in a big, brown paper bag. A certain amount of each herb is measured out for my particular prescription. I take it home and boil it in water for a period of 15 to 20 minutes, each time straining the water off. I have been drinking the tea since about November and I have not had a problem sleeping since that time. I have since decreased my tea intake and now only take it as necessary. I, for one, am a firm believer in qi gong and Chinese herbs.

Vicki on becoming centered

I learned qi gong about a year ago on the recommendation of a friend. I had practiced tai chi about 15 years ago for quite some time, but found the form quite complex, and didn't stick with it to learn it well. I became drawn to qi gong because you could learn the form in a much shorter period of time.

Mostly I take classes where I work with other students. I will practice parts of the form at home as well. I find that it helps me to become more centered, more clear about wherever I am at that time, more clear in myself, whether that means realizing that I am tired and need to rest or that I need to make a decision. The practice facilitates a sense of wholeness, which is very important.

Allison on centering

Last year, I learned the eight routines of soaring crane qi gong in a class. I find it to be a very useful technique for centering myself. I think it also gives improvement flexibility and tone. The centering is very important because it helps you pull energy in and blend your own energy with what's out there in the world. There's not a line delineating you from the outside world, which I find very helpful. It helps me move through life a little easier.

I use qi gong as a way of starting my day and as a way of getting my body warmed up. It also helps me to deal with whatever projects I have on hand. I am an actress, so I often use qi gong prior to a performance. I find that even using one or two of the routines in the soaring crane method helps me to generate my own internal energy and to have greater focus. Because it's a standing meditation, I don't space out. I actually keep a very sharp focus and the energy just sort of flows. Because of that, I feel energized and very clear. My mind is no longer a jumble. I benefit a lot from it.

Bob on relaxation from stress

I have been helped by qi gong in a lot of ways. It really helps me to relax after a stressful day of work. It gives me greater stamina for physical activities. The list goes on and on. More specifically, after doing qi going, I find that I am in a certain relaxed state and that I have a very clear thought process. It allows me to approach my work with new energy and insights. So it's very helpful in that way.

The benefits are difficult to put into words because the effects are personal. It is something that allows me to really relax.

Reconstructive Therapy

This little-known therapy has great potential for healing painful joint conditions, even after other modalities have failed. Reconstructive therapy actually builds new joints, ligaments, and tendons. By doing so, it gets to the root of the problem and provides freedom from pain.

Our bones and muscles can place undue stress on our ligaments, tendons, and cartilage. Joints in the knees, ankles, neck, wrists, and elbows and the entire spine, can become damaged as a result. Sometimes people are born with joint weaknesses; their joints are loose and unstable, causing them to be hypermobile or double-jointed. Reconstructive therapy helps either scenario by creating tighter joints. Ligaments become larger, stronger, and attach more firmly to bone.

During the course of treatment, low doses of nutritional substances are injected into the ligaments. The exact nutrients given differ, depending upon the needs of the area involved. These agents stimulate a slight irritation that promotes healing. New blood vessels grow into the area. More blood means greater oxygen and nutrients. Tissues heal as fibroblast growth factor puts more fibroblasts and collagen into the ligament, tendon and cartilage. As a result, ligaments become stronger, and better able to hold vertebrae and joints in place. This, in turn, eliminates pain.

Reconstruction therapy differs markedly from the conventional approach, which addresses symptoms only. Usually, doctors begin by giving anti-inflammatory medications, which only help temporarily. These drugs cause inflammation of the GI tract, and inhibit collagen formation, which prevents true healing. The next step is often exercise or physiotherapy. If that does not work, cortisone shots are given. Next in line is an arthroscopy or mini-surgery. Then more cortisone and more anti-inflammatory treatments may be given. Finally, joints are replaced. The person gets a new knee or hip. Or a laminectomy may be performed to remove a disk from the neck or low-back area. This type of operation adversely affects structure, and makes the person weaker and more prone to pain.

With reconstructive therapy, by contrast, ligaments actually strengthen and results are permanent. This therapy is used to treat any number of musculoskeletal conditions, including low back pain, arthritis, bursitis, carpal tunnel syndrome, disk problems, sciatica, tendinitis, frozen shoulder, and athletic injuries. Reconstructive joint therapy is also useful for people with torn ligaments and cartilage problems. Candidates for treatment are people on anti-inflammatory drugs, such as aspirin, cortisone, Motrin, and Naprosyn. Also people who have joint sounds—grinding, pops or clicks—when they move their neck or knee may benefit. This technique is also for people who continue to go to chiropractors because they can't stay in alignment, as well as for people who feel worse with exercise, and people who have undergone surgery. People who are not candidates for reconstructive therapy are those who have a marked impairment in their immune system. This includes those with cancer and AIDS.

A big advantage to the treatment, as opposed to surgery, is that there is no down time after treatment. A person can return to work immediately. Also, there is an amazingly high success rate: 88 percent of patients respond, and the results are permanent.

Patient Stories

Al on knee injury

Approximately eight months ago, I suffered a fall which resulted in a completely severed, interior cruciate ligament, several other partially torn ligaments, and injury to the medial meniscus. Within three to four weeks of that injury, I came to Dr. Calapai for reconstructive therapy injections into the area. This resulted in almost immediate relief of terrible, severe pain.

Now my knee is almost normal. As a matter of fact, a result of having a completely severed interior cruciate ligament is that one can no longer straighten out the knee unless one has surgery to sew the interior cruciate back together. Miraculously, after a number of reconstructive therapy injections, I can almost completely straighten out my knee without any surgery whatsoever.

George on back injury

I have been in construction all my life, and somewhere along the line, I injured my back, although I didn't realize it until I started getting aches up the back of my left leg. I heard about reconstructive therapy, so I started getting treatments for my back. Then I treated my hip, knee, and shoulder. All these areas improved and feel great at present.

Ann on sprained ankle

Over a period of years, I sprained and resprained my ankles. I tried lots of therapies, including massage and orthotics, but nothing helped.

Then I came to Dr. Calapai, who diagnosed me as having hypermobility of the joints. He treated my ankles with reconstructive therapy. Now I am able to participate in most activities without pain or stress. The podiatrist said he never saw anybody heal so fast. He called me his phenomenon.

Terri on arthritis

For years, I have been suffering with arthritis, and have been in severe pain most of the time. It really put a damper on my life.

Then I discovered reconstructive therapy. I'm starting to walk normally again, and there is a tremendous relief from pain. I'm looking forward to a complete cure. I'm 60 percent there already.

Reflexology

Reflexology is an ancient technique based on the premise that there are reflex points on the feet and hands that correspond to every muscle, nerve, organ, gland, and bone in the body. Pressing on these points breaks up congestion and helps the nerves to relax. This, in turn, reduces vascular constriction so that the blood and nerves flow more freely. As circulation improves, toxins are released.

There are roughly 7200 nerves in each foot. When the body becomes imbalanced, through the course of daily living, nerve impulses can become blocked. This means that nerve impulses to the muscles, organs and glands of the body are impeded to some extent. Reflexology stimulates nerve endings and starts up nerve communication. Reflexology also promotes endorphin release, enhancing one's sense of well-being.

The treatment can be performed by a therapist or it can be self-administered. There are several books on the subject, as well as workshops and courses that offer certification. After learning the basics, a person begins treatments with gentle finger pressure. Tenderness means there is a problem in the area corresponding to the reflex point. After resting for a day or two, the area can be reworked again. In time, there will be less tenderness as the problem heals.

Practitioners of this modality assert that performing reflexology once a week can catch most problems early and quicken recovery. This is because reflexology gets the circulation flowing so that the processes of nutrient absorption and waste elimination are improved. This is not to say that reflexology is a panacea. If symptoms are serious or prolonged, a doctor should be consulted.

Patient Story

Rochelle on ulcerative colitis

A while ago, I was in a bookstore, and I saw Laura Norman's book, *Feet First.* I read it through and it sounded very interesting. I decided that this might be something I should try, so I started seeing Laura.

After some months I started to notice some positive changes. My colitis symptoms abated—the diarrhea and bleeding have completely stopped—and I believe that reflexology has been a very, very important factor in accomplishing that. Laura also helped me to change my diet. All this has opened up my life magnificently. This has been the most positive step I have ever taken for myself.

I continue to get reflexology weekly. It helps to keep me healthy. It helps to reduce my stress levels, which I think is a factor in ulcerative colitis.

Reiki

Reiki is the Japanese word for universal life force. It is an ancient hands-on healing modality originally developed by the Tibetans and rediscovered by the Japanese in the 19th century. During treatments, energy is channeled and amplified from the universal life force through the Reiki practitioner to the client for the revitalization of body, mind, and spirit. Reiki can also be self-administered. By releasing physical and emotional blockages, and increasing energy, Reiki promotes total relaxation, which, in turn, enhances the body's ability to recover from stress and injuries.

Reiki is easy to learn and relaxing to both practitioner and recipient. It is usually taught in a one-day workshop where a Reiki master performs a series of attunements on students. Once the four upper energy centers, known as chakras, are opened, the student can channel energy.

Reiki can facilitate healing in a variety of circumstances. It works, practitioners explain, on the principle that the body recognizes this universal life energy and uses it to promote balance and total health.

Patient Stories

Nilsa Vergara on her clients's experiences

My first example is a 59-year-old woman, who came to our healing circle feeling old and tired. She suffered from aches and severe pain in her neck and knee from car accidents. She was also going through job changes, and her relationship with her adult son was estranged.

Each week, she received a 15-minute session and quickly began feeling better. She released a lot of emotional toxins via crying and verbal expression of what she was feeling. She decided to take a Reiki class so that she could give herself daily treatments.

Within a month, her changes were quite dramatic. She had a tremendous increase in energy and vigor. She told me she now feels like she is 28 years old.

With the Reiki, she now has very little pain. She feels emotional and vital. Her attitude has changed. She feels self-fulfilled and in control of her life. Her relationship with her son has greatly improved. To quote her, she says, "I feel like my whole life is as it should be."

As far as other modalities, she takes vitamin supplementation, food-grade hydrogen peroxide in her water to help oxygenate the body, and is about to receive acupuncture for her neck.

My next client is a 65-year-old woman. When she first came to see us, she was depressed. She had been in therapy for years but nothing seemed to lift the depression. She felt tired all the time and would catch colds easily. Emotionally, she felt like a victim, and others treated her as one.

After her first 15-minute session she felt immediately better. She knew that something powerful was happening. She returned and eventually studied Reiki. Today, she reports feeling much healthier. She has more energy and an optimistic outlook. She no longer feels like a victim and if anyone tries to put her in that role, she is no longer afraid to set limits. In addition, she is much better able to tolerate the cold weather, which indicates that her body has improved its oxygen intake.

My next client is a 60-year-old woman, who was feeling emotionally devastated when she first came to our healing circle. She had had cancer on her vocal cords, for which she received radiation therapy. Even though she was told that she was cured, she was still feeling pretty awful. She had lost her job and was feeling hopeless.

She had Reiki for five months and took a class. Now she feels totally different. Her hope has been renewed and she feels empowered. She is picking up a better sense of who she is internally. Her identity is not tied up with her job. She also has gotten better at eliminating physical toxins as well as people who tend to use her. On the physical side she had had a back problem with one of her disks, which she says is improving with Reiki. She says that Reiki has been a wonderful discovery for her.

This woman has an 83-year-old mom who fell and broke her hip bone as well as the bone in her wrist and arm. She decided to give her mother Reiki regularly and her mother responded quite well. She began feeling stronger and stronger. Within four weeks, she was out of her cast, walking with just the aid of a cane, and not a walker. This is pretty remarkable for an 83-year-old, because having a broken hip does not always hold a good prognosis. So, as you can see, Reiki really enhances the body's ability to recuperate.

A 45-year-old woman was diagnosed with lymphatic cancer in December 1994. She was feeling disconnected from herself, and working at a job that she hated. She had been given chemotherapy, which made her lungs less elastic. Then, she was given steroids to increase the flexibility in her lungs.

She heard about the healing circle, and she came to us in August 1995. She received 15-minute sessions about three times a month. Reiki was the first alternative healing method she ever tried.

She feels that Reiki helped her to reconnect with her inner self. It also helped her to slow down and not be such a hassled A-type personality. She is starting to pay much more attention to herself. Becoming conscious and aware of the self is one of the most important parts of healing. She is also more aware of her breath. She is beginning to investigate additional modalities, such as diet, exercise, and food supplements.

My next client is a 53-year-old woman who had some serious memory problems. Her thinking was scattered, she was fearful and guilt-ridden, and she was estranged from her adult children.

I recommended Reiki to her to see if we could work through some of these emotional blockages and change these negative patterns. She took a Reiki class. Six months later, her memory improved tremendously. She was much more focused in her thinking and her job performance improved greatly. She became more insightful, much less fearful. Now she can speak with her adult children, set limits, and no longer feel anxious and guilt-ridden. In addition to using Reiki, she uses herbal teas for detoxification, drinks vegetable juices, fasts, and gets colonics.

An 83-year-old friend of hers was terminally ill. He was suffering from severe respiratory problems and had been hospitalized. He was in intensive care for two weeks. After leaving the IC unit, she gave him Reiki every day for a week. A nurse who was observing her commented that the patient who had been agitated, miserable, and in a great deal of pain became quiet, peaceful, and pain-free. The nurse told her, "Please, whatever you are doing, keep on doing it." He passed on very peacefully.

Reiki is very effective in helping those who are close to death by releasing pain and fears. My client felt a great sense of empowerment that she could do something for him to ease his passage and to connect with him in a very caring way.

Rolfing

Rolfing is a bodywork technique that aims to realign the body through deep work on soft tissue and fascia surrounding muscles. The premise behind Rolfing is that people lose symmetry between the right/left and back/front planes of their bodies, and that these discrepancies get worse with time, and result in dysfunctions. Rolfing works to reduce these discrepancies. Also, people tend to lose touch with their natural centers of gravity, which Rolfing works to correct so that standing and moving become more comfortable and efficient.

Once structural changes are made, the system works to improve itself. Treatments follow a pattern and a whole series is usually 10 sessions long. Every part of the body is addressed, not just the area that hurts, so that lasting changes can be made. Sessions vary according to individual needs. And effects are cumulative. With each session, resultant changes last longer and longer. An aspect of this practice is that Rolfers often help clients improve their work habits, e.g., the way they sit at a desk or work on a computer, in order to ensure long-lasting health.

Patient Stories

Elizabeth on body trauma

When I was two years old, I had bad pneumonia and I was in the hospital for about three months. I just about died. As a result of that, my body had a lot of trauma. I was very weak when I was growing up. I had a collapsed chest and rounded shoulders.

Initially, I started to go for Rolfing at age 20. Then I met Beth a bit later. Although I had 10 different Rolfers work on me, when I started working with Beth, it was the first time that I really started to experience a lot of changes. At the same time, I was working with some equestrian instructors, trying to make some progress riding. It was a marvelous thing to be able to work with Beth while I was also working at this new physical skill, learning to jump horses. We worked a great deal with my hips and the rotation in my femurs, the rotation in my legs, also with the chest and shoulders, and a great deal with my back. Her work is hands directly on the body, going deep into the tissue, doing basically the Rolfing movements.

I found it to be extremely helpful. I found that I was able to move out of movement patterns and go into using my arms and legs in ways I could never do before. My coordination increased a great deal as well.

Jeanne on lack of flexibility

I had gone for several years without an enormous amount of exercise. I had some pain in my lower back. And basically, the problem was that I was very stiff. I had some tendinitis and some problems with my knees. I started to work with a personal trainer, but my flexibility was really awful.

I had known about Rolfing for a long time. I remembered reading about it long ago. I saw Beth's name in a magazine that listed practitioners so I called her.

I have had eight sessions with her now. The first session, she worked all over my body. Then she did my lower legs, my knees, my hamstrings, my shoulders, my back, even my head actually. Some of the changes have been really dramatic. There have been dramatic increases in the flexibility in my legs. When my trainer and I stretched out after a session of work on my hamstrings, I got a 3- or 4-inch increase in the stretch in my legs. The week after that, she did my lower leg, and the alignment of my knee changed dramatically. I normally was knock-kneed. When I bent my leg, my knee went out over the arch of my foot. It now tracked straight over my toe, which is where it is supposed to be. That hasn't changed back since I have been going to her. I had very tight trapezius muscles around my neck. Since Beth has been working with them, they have notably started to relax down. I don't have the bulging around my neck that I used to have. The changes have been dramatic and beyond what I expected to have happened.

Shiatsu

Shiatsu is a Japanese system of bodywork that translates to mean finger pressure. During treatment, various degrees of pressure are used to balance energy along energy pathways (meridians) of the body. Different styles of shiatsu use varying degrees of pressure.

Shiatsu is both a diagnostic tool and a method of treatment. Practitioners diagnose from the abdomen, where centers representing each of the meridians are present. During a typical session, a client will come in and give the therapist an idea of how he or she is feeling physically and emotionally. The person then lies down on a floor mat or a massage table, with clothing on. The session begins with palpations to the abdomen to feel energy imbalances. Then the therapist works different meridians throughout the entire body that correspond with imbalances in the abdomen. Shiatsu practitioners look for tsubos along the meridians; this refers to points that either have too little or too much energy. By applying a certain type of pressure, shiatsu either brings energy to those points or disperses energy, thereby bringing the body into greater harmony. In sum, the therapist's role is to observe the way energy moves in the body and to guide energy to make the shift toward greater balance. At the end of a session, the therapist will once again palpate the abdomen to see if any changes have been made.

Shiatsu realizes that each person is a unique entity; therefore, different people with the same symptoms may respond differently to a session. Some people will experience great benefit right away while others will need several sessions in order to feel better.

Shiatsu is similar to acupuncture in that it works with meridian systems; however, the main difference is the use of hands and finger pressure in the first therapy, and the use of needles in the latter. Shiatsu is also less concerned with specific points and more involved with the whole meridian. Shiatsu is even more dissimilar to Western allopathic medicine, since shiatsu is a holistic, noninvasive therapy. Also, shiatsu realizes that getting ill is a process and that getting well must take time, whereas Western medicine often takes a quick-fix, silver-bullet approach.

Patient Stories

George on hypertension and emphysema

My wife was at a bookstore in Greenwich where she saw Ken giving someone a partial treatment. She was impressed by his talk and by what he did, and thought it might be good for me. So three years ago I went to see him. Shiatsu helped me in so many ways that I just continued.

In general, I feel much, much better. Ken has a technique of working on the lungs to increase their capacity. I also become more relaxed, which helps the blood pressure go down for a while.

I find Ken a truly sincere guy who cares about how you feel, unlike a doctor who can't get you out of his office fast enough. I look forward to my weekly shiatsu sessions. It makes me feel good in many, many ways. My wife tells me I look better, which makes me feel better too. My blood pressure went down, but not enough to get off medication, although my dosage is lower than it was. My breathing capacity is much improved, too. I'd recommend it for everyone.

Lilly on stress

My desire for shiatsu was not due to any medical condition; I just carry a lot of stress in my body. I work in the television business, which is stressful and has long hours. I went for shiatsu hoping to alleviate some of the stress so that I wouldn't feel so tense. I began to go once every 12 days.

The first time I went, I honestly didn't notice anything. I also happened to have a cold and was really out of it. The third time and the remaining times, I began to feel much more relaxed throughout my whole body. It's not just relaxation, like regular massage; this really works on the meridian points in the system. After this, I felt less fractured. I felt like my head and my body were connected and I was calm and relaxed. But it wasn't as though I was sleepy. It was as if all the energy was flowing better throughout my whole system.

Now, I don't carry tension in my body in the same way. If I was under a lot of tension, I would hold it from my neck down. With the bodywork, I don't carry it there. It really releases the stress in my back. My body is a lot more aligned.

Tai Chi Chuan

Tai chi chuan, usually called tai chi, is a Chinese martial art and meditation that combines a choreographed series of slow movements with mental concentration and coordinated breathing. Practitioners learn how to align their bodies with gravity, which creates a profound sense of relaxation that benefits the individual on all levels: physically, emotionally, mentally, and spiritually.

On a physical level, tai chi improves health as gentle movements massage internal organs and enhance their functioning. This deepens breathing and gets more blood and energy flowing throughout the whole body. One way in which tai chi helps circulation is through shifts in weight. With each posture, the weight of the body alternates between the right and left side, causing the leg muscles to contract and expand. That helps pump blood back up into the heart, making tai chi a wonderful practice for people with heart disease. Tai chi also increases joint flexibility, making it an excellent practice for arthritics. Also, by aligning the body with gravity, tai chi helps the spine straighten, which alleviates tension, especially in the lower back. This is why many chiropractors and other doctors who deal with pain recommend tai chi to their patients. Many other conditions can be ameliorated in that tai chi releases stress, and most diseases have a stress component.

Tai chi can provide greater emotional stability and a better sense of self. When you practice this art, everything slows down and you see your life in a different perspective. Tai chi allows people to see the big picture, to step away from anxieties and irritations, immersing themselves instead in something quiet and slow. Breathing deeply fosters relaxation as well.

People who practice tai chi report that as the mind becomes balanced with the emotional and physical centers in the body, it stops dominating their awareness with plans, calculations, details, decisions, and worries. As greater awareness moves into the body, the mind empties and calms down enough so that clearer thinking prevails.

On a spiritual level, tai chi can be a beautiful meditation in movement that takes you on a journey of self-discovery. It helps people to improve awareness and let go of blocks. As one works in silence, the spirit has the opportunity to open up and grow.

Finally, tai chi can be used as a nonaggressive form of self-defense. When one can relax in the face of danger, one becomes more alert and better able to deal with whatever is happening in the moment. Tai chi teaches practitioners how to overcome muscular strength with softness. So, without resisting or running away you learn to yield to incoming forces by listening and interpreting energy rather than opposing or fighting it. This is called cultivating strength through softness.

Patient Stories

Carol on Crohn's disease

My condition hasn't gone away, but tai chi is one of the things that helps me to manage it and reduce stress without any toxic side effects. I can't say whether or not there is a physical difference in my intestines before and after beginning tai chi. I can only tell you that my experience of it is that the complete concentration that it takes to do the form helps to get rid of all the junk in my head. It gives me a vacation from concern. Tai chi is one of the things I do in my life where I'm not aware of myself every second as a person with an illness. That's a tremendous gift.

Christiana on aggression

I was introduced to tai chi by a Chinese friend of mine about a year ago. We were talking about the meaning of suffering, violence, and aggression and I told her that I didn't want to react to aggression with aggression because I believe that gets you stuck in a vicious circle. Physical violence doesn't happen every day, but verbal violence is something that concerns me a lot. I was looking for a way to get out of that.

My friend does tai chi and he introduced me to a form. I realized there was something more there than just intellectual knowledge. There was something that went through his whole being. That fascinated me because it showed me a side of him I had never seen before. It was so serene and serious and deeply human that I yearned to have this experience myself also.

Since starting tai chi, I accept life more and I live more through my body than my intellect. It has also influenced my body posture. I realized that I used to often carry my shoulders up and now I am able to relax them. Just because of that, my presence has changed, and people react differently towards me. I have become more aware of my surrounding. I watch animals and children more, and they are more dear to me now, because I realize that they are doing tai chi all day long. They have this basic life force in them, and I am trying to learn from them. Tai chi has brought more spirituality into the most ordinary things, for instance house cleaning, and being with strangers on the subway.

Eric on creativity

I am a creative artist who was in a certain space when I was being creative, and I wanted to have that feeling of creativity more throughout my life. What I found with tai chi was that it allowed me to have creativity in my everyday actions. So, I went from a place I was creative for short periods of time in my artwork to a place where everything I did became connected. Tai chi is a moving meditation. When you meditate, you see yourself more clearly; there's more energy available. Doing tai chi in a group helps you become more aware of energy. You can feel everyone moving together, even if you are not seeing them. You become very aware of everyone being connected. That feeling stays with you after class, when you go outside.

Vitamin Drips

A vitamin infusion usually combines measured amounts of vitamin C, with other nutrients such as B-complex vitamins and botanicals, to improve the immune system and overall functioning. Much higher dosages of vitamins are absorbed intravenously than orally. Optimal vitamin dosages help reverse many serious conditions, including AIDS, cancer, and chronic fatigue syndrome. Well people benefit from the therapy in that it keeps the body functioning at its best.

Patient Stories

Mildred on fractured nose

My problem started on New Year's Day 1994 when I skidded on some ice coming home from work. As I was stopping for a light, I hit a tree head-on. I had multiple bruises but my main injury was a nasal septic fracture, telescope septum, a deep vertical laceration, and a piece of the nose was just gone. The fracture was so comminuted that the doctor had to press the splinted pieces of bone in place. It was probably the only time in my life I was glad I had a big nose.

The surgeon had one other patient in his practice with a similar injury. He didn't mention the outcome or follow-up treatment, but he did say that if the integrity of the cartilage was compromised that it could be replaced with a synthetic material. That didn't sit too well with me. It put up a signal for me to do something more aggressive.

I did get some supplementation. I got some collagen, homeopathic medicine, and magnets, but somehow I felt I could do more.

Then I saw Dr. Robbins for a podiatric routine examination. He suggested that vitamin C therapy could help. . . . I've continued on a fairly steady basis with a hiatus of about six months. I have resumed treatment and am now up to about 100,000 units.

It was during my last visit that the doctor showed me photos of my face right after the accident. It was swollen and deformed. He seemed somewhat pleased and surprised at my progress and took follow-up pictures.

I really think that he didn't want to frighten me earlier on but is now confident enough to show me the earlier pictures because he feels that the healing process is sufficiently on its way. I really feel that a miracle happened. The scaring is hardly visible, which I wasn't even concerned about. It can be smoothed out in the office next visit and there will be no visible signs of the accident.

Sam on mercury poisoning

I had a car accident and chipped my tooth. This was just before the New York City marathon. I ran the marathon and was absolutely drained.

I went to a holistic dentist, Eli Stern, and discovered that I had mercury in my mouth which was weakening my immune system. I was very surprised.

I gradually had the mercury removed. After each dental visit, I would have chelation therapy to get the mercury out of my body. Then I would take 100,000 mg of vitamin C and other nutrients in a drip to build my immune system. I did this religiously three days a week for a month.

I think it is important for athletes to know that silver amalgam fillings are draining to the immune system.

I plan to continue taking vitamin C drips after races to keep my immune system 100 percent strong and to make sure that nothing weakens my immune system and that no illnesses happen. This is one way that I can do it.

Marisa on HIV, cytomegalovirus, Epstein-Barr virus, and herpes 6

I didn't know I was in such serious shape. I thought I just had colds. The cold that I had prior to taking the drips stayed with me for about a month and I was very sick with it. I was totally nonfunctional, but I thought it was just a cold.

I watched a program on alternative medicine and called up to make an appointment. I went to Dr. Calapai who put me on a diet and vitamin C drips. The protocol he put me on called for drips three times a week in the beginning. I could feel my body getting a lot stronger. It didn't stop me from getting colds but if I got a cold, it did not stop me from being able to function.

He also took a blood test. My blood work showed that I had CMV, EBV, and herpes 6. After a series of vitamin C drips, all of these decreased to normal levels. I am definitely an advocate of alternative medicine and vitamin C drips. I think everybody should take them, especially those of us who get a "death sentence" when they are HIV-positive. To me it is more of a wake-up call to take care of your body.

I feel great today. I have two jobs and take care of my three-year-old son. My son is also HIV-positive. I can't give him drips but I do give him large amounts of vitamin C. As a result, he is very stable. I don't want the doctors to suggest that he go on anything. So far, they are very pleased with his blood work. One day, the nurse said to me that his health is nutritionally related. He hasn't dropped down and doesn't need to go on any toxic drugs.

I have preached about vitamin C drips to quite a few friends. A very close friend of mine did not go the alternative route. She chose to take AZT, DDI, and some other toxic drug, and has since died.

When I went to Dr. Calapai, I met a friend there. When I first met her, they literally carried her in. She was like a stick. She has been taking the drips and has since moved into her own apartment. She takes care of her daughter, is working at a job, and is in excellent health now.

Aaron on asthma

I started taking vitamin C drips almost a year ago. At first, I was very consistent and would go about three times a week. Then due to business, I went less consistently but as often as possible. I began to notice improvement immediately. As the dosage increased, so did the improvement.

I can't say that I've cured asthma yet, although I believe I will. I have had a lot more relief. In general, I have a lot more energy. Specifically, regarding the asthma, I don't have as many attacks as I used to have, and the severity of the attacks is much less than it used to be. That alone has been tremendous. It's a great change and a real important part of my life. I believe in the vitamin C drips and continue with it, as well as an improved diet and exercise.

Lynn on chronic fatigue syndrome

Chronic fatigue syndrome is a nightmare. You have viral symptoms, swollen glands, mental confusion, memory loss, paranoia, and no one in the medical profession knows how to help you.

Fortunately, I had a holistic physician in 1986 who diagnosed it and started me on low-level IV vitamin C drips. I followed that protocol for a few years and it helped to stabilize me. I was able to continue working at a reduced level.

Because my immune system was so compromised, on a trip to Mexico, I ended up picking up three parasites and candida in one fell swoop. My doctor had me on Flagyl for two years, and that debilitated me even more. Eventually, he didn't know what to do for me. I developed a terrible cough and was continually coughing green phlegm. My muscles were so sore that it felt like I had broken my ribs on three different occasions.

I came to the Healing Center in March 1993. That's when I tested positive for four viruses. Before I didn't even know what I had other than chronic fatigue immune dysfunction. The doctors started me on an IV vitamin C protocol. The vitamin C drip also included glutathione, liquid vitamin A, and glycyrrhiza. I continued the drips three times a week. At first I received 100,000 mg and eventually worked up to 200,000 mg because I wasn't really getting that much better on the lower dosage. I was functioning but I still had colds. Without the higher dosage, I would still be sick today. There is no doubt in my mind about that.

I also take [supplements]. I eat organic vegetarian foods. I took ozone a few times. I had the silver removed from my teeth. I took colloidal silver, which helped my pneumonia tremendously.

After almost two years of drips, I definitely feel significantly better. The virus has abated or been reduced. I no longer have swollen glands, mental confusion, skin funguses, body aches, or arthritis. My pneumonia is minor. Now, instead of having colds for two to three months, they last only a few days. I am mentally clear and much more productive. I'm a happy person and I'm able to exercise three times a week, as I was prior to this illness.

The male ego in the medical establishment is very frustrating to work with. When I first told my physician about the vitamin C/glutathione therapy, he screamed at me. He said I was crazy and that the treatment was dangerous. As I said, if it weren't for the 200,000-mg IV vitamin C program with all the extra things in it, I'd still be sick today. There's no doubt in my mind about that. . . .

Toni on Epstein-Barr virus

I was a very energetic person until six months ago. Then I could hardly walk to my chiropractor's office, which is about a mile away. I told her that I was extremely tired and she did a blood test. Epstein-Barr showed up.

The regular medical establishment just doesn't want to deal with it because EBV has such a mishmash of symptoms. You have a sore throat, a stiff neck, tiredness, swollen feet, diarrhea, and muscle aches. They tell you that you are just working too much or that you have the flu and need antibiotics. They basically ignore you because they don't want to deal with it.

Then I heard you talking about a doctor at the Healing Center. I went to him and got a very thorough blood test which demonstrated four viruses, not just the Epstein-Barr.

He started me on vitamin C drips with the glutathione. I didn't have an immediate result. I got disgusted with it and almost decided to quit. I stayed with the treatments and am glad that I did. By the time I hit 100,000 units I started to feel great. It was like a light switch going on. I had 15 symptoms and 80 percent of them are totally gone. The remaining symptoms are alleviated. I am almost 100 percent back to normal. It's just wonderful.

One pleasing effect is how dramatically my skin improved. I'm 48 years old and beginning to get lines and wrinkles like everyone does. The lines around my mouth, which had started to appear, totally disappeared from the treatments. My skin is as soft as a baby's skin.

Ethyl on metastatic breast cancer

I was originally diagnosed in November 1987. Since that time, it spread to my bones and liver. I was on chemotherapy for two years, on and off, and was experiencing tremendous fatigue during and after chemotherapy. I had reactions where I had sores in my mouth, bleeding in my nose, and general malaise.

Since starting direct ozone and vitamin drips, I have no more bleeding, no more sores, and no fatigue.

The last time I was in the hospital for chemotherapy, my doctor said to me, "We'll probably have to give you a tranfusion." I replied, "I don't think you're right." He did some blood work and then told me that I was much stronger than he had thought I was.

I really feel a tremendous, tremendous difference. I can't wait until tomorrow to get my vitamin C drip because it is very healing for me. When I start getting ozone next week, I'm going to be a new person.

Patients Speak Out on Cancer Therapies that Work

To demonstrate the power of natural approaches to healing cancer, this section offers firsthand accounts of people who have used them. Approaches to treatment vary, but one factor remains constant: these people, who had life-threatening illnesses, are now alive and well.

714-X[1]

Susan on son's Hodgkin's disease

Last summer, Billy was diagnosed with Hodgkin's disease. We didn't know any better so we went with chemotherapy. Billy had five treatments from August until October. Although he did fairly well compared to some people, he did have the typical side effects. He got nauseous and tired, he lost his hair, and he had some jaw pain. His main concern with the chemotherapy was that it was poisonous. He would look at the drugs dripping into his body and realize how toxic they were. That, in a nutshell, is why he ran away.

When we started to talk about using other forms of treatment, the doctors began to use scare tactics on us. They told us that Billy would die if he went off chemotherapy and they described to Billy, in detail, exactly how he would die. They said that in addition to the chemotherapy, Billy would have to have radiation at the end of the treatment program. Billy refused any more treatment.

We were contacted by many people about many therapies. One of these people, Charles Pixley of Writers and Research in Rochester, New York, told us about a therapy called 714-X. Initially, he sent us a booklet about the treatment. Eventually, Billy, my husband, and I, decided to use it. That was in January and he has since flourished. His cancer is gone. Last December, he was tested and there was some cancer at that point. In March, he was tested

[1]Author interview with patients, 6/12/95

again and the cancer was totally gone. He continues with the treatment. They recommend a six month minimum treatment. We're almost at the end of that.

Billy is flourishing with this therapy. His hair has come back. He has gained weight. He has grown. He is like a vacuum cleaner as far as his appetite goes. He is a very active young man. He loves skateboarding, and skateboards every day if the weather permits.

The doctors who originally said he would have been dead more or less pat us on the back and say, that's nice. Instead of expressing an interest, they tried to force us into continuing with chemotherapy by reporting us to the Department of Social Services. However, no action was ever taken and we were able to pursue the treatment of our choice.

I have informed the media about our story in an attempt to get on national TV again. I want to tell them about 714-X and where to get it because we get hundreds of calls from people all over who have searched for it. The media is apparently afraid because they all appear interested when I call them but I never hear back from them.

Harry on massive tumor outside the colon

I was given six months to a year to live. The surgeon said for me to live it up, eat and do anything I wanted to do. He sent me to the oncologist who told me that they could give me treatments but that I had about a 15-percent chance of being helped, and even if I was helped, the treatments would only increase my longevity by a couple of months. I was discouraged with that so I made some trips to Mexico to study various alternative treatment approaches. Then I got a newsletter from a friend of mine about 714-X and I decided to try it because it was something I felt I could continue on.

My son gave me the injections, which were painless. We followed this program for six months. The total program consisted of 168 shots. Right after I started taking the 714-X I felt better. I feel just fine now.

When I started on this program, my son turned my way of living around 180 degrees. He prepared an organic diet for me. I cut out alcohol and cut down on cigar smoking to one in the morning and one at night.

Since then, I have felt much better than I have in years. The 714-X stimulated my immune system back to normal.

I went back to my doctor two years later and was given a colonoscopy and some other tests. Tests showed that the tumor had not enlarged and that the growth had stopped. It became dormant. The oncologist wanted to see me, I guess, out of curiosity. He told me that I have a 60-percent better chance of survival. He said that, eventually, the tumor will shrink and then disappear.

Rick on leukemia

At first, I tried chemotherapy, but it failed to work five times. After each treatment I would experience a relapse because my leukemia was so aggressive. I was working on my next option, a bone marrow transplant. Iowa City had a few matches for me. The first one they tested was almost a perfect match so I went in and had the transplant done. They gave me a 5-percent chance of actually making it through the transplant. Even if I made it through the transplant, I only had another 5-percent chance of cure. I survived the transplant but, three months later, my blood tests were really bad. My platelets never did recover completely.

I continued looking for answers. I was very familiar with Reich's technology and felt strongly that something along those lines could help me. The only problem was that nobody was using or dealing with this technology.

I had a live cell blood analysis done, which tells you more than a CBC or any test given in conventional medicine. According to my test, it was obvious that I was relapsing from the transplant. My relapse wasn't documented by conventional medicine but, of course, they don't use this method so it doesn't matter. I knew and other people knew.

Eventually, I found a group that was duplicating what Reich did with his ray tube. I found this machine, got the 714-X again, and went back on these alternative therapies. Three weeks after getting this machine and getting back on the 714-X, my blood counts, every single one of them, returned to within the normal range. It was amazing. Everybody was astounded by it. I don't know what to attribute it to but I do know that something helped me. I had my transplant in January 1994. I relapsed around April, and here it is May 1995. I've had normal blood tests ever since.

Combination Therapies and Lifestyle Changes[2]

Ed on prostate cancer

I had a radical prostatectomy. Afterwards, my PSA kept going up. It got to 9.1. They thought it would be in the lymph nodes and they wanted to do chemo and radiation. At that point, I was pretty disgusted.

I wanted to try some alternative approaches. I went for hypnotherapy . . . I also started working with a dietitian to change my diet. I started eating whole foods: fruits, vegetables, foods that weren't processed. I ate more organic foods.

This was a big change for me because I was brought up on meat and potatoes. It was also difficult for me because I grew up not liking vegetables. As a

[2]Author interview with patients 6/21/95

child, my mother forced us to eat what was on our plates, which included spinach and Brussels sprouts and broccoli and I didn't even like being in the same room as a Brussels sprout. So, I had a lot of changing to do.

I also started Essiac tea. When I started on the tea and the diet, it started moving my PSA down. It's down to 0.1 now, the normal range. I feel as healthy as a horse.

Cathy on stage IV Hodgkin's disease

I was in such bad shape that I couldn't lay down or walk. There was fluid in my lungs and tumors around my heart, which advanced into my abdomen. I had been on chemotherapy for about 10 months. At first, the chemo got me back on my feet but after a while it stopped working. That's when the doctors recommended a bone marrow transplant. They said it was my only hope for long-term survival.

At that point, I simply could not tolerate any more chemotherapy and the thought of a bone marrow transplant was out of the question. I had heard about 714-X from a very well-respected physician in British Columbia and I decided to start it. At the same time, I began to follow a holistic program.

I made quite a few changes. I always thought that I had a healthy lifestyle but I learned that, in fact, it really wasn't. I started doing everything that I could do to strengthen my immune system. That included a completely chemical-free lifestyle and an organic diet, with no white sugar or flour and very little dairy. The little dairy that I did have was unpasteurized and organic. I also had a lot of fresh vegetable juice and used only distilled water. I was also very careful about using chemical-free skin and hair products and about avoiding toxins such as household cleaners and pesticides. Along with that, I was on a very strict detoxification program which included cell cleanses, gallbladder flushes, and coffee enemas. I exercised using a trampoline and took pancreatic enzymes and glandulars that were specifically prescribed for me by a holistic physician. All together, it did the trick, and now I'm completely clear.

I began to notice improvement two to three weeks into the program. My energy level increased and I had less pain. The best way to describe it is to say that I started to feel like my old self again. Two months after starting the 714-X, I had a CT scan done and it showed marked improvement so I knew I was on the right track. I was very excited. On my latest scan, which I just had last month, it showed that there was no sign of disease at all. I feel wonderful.

The most important thing is to have hope no matter what your physician tells you. You have to believe that there is more out there. You can fight for your life. I did and it worked. It's just a matter of getting the right information. I think it's important to get information from both the medical side as well as the holistic side and find out what is best for you and what you believe in. Then go for it. Put everything into it that you can and it will work.

Orville on lymphoma that had metastasized

I am 66 years old and had always enjoyed good health until two years ago when a bump appeared over my right temple. It started growing fast and was about the size of a marble. It was removed and I was told that I had aggressive non-Hodgkin's small cell lymphoma.

I was interested in alternative medicine and that's the route I took. First, I went to Mexico for treatment and it disappeared in about three weeks. I thought that was fantastic since I had arrived with cancer all over my body.

A few months later it began to appear again. I went to Dr. Michael Schachter's clinic in Suffern, New York. After a couple of weeks of treatments there, it vanished again.

Then it came back a third time, months later. At one point, the cancer got as large as a golf ball on my jawbone. It was pulling at my cheek and I could hardly talk or swallow. It was just a bad-looking thing and a bad-feeling thing, and it caused me a lot of pain.

This time I combined the therapy Dr. Schacter had me on with homeopathy. Basically, the therapies I used included eating organic foods and adding such things as laetrile, shark cartilage, homeopathic remedies, and a well planned, well thought out vitamin and mineral program.

The bottom line is, it worked. Utilizing all the different therapies made the cancer shrink and vanish. My medical records show that it disappeared in two months and 11 days. That was little over a year ago. Any time I get an examination, everything is clean. I don't seem to have any sign of cancer. There is nothing like the alternative way of treating cancer.

Lucinda on advanced breast cancer

I had severe breast cancer that metastasized to my ribs and throughout my whole spine. My prognosis was poor. Basically, I was told there was nothing they could do for me. Still, they wanted to try by putting me through the trauma of chemo and radiation even though it wasn't going to cure me. It could only possibly prolong my life a little bit. I refused treatment and they just sent me home to die with a box full of drugs.

Something inside of me said, no, wait a minute, I choose not to do this. There's some other reason I'm supposed to be here. Through the grace of God, or the universe giving me another chance, I was put in contact with a clinic down in Mexico called Genesis West. I went down in a wheelchair on just about every drug you could possibly name. I was totally nonfunctional, mentally and physically.

In the clinic, I received a wide variety of treatments. A few of them involved ozone therapy and hyperthermia. Of course, diet and supplementation to build the immune system were used. The whole basis of this is that the body is built to repair itself and that it has that capability.

I came back a total fighter. Now I'm walking, talking, and living my life completely and fully. I'm fighting every day and I'm determined to beat this.

The change is nothing short of miraculous. In fact, the medical doctors are amazed. Of course, they don't want to admit it but it's real concrete proof for them. I haven't gone in for any tests, like bone scan or MRI or anything like that yet but they look at me and can see that I'm clear-eyed, walking, and functioning. Nobody can tell anything is wrong with me. Obviously, something I'm doing is working.

This experience has been a blessing for me. I want people to know that they have a lot more power and control within themselves than they know and they need to learn that because there is always hope. You've got to always keep fighting if that's what you want.

Leslie on metastatic breast cancer

I have been treated at Dr. Schacter's office for a little over a year. I came from Sloan Kettering in Manhattan where I was treated with radiation and chemotherapy. I was there for nine months. None of those treatments worked and the cancer kept spreading. It finally spread to my liver and I was given six months to live.

When I came to see Dr. Schacter, I was in pretty bad shape. When I started on his oral supplements, and later on his IV supplements, I started to get better. At the same time, I cut out dairy products and red meat and increased my intake of fresh fruits and vegetables. I made sure that I had no refined foods or sugar. If I did have something it would be from the organic food shelf rather than from a fast food chain. I started juicing and that gave me a tremendous lift in energy. My body was telling me that it was very happy. That was a turning point for me in knowing how important nutrition is in battling cancer.

I started to lose the cancer from my body. The tumor markers improved and I started gaining weight. I had much more energy. At this point in time, my blood tests are back to normal. If you looked at me, you would not know I was a cancer patient.

What happened to me is amazing. I feel that it was a combination of the right treatments for me and a lot of prayer, creative visualization, and meditation. I continue to live that way now.

Essiac Tea[3]

Marilyn on breast cancer

My husband brought home an article out of the newspaper about Essiac tea just before I had my lymph nodes removed. They figured for sure that the lymph nodes were invaded with it. I started on this tea 10 days before going back into the hospital. I went in and the lymph nodes and the rest of the surrounding tissues were clean. Three specialists were very surprised and kept remarking what a miracle it was because of the stage III cancer that had already broken free of the tumor and was already invading the rest of the breast.

Although I opted for a traditional approach to treatment, I attribute the lack of hair loss and the ability to handle radiation and chemotherapy without side effects to the benefits of the tea. I feel wonderful today. I've got a new lease on life. I drink the Essiac tea twice a day faithfully. This has been two years now.

Lynette on bone cancer

The prognosis was really bad. I went to see a bunch of specialists and they basically all said the same thing: If I lived I wouldn't want to because everything was just disintegrating. It was a big old mess and I wasn't real happy because I wasn't able to get any answers.

I went to the health food store and started reading different books and talking to some people. That's how I learned about Essiac tea. I was kind of skeptical but got a number to find out what the deal was on this tea. I spoke to someone who told me that she had come across an all-natural herbal tea that doesn't affect any other medication that you're on. I said, what the heck. I'll try it.

At the time, I could barely walk. I have total shoulder replacements and a hip replacement. They tried doing bone grafts but that didn't take. The disease was in my ankles, wrists, and knees. They wanted to do knee replacement surgery on me. In my situation, there is no stopping the disease and there is no treatment for it. What they do is cut out the dead bone and try to put metal in there. I'm basically all bionic.

When I started taking the tea, I could barely walk. I was on crutches and my legs were swollen. I had them wrapped. I drank the tea three times a day. Within three to four days, I didn't have any pain.

I had some x-rays done before starting on the tea and afterwards. Before the tea, they were really bad. My bones were fractured and broken and that all the ligaments were eaten away. Four weeks later, I had x-rays taken again. The

[3]Author interview with patients 6/21/95

doctor was amazed. The x-rays showed some bone damage, but not as much as before. A week later, I went to another doctor and had x-rays taken again. This was six weeks after taking the stuff. All the bone damage was gone. There was nothing there. They thought they mixed up my x-rays.

Today I'm great. I go biking and study martial arts. This stuff is great.

Hippocrates Health Center[4]

Mike on kidney cancer

I'm a high school teacher from Los Angeles. In February of 1993, I had a kidney stone. After some x-rays and a CT scan, I was diagnosed with kidney cancer in my right kidney. I had two or three tumors. My doctor told me bluntly that if I didn't have a radical nephrectomy, which meant the extraction of all my lymph nodes underneath my arm all the way down to my hip, if I didn't take out my adrenal glands and kidney completely, and if I didn't have that operation by November of that year, I would be dead, no question about it. I told him that I wanted to get a second opinion and he told me that it would be useless because it's cut and dried; there was no other thing that I could do.

My brother, Ronnie, was diagnosed as having cancer of the bone marrow by Sloan Kettering and Johns Hopkins University. I called him to say that I had cancer too. He told me to do what he did. He went to the Hippocrates Center and went on a fast. I went on a 32-day water fast. Then I went on a 7-day juice fast. After that, I became a vegan. In other words, I didn't eat any meat, chicken, fish, or dairy products. I maintain that diet.

I go in for a CT scan every six months. The last one showed that the smallest tumor shrunk a very small amount. I've had every kind of blood test and analysis that you can possibly think of. I just recently had one, and I sent it over to the Hippocrates Center because I'm going back there. They found that everything with my blood is 100 percent normal. I'm in great health.

The Hippocrates Center looks at you as a whole person. They don't threaten you; they just treat you like a human being. They use a natural diet. In other words they don't heat anything up. Everything is raw food and raw grains, slightly cooked.

From that, I have maintained a phenomenal lifestyle. I'm active. I have three children. I'm not dead. I teach every day and it's pretty hectic teaching in the barrios of Los Angeles. Yet I maintain a high activity in life. What can I tell you? Things look great; I'm alive and I'm here.

[4]Author interview with patients 8/22/96

George on prostate cancer

I went to a Hippocrates program for three weeks. about two years ago, and as a result of that my prostate cancer went into remission. It was a program which consisted of organic, fresh, raw vegetables. It also consisted of green drinks which were taken twice a day. In addition to that, there was a great deal of wheatgrass, which I drank—also enemas. I did that for three weeks, and then I stayed on that program after I left the group. I went to the doctor about a week ago, and the doctor said that my cancer has disappeared; it is no longer there.

Patients of Dr. Nicholas Gonzalez[5]

Edmund on kidney cancer

Four-and-a-half years ago, I had major surgery. The doctors removed my left kidney, a large tumor, and one lymph node. I followed this with an interferon program for nine months to prevent any recurrence of the tumor. Unfortunately, this did not work for me because a second tumor came back. At that time, the doctor said that even though kidney cancer does not respond to radiation or chemo, we should try radiation. The radiation stabilized the second tumor but it did not make it disappear. At that time, I realized that the interferon was not going to work.

A friend of mine was on an aggressive nutritional program with Dr. Nicholas Gonzalez, in New York City. I started this program in January 1992, which was three-and-a-half years ago. Three months after I began the program, the second tumor disappeared. My weight, which was way down to 105, is now back to normal at 135. I'm feeling good. My color is back. And recent CT scans and bone scans have been negative. I'm 70 years old.

Henrietta on breast cancer with metastases to the lung

My original cancer was discovered in 1988. I had lymph node involvement and went through surgery. After six months of chemotherapy, I had a 50-percent chance of surviving five years. They never say anything about getting totally well, just five years. After three years, it metastasized around my left lung. At that point, the prognosis was not good. I was told that my life expectancy was two to three months.

At that point, I found Dr. Gonzalez in New York City. His treatment is a three-part program consisting of supplements, diet, and detoxification. I have been going to Dr. Gonzales for three years and nine months.

[5]Author interview with patients 6/21/95

The program has been very successful for me. I can't say it is an easy program. It requires a lot of self-discipline because the diet is rigorous. I'm not saying that you just start on this program and feel great. You don't. If anything, I felt worse before I felt better because of the toxicity that was built up in my body. But it has worked for me and I believe so strongly in the program that it has taken the fear of cancer away. I think this may be a major key because when you believe in something that strong it takes fear away.

At this point, I am stabilized. My cancer level is down to a safe zone and I am functioning normally. I feel great.

The clinic I went to originally was contacted. My oncologist said that if indeed I was still alive, I was a very lucky woman. They didn't give me any hope of living with the traditional medicine.

Dr. Max Gerson's Therapy[6]

At the beginning of the 20th century, Dr. Max Gerson was a specialist in internal medicine living in Germany. Early in his career, while working at a sanitarium, he made a link between food and illness. He noticed that on Mondays, patients would have a gross exacerbation of their symptoms. Having a curious mind, he wanted to find out why. He found that patients ate diets from home rather than the hospital during the time their families visited them. These foods were high in saturated fats, salt, preserved, pickled goods, and alcohol. During the week, by contrast, they were on a bland diet.

He started looking for an ideal dietary approach for patients with lupus and tuberculosis. There was no treatment of any value for lupus at that time. Yet, he was able to reverse a lot of the disease process by putting people on a diet of grasses and vegetables that he would juice. In fact, he became so well known for his success in treating these conditions that the German physicians made him director of the clinic. Later, he would go on to write several textbooks on the subject of natural approaches to reversing conditions previously considered irreversible. Dr. Gerson was something of a superstar in Europe until the 1930s.

He later came to the U.S., where he started using the same therapy, but for cancer. He found he was able to successfully treat many people by giving them 13 glasses of fresh vegetable juice a day, and by eliminating from the diet extra sodium and all animal proteins except for yogurt and a cultured buttermilk. He also gave potassium supplementally. He was able to provide treatments for cancer that no one else could match. In fact, so impressive was his work that early on in his career the *Journal of the American Medical Association* published an article of his. This very same journal later attacked Gerson and called him a quack.

---

[6]Author interview with patients 7/11/95

By the time he reached the height of his career, there was a special Senate investigation of his work headed by Senator Claude Pepper of Florida. Pepper invited Gerson to bring forward medical documentation and patients. Gerson brought forth 50 patients who had suffered from what had been considered terminal illness but who, five years after Gerson's treatment, were alive and well.

Pepper and his committee were so impressed that not only did they not condemn him, but they actually commended him.

Today, his work is continued in Mexico by his daughter Charlotte Gerson Strauss.

Tom on skin melanoma

In March 1982, I found a mole on the right side of my forehead. It didn't concern me much because it wasn't big; it was about half the size of my little fingernail. I talked to my family physician about it, not thinking much of it, but when he saw the thing he was concerned. He said, we'd better take this off and biopsy it.

They did that and the report that came back really shocked me because I had been eating organic foods and a right diet for many years. The news was all bad. It was malignant, it was Clark Level 4. . . .

After the surgery, the cancer returned within 10 days to the site of the incision. I guess that was because they didn't get it all. Then I began to have tumors appearing all over my upper body, chest, and arm. This all happened within a matter of days.

Initially, they wanted to do extensive surgery at the site of the original appearance, but when the thing spread, four different doctors started giving me different advice. Basically, they were all saying that nothing was going to cure this cancer.

At that point, I declined the radical surgery that they wanted to do on the site of my head, and I started looking for different approaches. I knew something about alternative methods, but nobody was at all hopeful, until we talked to the Gerson people. We called the Gerson Institute, and they said that the Gerson therapy was very effective with melanomas. They said that the fact that I hadn't had other treatments which would tend to suppress the immune system was in my favor. Also, the fact that I was fairly young, 42 at the time, was in my favor. I knew something about the therapy, so it wasn't a complete shock. I had some belief in Dr. Gerson and his therapy, so I tried it.

I talked to Charlotte [Gerson Strauss], and she said that melanoma patients detoxify rapidly. She said my chances of recovery were good, but that I would have quite a bit of nausea in the beginning. Everything she told me came true. I got quite ill initially, the type of illness that you'd have if you had a stomach flu. But I was nervous enough about my situation that after I had been on the therapy for a week or so, I thought, my God, I'm not going to be able to do this.

The family had a council of war. We all talked it over with the Institute. They calmed me down and told me they'd cut back the juices a little bit, and cut back the medicine a little for a few days, and just keep trying it. We got through that period and I felt better again.

The heart and soul of the Gerson therapy is that every hour of the day, from 8 in the morning to 7 at night, you have an 8-ounce glass of fresh-squeezed vegetable and fruit juice. It alternates. Basically, one hour you have a juice that's half carrot juice mixed with apple juice, and the next hour you have green juice, which I think is three different types of lettuce, plus green pepper, red cabbage, and then apple with that also. The juices are laced with potassium salts. In addition, you have three meals. The Gerson therapy is not a fast at all, but your diet is specified.

In the beginning of the therapy, you start digesting the cancer and putting it out of the body in the form of metabolic toxins. If your body is full of cancer, the way mine was, you're going to have a lot of toxins to process. To help that out, in the beginning . . . you take a coffee enema every four hours when you're up: 6 a.m., 10 a.m., 2 p.m., 6 p.m., and 10 p.m. The coffee enemas put the drug caffeine directly into the portal vein. That enables the liver to detoxify a lot more efficiently than it could otherwise. The coffee enema is a great help. It relieves pain, it relieves digestive discomfort, and it is a crucial part of the therapy. That's basically how it went in a day.

Within two months, every visible tumor on my body had regressed. It had shrunk, dried up, and fallen off. It all happened so quickly. I started out in March 1982 thinking I was a healthy guy. Then, in early May 1982, I was told that I had cancer and very little chance to live. In July 1982, I was on the Gerson therapy and everything cancerous that could be seen had regressed and disappeared.

The Gerson people said that even though everything that could be seen was gone, there was more of a problem under the surface. They recommended that I stay on the therapy for 18 to 24 months, which I did. I stayed on the therapy for 20 months, and in the subsequent 13 years, I've had no recurrence of the cancer.

Over the years, I've talked to hundreds of people with cancer of various types and I try to share my experience with them. You can pretty much see who will succeed with this type of therapy and who will not. People used to the passive mode, where professionals do things to them—they cut, they burn, and they put chemicals in, and the patient sits there and it happens to them—are generally horrified when they find out the extent to which the patient has to cooperate in his own recovery on one of these metabolic programs. But people who can take that aboard have a very, very high success rate on this therapy. The exceptions are people who have been bombed with chemotherapy before they get on it. In order to do the Gerson therapy you have to be motivated and open to a radical change in lifestyle that a diet change like this imposes.

Joan on breast cancer

I had a radical mastectomy. One year later, I had a recurrence. It was not biopsied, however. The surgeon said that he would monitor this mass.

My husband and I did a lot of research and decided to try the Gerson therapy. I began the program in August 1977. By May 1978, when I saw the surgeon again, the mass was gone. Since that time, I have remained completely clear. It has been 18 years, and I have never had any recurrences. I have had myself closely monitored over the years by surgeons and lab work.

The Gerson therapy is intensive and comprehensive. It consists of nutritional treatment through diet and 13 juices per day. It consists of medication: potassium, niacin, thyroid, lugol solution, pancreatin, acidol pepsin, and liver and B12 combined as daily injections. It also consists of detoxification in the form of coffee enemas to help the liver. It's a very comprehensive therapy.

I still continue with my diet of organically grown fruits and vegetables. I also continue with almost daily coffee enemas. I have not eaten meat, except for poultry and fish, for these 18 years. That was a decision I made on my own. Some people go back to their former diets, but I realized that my former diet was too high in fats, and could be a possible problem again.

I did not tell the surgeon that I was doing the Gerson therapy. Nor did he ask me any questions. I wanted to keep the surgeon monitoring me, so I decided not to make him angry by telling him what I had done.

At that time, there was not the knowledge and the education about any options as far as treatment was concerned, except for the orthodox establishment options. I had been told at the beginning about the American Cancer Society's statistics and what their thoughts on treatment were. I was an RN who saw that much of this treatment was ineffective with the cancer patients, so I did not feel that the American Cancer Society was credible. Having seen this in my profession, I decided that I was going to do a different therapy. I had read about Gerson's therapy in Dr. Gerson's book. I felt it was credible and the thing to do for myself.

George on pancreatic cancer

I went to the Gerson therapy center in February 1983. Prior to going there, my wife and I were on the way to Hawaii. We were in Seattle and preparing to leave for Hawaii the next morning. I got very sick and had a lot of pain in my stomach and back. We phoned the doctor who was listed in the hotel directory, and took a taxi to the hospital. I had a blood test, an x-ray, and examination by a doctor there. The doctor said that he wasn't sure what the problem was, but he suggested that we not go to Hawaii. He said we should go home instead and get further tests done. That's what we did.

My doctor sent me to a specialist in Victoria. I went through a lot of tests that I never heard of before. On January 21st, he took some blood tests and said that the amylase in my blood was high. A normal level was between 70 and 320, and mine was 627. It proved that there was a very bad infection in my body.

I finally took a CT scan, which showed a mass in the head of the pancreas. The specialist said that there was absolutely no question about it. I had cancer of the pancreas.

We had heard about Gerson's therapy through somebody that my daughter knew. We phoned the Gerson Institute and went down there in February 1983. We spent one month there.

Afterwards, we stayed in our condo in Escondido for eight months because that was the only place we could get organic foods. We had our organic vegetables delivered by a lady who got her vegetables from the same source as the Gersons.

When we came home, I had put weight on and I felt good. My blood tests were also good. I took another CT scan and it showed no tumor. I phoned the head doctor at Gerson's in April 1984, and he told me to stay another four months on the program . . . That's 11 years ago, and I have had absolutely no problem since.

Patricia on pancreatic cancer

I had pancreatic cancer that spread to my liver, gallbladder, and spleen, and was told that I had less than three months to live. My doctors were doing nothing. They said that chemotherapy and anything else would not help me, and that I should prepare my family and get my affairs in order. I was in the process of doing that. Then one morning, my husband and I heard about the Gerson clinic in Mexico. My husband got up and said, "That's it. Pack your clothes. We're going."

We went down on March 7, 1986, and started the therapy that day. Before I started the therapy, I had been throwing up mouthfuls of blood. I was just about finished. Ten days later, I stopped bringing up blood and the pain was gone. I said to my husband, "I don't know if I'm going to live, but I feel better than I have in a year."

Six months later, I went to see my doctor, who wondered why I was still around. He asked if I would have a CT scan, which I did. The test showed that the masses of cancer had gone. My doctor said, "I don't know what you're doing, and I don't want to know what you're doing, but just keep doing it." I think he was shocked to see that I was still around.

Another six months down the road, he asked me to take another CT scan, which I did. He said, "Patricia, there's no sign of cancer at all." That was nine years ago. Today, I feel wonderful. I have no sign of cancer at all.

I took the two Gerson books to my doctor, and he read them, but he said that it was just too deep for him. He just calls me his miracle now.

Marilyn on melanoma and cervical cancer

I developed these conditions in 1979 when I was 36 years of age. My prognosis from my physicians was not good. The melanoma, in particular, was very virulent. They didn't come out and tell me how long they thought I had to live, but they tactfully tried to tell me that my chances weren't good. I read and did some of my own research and found that with stage 4 melanoma, the patient tends to expire in one to five years. It's now been 15 years. I'm not a typical patient.

I did a lot of research and picked Dr. Max Gerson's therapy because I felt that it was the hardest and the most curative. It had the best results with melanoma. I was inspired by the fact that Dr. Gerson had worked with Albert Schweitzer, and that he was a pioneer. He just was an incredible physician with a wonderful answer, but not many people were willing to use this therapy for their problems.

I found after the first six months of the therapy I began to feel really normal. I didn't have reactions and feelings that come when you do a metabolic therapy. I started to feel intuitively that I wasn't going to die, that I was never going to have a recurrence. I know that the mind has a great deal to do with healing. I just knew because this diet was building my cells that my mind was stronger. It felt that I had turned the corner. It's been almost 16 years, and I feel better than I ever have in my life. I attribute that to his work and, of course, my participating in it.

Sharon on non-Hodgkin's lymphoma

I did not have chemotherapy. I went directly to the Gerson Hospital. I was there for two weeks, and in five days I lost 28 pounds of fluid. I had been very swollen with edema. When I got back, I continued on the therapy, and in six months I went back to the doctor. I had an MRI, and my tumor was gone. I am not on a modified therapy. It's been three years.

For more information call 212-787-2404.

Dr. Emanuel Revici's Therapy[7]

Dr. Revici, a man who has hit the century mark, has practiced medicine for over 70 years. In that time, he has saved numerous lives and has been acknowledged by some of the world's greatest scientists. Dr. Revici has received many rewards for his unique and spirited approach to science. He has also been slandered by the American media, who have no knowledge of the thousands of patients he has cured. As a result, he was put on trial, but he was completely exonerated. To date, Revici is totally acquitted of every charge made against him.

Norman on colon cancer

Over six years ago, I had surgery for colon cancer. The doctors didn't have any recommendations; they said I was on my own.

I heard about Dr. Revici and decided to see him. It's probably the best thing I have done in many, many years. I went on his program which consists mostly of minerals. At first, it was rather intense in that I had to use them four times a day, but like everything else, you get used to it.

Now I'm on a maintenance program where I use his prescribed minerals one month on and six months off. My CEA test, which is the test that they use for colon cancer, comes in below 0.5. I only need to have a colonoscopy every two years because I've been clear for several years. I'm just happy to be here. I only have praise for him.

I personally feel Dr. Revici's therapy has made a difference in my life. He's so positive that when he tells you something you almost walk out feeling you have a white shield around you that will protect you. I wouldn't think of not using his program. I wouldn't consider it. In point of fact, I recommended it to one person who was very far gone, and he helped that person. I can't say enough about him.

Charlotte on ovarian and oat cell lung cancer

My story started in 1980 when I was diagnosed at New York Hospital with oat cell lung cancer. I walked out of there not wanting to take their treatments. A little while later, I went to Mt. Sinai Hospital and was diagnosed with ovarian cancer as well. I had a hysterectomy there and was put onto the lung cancer ward where I received chemotherapy. I took two more chemotherapy treatments after that.

During that time, I got on the Kelly nutritional program, which was available at that time. I started to make a lot of changes in my lifestyle. I had a clean x-ray after the first chemo and thought that was it. I shook hands with the doc-

[7]Author interview with patients 7/10/95

tor to say good-bye. He held onto my hand and said that this happens to 50-percent of the people who use chemo. Unfortunately, he said, it's not a cure. He told me that if I didn't continue to take chemo every month, the disease would be back in three weeks, and that I'd be dead within six months. That was frightening, but I also felt that chemo was not going to help me live a long time. He wanted me to take chemo for two years. I asked him if at the end of two years if I would be free of cancer and cured. He said, if I lived that long we would talk about it then.

I got help from a psychiatric nurse who got me some statistics, and I found out that I had less than a 1-percent chance for survival. I figured that that wasn't a very good record. I wanted to look around and thought I could do better myself if that was all that they were going to be offering me. Also at that time, they were telling me that they wanted to radiate my brain because oat cell lung cancer usually metastasized to the brain, and I would die a horrible death.

With that prospect looming on the horizon, I figured I had to make some changes. I went to see Dr. Revici and explained my situation to him. I said that I didn't want to continue with the chemotherapy because I didn't believe it would help me. He gave me a complete examination, and said that he thought he could help me. My impression of Dr. Revici was that he was a pure healer, innocent in spirit. He is a lovely individual. When you meet him, you feel complete trust and sincerity, and you believe that you can do well in his hands.

I took his medicine which I understand is toxic except for the way that he delivers it. And being delivered on the lipids, that it goes directly to the tumor. I went along with his program. It really was not devastating in any way. It was just one capsule a day.

After three months, I had another x-ray taken, and it was clear. I stayed on his program for a year. I've always had clear x-rays since I've been with him, and have never had any signs of disease since that time. I go for a lung x-ray from time to time, and the doctors ask what I am there for. I say that I'm checking up to see how my lungs are doing. They look at my lungs and say that I have absolutely no sign of ever having had lung cancer. Now, I do have my former x-rays and my pathology slides, so I can prove that I did indeed have lung and ovarian cancer. I have no doubt that it was Dr. Revici's treatment that helped me.

What a shame that people go at the end of a disease rather than at the beginning when they have a better chance of getting help. They tend to think that alternatives should be saved as a last-ditch effort. I've seen people even at the end do very, very well indeed with him, but I think we need to let people know that for best results they should seek out alternative therapy at the beginning when they have the best chance to support their own innate healing ability, rather than going against it with chemotherapy, surgery, and radiation. If people would like to reach me, I am at 212-777-0111.

Robert on angiosarcoma

In early 1987, I discovered that I had a lump in my jaw. I went through a series of extensive tests, including two biopsies, one in the hospital and one outside. It included MRIs, CT scans, x-rays, and that sort of thing. Out of that came the diagnosis of angiosarcoma. Basically, the doctor who was associated with Georgetown Hospital told me that with this diagnosis I had about one chance in 10 of being alive in five years. He said that that particular kind of cancer was not treatable by any of the usual techniques, namely surgery, radiation, or chemotherapy.

Given that kind of prognosis, and given the lack of treatment options . . . I decided it was time to look elsewhere for treatment. My wife had worked with a lady who was a former patient of Dr. Revici, so I knew of Dr. Revici through her, and contacted the doctor. I became a patient of his in 1987. I was actively under his care for about six years. By that I mean I went to see him in his office approximately once a month. The treatment consisted primarily of capsules that I took orally. He put me on a number of different medications.

What struck me about his treatment is that he tailors it to the person. He would sometimes have me on two or three medications. He would tell me to call him in three or four days, and he might change the medication, depending upon how I was reacting to it. Over that period, he probably had me on a couple dozen different things. I have not been receiving treatment for a little over a year.

His office asked me to have an MRI done, which I did a couple of months ago. I sent them the results. Basically, the MRI shows that in the last three years, there has been no growth at all in the tumor.

Jay on squamous cell carcinoma

I had a squamous cell carcinoma in the throat and was given two to six months to live in 1982. They wanted to operate and remove my entire voice box—my vocal cords and everything—and give me chemo, which I wouldn't allow.

I immediately got on Dr. Revici's therapy, and studied his entire program relating not only to his medication, but the nutrition, vitamins, minerals, enzymes, even some bioactive frequencies later on.

That was 13 years ago. Today, I feel like a million dollars. I have never spent a night in the hospital. I'm very active. At the time I started on his program, you couldn't understand me. I sounded like the godfather's godfather. In a period of about 4 months, my voice was back to normal and I've never had a sick day.

I spoke with my original diagnosing physician many, many times. I happened to know one in New York, and one in California, who are top guys in the allopathic field in otolaryngology. About two years later, I finally agreed to let them do a second in-depth biopsy on my throat, just to get them off my back, because they were friends of mine. When my right vocal cord was originally diagnosed, it was over ¾ of an inch in diameter. They couldn't understand why all of this cleared up in such a short period of time. It was all 100 percent clear.

Arthur on Kaposi's sarcoma

I was diagnosed at the VA hospital. The doctors there suggested operating to cut out the sores on my foot. I did not agree. I had a problem with the medical professional who attended to me. He asked me if I was homosexual and I said I wasn't. He told me that those were the kinds of people who get this. He also told me I could die from this. I didn't like the approach they had there.

I decided I would try another method. Fortunately, I listened to you and learned about Dr. Revici. I began treatment with him back in 1991. I successfully overcame my condition.

Lee on breast cancer

My cancer started in 1986. I felt a lump in the right breast, and had a mammogram, which was negative. The doctor said that the lump was benign, and that I shouldn't worry. In 1988, the lump seemed bigger and harder, and I was advised to get a mammogram. This time, it showed a mass. I then had a biopsy at Beth Israel Hospital, which diagnosed a 4-cm infiltrating ductal carcinoma in my breast. I saw a number of doctors and surgeons who advised a modified, radical mastectomy, with chemotherapy and radiation.

I knew that there were other options from listening to your program and reading. I decided to try Dr. Revici's nontoxic individualized cancer therapy, even though I was warned by all the doctors that he was a quack, and that I could die without conventional treatment. I called Dr. Revici, and he told me to have a lumpectomy if I didn't want the mastectomy, and then to come for treatment. I had the lumpectomy in December 1988, and I began treatment with Dr. Revici in January 1989.

I found him to be very caring and considerate. He encouraged me to call him often to tell him how I was feeling. His own phone number was given to me.

In July 1989, I stopped the treatment because I felt that six months of it was sufficient. About nine months later, I felt another hard lump in the same breast. A mammogram revealed another mass, approximately 1.5 cm, and the tumor marker for breast cancer was high.

I returned to Dr. Revici in May 1990, and he urged me to have the lump removed. I didn't want another operation, and Dr. Revici was understanding. He said that he would try to help me anyway.

I was given a variety of Dr. Revici's medicine. At times I became discouraged, but Dr. Revici kept reassuring me that the lump would go away. Gradually, it did become softer, and after about two years I no longer felt the lump.

The last mammogram I had was negative, and the tumor marker for breast cancer was normal. I still take Dr. Revici's medicine about every two months. I also take vitamins and herbs. I changed my diet. I don't have meat or chicken, and I eat very little sugar or dairy. I drink bottled water and take exercise classes in yoga and low-impact aerobics. I am very grateful to Dr. Revici.

Fred on prostate cancer

I was given this diagnosis about three years ago. I went to see a urologist who biopsied me. It was a very unpleasant procedure. He immediately suggested that I undergo a radical prostatectomy, but the operation itself and all of its side effects were most unappealing. I went to see a radiologist who suggested radiology. Each special branch seems to have their predilection. I was somewhat turned off by what I was beginning to know were the side effects of that invasive approach also: the incontinence, the impotence, and the lowering of the immune system's abilities to take care of the body.

I finally called Dr. Revici, and decided to go with him. I've been seeing him for three years. I cannot say, unfortunately, that my tumor has completely disappeared, as has been the case for other of his patients, but it certainly seems stabilized. Furthermore, my general well-being is terrific. I feel very, very energetic, both mentally and physically. Most of that I attribute to Dr. Revici's ministrations. I do other things to enhance my immune system, but I think that Dr. Revici's approach is key to what I hope is a stabilized situation.

Ronald on bone, lung, and kidney cancer

My experience with cancer began in 1976 when a large tumor was discovered in my pelvis just above the knee. It resulted in an amputation in 1977. In 1979, the cancer metastasized to the lung, and I had an operation on my right lung to remove a couple of nodules. To my regret, in 1980, I was diagnosed with renal cell carcinoma. At that time, they told me that I had six months to two years to live. There was no treatment available. Surgery wasn't possible. Neither was chemotherapy expected to be of any benefit.

At that point, I heard about Dr. Revici, and went to see him. I started on his therapy in October 1980. To my surprise, within about a month or so, I began to feel my energy return. My appetite began to increase, and my condition improved. I continued on his therapy for a while. Then I returned to work.

I had another episode of metastatic cancer in 1987. Again the bone cancer was active in my left hip. I went back to Dr. Revici. With his help, I went into remission. Unfortunately, in 1991, I had another episode of bone and lung cancer. I went back to Dr. Revici again and continue on his therapy until today. The tumor in the right lung was a little resistant to the treatment, but after a couple of years of treatment, it appears that the tumor is going into remission. I'm very happy about that.

I've been able to enjoy a reasonable quality of life over these years, thanks to Dr. Revici's treatment. My life certainly has been extended beyond the six months to two years that was expected by the traditional medical community.

Dr. Stanislaw Burzynski's Therapy[8]

Since 1977, Stanislaw Burzynski, M.D., Ph.D., of Houston, Texas, has helped thousands of patients recover from advanced cancer. Originally from Poland, where he was considered one of the brightest scientists and physicians, he later came to this country, and worked with Baylor University. Here he was a shining star, with over 60 articles printed in peer-reviewed journals. His amazing research showed that cancerous cells could be reprogrammed back into normal tissue.

Dr. Burzynski's treatment consists of a series of substances called antineoplastons, which help reprogram cancer cells into normal cells. Antineoplastons are part of a larger group of chemical compounds called *peptides,* that exist in every human body. Simply stated, antineoplastons are a special class of peptides, found in the body, that combat neoplastons—abnormal cells or cancer cells. Cancer patients have a severe shortage of these cancer fighters. Antineoplastons could be the vehicle needed by the body to ward off and even reverse the development of these cancerous cells.

Dr. Burzynski put this theory into action, treating patients by reintroducing antineoplastons into the bloodstream either intravenously or orally with capsules. In many cases, tumors shrank in size or actually disappeared. Some patients even experienced a complete remission of the cancers, and years of follow-up study reveal no sign of any return.

Unfortunately, Dr. Burzynski has been targeted by the medical establishment. His clinic may be closed permanently.

Venuta on breast cancer

One week after diagnosis, I had a mastectomy. Then they wanted to give me chemotherapy but I didn't want it. I decided to go to Dr. Burzynski. He connected me to an IV for 5 months, nonstop, 24 hours a day with his antineoplaston medication. During that time, I was never sick. I had a normal life. I have a 7-year-old child. I've been going to meetings at school. I've been driving my car. I have chemotherapy, and I can drive my car. I never even lost my

[8]Author interview with patients 7/13/95

hair. Nobody in the whole world knew that I was having chemotherapy. After 5 years, I am talking with you.

Currently, I'm perfect. I have no cancer. I feel good and I run my own business. I go to Dr. Burzynski for check-ups, and everything looks good.

Theresa on stage 4 lymphoma

In 1984, after the birth of my daughter, I had a biopsy which showed that I had stage 4 lymphoma. My doctors said that I should go on chemotherapy right away, even though I wouldn't be able to get rid of the lymphoma. They said it was incurable.

I had a second opinion . . . and they said the same thing, but they said they could check it for a while and not give me any chemo right away. I never did end up having chemotherapy or radiation.

Today I'm great thanks to Dr. Burzynski. He gave me the antineoplaston therapy, which means anticancer. It's a peptide that he discovered. Apparently, most peptides are growth-enhancing peptides. Peptides are the precursors to amino acids which are the precursors to proteins. The peptides that he found are peptides that inhibit the growth of certain types of cells. Rather than killing the cancer cells along with a lot of other healthy cells, peptides just keep the cancer cells from growing. They live out their lifespan and then they die off. Eventually, whatever organ is affected is turned back into a healthy organ. That's what happened with me.

While I was healing, I made a lot of changes. I realized I had a lot of anger that I wasn't dealing with. I was taught that anger is bad and hurtful, and I developed a way of suppressing my anger and not even knowing that I had it. So one part of getting well, a big part, was coming more to terms with my anger, accepting it, and expressing it appropriately, rather than stuffing it inside and turning it into cancer.

Another aspect was learning to visualize my cancer going away, and holding a more positive view of my future. I did change a lot of things. I changed my job, and I changed a lot of my relationships. I went through a lot of changes.

Today, I feel a lot different than I did then. I'm much more aware of my feelings, and physically I feel a lot better. Over the months that I worked with Dr. Burzynski's medicine, I saw my cancer gradually disappear. I was grateful to be able to deal with my healing process in a nontoxic way, and I'm really grateful to be alive.

Ellen on intestinal asbestos cancer

This is the same type of cancer that Steve McQueen died of. It was a slow-growing cancer. I was on 250 pain pills a month for ten years. Finally, Sloan Kettering gave me two years to live.

I called Dr. Burzynski and asked him if he could help me. After the first week of treatment, I was off the pain pills. I had no side effects. I was on his program for nine months and I got cured.

Tessie on lymphoma

I was advised to get chemotherapy, which I started in June 1992. In July 1993, it reappeared in my neck. My doctor said that with my condition, chemotherapy might help. But the second time that I started chemotherapy, the tumor was not getting smaller.

I had the feeling that I had to do something different. I decided to go to Dr. Burzynski because I got tired of the chemotherapy. I told my doctor that I was going to stop the chemotherapy and get a second opinion. My doctor was shocked, and he started putting pressure on me to go back on chemotherapy. He said I would lose ground, but I didn't. Today, I am free of cancer.

Actually, the chemotherapy was causing me to lose ground. I was so weak from it that I was running a fever. I had bronchitis, and I had pneumonia. My heart was also damaged from the chemotherapy. After getting well, I went back to my doctor for blood tests to send to Dr. Burzynski, and he was ignoring me.

Mary Jo on low-grade non-Hodgkin's lymphoma, stage 4

I was told that I needed a bone marrow transplant, massive chemotherapy, total body irradiation, and six weeks of total isolation in a hospital. My doctor gave me no guarantee, but he said that this was my only chance for a cure. My other option was to take chemotherapy and radiation every two years. I already had a tumor on the side of my neck, which was growing. If I didn't follow his advice, he said it would press against my organs and I would die.

I did some more research. That's when I heard about Dr. Burzynski's totally nontoxic treatment. I took the next flight to Houston, and met with him. Immediately, I had a wonderful feeling. He gave me names of other patients he treated with my condition, and I called them right away. These people were in remission from non-Hodgkin's lymphoma for over five years. I thought I would be foolish not to try it. When I called my doctor at UCLA, he was adamant that I not start Dr. Burzynski's treatment, but I did it anyway.

My medical records are open to everybody. Every CT scan I had showed a reduction. I have maintained my doctor at UCLA who says, over and over again, "I can't say it's not working, but I don't know why it's working." He calls me a spontaneous remission.

One thing that is so important about Dr. Burzynski's treatment is that it is totally nontoxic. I lived a completely normal life while I was on it. I was able to do grocery shopping, drive my kid's car pools, everything.

Dr. Lawrence Burton's Therapy[9]

I have followed Dr. Burton's work from the 1970s up until his recent death. I was always amazed at the challenges that he offered the National Cancer Institute and medicine in general. He would say, essentially, if you feel my non-toxic, noninvasive, Immuno-Augmentative Therapy (IAT), which uses the immune system to fight off cancer, is fraudulent, then what are you doing that is better? No one ever accepted his challenge. And of course, orthodox medicine can show very few successes.

The man who made such startling progress in the treatment of cancer had a long career in research. Burton decided to go into cancer research after witnessing the horrors of cancer treatment at the U.S. Navy's Cancer Center at Brooklyn Naval Hospital in the 1940s. In those days, the accepted procedure for cancer treatment was radical surgery. If you had a cancer of the foot, the leg was removed at the hip. After World War II, Burton continued his cancer studies and gradually moved up to become a senior investigator and oncologist at St. Vincent's Hospital, a noted teaching hospital in New York.

Burton's IAT has its roots in this period of his career. In 1959, Burton and a team of cancer researchers accidentally discovered a tumor-inhibiting factor that reduced or eliminated cancer in a special breed of leukemic mice. Their research progressed well enough so that, in the November 1962 issue of *Transactions of the New York Academy of Sciences*, they reported on certain substances that were capable of causing remission in over 50 percent of the leukemic mice treated.

The studies were repeated in the presence of numerous scientists and science writers, and once again the tumors almost completely disappeared. This resulted in positive publicity at first, but the findings were soon discredited by disbelieving physicians as trickery.

Despite this, Dr. Burton's team treated patients with IAT at St. Vincent's Hospital. They were working under Dr. Antonio Rottino. In 1972, Dr. Rottino announced that the IAT treatments had to cease. The treatments were considered experimental and therefore unproven and so were not appropriate to use as part of regular medical care. The actual reason for the funds being stopped was the team's refusal to give over their work to other organizations that fund cancer research, which wanted to take credit for the work. The group was forced to disband.

During this time, Long Island psychologist Martin Goldstone's wife was being treated with IAT (the Burton-Friedman technique). She had enjoyed such promising results that, when they learned that the treatments had been stopped at St. Vincent's, she and her husband and other prominent people in the Great Neck, New York, community raised enough funds to establish the

[9]Author interview with patients 7/18/95

Immunology Research Foundation to continue the work of Doctors Burton and Friedman, Burton's associate.

The Immunology Research Center moved from Great Neck, New York, to Freeport on Grand Bahama Island in 1977. Since then, over 2,500 terminal cancer patients have undergone treatment there. According to Dr. Burton, 50 to 60 percent of these patients experience tumor reduction. Many are able to resume normal lives; frequently they survive five years and more beyond the initial diagnosis of cancer (usually made by a traditional attending physician prior to Burton's involvement in the case). The five-year survival period is sufficient for the American Cancer Society and the National Cancer Institute to consider a patient cured.

Dr. John Clement, an internationally renown cancer specialist now running the center, explains how IAT fights cancer:[10]

"IAT is a nontoxic, immune-modulation method of controlling cancers. The intellectual basis of the treatment is that many cancers can be controlled by restoring the competence of the patient's own immune system. The body's complex immune-fighting system may well be the first, best, as well as the last line of defense against many cancers. We are not dealing with toxic chemicals in any way. We are giving people solutions from the blood of healthy people, obviously screened to be completely safe and free from any type of cross-infection. We are giving humeral cytokines. Cytokines are well known by the names of various types, such as interferon and interleukin. And the substance that we are using most is called tumor necrosis factor. The method we use is similar in any type of cancer we treat. This method is recognized by some people but is completely different from most accepted types of cancer treatment.

"The way in which we use our method is that we take blood from the cancer patient and assay the blood for the factors we believe are aiding the patient's own cancer to destroy the patient. We try to correct and improve the factors in the blood by giving the patient small injections on a daily basis of the factors we are concerned with. By identifying these factors, we are able to control them, put them back into balance, and often destroy the patient's own cancer.

"The cancer patient has in their blood a system of blocking proteins. These blocking proteins prevent the patient from rejecting the cancer as a foreign body. These can be determined, defined, analyzed, and removed. If you put a kidney from some other person into a patient, the kidney will be rejected, because of these blocking proteins. These proteins have been determined. Their molecular weight is known, and they are known to be present, circulating in the blood of patients with cancer. It is our aim in our treatment to prevent these blocking proteins from preventing the patient from curing himself or herself. We measure these blocking proteins on a daily basis. We give similar

[10]Author interview with Dr. John Clement, 12/31/95

proteins which, in fact, knock the blockers out, and allow the patient's own immune system to reject the patient's cancer."

Craig on lymphoma

I was originally diagnosed in 1979 with a malignant lymphoma. By the time it was diagnosed, it was already stage 4, which meant that it was in my bones.

I was given radiation and three different series of chemotherapy . . . in early 1980. When they saw how my liver was, they gave me a 10-percent chance of seeing Christmas day. I continued on more radiation and chemotherapy.

In the meantime, I saw a program on "60 Minutes" about Dr. Lawrence Burton in the Bahamas and how he was blackballed from the medical establishment. He was being recognized as a viable cancer researcher. I kept it in the back of my mind.

I kept getting worse and worse and worse. Finally, I went to the Bahamas as a last resort. The treatment I received was a daily injection of four different proteins . . . There were absolutely no side effects whatsoever. I began to feel better right away. Of course, I'd been through a lot of chemotherapy and I was coming out of that. It took me about a year to really start coming back, but everything has been fine. I've had a lot of check-ups ever since and there's absolutely no sign of cancer in my body.

Jill on multiple myeloma

I was diagnosed in October 1981. I was told to go on chemotherapy and radiation, which I took for three years. In March 1984, I was told by my doctor to go home and die. He said that I should make out my will, and that he would supply me with enough morphine to keep from being in too much pain.

At that point, I weighed 85 pounds. I could not lay down or sit down without a great deal of pain.

While I was waiting to die at home, I had 24-hour-a-day nurses taking care of me. During this time, I assembled quite a library of literature about cancer. One of the books I had was called *Cancer Survivors and How They Did It*. In that book is a chapter about Dr. Burton and IAT. A nurse who was taking care of me read the chapter and suggested that we call these people. We did, and we talked to a woman who survived pancreatic cancer. The nurse was terribly impressed, and we sent for the brochure. It was the end of May, and my daughter was just getting out of college. I called her and asked, "Do you want to go to the Bahamas?" Off we went. She pushed me through airports in a wheelchair.

When we reached our destination, we talked to Dr. Burton, and I started the program immediately. About six weeks into it, I turned over in bed by myself for the first time. Eventually, I was able to walk on crutches to the bathroom. The doctor in Los Angeles told me that I would never walk again. The rest is history. Here I am 14-plus years later.

Mine was not a miraculous recovery. I made progress in very small increments. When I look back on a day-to-day basis, I cannot report much change, but on a month-to-month basis, I could tell that I was definitely getting better. I began feeling a lot stronger, with less pain. Every six months, I returned to the Bahamas for a tune-up. Again, I had my blood checked daily. I got the new series of shots daily, and stayed for a month or more. Then I would once again come home, and the same sorts of things happened. I noticed that I was very gradually feeling stronger and getting better. That has continued until now.

I must interject this. At one point, I was in a very, very serious car accident, where I broke every bone in my body. Multiple myeloma is bone marrow cancer, which compromises your bones tremendously. The orthopedic doctor in the hospital put me back together. While he was in there, he said that he scraped all the old cancer cells off, but he couldn't see any new ones that developed. He didn't want to go way out on a limb and say that IAT was helpful, but he said that something had stopped the cancer growth. I think that's rather significant, and I attribute it to IAT and the good Lord above. I don't know what else I have done. It certainly wasn't the chemo and the radiation kicking in after all those years, which they like to say. Even though this accident set me back a great deal, I continue to go back to the Bahamas about every six months, and continue doing the program at home, taking shots every day.

Jesse on lymphoma

In 1980, I was diagnosed with lymphoma. I had 20 treatments of radiation, and 11 months of chemotherapy. During this time, the cancer continued to spread. It spread to both lungs, and to the bone marrow. During this two years of treatment, I had many biopsies done, which all turned out to be malignant tumors. After the two years, they told me to come back in two weeks, and they would tell me what they were going to do next, but that I had very little time left, and they were going to try to make me as comfortable as they could.

When I came home, I knew I was not going back because I had heard of this place in Freeport, Bahamas. I called a lady, and she gave me a phone number to reach the Bahamas. I called and they took me. I had to bring my records, which the doctors did not want me to have, but they couldn't hold me, so they gave me very little information to take with me.

I went to Freeport in June 1982. When I went, I really didn't go for a cure because I had been told that I had a very short time left. I could look at myself and I knew that because I had tumors all over my body and on my face. I was covered from top to bottom.

After going to Freeport, Dr. Burton told me that the lymphoma that I had, chemo would not even treat. After he told me that, I knew that he was telling the truth because it had continued to spread.

After being in Freeport for just a very few days, I had a talk with Dr. Burton, and after talking with him, I knew that he had the cure. He said to me, Mrs. Pennington, you don't have a problem. That, in itself, did so much for me because you will have a tendency to believe what a doctor tells you. There I sat, barely able to hold my head up, and Dr. Burton was telling me that I didn't have a problem.

After two weeks, all of the visible tumors were gone. After one week, I could see a great difference in the way that I felt. And after five weeks, I was sent home. It was in July 1982.

When I came back, I saw my treating physician. He said that I was cured, but that it was the chemo that cured me. He twisted his story because I had five biopsies just before leaving his care and going to the Bahamas, and they were all malignant. He did the biopsies, and he gave me the reports, telling me that he was going to make me as comfortable as he could before I died. Yet, when I came home from Freeport, he told me that I was cured.

That, in itself, makes me very bitter, knowing that a doctor will lie to you, and tell you just anything. I really don't appreciate that. To me, cancer in the United States is just a money racket. I know what they took from me, and they gave me nothing. I would love to have a refund.

Index

abortion, 254, 333
abrotanum, 466
abscesses, 462
accidents, 642–43, 658–59, 659–60
acetaldehyde, 42
acetaminophen, 278
acetylcarnitine, 25, 59, 191, 199
acetylcholine, 61, 191
acid indigestion, 202–3
acidic vs. alkaline foods, 110, 155, 165–66, 400,
    458, 497
acidophilus, 25, 100, 167, 293, 421; lactobacillus,
    128, 167, 222, 229, 498
acne, 461, 464, 466
aconite, aconitum, 175, 184, 252
aconitum napellus, 78, 175
acquired immune deficiency syndrome. See AIDS
    and HIV
acupressure, 249–50, 414
acupuncture, 19, 39–40, 88, 136, 162–63, 249– 50,
    259, 338, 352,; 391, 432, 455, 575–80
adapton, 413
ADD (attention deficit disorder), 81
Adderall, 342, 344–45
adrealinum, 448
adrenal system, 47, 326
adrenaline, 11
Adriamycin, 118
aerobic exercise, 297, 389
affirmations, 414–15
aggression, 706–7
aging, 3–20; antioxidant supplements and, 14–15;
    aromatherapy and, 17–18; chelation therapy
    and, 6; detoxification, 4–8; diet and, 9–10;
    herbs and, 16–17; juice fasting and, 4–6;
    minerals and enzymes, 15–16; personal expe-
    riences with, 629; rebuilding and, 8–19; stress
    reduction and, 18–19; what to avoid with, 19
Agrimony, 464
AHT (autohemotherapy), 678
AIDS and HIV, 21–40, 709–10; aqueous penicillin
    treatment for, 38; diet for, 22–24; herbs for,
    28–34; homeopathy for, 36–38; ozone ther-
    apy for, 38; peripheral neuropathy and, 261;
    phytochemicals and, 34–35; supplements
    for, 24–28; symptoms of, 22; treatment of,
    22–38; what to avoid with, 40
air; filtration systems, 48–49; quality, 241
AL–721, 26
alanine, 437

alcohol; breast cancer and, 98; cancer and, 123;
    digestive disorders and, 213; headaches and,
    277, 284; heatstroke and, 302; osteoporosis
    and, 392; stroke and, 470
alcoholism, 41–43
Alexander technique, 89, 136–37, 422–23, 581–82
alfalfa, 67, 73, 111, 269, 294, 309, 369
algae, 10, 111, 168; blue-green, 111, 472; green,
    168
alkaline vs. acidic foods, 110, 155, 165–66, 400,
    458, 497
allergies, 44–55; arthritis and, 70, 76–77; autism
    and, 81–82; chemical sensitivity, 45; diabetes
    and, 198–99; ear infections and, 222; fixed
    vs. cyclic, 44–45; food, 44–45, 76–77, 81–82,
    204, 342–43, 444, 463, 667–68; headaches
    and, 282; learning disorders and, 342–43;
    personal experiences with, 575–77, 607, 629,
    670–71; phobias and, 411; protease and,
    157; respiratory illnesses and, 442, 444, 449;
    self-diagnosis of, 46–48; sinusitis and, 453,
    455; supplements in treatment of, 51–53;
    symptoms of, 48; tests for, 45–46; treatment
    of, 48–54; types of, 44–45; UTI and, 495–96;
    what to avoid with, 55
allium cepa, 175
allspice, 207
almond oil, 83
aloe vera; for AIDS, 32; for allergies, 671; for ane-
    mia, 68; for arthritis, 73; for cancer, 117; for
    cold and canker sores, 168; for digestive
    disorders, 208; for dysmenorrhea, 217; for
    foot and leg problems, 265; for headaches,
    281; for hemorrhoids, 304; for hepatitis,
    309; in juice, 5; for lupus, 352; for skin con-
    ditions, 464
alpha-lipoic acid, 14, 25, 52, 100, 113, 133, 147,
    158, 173,; 199, 308, 446–47
Alzheimer's disease, 56–63; causes of, 56–57; herbs
    for, 61–62; supplements for, 58–61; treat-
    ment of, 57–62; what to avoid with, 62–63
American angelica, 54
American Cancer Society, 108, 725, 737
American creosote bush, 30
American ginseng, 439
amino acids, 42, 229
ampalaya, 200
amphetamines, 469
anacardium, 150, 467
anas barbariae, 223

anchoring, 413
andropause, 364, 369
anemia, 64–68; sickle cell, 451–52
angelica, 30, 54, 68, 173
angelica sinensis, 158
anger, 689–90
angina, 289, 290, 612, 614
angina pectoris, 286
angiosarcoma, 730
anise, 338
ankle, sprained, 695
ankylosing spondylitis, 69–70
anorexia nervosa, 226–31
antibiotics, 81, 123, 126, 212, 357
antifungals, 129, 209
antigens, arthritis and, 77
antimonium tartaricum, 176–77
antineoplaston therapy, 121, 733–35
antioxidants; aging and, 5, 13, 14–15, 16; arthritis
    and, 74; back and neck pain and, 93; breast
    cancer and, 100; cancer and, 112–15, 118;
    carpal tunnel syndrome and, 133; cerebral
    palsy and, 137; CFS and, 147–48; depression
    and, 190; diabetes and, 199; digestive disor-
    ders and, 209–10; for ear infections, 222; for
    heatstroke, 301; hepatitis and, 308; lupus
    and, 351; Parkinson's disease and, 401; for
    skin cancer, 459; for skin conditions, 465; for
    stroke, 471; for trauma, 489
apis, 314, 646
apis mellifica, 184, 252
apis mellwiga, 440
apis mollifica, 466
apple, 68
apple juice, 5
applied kinesiology, 46, 583–85
aqueous penicillin treatment, 38
arabinogalactan, larch, 121
arginine, l-arginine, 117, 292
arjuna, 294
Armour Thyroid, 83
arms, lymphedema in, 360–63
arnica, 184, 223, 373, 425
aromatherapy; aging and, 17–18; for chronic pain,
    165; colds and flu, 177–78; for depression,
    193; description of, 586; for dysmenorrhea,
    219; for fever, 253; for headaches, 281; for
    lupus, 353; menopause and, 370; for Parkin-
    son's disease, 402; pregnancy and, 424; for
    respiratory illnesses, 448; for stroke, 474
arrhythmia, cardiac, 287
arsenicum, 643
arsenicum album, 37, 150, 176, 184, 314
arsenicum iodadum, 37
arteriosclerosis, 286, 288, 610, 611, 612, 616
arthritis, 15, 18, 69–80, 161; allergies and, 70;
    causes of, 70; gouty, 69; herbs for, 73–74,
    159–60; juvenile rheumatoid, 69–70; osteo-,
    69, 78; personal experiences with, 27, 598,
    614, 621, 624–25, 626,; 673–74, 682, 695;
    psoriatic, 69; rheumatoid, 69–70, 266,
    673–74; symptoms of, 71; treatment of,
    71–80; what to avoid with, 80
artichoke, 211, 319
ascorbic acid. *See* vitamin C
ash, prickly, 7, 74;

Ashwagandha, 54, 415
aspartame, 278, 285
aspirin, 71, 159, 252, 278, 694
asthma, 53, 442–43, 444–45, 446, 448, 647, 710
astragalus, 17, 30, 53–54, 68, 101, 117–18, 148, 149,
    171, 309,; 325
atherosclerosis, 56, 293
athlete's foot, 265, 462
attention deficit disorder (ADD), 81, 340
attention deficit hyperactivity disorder (ADHD),
    340–50
aurum metallicum, 192, 425
aurum muriatium, 259
autism, 81–84
autohemotherapy (AHT), 678
autoimmune disease; UTI and, 495; *See also* AIDS
    and HIV; multiple sclerosis
avocado, 326
Ayurvedic medicine, 371, 415; personal experi-
    ences with, 587–91

Bach Flower remedies, 90
back and neck pain, 85–95, 161; dysmenorrhea
    and, 219; pain relief techniques, 89–90; per-
    sonal experiences with, 582, 592–93, 620–21,
    622, 654–55,; 694; preventing reinjury,
    93–94; what to avoid with, 94–95; profes-
    sional assistance for, 87–89; seeking treat-
    ment for, 86–87; self-help for, 91–92;
    symptoms, 86
bad breath, 181, 203, 408
baibu, 396
baineiting eye drops, 248
baking soda, 407, 605
balanced hormonal treatment, 77–78
baldness, 635
banaba, 200
baptista, 38, 252
barberry, 159, 309, 454, 464
barley grass, 10, 111, 400
baryta carbonica, 150
basal cell carcinoma, 457
basil, 30
bay, 18
bee pollen, 17, 66, 83, 168, 269, 437, 444, 486
bee propolis, 30, 167, 172
beet juice, 5, 6
belladonna, 175, 185, 223, 235, 252, 302, 448, 466
Bell's palsy, 621, 687
benign prostate hypertrophy, 13
bentonite, 48, 630
berberine, 119, 129, 159, 183, 309, 395, 454
bergamot, 18
beta carotene; aging and, 9, 14; for AIDS, 25;
    breast cancer and, 100; for cancer, 113; for
    cervical dysplasia, 139; for cold and canker
    sores, 167; for colds and flu, 174; for ear
    infections, 222; for endometriosis, 235; for
    osteoporosis, 388; for periodontal disease,
    407, 606; for respiratory illnesses, 445; for
    sinusitis, 454; for skin conditions, 465; for
    stroke, 473; for trauma, 489, 490; for UTI, 498
beta interferon, 374
Betadine, 499
betaine hydrochloride, 275
bifidus, 25

bilberry, 119, 183, 200, 248, 295, 459
bindweed, 117
biofeedback; for cerebral palsy, 137; for chronic pain, 163–64; description of, 592; for eye disorders, 250; personal experiences with, 592–93; for stress, 19; for tinnitus, 479; for trauma, 490
bioflavonoids, 14, 25, 168, 173, 182, 210, 269, 291, 401, 459
biological dentistry, 45–46, 184, 376, 594–607
bio-oxidative therapies, 358
biotin, 129, 200
bitter melon, 31, 32
bitter orange, 18
black cohosh, 14, 218, 294–95, 325, 369, 422
black currant, 75, 100, 111, 183, 368, 445
black haw (viburnum, cramp bark), 158, 218, 422, 430
black locust, 68
black salve, 459
black walnut, 17, 129, 352, 395, 396
bladder, 259; UTI and, 493–501
blessed thistle, 369
blisters, 263
blood; pH of, 458; sickle cell anemia and, 451; sugar *See* hypoglycemia; type, arthritis treatment, 72–73
bloodroot, 119, 183, 459
"blue babies," 287
blue cohosh, 422
blue-green algae, 111, 472
blue vervain, 160, 369
blueberries, 111, 270
blueberry (huckleberry) leaves, 200, 325, 474
bone cancer, 719–20, 732–33
bone spurs, 269
bones. *See* osteoporosis
borage, 75, 100, 111; oil, 183, 200, 368, 445
borax, 373
boric acid, 50
boron, 13, 25, 75, 266, 368, 388, 408
boswellia, 54, 74, 133, 266
bovine cartilage, 627
bovista, 431
bowel. *See* colon; intestines
brain; allergies in, 47; cancer of, 420–21, 652–54, 668–70; dementia and, 56–63; stroke and, 468–76
breast cancer, 96–103, 368, 387; causes of, 96–98; lymphedema and, 360; personal experiences with, 632, 681–82, 712, 717–18, 719,; 721–22, 725, 731–32, 733–34; supplements for, 99–101; symptoms of, 98; treatment of, 98–102; what to avoid with, 102
breast-feeding, 448–49
breasts; implant reactions in, 104–5; tenderness, 419, 431
breathing exercises, 68, 362, 383
brewer's yeast, 168, 487
bromelain, 5, 25, 53, 93, 157, 275, 444
bronchitis, 443
bruxism, 180
bryonia, 252
buchu, 422, 464, 498, 499
buckthorn, 309
bugleweed, 294

bulimia, 226–31
bunions, 266–67
bupleurum, 158, 224
bupleurum falcatum, 30
burdock, 8, 30, 67, 74, 101, 150, 168, 200, 309, 464, 498
Burkitt's syndrome, 22
bursitis, 612
Burton-Friedman technique, 736–37
butcher's broom, 62, 270, 295, 304
butterbur, 54, 283–84
butyric acid, 25

cabbage juice, 5, 6, 73, 111
caffeine, 100, 144, 325
calamus, 192
calcarea carbonica, 78
calcarea fluorica, 408
calcarea phosphorica, 388–89
calcium; for allergies, 53; for arthritis, 75; for autism, 83; for back and neck pain, 93; for breast cancer, 100; cholesterol and, 321; for chronic pain, 158; for dental disorders, 182; for endometriosis, 235; for foot and leg problems, 269; for heart disease, 293; for learning disorders, 347; menopause and, 367–68; osteoporosis and, 388; for parasites, 396; for periodontal disease, 407, 408, 606, 675; for phobias, 415; pregnancy and, 421; for respiratory illnesses, 445; for tinnitus, 478; for TMJ, 483
calcium carbonate, 368
calcium chelate, 53
calcium citrate, 14, 53, 368, 388
calcium sulphide, 169
calculus, 408
calendula, 168, 183, 185, 406, 464, 467
calgarea sulphurica, 466
cali corbonicum, 408
calluses, 264
camphorus, 643
cancer, 106–25, 286; AIDS and, 22; bone, 719–20, 732–33; brain, 420–21, 652–54, 668–70; causes of, 106–8; cervical, 123, 727; colon, 685–86, 714, 728; colorectal, 680–81; combination therapies for, 715–18; Emanuel Revici's therapy for, 728–33; Essiac tea for, 101, 119, 439, 716, 719–20; herbs and, 101, 117–19; heredity and, 107–8; Hippocrates Health Center, 720–21; Hodgkin's disease, 683–84, 713–14, 716–17; intestinal asbestos, 734–35; kidney, 720, 721, 732–33; Lawrence Burton's therapy for, 736–40; leukemia, 106, 715; liver, 642, 680–81; lung, 721–22, 728–29, 732–33; lymphoma, 106, 717, 734, 735, 738, 739–40; Max Gerson's therapy for, 459, 722–27; Nicholas Gonzalez's therapy for, 721–22; ovarian, 728–29; pancreatic, 725–27; personal experiences with, 713–40; prostate, 12–13, 434, 435, 436, 679, 682, 715–16, 721, 732; psychology and, 101–2, 108; 714–X for, 120, 713–15; skin, 457–60, 723–25; Stanislaw Burzynski's therapy for, 121, 733–35; symptoms of, 108; thyroid, 690; treatment of, 108–22; what to avoid with, 122–25; *See also* breast cancer; chemotherapy

candida, candidiasis, 26, 126–31, 493, 497; personal experiences with, 577, 597–98
canker sores, 167–70
cantharis, 499
caprylic acid, 83, 129
capsicum, 54, 395, 396
caraway, 18; oil, 183
carbidopa, 190
carbohydrates; diabetes and, 195, 197; hypoglycemia and, 323; intolerance of, 377, 379; obesity and, 379; *See also* complex carbohydrates
carcinoma, 106
carcinoma, squamous cell, 457–58, 730–31
Carciviren-V (C-1983), 36
cardiac arrhythmia, 287
cardiovascular system; allergies in, 47–48; *See also* heart disease
carnitine, l-carnitine, 42, 292, 325, 336, 380
carnivora (Venus flytrap), 32–33, 101, 121
carnosine, 60, 83
carotenoids, 113–14, 247
carpal tunnel syndrome (CTS), 132–34, 611–12, 645–46
carrot juice, 5, 6, 111
carsinonima, 38
cascara sagrada, 395
cassia, 158
castanospermine, 30
castor oil, 219, 236, 259, 269
catalase, 16, 114
cataracts, 244
caterpillar fungus, 32
cat's claw, 33, 101, 265, 352
cavitations, 180
cavities, 179–80
cayenne, 5, 74, 119, 160, 168, 248, 294, 301, 321, 446, 454,; 474, 486
celandine, 121
celery, 5, 6, 464
centering, 691–92
Centers for Disease Control, 21, 142, 474–75
central nervous system, 47
cerebral palsy, 135–37
cerebrovascular accident (stroke), 468–76, 614–15
cervical cancer, 123, 727
cervical dysplasia, 138–41
CFS. *See* chronic fatigue syndrome (CFS)
chalazions, 670–71
chamomile, chamomilla, 183, 208, 218–19, 223, 236, 415, 464,; 644
chaparral, 168, 396, 454, 459
chaste berry, 369, 430
chelate, 368
chelation therapy, 6, 77, 200, 295–96, 401, 440, 449, 471; description of, 608–9; personal experiences with, 609–16
chemical sensitivity, 45
chemicals, environmental, 238–43
chemotherapy, 108–9, 642, 668–69, 670, 713, 714, 715, 719, 721,; 726, 728–29, 733–34, 735, 738
cherry, wild, 54, 446
chestnut, horse, 304
chewing, improper, 213
chickweed, 7
chimaphilia, 440
China remedy, 369

chiropractic; for arthritis, 78; for back and neck pain, 88; for chronic pain, 162; description of, 617; personal experiences with, 618–27; for TMJ, 483
chitosan, 319
chlamydia, 333
chlorella, 10, 31, 111, 182–83, 400
chlorhexadine, 606
chlorophyll, 10, 73, 111, 129, 445
cholesterol levels, 317–22, 598; *See also* heart disease
choline, 52, 61, 83, 191, 235, 274, 347, 375
chondroitin, 352
chondroitin sulfate, 75, 266, 627
chromium, 42, 100, 117, 147, 321, 325, 408, 464, 489
chromium picolinate, 199, 380
chronic fatigue syndrome (CFS), 142–53, 634–35, 710–11; causes of, 143–44; symptoms of, 145; treatment of, 145–52; what to avoid with, 152
chronic obstructive pulmonary disease (COPD) (emphysema), 443,; 704
chronic pain. *See* pain, chronic
chronic sickness, 590
chrysin, 13
cimifuga, 218, 236, 425
cinchana, 395
cinnamon, 158, 325
circulatory problems; in feet and legs, 269–70; personal experiences with, 684–85
citrus seed extracts, 25–26, 83, 129
clary sage, 18
claudication, intermittent, 270, 610
cleansers, 51
cleavers, 464
clove, 18, 395, 454
clover, red, 8, 101, 119, 168, 172, 309, 464
CMV (cytomegalovirus), 709–10
Coca test, 46–47
cocaine, 344, 469, 470
cocculus, 373, 425
cod liver oil, 75, 498
coenzyme 1 (NADH), 15, 61, 100, 148
coenzyme Q10. *See* Q10, coenzyme
coffea cruda, 185
coffee; enema of, 725; *See also* caffeine
cohosh; black, 14, 218, 294–95, 325, 369, 422; blue, 422
colcynthis, 218
cold sores (fever blisters), 167–70
colds and flu, 171–78; fever, 251–53
Coley's toxins, 120
colitis, ulcerative, 206, 697
colloidal silver, 352–53
colon, 77, 130, 384, 397; cancer of, 685–86, 714, 728; *See also* intestines
colon therapy, 352, 384; description of, 628; personal experiences with, 629–35
colonic irrigation, 7
colonics, enemas, 352, 397, 465
colorectal cancer, 680–81
combination therapies, 715–18
comfrey, 67, 74, 119, 445
complete decongestive physiotherapy (CDP), 361
complex carbohydrates; aging and, 9–10; AIDS and, 22; diabetes and, 197; hypoglycemia and, 324
compound Q, 31

confidence, 652
congenital heart disease, 287
congestive heart failure, 287
conium maculatum, 440
conjugated linoleic acid (CLA), 116, 199
constipation, 203, 418, 495, 633–34, 635
contact dermatitis, 462, 466
contraceptives, oral, 124, 333
Coolmax, 265
COPD (chronic obstructive pulmonary disease)
    (emphysema), 443,; 704
copper, 67, 75, 76, 352, 388
coptis, 159
coriander, 18
CoQ10. *See* Q10, coenzyme.
corn silk, 7, 216, 439, 464, 498
corns, 264
corticoid, 389
cortisone, 52, 71, 694
corydalis, 158, 159
counseling, 415
cramp bark (black haw, viburnum), 158, 218, 422,
    430
cranberry, 497
craniosacral therapy, 282
creativity, 707
Creutzfeld-Jakob disease, 56
Crohn's disease, 203–4, 706
croton tiglium, 467
CTS (carpal tunnel syndrome), 132–34, 611–12,
    645–46
cumin, 18
curcumin, 61, 76, 99, 118, 133, 160, 174, 308, 319,
    401
currant, black, 75, 100, 111, 183, 368, 445
curry, 293
Cushing's disease, 577–78
cyanosis, 287
Cylert, 344
cypems, 158
Cyprus, 304
cysteine, l-cysteine, 325–26, 375, 401, 445
cystic fibrosis, 660
cystitis, 493; interstitial, 495–96
cysts, 462
cytomegalovirus (CMV), 709–10

Daflon, 303–4
dairy products, 205, 667, 671; cancer and, 122–23
danazol, 234
dance injuries, 659
dandelion, 8, 217, 270, 325, 388; leaf, 7; root, 43,
    67, 119, 158, 200, 309, 464
DASM (dehydroandrographolide succinic acid
    monoester), 31
deep breathing, 19
deer ticks, 355–59
deglycyrrhizinated licorice (DGL), 209
dehydroandrographolide succinic acid monoester
    (DASM), 31
dehydroepiandrosterone (DHEA), 11; for AIDS,
    26; for Alzheimer's and dementia, 59–60; for
    anemia, 67; for arthritis, 76; for cancer, 115;
    for colds and flu, 173; for depression,
    190–91; for diabetes, 199; for learning disor-
    ders, 348; for lupus, 352; for menopause,

368; for obesity, 381; for osteoporosis, 388;
    replacement therapy, 12–13
dementia, 56–63
demulcents, 498
denatured foods, 124–25
dental disorders, 179–86; biological dentistry,
    45–46, 184, 376, 594–607; causes of, 180–81;
    common problems, 179–80; mercury amal-
    gam fillings, 46, 343, 376, 594–607, 709;
    periodontal disease, 180, 404–9, 597, 602–3,
    605–6, 675; personal experiences with,
    594–607, 644; proper dental hygiene,
    183–84; symptoms of, 181; treatment of,
    181–85; what to avoid with, 185
depression, 187–94; causes of, 188; eating disor-
    ders and, 229; homeopathy for, 192–93;
    menopause and, 369; personal experiences
    with, 604; postpartum, 424–25; stroke and,
    474–75; symptoms of, 188–89; treatment of,
    189–93; what to avoid with, 193–94
dermatitis, 462–63, 466–67; contact, 462, 466; seb-
    orrheic, 463
desensitization, 412
Desoxyn, 344
detoxification; for allergies, 48–49; antiaging prop-
    erties of, 4–8; for arthritis, 77; of bowel, 211;
    for breast cancer, 101; for CFS, 152; for envi-
    ronmental illness, 240; for parasites, 397; of
    respiratory system, 447–48; for skin condi-
    tions, 465; of specific systems, 6–8
devil's claw, 74, 269
Dexedrine, 344
dextroamphetamine, 344
DGL deglycyrrhizinated licorice), 209
DGLA (di-hommo-gamma linoleic acid), 449
DHA (docosahexaenoic), 67, 133, 200
DHEA (dehydroepiandrosterone), 11; for AIDS,
    26; for Alzheimer's and dementia, 59–60; for
    anemia, 67; for arthritis, 76; for cancer, 115;
    for CFS, 148; for colds and flu, 173; for de-
    pression, 190–91; for diabetes, 199; for learn-
    ing disorders, 348; for lupus, 352; for
    menopause, 368; for obesity, 381; for osteo-
    porosis, 388; replacement therapy, 12–13
di-hommo-gamma linoleic acid (DGLA), 449
diabetes, 195–201, 610–11; candidiasis and, 127;
    foot and leg problems with, 261; gestational,
    418–19; pregnancy and, 421
diabetic retinopathy, 245
Diabinese, 197
diagaku eye drops, 248
diarrhea, 204, 418
diet, nutrition; acidic vs. alkaline foods, 110, 155,
    165–66, 400, 458, 497; in alcoholism treat-
    ment, 42–43; for allergies, 49, 671;
    Alzheimer's, dementia and, 58–61; for ane-
    mia, 65–66; anti–aging diet, 9–10; for arthri-
    tis, 72–73, 626–27; for autism, 82–84; back
    and neck pain and, 93; for breast cancer,
    99–101; for cancer, 110–12; candidiasis and,
    128; CFS and, 145–46; cholesterol and,
    318–19; chronic pain and, 155; for colds and
    flu, 171; denatured foods, 124–25; for de-
    pression, 190; for diabetes, 197, 198; for
    digestive disorders, 207–8, 212, 213–14; for
    dysmenorrhea, 216; endometriosis and, 234;

diet, nutrition; acidic vs. alkaline foods, (*cont.*)
for environmental illness, 240–41; for eye disorders, 246–47; for fibroids, 257–58; foods with flora, 207; for gallstones, 274; for heart disease, 289–90; for hemorrhoids, 303; for hepatitis, 307–8; for herpes, 312–13; high-fiber, 207; Lyme disease and, 357; for lymphedema, 361; for menopause, 367–68; MS and, 375; obesity and, 379; organically grown food, 669–70; osteoporosis and, 387; for parasites, 396–97; Parkinson's disease and, 400–401; periodontal disease and, 407; personal experiences with, 663–76; PMS and, 428–30; pregnancy and, 420; prostate conditions and, 436; respiratory illnesses and, 443–44; rotation, 49, 76–77, 671; for sinusitis, 453–54; skin cancer and, 458–59; skin conditions and, 463; tinnitus and, 477–78; trauma and, 488–90; for TSS, 486; for UTI, 497–98; vegetarian diet, 66, 99

Diflucan, 83

digest RC, 210–11

digestive disorders, 202–14; eating disorders and, 229; herbs for, 208–9; personal experiences with, 667–68; treatments of, 207–12; what to avoid with, 212–14

digestive enzymes, 53, 174, 210

digestive harmony, 130

dill, 18

dimethyl sulfoxide (DMSO), 115, 168, 683, 685

dimethylaminoethanol (DMAE), 58, 191, 347

dimethyl glycine (DMG), 83, 100, 375, 445

dinitrochlorobenzene (DNCB), 36

dioscorea (wild yam), 158, 218, 294, 309, 368, 369, 622

dioxychlor, 26

dithiolethione, 31

diverticulitis, 204, 629–30

dizziness, 666–67

dL-phenylalanine (DLPA), 156, 352

DLPA (dl-phenylalanine), 156, 352, 401

DMAE (dimethylaminoethanol), 58, 191, 347

DMG (dimethyl glycine), 83, 100, 375

DMSA, 84

DMSO (dimethyl sulfoxide), 115, 168, 683, 685

DNCB (dinitrochlorobenzene), 36

dock, yellow, 8, 17, 67, 137, 309

dolphin-assisted therapy, 137

dong quai, 14, 67, 158, 159, 218, 369, 431

dopamine, 188, 400, 401

dowager's hump, 390

doxorubicin, 118

Doxycycline, 585

Dramamine, 372

drips, vitamin, 708–12

dulcamara, 169, 177, 314, 466–67

dysidia, 36

dysmenorrhea, 215–20

dysplasia, cervical, 138–41

E. coli, 493, 497

ear; infections, 221–25, 618, 648; tinnitus, 477–80

Easter lily, 445

eating disorders, 226–31; *See also* obesity

echinacea; aging and, 7, 8; for AIDS, 33; for allergies, 54; for arthritis, 626–27; for breast can-

cer, 101; for cancer, 118; for CFS, 149; for cold and canker sores, 168; for colds and flu, 171–72; for foot and leg problems, 265; for hemorrhoids, 304; for periodontal disease, 407; for respiratory illnesses, 446; for sinusitis, 454; for skin conditions, 464

eclipta alba, 31

eczema, 464, 630; irritant, 463

EDTA (ethylene diamine tetraacetic acid), 6, 608

educational kinesiology, 414

EFT (Emotional Freedom Technique), 19

egg lipids, 26

elder, 68

elderberry, 454

elder flower, 172, 301

elecampane, 172, 395; ; electromagnetic pollution, 242

electromagnetic radiation (EMR), 124

eleutherococcus senticosus, 168

elimination test, 47

elm, slippery, 159, 172, 304, 446, 498

Emotional Freedom Technique (EFT), 19

emphysema (chronic obstructive pulmonary disease), 443, 704

EMR (electromagnetic radiation), 97–98, 124

encephalitis, 22

endometriosis, 232–37

endorphins, 155–56, 413

enemas, colonics, 352, 397, 465; coffee, 725

energy; increased, 671–72; lack of, 635; maximizing, 588–89

environmental illness, 238–43; personal experiences with, 583–84

environmental toxicity, 70

enzyme therapy, 636–38

enzymes; aging and, 15–16; cancer and, 115; digestive, 53, 174, 210; pancreatic, 120; protein-digesting, 133; proteolytic, 438

episiotomy problems, 419

Epsom salts, 304

Epstein-Barr virus, 311, 590–91, 611, 709–10, 711–12

essential fatty acids. *See* fatty acids, essential

essential oils, 90, 177–78, 193, 253, 315; *See also* aromatherapy

Essiac, 101, 119, 439, 716, 719–20

estradiol, 99, 368

estriol, 14, 99, 368

estrogen, 13, 99, 100; for Alzheimer's and dementia, 60; fibroids and, 255, 256; headaches and, 278; infertility and, 333; menopause and, 364, 368; natural estrogen therapy, 14; obesity and, 381; plant, 366, 367; PMS and, 428, 433; UTI and, 494

estrogen replacement therapy, 387

estrone, 368

ethylene diamine tetraacetic acid (EDTA), 6, 608

eucalyptus, 18, 454

eupatorium perfoliatuin, 176

euphrasia, 175

Euphytose, 483

evening primrose oil; for arthritis, 75; breast cancer and, 100; for dental disorders, 183; for diabetes, 200; for dysmenorrhea, 216; for fibroids, 258; for headaches, 282; for hepatitis, 309; menopause and, 368; for MS, 375; for respiratory illnesses, 445; for UTI, 498

exercise; aerobic, 297, 389; for AIDS, 39; for arthritis, 79; for back and neck pain, 91–92; for breast cancer, 101; for CFS, 151; cholesterol and, 321; for chronic pain, 160–61; for depression, 189–90; for diabetes, 198; for dysmenorrhea, 219; for eye disorders, 249; for heart disease, 296–97; hormonal imbalance and, 11; lungs and, 7; for lupus, 352; menopause and, 370–71; for obesity, 382–83; for osteoporosis, 389–91; Parkinson's disease and, 402; for PMS, 430; pregnancy and, 422; sinusitis and, 456; stroke and, 475; for UTI, 499; weight, 296
eye problems, 244–50; diabetes and, 196–97, 199; eye crossing, 248; personal experiences with, 610, 687–88
eyebright, 17, 54, 172, 200

Fargelin, 304
farsightedness, 245, 246
fasting, 674; aging and, 4–6; for allergies, 48
fat, dietary, 23, 100
fatigue, 419, 607, 665–67, 688–89
fatty acids, essential; for AIDS, 26; in alcoholism treatment, 42; for allergies, 53; for arthritis, 75; for autism, 83; for cancer, 113; for candidiasis, 129; for carpal tunnel syndrome, 133; for CFS, 148; for chronic pain, 158; for dental disorders, 182; for depressipn, 190; for diabetes, 200; for digestive disorders, 210; for ear infections, 222; for gallstones, 274; for headaches, 284; for heart disease, 291; for hepatitis, 308; for learning disorders, 347; for lupus, 351, 352; menopause and, 367; for obesity, 380; for osteoporosis, 388; for periodontal disease, 408; for PMS, 429; *See also* omega-3 fatty acid
fennel, 7, 18, 208, 338, 498
fenugreek, 446
ferrum phosphoricum, 175, 185, 223, 252, 646
ferrum picricum, 440
fever, 251–53; flu and, 171–78
fever blisters (cold sores), 167–70
feverfew, 31, 119, 159, 284
fiber, 110–11, 325, 367
fibroids, 254–60
fibromyalgia, 278, 587–88
fibromyoma uteri, 254
fibrosis; cystic, 660; idiopathic pulmonary, 587–88
filtration systems, air, 48–49
fish oil, 83, 320
Flagyl, 395, 710
flatulence, 204, 418
flavonoids, 114, 465
flaxseed, 499; oil, 60, 83, 111, 274–75, 352, 429
flu and colds, 171–78; fever and, 251–53
fluoridation, 182
fluoride, 182, 188
flushes; gallbladder, 274; for lupus, 352–53
Flutamide, 436
fo-ti tieng, 16
folic acid; in alcoholism treatment, 43; anemia and, 64–65, 67; cancer and, 116; and cervical dysplasia, 139; CFS and, 148; depression and, 190; heart disease and, 291–92; infertility and, 337; menopause and, 367; osteoporosis and, 388; pregnancy and, 420

folliculinum, 432
food allergies, 44–45, 76–77, 81–82, 204, 342–43, 444, 463,; 667–68
foot and leg problems, 161, 261–72; circulatory problems, 269–70, 684–85; external, 263–65; infections, 686; internal, 268–69; joint pain, 266, 688–89; knee pain, 621–22, 623, 694; lymphedema and, 360–63; personal experiences with, 621–22, 623, 662, 684–85, 686,; 694, 695
footwear, 266, 267, 270–71
FOS (fructooligosaccharides), 43
fragaria, 408
frankincense, 18
fructo-oligosaccharides (FOS), 43, 293
FSH, 367
fungal rashes, 462

GABA, 347, 415
gallbladder flush, 274
gallstones, 273–76
gama-amino butyric acid (GABA), 347, 415
gamma linoleic acid (GLA), 75, 100, 133, 158, 173, 183, 200,; 368, 380, 429, 438, 449
ganoderma (reishi) mushrooms, 17, 33, 112, 149, 309, 321, 336
gardenia, 216
garlic; aging and, 8, 10, 16; for AIDS, 23, 31; in alcoholism treatment, 43; for allergies, 53; for arthritis, 626; for autism, 83; breast cancer and, 100; for cancer, 118; for candidiasis, 129; for CFS, 149; cholesterol and, 319, 321; for cold and canker sores, 168; for colds and flu, 174; for dental disorders, 182–83; for eye disorders, 248; for headaches, 672; for heart disease, 293; for hepatitis, 309; for MS, 375; for parasites, 395; for periodontal disease, 407; for respiratory illnesses, 446, 447; for sinusitis, 454; for stroke, 474; for UTI, 498
gastric reflux, 204–5
gastrointestinal system; allergies in, 48; bladder and, 259, 493–501; indigestion and, 18, 202–3; parasites in, 393–98; PMS and, 431; pregnancy and, 417–18, 419; *See also* colon; digestive disorders; intestines
GastroPro, 211, 308
GE-3-S, 36
ge xia zhu yu wan, 158
gelsemium, 37, 150, 176, 252
general health and wellness, 623–24
general practitioners, 87
genetic predisposition, cancer and, 107–8
genistein, 117
gentian, 67, 173, 325
German chamomile, 130
germanium, 100
Gerson therapy, 459, 722–27
Gestalt therapy, 655
gestational diabetes, 418–19
GHRH (growth hormone releasing hormone), 12
giardia lambia, 395
ginger; for arthritis, 74; for cancer, 118; for carpal tunnel syndrome, 133; for cerebral palsy, 137; cholesterol and, 321; for cold and canker sores, 168; for colds and flu, 172; for depression, 192; for digestive disorders, 208;

ginger; for arthritis, (*cont.*)
for eye disorders, 248; for heart disease, 293; for hypoglycemia, 325; for motion sickness, 372; pregnancy and, 422; for respiratory illnesses, 446; for sinusitis, 454; for TSS, 486
ginger, wild, 159
gingivitis, 180, 404–5
ginkgo biloba; aging and, 16; for AIDS, 31; for allergies, 52; for Alzheimer's and dementia, 61–62; for autism, 83; cancer and, 118; for cerebral palsy, 137; for chronic pain, 160; for depression, 192; for eye disorders, 247, 248; for headaches, 284; for heart disease, 294; for infertility, 338; for learning disorders, 347; for Parkinson's disease, 401; for PMS, 430–31; for respiratory illnesses, 446; for skin cancer, 459; for stroke, 471, 474; for tinnitus, 478
ginseng, 16–17; AIDS and, 31; for allergies, 54; for Alzheimer's and dementia, 62; American, 439; for anemia, 67; cancer and, 118; Korean, 62; for menopause, 369; panax, 148, 149, 325; Siberian, 43, 148, 149, 325, 439; for TSS, 486
GLA (gamma linoleic acid), 75, 100, 133, 158, 173, 183, 200,; 368, 380, 429, 438, 449
glandular polypeptide extract, 36
glaucoma, 245, 610
glonoinum, 302
glucosamine, 75, 284, 352
glucosamine hydrochloride, 75
glucosamine sulfate, 75, 158, 266
glutamic acid, 42, 437
glutamine, l-glutamine, 42, 52, 60, 83, 115, 210, 308, 325, 326,; 347, 358, 490
glutathione, 16, 42, 52, 60, 83, 118, 147, 148, 308, 401
glutathione peroxidase, 27, 114, 445
glycemic index, 379–80
glycine, 437
glycosylation, 60
glycyrrhizin (licorice root), 34, 52–53, 148, 159, 168, 172,; 325, 439, 446
gold injections, 71
goldenrod, 464, 498
goldenseal; for AIDS, 31–32; for allergies, 52; for anemia, 67; for cancer, 119; for candidiasis, 130; for cold and canker sores, 168; for colds and flu, 172; for dental disorders, 183; for hypoglycemia, 325; for parasites, 395; pregnancy and, 422; for sinusitis, 454; for UTI, 159, 498, 499
gotu kola, 17, 248, 270, 352
gout, 267
gouty arthritis, 69
grape seed extract, 52, 75, 115, 401
grape seed oil, 14
grapefruit seed extract, 396
green algae, 168
green tea, 99–100, 111, 172, 209, 217, 319, 401, 447, 465, 474
greens; aging and, 10; AIDS and, 23–24; cancer and, 111; eating disorders and, 230; juices, 73, 486
growth hormone releasing hormone (GHRH), 12
gugulipid, 319

Gulf War syndrome, 143–44
gum disease. *See* periodontal disease

Haldol, 402
halibut oil, 498
hamstring tear, 662
haw, black (viburnum, cramp bark), 158, 218, 422, 430
hawthorn, 401, 459, 474, 486; berry, 248, 294
hay fever, 44
HCA (hydroxy citric acid), 381
HDLs (high-density lipoproteins), 317–18, 475
headaches, 277–85, 431, 432; herbs for, 159, 281–82; personal experiences with, 593, 601–2, 607, 619, 624, 672,; 676; sinus, 280; treatment of, 279–84
hearing, 688–89; tinnitus, 477–80
heart attacks, 614, 632–33; stroke vs., 468
heart disease, 286–99; diabetes and, 196; eating disorders and, 227; herbs for, 293–95; personal experiences with, 603–4, 609, 610, 611, 612, 613–14,; 615–16; power of the mind with, 297–98; stroke and, 469; symptoms of, 288; treatment of, 288–98; types of, 286–88; what to avoid with, 298
heartburn, 419
heat exhaustion, 300–302
heatstroke, 300–302
heavy metal toxicity, 57, 262, 349, 402
heel imbalances, 268–69
Hellerwork, 236
hemorrhoids, 303–5
hepar sulphuris, 169, 176, 185, 223
hepar sulphuris calcareum, 440, 466, 644
hepatitis, 306–10; personal experiences with, 580, 663–64, 681, 685, 686
herbastatin, 130
herbs, 16–17; adaptogenic, 148; for AIDS, 28–34; in alcoholism treatment, 43; for allergies, 53–64; for Alzheimer's and dementia, 61–62; for anemia, 67–68; for arthritis, 73–74; for back and neck pain, 90; breast cancer and, 101; for cancer, 101, 117–19; for candidiasis, 129–30; for cerebral palsy, 137; for CFS, 148–50; Chinese, 158, 159–60, 217, 224; for cholesterol, 321; for chronic pain, 158–60; for cold and canker sores, 168–69; for colds and flu, 171; for dental disorders, 183; for depression, 192; description of therapy with, 639–40; for diabetes, 200; for digestive disorders, 208–9; for dysmenorrhea, 216–17; for endometriosis, 235; for eye disorders, 248; for fibroids, 258–59; for foot and leg problems, 270; for gallstones, 275; for headaches, 159, 281–82; for heart disease, 293–95; for heatstroke, 301; for hemorrhoids, 304; for hepatitis, 308–9; for hypoglycemia, 325; for infertility, 338; for lupus, 352; for lymphedema, 361; menopause and, 369; for osteoporosis, 388; for parasites, 395–96; for Parkinson's disease, 401; for phobias, 415–16; for PMS, 430–31; pregnancy and, 421–22; for prostate conditions, 438–39; for respiratory illnesses, 446; for sinusitis, 454; for skin cancer, 459; for skin conditions, 464;

for stroke, 474; suppositories, 140; for TMJ, 483; for TSS, 486; for UTI, 498–99
heredity; cancer and, 107–8; stroke and, 470
herpes, 167–69, 311–16, 493, 709–10
HGH (human growth hormone), 11; replacement therapy, 12
high blood pressure. See hypertension
high-density lipoproteins (HDLs), 317–18, 475
hip pain, 622
Hippocrates Health Center, 720–21
HIV. See AIDS and HIV
ho shou wu, 17
Hodgkin's disease, 683–84, 713–14, 716–17
homeopathy; for AIDS, 36–38; for anemia, 68; for arthritis, 78; for back and neck pain, 90; for candidiasis, 130; for CFS, 150–51; for colds and flu, 175–77; for dental disorders, 184–85; for depression, 192–93; description of, 641–42; for diabetes, 200; for dysmenorrhea, 218–19; for ear infections, 222–23; for endometriosis, 235–36; for fever, 252; for fibroids, 259; for heatstroke, 301–2; for herpes, 169, 313–15; menopause and, 369–70; for motion sickness, 372–73; for osteoporosis, 388–89; for periodontal disease, 408; personal experiences with, 642–48; for PMS, 431–32; pregnancy and, 424–25; for prostate conditions, 439–40; for respiratory illnesses, 448; sequential, 646–47; for skin conditions, 466–67
honey, 444
hops, 192, 401, 415
horehound, 54, 173
hormonal imbalance, 11–12, 622
hormonal treatment, balanced, 77–78
hormone rebalancing, aging and, 11–14
hormone replacement therapy, 13–14, 124, 366
horse chestnut, 270, 304
horseback riding, therapeutic, 137
horseradish, 68, 446
horsetail, 68, 388, 422
hoxsey herbs, 119
HPV (human papilloma virus), 138
huckleberry (blueberry) leaves, 200, 325, 474
human growth hormone (HGH), 11; replacement therapy, 12
human papilloma virus (HPV), 138
huperzine A, 62
Hydergine, 473–74, 489–90
hydrangea root, 439
hydrastinum muriaticum, 259
hydrazine sulfate, 120
hydrochloric acid, 67, 444
Hydrofloss, 605–6
hydrogen peroxide, 397, 407, 496, 605, 683, 685
hydrotherapy, 48, 219
hydroxy citric acid (HCA), 381
hydroxyurea, 451–52
hyperbaric oxygen therapy, 136, 471–72, 677
hypercholesterolemia, 318
hypericum, 185
hypericum perforatum, 314–15, 369
hyperopia, 245
hyperpyrexia, heat, 300–302
hypertension (high blood pressure), 287, 289, 469; personal experiences with, 592–93, 610, 612–13, 704

hyperthermia, 39
hyperthyroidism, 665
hypnotherapy, 19; description of, 649–50; personal experiences with, 650–57
hypoglycemia, 323–27, 665–66, 671
hypothyroidism, 57, 83, 144, 377–78, 382; treatment of, 328–31
hyssop, 18, 173
hysterectomy, 233, 254, 255–56, 728

IAT (Immuno-Augmentative Therapy), 736–40
ibuprofen, 234
idiopathic pulmonary fibrosis, 587–88
IgG ELISA, 442
ignatia, 37, 177, 192, 425
Ilizarov technique, 137
imagery, 412
immunizations. See vaccinations
Immuno-Augmentative Therapy (IAT), 736–40
immunoglobulins, 44
immunotherapy, neutralization, 50
implants, breast, 104–5
Indian snakeroot, 294
indigestion, 202–3; aromatherapy for, 18
indole-3-carbinol (I3C), 139
indomethacin, 234
indosin, 121
infections; arthritis and, 70; ear, 221–25, 618, 648; foot, 686; personal experiences with, 644, 648, 679–80; prostate, 435; UTI, 159, 493–501; yeast, 257, 579, 636–38
infertility, 332–39
inflacin, 76
inflammation, 154
influenza and colds, 171–78
ingrown toenails, 267
injuries, 659, 659–60, 662, 694
inositol, 83, 191, 275, 375, 412, 415
inositol hexaphosphate (IP-6), 115
insomnia, 18, 661, 690–91
insulin, 195–201, 377–78
interferon, 120, 681, 737; beta, 374
interferon alpha, 307
interleukin, 737
intermittent claudication, 270, 610
interstitial cystitis, 495–96
intestinal flora, 27
intestines; cancer of, 734–35; detoxification of, 6, 7; twisted, 630–32; See also colon
IntraArticular Growth Hormone (IAGH), 79
iodadum, 37
iodine, 27
ipecacuanha, 448
iron, 66, 93, 182, 235, 421
iron deficiency anemia, 64
irritable bowel syndrome, 205
irritant eczema, 463
iscador, 121
isoflavones, 368, 387, 430

Jamaica weed, 309
jelly, royal, 33–34, 326, 486
jewel weed, 464
jock itch, 462
joint pain, 266–67, 646–47, 688–89

juice, 10; aging and, 4–6; for AIDS, 23–24; for arthritis, 73; for cancer, 111; for CFS, 146; for chronic pain, 155; for lymphedema, 361; for respiratory illnesses, 444; for sinusitis, 453; for skin conditions, 463; for tinnitus, 478
juniper, 18, 422, 498
juvenile rheumatoid arthritis, 69–70

kali bichromicum, 177
kali carbonicum, 425
kali muriaticum, 223
kali phosphoricum, 150
Kaposi's sarcoma, 29, 39, 731
Kaposi's syndrome, 22
kava kava, 160, 192, 415–16
kelp, 10, 295
kidneys; cancer of, 720, 721, 732–33; detoxification of, 6, 7; diabetes and, 197; skin conditions and, 461, 464, 466; stones, 610; UTI and, 493, 495
kinesiology; applied, 46, 583–85; educational, 414
knee injuries, 621–22, 623, 694
kola nut, 381
ku shen, 130, 396
kut, 62

l-arginine, arginine, 117, 292
l-carnitine, carnitine, 42, 292, 325, 336, 380
l-cysteine, cysteine, 325–26, 375, 401, 445
l-dopa, 27
l-glutamine, glutamine, 42, 52, 60, 83, 115, 210, 308, 325, 326,; 347, 358, 490
l-methionine, methionine, 42
l-tryptophane, tryptophane, 61, 415
l-tyrosine, 52
laccaninum, 431
lachasis, 431
lactobacillus acidophilus, 128, 167, 222, 229, 498
lactobacillus bifidum, 128, 222, 229, 498
lactoferrin, 116, 129
lady's slipper, 401, 415
lamivudine, 307
larch arabinogalactan, 121
lavender, 18, 464
LDLs (low-density lipoproteins), 317, 318
lead poisoning, 611
learning disorders, 340–50
lecithin, 43, 59, 292, 320, 380, 465, 473, 672
leg problems. *See* foot and leg problems
legustrum, 149
lei wan, 396
leiomyoma uteri, 254
lemon, 18, 304, 347
lentinan, 118
leptotania, 32
leukemia, 106, 715
LH, 367
licorice, 7, 208–9; deglycyrrhizinated, 209; root (glycyrrhizin), 34, 52–53, 148, 159, 168, 172, 325, 439,; 446
life plant (phyllanthius), 34
lifestyle factors; cancer and, 106–7; phobias and, 413; prostate conditions and, 440
light therapy, 192
lignosulfonate (LS), 36
ligustrum lucidum, 33

lily of the valley, 294
linden, 67
linseed oil, 269
lipids, egg, 26
lipoma, 671
lipoproteins, 317–18
live-cell therapy, 39
liver, 113; beet juice and, 5; cancer and, 642, 680–81; detoxification of, 6, 7; hypoglycemia and, 326; personal experiences with problems of, 619–20, 680–81; skin conditions and, 461, 462, 466; *See also* hepatitis
lobelia, 446
lodge, sweat, 490–91
lomacium, 150, 168, 173
lonicera, 148
low-density lipoproteins (LDLs), 317, 318
lungs; cancer of, 721–22, 728–29, 732–33; detoxification of, 6, 7
Lungtanxieganwan, 281, 430
lungwort, 445
Lupron, 256, 436
lupus, 351–54; *See also* allergies; arthritis
lutein, 114, 247
Luvox, 412
lycium rehmarinia, 248
lycopene, 9–10, 438
lycopodium, 150
Lyme disease, 355–59, 585, 611
lymphatic system; breast cancer and, 97; detoxification of, 8; manual drainage of, 361
lymphedema, 360–63
lymphoma, 106, 717, 734, 735, 738, 739–40

ma huang, 422
macrobiotic foods, 112
macular degeneration, 245, 256
mad cow disease, 56
magnesium; in alcoholism treatment, 42; for Alzheimer's and dementia, 59; for arthritis, 75, 626; for autism, 83; for back and neck pain, 93; breast cancer and, 100; for CFS, 147; cholesterol and, 321; for chronic pain, 158; for dental disorders, 182; depression and, 190; for diabetes, 199; for digestive disorders, 210; for dysmenorrhea, 216; for headaches, 278, 283, 284; for heart disease, 292–93; for hemorrhoids, 303; for hypothyroidism, 330; for learning disorders, 347; for obesity, 380; for osteoporosis, 388; for parasites, 396; for periodontal disease, 408, 675; for phobias, 415; for PMS, 429; for respiratory illnesses, 444–45; for stroke, 471, 472; for tinnitus, 478; for TMJ, 483; for trauma, 489, 490
magnetic healing; for back and neck pain, 90; for cerebral palsy, 136; for chronic pain, 164; for foot and leg problems, 265; for lymphedema, 362; for MS, 376; for respiratory illnesses, 449; for skin conditions, 465; for tinnitus, 479
magnetic molecular energizing therapy, 136
maidenhair fern, 68, 478
maitake mushrooms, 33, 459
malabsorption syndrome, 205
malaria, 673–74
malignant melanoma, 458

manganese, 42, 75, 182, 330, 388, 408
mantras, 19
manual lymphatic drainage, 361
marjoram, 18, 248
marshmallow, 304, 446, 498
massage therapy, 89; for chronic pain, 165; description of, 658; for headaches, 280; personal experiences with, 658–62; pregnancy and, 423–24; *See also* reflexology
masterwort, 173
maxepa, 293
meadowsweet, 68
meat, cancer and, 122
meclizine, 666
meditation, 19, 39, 193
medorrhinum, 37
melanoma, 106, 457, 723–25, 727
melatonin, 13, 19, 60, 67, 84, 115, 174, 372, 401, 473
melia, 158
Mellaril, 402
melon, bitter, 31, 32
melon juices, 5
memory loss, 18
men, testosterone rebalancing in, 13
meningitis, 22
menopause, 13, 364–71; candidiasis and, 126–27; depression and, 191; personal experiences with, 604; UTI and, 494
menstrual pain, 215–20; herbs for, 67, 158; personal experiences with, 590–91
menstruation; endometriosis and, 233; headaches and, 278; hypothyroidism and, 328; infertility and, 33; *See also* menopause; premenstrual syndrome
mercurius, 37, 223, 644
mercurius solubilis, 185
mercurius vivus, 176
mercury, in fillings, 46, 343, 376, 594–607, 709
methamphetamine, 344
methionine, l-methionine, 275, 321, 445
methylsulfonylmethane (MSM), 53, 76, 158
MGN-3, 112
migraine headaches. *See* headaches
milk thistle, 7, 43, 137, 270, 308, 464
minerals; aging and, 15; in alcoholism treatment, 42; allergies and, 53; for Alzheimer's and dementia, 57; arthritis and, 75; eating disorders and, 228–30
ming mu, 248
mint, 67, 159, 168
mistletoe, 33, 101, 294
modified citrus pectin (MCP), 116, 438
molasses; blackstrap, 67; unsulfured, 486
molybdenum, 53, 100
monosodium glutamate (MSG), 277, 284–85, 449
morning sickness, 417–18
motherwort, 294, 369
motion sickness, 372–73
Motrin, 71, 622, 694
MS (multiple sclerosis), 374–76, 625–26, 644–45, 648, 650–51
MSG (monosodium glutamate), 277, 284–85, 449
MSM (methylsulfonylmethane), 53, 76, 158
muira puama, 13
mullein, 54, 395, 446
multiple myeloma, 738–39

multiple sclerosis (MS), 374–76, 625–26, 644–45, 648, 650–51
muriaticum acid, 150
muscle tightness, chronic, 661–62
mushrooms; AIDS and, 23, 33; cancer and, 111–12, 459; for colds and flu, 174
myeloma, multiple, 738–39
myocarditis, 287
myoma coagulation, 255–56
myomectomy, 255
myopia, 245
myrrh, 183, 265, 407, 446

n-acetyl-cysteine (NAC), 13, 27, 42, 52, 60, 116, 147, 173, 199,; 308, 401, 445
NADH (nicotinamide adenine dinucleotide), 15, 61, 100, 148, 191
Naltrexone, 39
naoili, 18
Naprosyn, 234, 694
natmur, 169, 370, 425, 431–32
natrum muriaticum, 169, 175–76, 192–93, 314
natrum sulfuricum, 448
naturopathic medicine, 337–38
nearsightedness, 245, 246
neck pain. *See* back and neck pain
nervines, 401
nervous system balance, 591
nettles, 13, 67, 74, 208, 388, 446, 464; stinging, 54, 150, 229
neurolinguistic programming, 413–14
neuromuscular therapy, 79
neuropathy, peripheral, 261–62
neurosurgeons, 87–88
neutralization immunotherapy, 50
nexrutine, 76
niacin (vitamin B3), 190, 247, 293, 320, 375, 478
niacinamide (vitamin B3), 74–75, 147
nicotinamide adenine dinucleotide (NADH), 15, 61, 100, 148, 191
nicotine, 98, 325
non-Hodgkin's lymphoma, 22, 727, 735
nose; fractured, 708–9; runny, 676
Null, Gary, 634, 666, 670, 672; protocol, 505–72
nutmeg, 18
nutrition. *See* diet, nutrition
nux vomica, 151, 176, 373
Nystatin, 83, 129

oats, 149, 168, 192, 208, 369, 464
obesity, 377–85, 651, 664–65
O'Connor technique, 89
olive oil, 111, 224
omega-3 fatty acid; for arthritis, 75; for cancer, 113; for carpal tunnel syndrome, 133; for depression, 190; for digestive disorders, 210; for ear infections, 222; for eye disorders, 247; for gallstones, 274; for headaches, 284; for heart disease, 291; for lupus, 351, 352; for phobias, 415; for prostate conditions, 438
omega-6 fatty acid, 113, 190, 247, 291
onions, 10
oregano oil, 130, 396
Oregon grape, 130, 159, 309, 464
organically grown food, 669–70
origanum, 208

Orinase, 197
orthopedic doctors, 87
orthotics, 266
osha root, 32, 422
osteoarthritis, 69, 78, 266, 626–27
osteocalcin, 387
osteopathic physicians, 133
osteoporosis, 6, 7, 15, 386–92
ovarian cancer, 728–29
oxygen therapy, 677–86; hyperbaric, 136, 471–72, 677
ozone therapy, 262; for AIDS and HIV, 38; for cancer, 119; for foot and leg problems, 266, 270; for hepatitis, 309; for herpes, 315; for Lyme disease, 358; personal experiences with, 677–79; for sickle cell anemia, 452

pain, chronic, 154–66; acupuncture for, 162–63; biofeedback for, 163–64; causes of, 154; chiropractic for, 162; exercises for, 160–61; herbs for, 158–60; home remedies for, 162; magnetic healing for, 164; personal experiences with, 580, 585, 621–22, 623, 654–55; psychology and, 162; therapeutic touch for, 165; treatment of, 155–65; what to avoid with, 165–66; *See also* back and neck pain; joint pain
palmetto, saw, 13, 173, 438–39
panax ginseng, 148, 149, 325
pancreas, 11, 326; cancer of, 725–27
pancreatic enzymes, 120
pantothenic acid (vitamin B5), 52, 75, 445, 478
papain, 157
papayas, 83, 157
parasites, 212–13, 393–98, 493
parathyroid glands, 386
parathyroids, 389
Parkinson's disease, 159, 399–403
parsley, 67, 464, 498
passionflower, 192, 369, 415
pau d'arco, 7, 101, 119, 200, 309, 352, 459
PCO's, 401
pectin, 318
pemoline, 344
pennyroyal, 422
pentamidine, 36
pepper, 248
peppermint, 18, 33, 173, 301, 454; oil of, 253. 210
peptic ulcers, 205–6
perilla oil, 320
periodontal disease, 180, 404–9; personal experiences, 597, 602–3, 605–6, 675
periodontitis, 405
peripheral neuropathy, 261–62
pesticides, 123, 428, 460
petroleum, 314, 373
pets, 646–47
phenylalanine, 61, 401
philodendron, 216
phlebitis, 270
phobias, 410–16
phosphatidylcholine, 61, 275
phosphatidylserine, 27, 60–61, 347
phosphoric acid, 37, 151, 425
phosphorus, 182, 314, 370, 75.100
phyllanthius (life plant), 34
phyllanthus, 309

physiatrists, 88
physical handicaps, overcoming, 618–19
physical therapists, 88–89
phytochemicals, AIDS and, 34–35
phytoestrogens, 99, 364, 368, 369
phytosterols, 364
picamilon, 284
piles (hemorrhoids), 303–5
pine, white, 445
pineapple, 83, 157; juice of, 5, 73
plantain, 68, 183
plantar warts, 263, 465
pleurisy, 598–99
PMS (premenstrual syndrome), 158, 427–44
pneumonia, 22, 598–99
poison ivy, 169, 464, 467
poison oak, 464
polio, 665–66, 672
pollen, bee, 17, 66, 83, 168, 269, 437, 444, 486
polyphenol, 10
polyunsaturated phosphatidylcholine (PPC), 211, 308
poplar bark, tulip, 149
poria cocos, 150
Porpoise, 605
post-polio syndrome, 665–66
post-traumatic stress disorder, 490–91
postpartum depression, 424–25
potassium, 53, 75, 182, 191, 199, 293, 380, 478, 489, 490, 626
potato juice, 73
Prednisone, 71, 351, 374
pregnancy, 119; anemia and, 65; candidiasis and, 126–27; personal experiences with, 620; problems with, 417–26; TMJ and, 482; UTI and, 498
pregnenolone, 60, 61, 191
Premarin, 366
premenstrual syndrome (PMS), 158, 427–34
pressure point therapy, 132, 152, 280, 433
prickly ash bark, 7, 74
pimagedine, 199
primrose oil, 83, 111; *See also* evening primrose oil
probiotics, 43, 128, 210, 498
progesterone, 14, 60, 191, 368, 369, 388, 425, 428, 430, 434
progressive relaxation training, 483
prolactin, 14
promiscuity, 124
propolis, 17, 407; bee, 17, 66, 83, 168, 269, 437, 444
Proscar, 436
prostate; cancer of, 12–13, 434, 435, 436, 679, 682, 715–16, 721, 732; conditions of, 434–41
prostate glandulars, 437
prostate specific antigen (PSA), 12
prostatic hypertrophy, 434
prostatitis, 435
protease, 156–57
proteins, 23; digestive disorders and, 213–14; hypoglycemia and, 324–25; obesity and, 379; pregnancy and, 420; protein-digesting enzymes, 133; whey, 148, 174, 308
proteolytic enzymes, 438
protocol, Gary Null, 505–72
protozoa, 393, 395, 493
Prozac, 412, 427

PSA (prostate specific antigen), 12
psoriasis, 462, 464, 589, 618
psoriatic arthritis, 69
psychodrama, 655
psychological factors; Alzheimer's disease and,
    56–63; autism and, 81–84; cancer and,
    101–2, 122; chronic pain and, 162; eating
    disorders and, 230; hypnotherapy and,
    649–50; hypothyroidism and, 328; parasites
    and, 394; phobias and, 410–16; PMS and,
    427–34; psychological blocks, 650; qi gong
    and, 687–92; tai chi and, 705–7; trauma,
    488–92; *See also* depression
psychoneuroimmunology, 101–2, 108
psyllium, 210, 304, 319, 380, 630
puirogenium, 644
pulsatilla, 177, 193, 218, 223, 425, 431, 466
pulsed electromagnetic therapy, 136
pumpkin, 396, 436, 439
purification lodge, 490–91
pycnogenol, 168, 459, 473
pygeum africanum, 439
pygeum extract, 13
pyridoxine. *See* vitamin B6
pyrogenium, 37

Q10, coenzyme; for aging, 14; for AIDS, 26; for
    allergies, 52; for Alzheimer's and dementia,
    58–59; for autism, 83; breast cancer and,
    100; for cancer, 114–15; for CFS, 148; for
    cold and canker sores, 168; for dental disor-
    ders, 182; for diabetes, 199; for digestive
    disorders, 210; for headaches, 283; for heart
    disease, 291; for MS, 375; for Parkinson's
    disease, 401; for periodontal disease, 408,
    602, 606, 675; for respiratory illnesses, 445;
    for sinusitis, 454; for skin cancer, 459; for
    stroke, 473
qi gong, 19, 687–92
quassi chips, 395
quercetin, 42, 168, 444, 445, 454, 459

radiation, 97, 124, 719, 721, 729, 738
radiofrequency ablation (RFA), 121–22
rashes, 264–65, 462, 466, 598
raspberry leaf, 421–22
Rauwolfia, 294
reconstructive therapy, 78–79, 133–34, 693–95
recreational therapy, 137
red clover, 8, 101, 119, 168, 172, 309, 464
red eyebright, 54
red raspberry leaf, 67, 338
red tea, 465
reflexology; for AIDS and HIV, 39–40; for eye dis-
    orders, 250; for headaches, 281; personal
    experiences with, 696–97; for PMS, 432; for
    prostate conditions, 440; for sinusitis, 455;
    for skin conditions, 466
regression, 655
Reich's technology, 715
reiki, 19, 698–700
reishi (ganoderma), mushrooms, 17, 33, 112, 149,
    309, 321, 336
relaxation; for CFS, 151–52; for depression, 193;
    for TMJ, 484
resentment, 651–52

respiratory illness, 442–50; asthma, 53, 442–43,
    444–45, 446, 448, 647, 710
respiratory system; allergies in, 47; detoxification
    of, 447–48
rest, 174–75
resveratrol, 116–17
Reye's syndrome, 252
rheumatic fever, 287
rheumatic heart disease, 287
rheumatoid arthritis, 69–70, 266, 673–74
rheumatologists, 88
rhododendron, 78
rhubarb, 33
rhumex crispus, 177
rhus toxicodendron, 78, 169, 467
riboflavin, 283
ricin, 36
ringworm, 462
Ritalin, 340, 344
Rolfing, 89, 136, 701–2
Roman chamomile, 18
root canal therapy, 46, 182
rose, 18
rose hips, 183
rosemary, 18, 137, 160, 207, 269
rotation diet, 49, 76–77, 671
Rovital-V (R-1103), 36
royal jelly, 33–34, 326, 486
runny nose, 676
rutin, 303

s-adenosylmethionine (SAMe), 43, 58, 76, 148,
    190, 308
sabal serrulata, 440
sabina, 369
SAD (seasonal affective disorder), 192
safflower oil, 264
sage, 158, 173, 269; oil, 183
salicylic acid, 159, 264
saline implants, 104
salvia, 158
SAMe (s-adenosylmethionine), 43, 58, 76, 148,
    190, 308
sanguinaria, 459
sarcoma, 106; Kaposi's, 29, 39, 731
sarsaparilla, 17, 173, 218, 369, 464
sassafras, 7, 101, 464
sauna, 8, 174
saw palmetto, 13, 173, 438–39
schizandra, 34, 54, 192
sciatica, 161, 620, 621–22, 624–25
sea buckthorn, 183
sea vegetables, 10, 23, 229
seasonal affective disorder (SAD), 192
seaweed, 36, 112
seborrheic dermatitis, 463
secale, 369–70
selenium, 15, 27, 43, 59, 67, 83, 100, 114, 133, 139,
    182, 235,; 293, 308, 321, 347, 388, 408, 445,
    473
self-hypnosis, 19, 655, 656
sepia, 169, 193, 370, 373, 425
sequential homeopathy, 646–47
serotonin, 188
sesame oil, 83
714-X, 120, 713–15

sex hormone binding globulin (SHBG), 13
sexual relations, 124; hypothyroidism and, 328; infertility, 332–39; menopause and, 365; UTI and, 494, 500
sexually transmitted diseases. *See* AIDS and HIV; herpes
shao fu zhu yu wan, 158
shark cartilage, 28, 116, 269, 627
shark liver oil, 116, 129, 173
SHBG (sex hormone binding globulin), 13
shiatsu, 89, 703–4
shingles, 167, 169, 314–15
Siberian ginseng, 43, 148, 149, 325, 439
sickle cell anemia, 451–52
silibinin, 114, 200, 308
silica, 182, 185, 258, 388
silicon, 408
silicone implants, 104
silver, colloidal, 352–53
silymarin, 43, 308
sinus problems, 280, 453–56, 598; *See also* allergies; headaches
sitz baths, 338, 499
skin; athlete's foot, 265, 462; brushing of, 8; detoxification of, 6, 8; dry skin, 264, 466
skin conditions, 461–67; acne, 461, 464, 466; allergies, 47; cancer, 457–60, 723–25; dermatitis, 462–63, 466–67; personal experiences with, 577, 578–79, 589, 598, 618, 620,; 630; psoriasis, 462, 464, 618; rashes, 462, 466
skullcap, 43, 159, 192, 301, 369, 401, 415, 446
sleep disorders, 144, 145, 188
slippery elm, 159, 172, 304, 446, 498
smoking, 140–41, 470
snakeroot, Indian, 294
SOD (superoxide dismutase), 10, 16, 75–76, 101, 114
sodium, 5
sodium nitrate, 277–78, 285
sodium selenite, 375
soidago virgaurea, 448
Solu-Medrol, 374
soy products, 111, 257, 320; menopause and, 364, 367, 368
spasmodic torticollis, 659
spirulina, 10, 67, 68, 111, 347, 381, 400
spleen, UTI and, 495
spondylitis, ankylosing, 69–70
spongia tosta, 448
sports, 675; injuries in, 167–68, 662; medicine specialists, 88
spruce, 445
squamous cell carcinoma, 457–58, 730–31
St. John's wort, 7, 34, 192, 229, 369, 431
staphisagria, 185, 440
Staphylococcus aureus, 485–87
star fruit juice, 73
Stelazine, 402
stem cell research, 136
stilingia, 7
stinging nettles, 54, 150, 229
stomach problems, pain, 159, 689–90
Strattera, 340
stress; aging and, 18–19; asthma and, 442; cholesterol and, 321; dental disorders and, 180–81; digestive disorders and, 211–12, 213; dysmenorrhea and, 219; eating disorders and, 227; headaches and, 284; lupus and, 353; massage and, 660, 662; obesity and, 384; personal experiences with, 692, 704; respiratory illnesses and, 448; skin conditions and, 462, 467; tinnitus and, 479; TMJ and, 481–82; trauma and, 488–90
stretching, 161, 219, 268
stroke, 468–76, 614–15; heart attacks vs., 468
strontium, 388
subprostrata, 301
success, obstacles to, 656–57
sudden infant death syndrome (SIDS), 341
sugar, 409; addiction to, 655–56; candidiasis and, 128; hypoglycemia and, 324; PMS and, 433; pregnancy and, 418–19
sulforaphane, 114
sulfur amino acids, 347
sulphur, 466
suma, 119
sunstroke, 300–302
superoxide dismutase (SOD), 10, 16, 75–76, 101, 114
Superskin, 263
supplements. *See specific diseases and supplements*
suppositories, 139–40
sweat lodge, 490–91
sylimarin, 200
syphilinum, 37

Tabebuia heptaphylla, 7
tai chi chuan, 19, 39, 705–7
tannins, 34, 474
tansy, 294
tardive dyskinesia, 625
taste, loss of, 227
taurine, 61, 83, 275, 293
TB (tuberculosis), 21
tea tree oil, 131, 168, 183, 265, 356, 407
teeth. *See* dental disorders
temporomandibular joint (TMJ) dysfunction, 479, 481–84
TENS (transcutaneous electrical nerve stimulation), 89, 132, 479
testimonials, participant, 505–72
testosterone, 13, 60, 191, 381
tetracycline, 464
theamine, l-theanine, 118, 347, 413, 431
therapeutic touch, 165
Thermax, 265
Thermostat, 265
thiamin (vitamin B1), 478
Thimerosal, 81
thistle, milk, 7, 43, 137, 308, 464
Thorazine, 402, 624, 625
thuja, 37, 440
thyme, 68, 395, 446
thymosin alpha-1, 307
thymus extract, 120–21
thyroid, 227, 262; cancer of, 690; hypothyroidism, 57, 83, 144, 377–78, 382; supplements, 8
TIAs (transient ischemic attacks), 470
ticitum acid, 151
ticks, deer, 355–59
tinea cruris, 462
tinea versicolor, 462
tinnitus, 477–80
TMG (trimethyl-glycine), 43

TMJ (temporomandibular joint) dysfunction, 479, 481–84
tobacco products, 98, 123
tobaccum, 372–73
tocopherol, 13, 15, 100, 147, 445
tocotrienol, 100–101, 147
toenails, ingrown, 267
Tolinase, 197
torticollis, spasmodic, 659
toxic shock syndrome (TSS), 485–87
toxins, aging and, 11
TPA, 472
transcutaneous electrical nerve stimulation (TENS), 89, 132, 479
transient ischemic attacks (TIAs), 470
trauma, 488–92, 646–47, 701–72
tremors, 399
triglycerides, 317, 320
trimethyl-glycine (TMG), 43
tryptophane, l-tryptophane, 61, 415
TSS (toxic shock syndrome), 485–87
tuberculosis (TB), 21
tulip poplar bark, 149
tumors, 420–21, 652–54, 668–70; See also cancer
turmeric, 34, 54, 93, 118, 133, 209, 218, 293, 459
tylophora asthmatica, 54
tyramine, 277, 285
tyrosine, l-tyrosine, 61, 352, 401

ukrain, 121
ulcerative colitis, 206, 697
ulcers, 684–85; peptic, 205–6; varicose, 270
uncaria tomensoa, 439
urinary tract infection (UTI), 159, 493–501
usnea, 150, 173
uterus, 232–37; bleeding in, 254–60
UTI (urinary tract infection), 159, 493–501
utica urens, 466
uva ursi, 325, 439, 498, 499

vaccinations, 81; allergy, 77; CFS and, 143; individualized, 120
vaginitis, 496
valerian, 43, 159, 192, 282, 295, 347, 369, 401, 415
Valium, 427, 615
vanadium, 408
vanadyl sulfate, 199
varicose ulcers, 270
varicose veins, 269–70
vascular endothelial growth factor (VEGF), 99
vegetables; AIDS and, 22–23; cruciferous, 99, 110; juices, 5, 73; menopause and, 367; sea, 10, 23, 229
Venus flytrap (carnivora), 32–33, 101, 121
vervain, blue, 160, 369
viburnum (black haw, cramp bark), 158, 218, 422, 430
viburnum opulus, 158
Vietnam War, 491
violet, 34
vision problems. See eye problems
vision therapy, 248–49
vitamin A, 262; aging and, 5, 14; in alcoholism treatment, 42; for allergies, 51; for arthritis, 74; for back and neck pain, 93; for cancer, 113; for carpal tunnel syndrome, 133; for

cervical dysplasia, 139–40; for cold and canker sores, 168; for dental disorders, 183; for endometriosis, 235; for eye disorders, 246; for fibroids, 258; for foot and leg problems, 263, 264; for herpes, 313; for hypothyroidism, 330; obesity and, 379; for periodontal disease, 407; pregnancy and, 421; for prostate conditions, 437; for skin cancer, 459; for skin conditions, 464–65; for tinnitus, 478; for UTI, 498
vitamin B complex; in alcoholism treatment, 42; for allergies, 52; for Alzheimer's and dementia, 58; for arthritis, 75; for back and neck pain, 93; for candidiasis, 129; for CFS, 147; for chronic pain, 156; for cold and canker sores, 168; for dental disorders, 183; for depression, 190; for ear infections, 222; for eye disorders, 247; for hepatitis, 308; for herpes, 313; hypoglycemia and, 324, 325; for hypothyroidism, 330; menopause and, 367; for periodontal disease, 602; for phobias, 415; for PMS, 429; for respiratory illnesses, 444; for stroke, 472–73; for tinnitus, 478; for TMJ, 483; for trauma, 489
vitamin B1, 326, 478
vitamin B3; niacin, 190, 247, 293, 320, 375, 478; niacinamide, 74–75, 147
vitamin B3 (niacinamide), 74–75, 147
vitamin B5 (pantothenic acid), 52, 75, 445, 478
vitamin B6 (pyridoxine); for acne, 465; for AIDS, 25; for allergies, 52; for Alzheimer's and dementia, 58; for arthritis, 75; for autism, 83; for carpal tunnel syndrome, 133; for cervical dysplasia, 139; for CFS, 147; cholesterol and, 320, 321; for endometriosis, 234–35; for headaches, 282; for hypoglycemia, 325; for infertility, 337; for learning disorders, 347; menopause and, 367; for MS, 375; for PMS, 429; for prostate conditions, 437; for skin conditions, 465; for tinnitus, 478; for UTI, 498
vitamin B12; for AIDS, 25; for allergies, 52; for Alzheimer's and dementia, 58; anemia and, 64–65, 66–67, 67; for CFS, 148; for chronic pain, 156; for heart disease, 291–92; for hepatitis, 308; for hypothyroidism, 330; for MS, 375; for parasites, 396; pregnancy and, 420, 421; for tinnitus, 478
vitamin C (ascorbic acid); aging and, 5, 14; for AIDS, 24; in alcoholism treatment, 42; for allergies, 51; for Alzheimer's and dementia, 59; for arthritis, 74, 626; aspirin and, 71; for autism, 83; for back and neck pain, 93; breast cancer and, 100; for cancer, 112–13; for candidiasis, 129; for carpal tunnel syndrome, 133; for cervical dysplasia, 139; for CFS, 147; cholesterol and, 320; for chronic pain, 156; for cold and canker sores, 167–68; for colds and flu, 173; for dental disorders, 182; for depression, 190; for diabetes, 200; for digestive disorders, 209–10; for ear infections, 222; for endometriosis, 234; for eye disorders, 246, 247; for fibroids, 257, 258; for foot and leg problems, 263, 266, 269, 270; for gallstones, 275; for heart disease, 290; for hemorrhoids, 303; for hepatitis, 308, 681; for herpes, 312; hypoglycemia and,

vitamin C (ascorbic acid); aging and, (*cont.*) 326; for hypothyroidism, 330; for infertility, 337; for learning disorders, 347; menopause and, 367; for MS, 375; for obesity, 380–81; for osteoporosis, 388; for Parkinson's disease, 401; for periodontal disease, 407, 602, 675; for PMS, 429; pregnancy and, 421; for prostate conditions, 437; for respiratory illnesses, 444, 445, 447; for sinusitis, 454; for skin cancer, 459; for skin conditions, 465; for stroke, 473; for trauma, 489, 490; for UTI, 498

vitamin D, 13; for AIDS, 27; for allergies, 51; breast cancer and, 100; for carpal tunnel syndrome, 133; for dental disorders, 182; for depression, 191; for eye disorders, 246; for foot and leg problems, 263, 264; for menopause, 367; for MS, 375, 376; for osteoporosis, 388; pregnancy and, 421; for prostate conditions, 437; for tinnitus, 478

vitamin E; aging and, 5, 14–15; for AIDS, 27–28; in alcoholism treatment, 42; for allergies, 52; for Alzheimer's and dementia, 59; for arthritis, 74; for autism, 83; for back and neck pain, 93; breast cancer and, 100; for cancer, 114; for carpal tunnel syndrome, 133; for cervical dysplasia, 139; for CFS, 147; cholesterol and, 320; for dental disorders, 182, 183; diabetes and, 200; for digestive disorders, 209; for endometriosis, 235; for eye disorders, 246, 247; for fibroids, 258; for foot and leg problems, 263, 264, 266, 270; for headaches, 672; for heart disease, 290–91, 293; for hemorrhoids, 304; for hepatitis, 308; for herpes, 312; for hypoglycemia, 325; for hypothyroidism, 330; for infertility, 336; for MS, 375; obesity and, 379; for Parkinson's disease, 401; for periodontal disease, 407, 602, 675; for PMS, 429; pregnancy and, 421; for prostate conditions, 437–38; for respiratory illnesses, 445; for skin cancer, 459; for skin conditions, 465; for stroke, 473; for tinnitus, 478; for trauma, 489

vitamin K, 5, 28, 67, 76, 100, 121, 200, 291, 352, 388

vitamins; Alzheimer's, dementia and, 57; autism and, 82; personal experiences with, 708–12; stroke and, 472–73

Vitex, 14, 259, 369

walnut, 68; black, 17, 129, 352, 395, 396; oil, 83

warts, 263–64; plantar, 263, 465

water, 10; chronic pain and, 155; pregnancy and, 418, 420; purification, 241; skin conditions and, 463; UTI and, 497, 499

watercress, 137

weight-bearing aerobic exercise, 389

weight exercises, 296

weight loss, 654

wheat bran, 210

wheat germ, 183, 486

wheat products, 205, 667, 671

wheatgrass, 10, 111, 400, 486

whey protein, 148, 174, 308

white pine, 445

white willow bark, 74, 159

whole grains, 474

wild cherry, 54, 446

wild ginger, 159

wild yam (dioscorea), 158, 218, 294, 309, 368, 369, 622

willow bark, 301

wintergreen, 439

witch hazel, 304, 464

women; anemia in, 64, 65; natural hormone replacement in, 13–14; osteoporosis in, 386–92; parasites in, 394; phobias in, 410; TMJ in, 482; UTI in, 493–501; *See also* menopause; menstruation; pregnancy; premenstrual; syndrome

wood betony, 7, 160, 173, 309

worms, 393, 493

wormseed, 396

wormweed, 395

wormwood, 67, 396

wounds, 263

wrinkles, 9

X-rays, 97

xenoestrogen, 257

Xiao Yao Wan, 101, 217, 281–82, 430

yam extract, 368

yam, wild (dioscorea), 158

yarrow, 173

yeast; brewer's, 168, 486; candidiasis and, 126, 128–29

yeast infections, 257; personal experiences with, 579, 636–38

yellow clock, 464

yellow dock, 8, 17, 67, 137, 309

yellow dye #5, 449

yerba mate, 17, 54, 381

yerba santa, 445

ylang ylang, 18, 193

yoga, 19, 39, 137, 193, 219, 296–97, 390–91, 660

yogurt, 128, 167, 497

yucca, 74, 269

yudaiwan, 130

Yunnan pai yao, 217

zeaxanthin, 247

zhang yan, 248

zinc; aging and, 15; for AIDS, 28; in alcoholism treatment, 42; for allergies, 53; for Alzheimer's and dementia, 59; for anemia, 67; for arthritis, 75; for back and neck pain, 93; for cancer, 117; for cervical dysplasia, 139; for CFS, 147; cholesterol and, 321; for cold and canker sores, 167; for colds and flu, 173, 174; for dental disorders, 182; for diabetes, 199; for ear infections, 222; eating disorders and, 227, 228–29; for endometriosis, 235; for hepatitis, 308; for hypoglycemia, 325, 326; for hypothyroidism, 330; infertility and, 333, 336; for learning disorders, 347; menopause and, 367; for osteoporosis, 388; for periodontal disease, 408, 602; for PMS, 429; for prostate conditions, 436–37; for respiratory illnesses, 445; for sinusitis, 454; for skin cancer, 459; for skin conditions, 464; for tinnitus, 478; for trauma, 489, 490

zinc picolinate, 83, 454

Zovirax, 312